VOLUME **8**

DISEASE CONTROL PRIORITIES • THIRD EDITION

Child and Adolescent Health and Development

DISEASE CONTROL PRIORITIES • THIRD EDITION

Series Editors

Dean T. Jamison
Rachel Nugent
Hellen Gelband
Susan Horton
Prabhat Jha
Ramanan Laxminarayan
Charles N. Mock

Volumes in the Series

Essential Surgery
Reproductive, Maternal, Newborn, and Child Health
Cancer
Mental, Neurological, and Substance Use Disorders
Cardiovascular, Respiratory, and Related Disorders
Major Infectious Diseases
Injury Prevention and Environmental Health
Child and Adolescent Health and Development
Disease Control Priorities: Improving Health and Reducing Poverty

DISEASE CONTROL PRIORITIES

Budgets constrain choices. Policy analysis helps decision makers achieve the greatest value from limited available resources. In 1993, the World Bank published *Disease Control Priorities in Developing Countries* (*DCP1*), an attempt to systematically assess the cost-effectiveness (value for money) of interventions that would address the major sources of disease burden in low- and middle-income countries. The World Bank's 1993 *World Development Report* on health drew heavily on *DCP1*'s findings to conclude that specific interventions against noncommunicable diseases were cost-effective, even in environments in which substantial burdens of infection and undernutrition persisted.

DCP2, published in 2006, updated and extended *DCP1* in several aspects, including explicit consideration of the implications for health systems of expanded intervention coverage. One way that health systems expand intervention coverage is through selected platforms that deliver interventions that require similar logistics but deliver interventions from different packages of conceptually related interventions, for example, against cardiovascular disease. Platforms often provide a more natural unit for investment than do individual interventions. Analysis of the costs of packages and platforms—and of the health improvements they can generate in given epidemiological environments—can help to guide health system investments and development.

DCP3 differs importantly from *DCP1* and *DCP2* by extending and consolidating the concepts of platforms and packages and by offering explicit consideration of the financial risk protection objective of health systems. In populations lacking access to health insurance or prepaid care, medical expenses that are high relative to income can be impoverishing. Where incomes are low, seemingly inexpensive medical procedures can have catastrophic financial effects. *DCP3* offers an approach to explicitly include financial protection as well as the distribution across income groups of financial and health outcomes resulting from policies (for example, public finance) to increase intervention uptake. The task in all of the *DCP* volumes has been to combine the available science about interventions implemented in very specific locales and under very specific conditions with informed judgment to reach reasonable conclusions about the impact of intervention mixes in diverse environments. *DCP3*'s broad aim is to delineate essential intervention packages and their related delivery platforms to assist decision makers in allocating often tightly constrained budgets so that health system objectives are maximally achieved.

DCP3's nine volumes are being published in 2015, 2016, 2017, and 2018 in an environment in which serious discussion continues about quantifying the sustainable development goal (SDG) for health. *DCP3*'s analyses are well-placed to assist in choosing the means to attain the health SDG and assessing the related costs. Only when these volumes, and the analytic efforts on which they are based, are completed will we be able to explore SDG-related and other broad policy conclusions and generalizations. The final *DCP3* volume will report those conclusions. Each individual volume will provide valuable, specific policy analyses on the full range of interventions, packages, and policies relevant to its health topic.

More than 500 individuals and multiple institutions have contributed to *DCP3*. We convey our acknowledgments elsewhere in this volume. Here we express our particular gratitude to the Bill & Melinda Gates Foundation for its sustained financial support, to the InterAcademy Medical Panel (and its U.S. affiliate, the National Academies of Science, Engineering, and Medicine), and to the External and Corporate Relations Publishing and Knowledge division of the World Bank. Each played a critical role in this effort.

Dean T. Jamison
Rachel Nugent
Hellen Gelband
Susan Horton
Prabhat Jha
Ramanan Laxminarayan
Charles N. Mock

VOLUME **8**

DISEASE CONTROL PRIORITIES • THIRD EDITION

Child and Adolescent Health and Development

EDITORS

Donald A. P. Bundy
Nilanthi de Silva
Susan Horton
Dean T. Jamison
George C. Patton

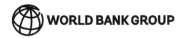 **WORLD BANK GROUP**

Softcover:
ISBN: 978-1-4648-0423-6
ISBN (electronic): 978-1-4648-0439-7
DOI: 10.1596/978-1-4648-0423-6

Hardcover:
ISBN: 978-1-4648-0517-2
DOI: 10.1596/978-1-4648-0517-2

Cover photo: © John Hogg/World Bank. Used with the permission of John Hogg/World Bank. Further permission required for reuse.
© Cover and interior design: Debra Naylor, Naylor Design, Washington, DC

Chapter opener photos:

Chapter 1: © Greatstock/Alamy Stock Photo. Used with permission. Further permission required for reuse; chapter 2: © Frank Spangler/Worldview Images. Used with the permission of Worldview Images. Further permission required for reuse; chapter 3: © Greatstock/Alamy Stock Photo. Used with permission. Further permission required for reuse; chapter 4: © Frank Spangler/Worldview Images. Used with the permission of Worldview Images. Further permission required for reuse; chapter 5: © Frank Spangler/Worldview Images. Used with the permission of Worldview Images. Further permission required for reuse; chapter 6: © Frank Spangler/Worldview Images. Used with the permission of Worldview Images. Further permission required for reuse; chapter 7: © Frank Spangler/Worldview Images. Used with the permission of Worldview Images. Further permission required for reuse; chapter 8: © Simone D. McCourtie/World Bank. Further permission required for reuse; chapter 9: © Scott Wallace/World Bank. Further permission required for reuse; chapter 10: © Greatstock/Alamy Stock Photo. Used with permission. Further permission required for reuse; chapter 11: © Frank Spangler/Worldview Images. Used with the permission of Worldview Images. Further permission required for reuse; chapter 12: © Frank Spangler/Worldview Images. Used with the permission of Worldview Images. Further permission required for reuse; chapter 13: © Simone D. McCourtie/World Bank. Further permission required for reuse; chapter 14: © Frank Spangler/Worldview Images. Used with the permission of Worldview Images. Further permission required for reuse; chapter 15: © Greatstock/Alamy Stock Photo. Used with permission. Further permission required for reuse; chapter 16: © Frank Spangler/Worldview Images. Used with the permission of Worldview Images. Further permission required for reuse; chapter 17: © Simone D. McCourtie/World Bank. Further permission required for reuse; chapter 18: © Frank Spangler/Worldview Images. Used with the permission of Worldview Images. Further permission required for reuse; chapter 19: © Frank Spangler/Worldview Images. Used with the permission of Worldview Images. Further permission required for reuse; chapter 20: © Frank Spangler/Worldview Images. Used with the permission of Worldview Images. Further permission required for reuse; chapter 21: © Scott Wallace/World Bank. Further permission required for reuse; chapter 22: © Simone D. McCourtie/World Bank. Further permission required for reuse; chapter 23: © Frank Spangler/Worldview Images. Used with the permission of Worldview Images. Further permission required for reuse; chapter 24: © Frank Spangler/Worldview Images. Used with the permission of Worldview Images. Further permission required for reuse; chapter 25: © Simone D. McCourtie/World Bank. Further permission required for reuse; chapter 26: © Frank Spangler/Worldview Images. Used with the permission of Worldview Images. Further permission required for reuse; chapter 27: © Frank Spangler/Worldview Images. Used with the permission of Worldview Images. Further permission required for reuse; chapter 28: © Scott Wallace/World Bank. Further permission required for reuse; chapter 29: © Frank Spangler/Worldview Images. Used with the permission of Worldview Images. Further permission required for reuse; chapter 30: © Frank Spangler/Worldview Images. Used with the permission of Worldview Images. Further permission required for reuse.

Library of Congress Cataloging-in-Publication Data has been requested.

Contents

Foreword

HEALTH AND EDUCATION DURING THE 8,000 DAYS OF CHILD AND ADOLESCENT DEVELOPMENT: TWO SIDES OF THE SAME COIN

Today, there is comfort to be found in returning to the inspired words of others. Until H. G. Wells' time machine is made, words are our emotional anchor to the past and, one hopes, our window to a brighter future. Speaking before the 18th General Assembly of the United Nations in 1963, it was President John F. Kennedy who noted that the "effort to improve the conditions of man, however, is not a task for the few." Development is a shared, cross-cutting mission I know well. For the breakthroughs we witness—from Borlaug's wheat to a vaccine for polio—are the products of cooperation, a clean break from siloed thinking, and a courage to work at the sharp edges of disciplines.

Working as a lecturer for five years in the 1970s and early 1980s, I came to see—in a way I never had as a student—that education unlocks talent and unleashes potential. And as Chancellor, Prime Minister, and most importantly a parent, education has remained a centerpiece in my life because of the hope it delivers. For when we ask ourselves what breaks the weak, it is not the Mediterranean wave that submerges the life vest, nor the food convoy that does not make it to the besieged Syrian town. Rather, it is the absence of hope, the soul-crushing certainty that there is nothing ahead to plan or prepare for—not even a place in school.

Two years ago, the International Commission on Financing Global Education Opportunity, composed of two dozen global leaders and convened by the Prime Minister of Norway and the Presidents of Chile, Indonesia, and Malawi, as well as the Director-General of UNESCO, set out to make a new investment case for global education. What resulted was a credible yet ambitious plan capable of ensuring that the Sustainable Development Goal of an inclusive and quality education for all is met by the 2030 deadline. While we continue to work today to ensure our messages become action—from increased domestic spending on schooling to an International Finance Facility for Education—we sought to produce an authoritative, technically strong report that would spend more time being open on desks than collecting dust on a shelf.

The *Disease Control Priorities* (*DCP*) series established in 1993 shares this philosophy and acts as a key resource for Ministers of Health and Finance, guiding them toward informed decisions about investing in health. The third edition of *DCP* rightly recognizes that good health is but one facet of human development and that health and education outcomes are forever intertwined. The Commission report makes clear that more education equates with better health outcomes. And approaching this reality from the other direction, this year's volume of *DCP* shows that children who are in good health and appropriately nourished are more likely to participate in school and to learn while there. The Commission report raises the concept of progressive universalism or giving greatest priority to those children most at risk of being excluded from learning. Here, too, the alignment with *DCP* is clear as health strides are most apparent when directed to the poorest and sickest children, as well as girls.

It is fitting that one of the Commission's background papers appears as a chapter in this volume. The Commission showed that education spending, particularly for adolescent girls, is a moral imperative and an economic necessity. Indeed, girls are the least likely to go to primary school, the least likely to enter or complete secondary school, highly unlikely to matriculate to college, and the most likely to be married at a young age, to be forced into domestic service or trafficked. And with uneducated girls bearing five children against two children for educated girls, the vicious cycle of illiterate girls, high birth rates, low national incomes per head, and migration in search of opportunity will only worsen so long as we fail to deliver that most fundamental right to an education.

Here is a projection to remember. If current education funding trends hold, by 2030, 800 million children—half a generation—will lack the basic secondary skills necessary to thrive in an unknowable future. In calling for more and better results-based education spending, the Commission estimated that current total annual education expenditure is US$1.3 trillion across low- and middle-income countries, an anemic sum that must steadily rise to US$3 trillion by 2030. A rising tide must lift all ships, and so as education spending at the domestic and international levels sees an uptick, the same must be witnessed for health. The numbers may seem large, but the reality is that this relatively inexpensive effort would do more than unlock better health and education outcomes; it would bring us closer to achieving all 17 Sustainable Development Goals and unlocking the next stage of global growth.

A key message of this volume is that human development is a slow process; it takes two decades—8,000 days—for a human to develop physically and mentally. We also know a proper education requires time. So the world needs to invest widely, deeply, and effectively—across education, health, and all development sectors—during childhood and adolescence. And while individuals may have 8,000 days to develop, we must mobilize our resources today to secure their tomorrow. Let us not forget that the current generation of young people will transition to adulthood in 2030, and it will be their contribution that will determine whether the world achieves the Sustainable Development Goals.

We have, to again draw on Kennedy's words, "the capacity to control [our] environment, to end thirst and hunger, to conquer poverty and disease, to banish illiteracy and massive human misery." We have this capacity, but only when we work together. Both the Commission report and this latest *Disease Control Priorities* volume seek to elevate cross-sector initiatives on the global agenda. In human development, health and education are two sides of the same coin: only when we speak as one will this call be heard.

Gordon Brown
United Nations Special Envoy for Global Education
Chair of the International Commission on
Financing Global Education Opportunity
Prime Minister of the United Kingdom, 2007–2010
Chancellor of the Exchequer, 1997–2007

Preface

More children born today will survive to adulthood than at any time in human history. This is true both in terms of the proportion of live births and of absolute numbers. The current cohort of children who have survived to age 5 years will transition to adulthood around 2030 and will be the Sustainable Development Goals (SDGs) generation. The health, nutrition, and education of these young people as they develop from ages 5 to 19 years will have lifelong consequences for the adults they become and for their role in the development of the next generation. Will the world have prepared them well for this task?

Our analyses in this volume show that although the education of this age group is the primary focus of public sector investment, their health is a much lower priority. Indeed, middle childhood and adolescence has historically received the least attention of any age group.

Health and development in middle childhood and adolescence is a new focus of the *Disease Control Priorities* series, which was first published in conjunction with the World Bank's *World Development Report 1993: Investing in Health*, and which has become a key reference for health policy makers in low- and middle-income countries (box 1.1). The earlier editions touched on human development; this third edition is the first to give a specific focus beyond health to issues of human development, including the special role of the education sector, and the first to give prominence to health in this age group. This volume complements volume 2, *Reproductive, Maternal, Newborn, and Child Health*, which focuses on health in the under-five age group.

This volume presents its analyses and conclusions in 30 chapters grouped into five parts:

- **Part 1. Estimates of Mortality and Morbidity in Children (Ages 5 to 19 Years)** explores mortality and morbidity in this age group, with a focus on low- and lower-middle-income countries. A new analysis of mortality is presented, with surprising conclusions, and morbidity is examined with respect to three selected issues: nutrition, education, and health in adolescence.

- **Part 2. Impact of Interventions during the Life Course (Ages 5–19 Years)** reviews development issues at different stages in the life course and presents a conceptual framework for health and development from birth, through middle childhood and adolescence, to young adulthood.

- **Part 3. Conditions and Interventions** describes the evolving age distribution of disease and how new understanding of interventions and epidemiology has transformed the ways in which health systems can contribute to health and development objectives.

- **Part 4. Packages and Platforms to Promote Child and Adolescent Development** explores how novel approaches to policy that deliver health and development interventions to children and adolescents are slowly being implemented in low-income countries. In many cases, the focus is on vertical programs as part of underdeveloped primary health care systems, with a particular emphasis on school-based delivery. Current health systems often fail children and adolescents, especially in the low-income countries and communities that most need them.

- **Part 5. The Economics of Child Development** assembles economic data and seeks to prioritize interventions within three age classes: early childhood, school-age, and adolescence. Each age group is considered in a separate chapter, and each chapter prioritizes interventions on the basis of cost-effectiveness, extended cost-effectiveness, benefit-costs, and returns on investment. Part 5 also includes age-specific economic analysis of important areas of development, including the role of education in delaying pregnancy and marriage, as well as public financing for mass deworming as an example of school-based intervention.

We would like to acknowledge the many thoughtful people who contributed to the content and conclusions of this volume. The 110 authors from 19 countries contributed most directly to the preparation of the 30 chapters presented here; the volume simply could never have happened without their substantial investment of time and effort in crafting and writing the chapters. We, and they, thank the more than 60 independent reviewers, selected and commissioned by the National Academy of Science, Engineering, and Medicine, who provided peer reviews of all of the chapters (see the section entitled "Reviewers" at the end of the volume for a detailed listing of these individuals).

As a further check on the policy implications of the conclusions, we sought input from those more directly involved in health policy making. A policy consultation was held in Geneva under the leadership of the Regional Director of the World Health Organization (WHO) Eastern Mediterranean Regional Office, with representation from 10 countries.[1] The African Union hosted a regional consultation of Ministry of Health representatives from five countries in Sub-Saharan Africa.[2] We also presented the main conclusions at a variety of fora, seeking feedback from practitioners—including the annual meeting of the European Society for Paediatric Infectious Diseases, in Brighton, United Kingdom; and the Bill & Melinda Gates Foundation, in Seattle, Washington, United States. We are grateful for the many thoughtful responses that we received.

We would also like to recognize our debt to all those who contributed to The *Lancet* Commission on Adolescent Health and Wellbeing. This volume was written in parallel with the report of the Commission and shares some common editors and authors. We support the conclusions of the Commission's report, published in May 2016 (Patton and others); we extend them in this volume to include further economic analysis, as well as an exploration of the health and development needs of children in middle childhood, an age group that may be even more neglected than adolescents in public health policy and planning.

The main conclusion of this volume is that human development is a process that extends over the first two decades of life; for individuals to achieve their full potential, there is a need for age- and condition-specific interventions throughout this 20-year period. The current focus on the "first 1,000 days" represents a failure to recognize the critical importance of subsequent development during middle childhood and adolescence. Although intervention during the first 1,000 days is indeed the essential foundation for subsequent development, it cannot serve as a substitute for continuing intervention during three key phases:

- The middle childhood phase of growth and consolidation (ages 5–9 years), when infection and malnutrition remain key constraints on development, and mortality rates are much higher than previously realized
- The adolescent growth spurt (ages 10–14 years), when the increase in muscle, bone, and organ mass approaches rates not seen since age 2 years, and there are commensurate demands for good diet and health
- The adolescent phase of growth and consolidation (ages 15–19 years), when major restructuring of the brain is associated with behavioral and social experimentation that has lifelong consequence.

We note the asymmetry between the public investment in formal education versus health during the age range of 5–19 years, and the lack of recognition that the developmental returns from education are themselves dependent on concurrent good health and diet. We argue that current policy on health and development has substantially neglected and underserved children in this age range, and that there is too little research on how to respond to the needs of middle childhood and adolescence. We propose packages of interventions for these crucial later phases of development that are in the same range of cost-effectiveness as interventions in the early years of life but of substantially lower cost. We also call for significantly increased investment in research into the health and development needs during middle childhood and adolescence.

Volume Editors
Donald A. P. Bundy
Nilanthi de Silva
Susan Horton
Dean T. Jamison
George C. Patton

Volume Coordinator
Linda Schultz

NOTES

1. Participants are listed at the end of this volume.
2. Participants are listed at the end of this volume, as well as online: http://www.dcp-3.org/CAHDEthiopia.

REFERENCE

Patton, G. C., S. M. Sawyer, J. S. Santelli, D. A. Ross, R. Afifi, and others. 2016. "Our Future: A *Lancet* Commission on Adolescent Health and Wellbeing." *The Lancet* 387 (10036): 2423–78.

Abbreviations

AIDS	acquired immune deficiency syndrome
AQ	amodiaquine
AS	artesunate
BCR	benefit-cost ratio
BMI	body mass index
CCT	conditional cash transfer
CHERG	Child Health Epidemiology Reference Group
CME	Child Mortality Estimation
CT	cash transfer
DALY	disability-adjusted life year
DCP1	*Disease Control Priorities in Developing Countries*, first edition
DCP2	*Disease Control Priorities in Developing Countries*, second edition
DCP3	*Disease Control Priorities*, third edition
DHS	Demographic and Health Surveys
DMFT	decayed, missing, and filled teeth
DOHaD	Developmental Origins of Health and Disease
DP	dihydroartemisinin-piperaquine
ECD	early child development
ECE	early childhood education
EFA	Education for All
EGRA	Early Grade Reading Assessment
ESP	education sector plan
FA	fractional anisotropy
FRESH	Focusing Resources on Effective School Health
FRP	financial risk protection
GBD	Global Burden of Disease
GDP	gross domestic product
GHE	Global Health Estimates
GIZ	German Development Cooperation
GNI	gross national income
GYTS	Global Youth Tobacco Survey

HAZ	height-for-age z-scores
Hb	hemoglobin
HBSC	Health Behaviour in School-Aged Children
HEADSS	home, education, activities/employment, drugs, suicidality, sex
HICs	high-income countries
HIV	human immunodeficiency virus
HIV/AIDS	human immunodeficiency virus/acquired immune deficiency syndrome
HLM	hierarchical linear model
HPV	human papillomavirus
HSV-2	herpes simplex virus-2
ICF	International Classification of Functioning, Disability and Health
IEA	International Association for the Evaluation of Educational Achievement
IEC	information, education, and communication
IHME	Institute for Health Metrics and Evaluation
INCAP	Institute of Nutrition for Central America and Panama
IPCs	intermittent parasite clearance in schools
IPT	intermittent preventive treatment
IQ	intelligence quotient
IRS	indoor residual spraying
IST	intermittent screening and treatment
ITN	insecticide-treated bednet
KMC	kangaroo mother care
LBW	low birth weight
LICs	low-income countries
LMICs	low- and middle-income countries
MDA	mass drug administration
MDGs	Millennium Development Goals
m-health	mobile health
MICs	middle-income countries
MICS	Multiple Indicator Cluster Survey
NCDs	noncommunicable diseases
NTD	neglected tropical diseases
OECD	Organisation for Economic Co-operation and Development
OOP	out of pocket
OTL	opportunity to learn
PDV	present discounted value
PIAAC	Programme for the International Assessment of Adult Competencies
PIRLS	Progress in International Reading Literacy Study
PISA	Programme for International Student Assessment
PFC	prefrontal cortex
PRIMR	Primary Mathematics and Reading
PT	planum temporale
QALY	quality-adjusted life year
RCT	randomized controlled trial
RDT	rapid diagnostic test
RMNCH	reproductive, maternal, newborn, and child health
RoR	rate of return
RSC	Rockefeller Sanitary Commission
RTI	road traffic injury

SABER	Systems Approach for Better Education Results
SSBs	sugar-sweetened beverages
SBM	school-based management
SDGs	Sustainable Development Goals
SES	socioeconomic status
SHN	school health and nutrition
SMC	seasonal malaria chemoprevention
SP	sulphadoxine-pyrimethamine
SR	self-regulation
STHs	soil-transmitted helminths
STI	sexually transmitted infection
TFR	total fertility rate
TIMSS	Trends in International Mathematics and Science Study
TT	tetanus toxoid
U5MR	under-5 mortality rate
UCT	unconditional cash transfer
UMICs	upper-middle-income countries
UN	United Nations
UNESCO	United Nations Educational, Scientific and Cultural Organization
UNICEF	United Nations Children's Fund
VLY	value of a life year
VSL	value of a statistical life
VWFA	visual word form area
WASH	water, sanitation, and hygiene
WAZ	weight-for-age
WG	Washington Group
WHO	World Health Organization
WHZ	weight-for-height
WPP	World Population Prospects
WRA	women of reproductive age
YLD	years lost to disability
YOURS	Youth for Road Safety

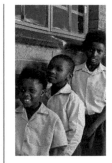

Child and Adolescent Health and Development: Realizing Neglected Potential

Donald A. P. Bundy, Nilanthi de Silva, Susan Horton, George C. Patton, Linda Schultz, and Dean T. Jamison

INTRODUCTION

It seems that society and the common legal definition have got it about right: it takes some 21 years for a human being to reach adulthood. The evidence shows a particular need to invest in the crucial development period from conception to age two (the first 1,000 days) and also during critical phases over the next 7,000 days. Just as babies are not merely small people—they need special and different types of care from the rest of us—so growing children and adolescents are not merely short adults; they, too, have critical phases of development that need specific interventions. Ensuring that life's journey begins right is essential, but it is now clear that we also need support to guide our development up to our 21st birthday if everyone is to have the opportunity to realize their potential. Our thesis is that research and action on child health and development should evolve from a narrow emphasis on the first 1,000 days to holistic concern over the first 8,000 days; from an age-siloed approach to an approach that embraces the needs across the life cycle.

To begin researching and encouraging action, this volume, *Child and Adolescent Health and Development*, explores the health and development needs of the 5 to 21 year age group and presents evidence for a package of investments to address priority health needs, expanding on other recent work in this area, such as the *Lancet* Commission on Adolescent Health and Wellbeing

(Patton, Sawyer, and others 2016). Given new evidence on the strong connection between a child's education and health, we argue that modest investments in the health of this age group are essential to attain the maximum benefit from investments in schooling for this age group, such as those proposed by the recent International Commission on Financing Global Education Opportunity (2016). This volume shares contributors to both commissions and complements an earlier volume, *Reproductive, Maternal, Newborn, and Child Health*, which focuses on health in the group of children under age 5 years.

There is a surprising lack of consistency in the language used to describe the phases of childhood, perhaps reflecting the historically narrow focus on the early years. The neglect of children ages 5 to 9 years in particular is reflected in the absence of a commonly reflected name for this age group. Figure 1.1 illustrates the nomenclature used in this volume, which we have sought to align with the definitions and use outlined in the 2016 *Lancet* Commission on Adolescent Health and Wellbeing. The editors of this volume built upon the commission's definitions to include additional terms that are relevant to the broader age range considered here, including *middle childhood* to reflect the age range between 5 and 9 years. The editors also refer to children and adolescents between ages 5 and 14 years as "school-age," since in low- and lower-middle-income countries these are the majority of children in

Corresponding author: Donald A. P. Bundy, Bill & Melinda Gates Foundation, Seattle, Washington, United States; donald.bundy@gatesfoundation.org.

Key Messages from Volume 8

1. It takes 21 years (or 8,000 days) for a child to develop into an adult. Throughout this period, there are sensitive phases that shape development. Age-appropriate and condition-specific support is required throughout the 8,000 days if a child is to achieve full potential as an adult.
2. Investment in health during the first 1,000 days is widely recognized as a high priority, but there is historical neglect of investments in the next 7,000 days of middle childhood and adolescence. This neglect is also reflected in investment in research into these older age-groups.
3. At least three phases are critical to health and development during the next 7,000 days, each requiring a condition-specific and age-specific response:
   - Middle Childhood Growth and Consolidation Phase (ages 5–9), when infection and malnutrition remain key constraints on development, and mortality rates are higher than previously realized
   - Adolescent Growth Spurt (ages 10–14), when there is a major increase in body mass, and significant physiological and behavioral changes associated with puberty

   - Adolescent Growth and Consolidation Phase (ages 15 to early 20s), bring further brain restructuring, linked with exploration and experimentation, and initiation of behaviors that are life-long determinants of health.
4. Broadening investment in human development to include scalable interventions during the next 7,000 days can be achieved cost-effectively at modest cost. Two essential packages were identified: the first addresses needs in middle childhood and early adolescence through a school-based approach; the second focuses on older adolescents through a mixed community and media and health systems approach. Both offer high cost-effectiveness and benefit-cost ratios.
5. Well-designed health interventions in middle childhood and adolescence can leverage the already substantial investment in education, and better design of educational programs can bring better health. The potential synergy between health and education is currently undervalued, and the returns on co-investment are rarely optimized.

Evolution of *Disease Control Priorities* and Focus of the Third Edition

Budgets constrain choices. Policy analysis helps decision makers achieve the greatest value from limited resources. In 1993, the World Bank published *Disease Control Priorities in Developing Countries* (*DCP1*), which sought to assess systematically the cost-effectiveness (value for money) of interventions addressing the major sources of disease burden in low- and middle-income countries (Jamison and others 1993). The World Bank's *World Development Report 1993* drew heavily on *DCP1*'s findings to conclude that specific interventions to combat noncommunicable diseases were cost-effective, even in environments with substantial burdens of infection and undernutrition (World Bank 1993).

DCP2, published in 2006, updated and extended *DCP1* in several respects, giving explicit consideration to the implications for health systems of expanded intervention coverage (Jamison and others 2006). One way to expand coverage of health interventions is through platforms for interventions that require similar logistics but that address heterogeneous health problems. Platforms often provide a more natural unit for investment than do individual interventions, but conventional health economics

box continues next page

Box 1.2 (continued)

has offered little understanding of how to make choices across platforms. Analysis of the costs of packages and platforms—and of the health improvements they can generate in given epidemiological environments—can help guide health system investments and development.

DCP3 introduces the notion of packages of interventions. Whereas platforms contain logistically related sets of interventions, packages contain conceptually related ones. The 21 packages developed in the nine volumes of *DCP3* include surgery and cardiovascular disease, for example. In addition, *DCP3* explicitly considers the financial risk–protection objective of health systems. In populations lacking access to health insurance or prepaid care, medical expenses that are high relative to income can be impoverishing. Where incomes are low, seemingly inexpensive medical procedures can have catastrophic financial effects. *DCP3* considers financial protection and the distribution across income groups as outcomes resulting from policies (for example, public finance) to increase intervention uptake and improve delivery quality. All of the volumes seek to combine the available science about interventions implemented in specific locales and conditions with informed judgment to reach reasonable conclusions about the effect of intervention mixes in diverse environments.

DCP3's broad aim is to delineate essential intervention packages—such as those for school-age children and adolescents, as outlined in this volume—and their related delivery platforms. This information is intended to assist decision makers in allocating often tightly constrained budgets and achieving health system objectives.

Four of *DCP3*'s nine volumes were published in 2015 and 2016, and the remaining five will appear in 2017 or early 2018. The volumes appear in an environment in which serious discussion about quantifying and achieving the Sustainable Development Goals (SDGs) for health continues (United Nations 2015). *DCP3*'s analyses are well-placed to assist in choosing the means to attain the health SDGs and assessing the related costs. These volumes, and the analytic efforts on which they are based, will enable researchers to explore SDG-related and other broad policy conclusions and generalizations. The final volume will report those conclusions. Each individual volume will provide specific policy analyses on the full range of interventions, packages, and policies relevant to its health topic.

Source: Dean T. Jamison, Rachel Nugent, Hellen Gelband, Susan Horton, Prabhat Jha, Ramanan Laxminarayan, and Charles N. Mock.

primary school, owing to high levels of grade repetition, late entry to school, and drop outs. As income levels rise and secondary schooling enrollment increases, children attending school will be older than age 14 years. Figure 1.1 also demonstrates the overlap between many of these terms. For example, the Convention on the Rights of the Child defines *child* as every human being younger than age 18 years, whereas this volume defines *adolescence* as beginning at age 10 years and continuing through age 19 years (United Nations General Assembly 1989). Figure 1.1 also shows the alignment between age groups and four key phases critical to development. These key phases are used as an organizing principle for intervention throughout this volume. Where possible, the editors have extended the analyses to include children through age 21 years; but standard reporting of age data is in quintiles, so for convenience the editors have accepted the upper age range as 15-19 years.

Some issues of potential importance to child development are examined in other volumes of *DCP3*. For example, environmental issues are examined in some depth in volume 7 (Mock and others 2017), which examines the impact of pollution on health and human development—especially the exceptional prevalence of lead poisoning, which affects the intellectual development of children.

A premise of this volume is that human development occurs intensively throughout the first two decades of life (figure 1.1), and that for a person to achieve his or her full potential, age- and condition-specific interventions are needed throughout this 8,000 days (box 1.3). We use four key tools—cost-effectiveness, extended cost-effectiveness, benefit-cost, and returns on investment—to identify and prioritize investments at different ages and to propose delivery platforms and essential packages that are costed, scalable, and relevant to low-resource settings. These analyses suggest that public investment in health and development after age 5 years has been insufficient.

Figure 1.1 Nomenclature Concerning Age and Four Key Phases of Child and Adolescent Development

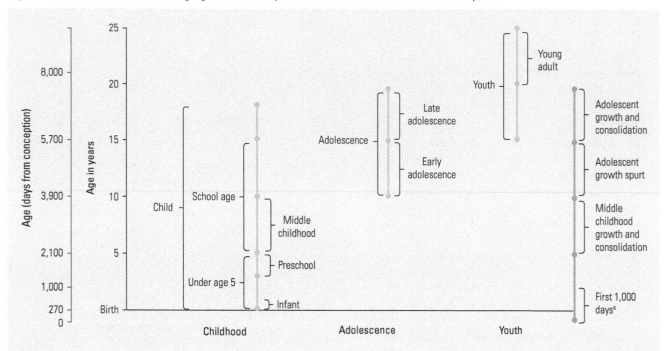

Note: a. The first 1000 days is typically measured from the time of conception, as is the 8,000 days that we discuss as the overall child and adolescent development period; other age-ranges presented here are measured from birth.

Box 1.3

Early Childhood Development

This volume takes a broad approach by examining child and adolescent health and development more generally, rather than focusing only on health. Therefore, although it focuses primarily on the 5–19 years age group, it also includes a discussion of early childhood development (ECD), which complements the discussion on early health in volume 2.

The existence of key synergies justifies the inclusion of ECD in a series focused on health. These include synergies in the outcomes of different investments in children and synergies in the delivery of both sets of interventions.

Synergies in investments in children. Elsewhere in this chapter, we discuss the synergies between health and education for those ages 5–19 years. These same synergies are also important for young children. A pathbreaking study in Jamaica (Grantham-McGregor and others 1991) demonstrated that health and nutrition interventions alone are insufficient to address developmental deficits in young children facing multiple deprivations. Combining health and nutrition interventions with responsive stimulation was found to have short-term developmental benefits for growth and cognitive development not only in childhood but also into adulthood (Gertler and others 2014), with long-term effects on adult earnings and social outcomes.

Violence against children (child abuse) is an extreme negative example of the same synergy.

A systematic review (Norman and others 2012) documented how this extreme form of poor nurturing adversely affects physical and mental health. Child maltreatment and neglect are associated with substantial medical costs in childhood and adulthood

box continues next page

Box 1.3 (continued)

(Brown, Fang, and Florence 2011; Fang and others 2015) and have negative impacts on adult economic well-being (CDC 2015; Currie and Widom 2010; Zielinski 2009). Although most of these studies are from high-income countries, similar results have been found in low- and middle-income countries.

Delivery platforms for early interventions at different ages. In the first 1,000 days, children's main contact with public sector institutions is with the health system, and it makes sense to use the health system to deliver education to parents about responsive stimulation. This education can be delivered through group sessions for parents at the local health facility or through home visits incorporating messages on responsive stimulation, as discussed in chapter 19 in this volume (Black, Gove, and Merseth 2017). Once children have received the required immunizations, they have fewer interactions with the health system; there are synergies then in using preschools and the school system to deliver health and nutrition interventions to children after age three years.

To date, the few published studies that have estimated the marginal additional cost of integrating programs for responsive stimulation into existing health services have found these costs to be modest (Horton and Black 2017, chapter 24 in this volume). However, these additional tasks cannot simply be loaded onto existing health workers without recognition of the need for additional training and supervision and for some increase in the ratio of health workers to population. Given the limited number of studies, it is not possible to estimate the economic returns to integrated programs.

An essential package for ECD. Chapter 24 in this volume (Horton and Black 2017) develops a basic ECD package relevant for low-income countries; the package focuses on parenting programs and encourages "responsive stimulation" (the positive interaction between a young child and his or her caregiver, with mutual benefit). These programs are estimated to cost US$6 per child and are delivered in the first 1,000 days. As per capita incomes rise, preschool programs for children ages three to five years might be added.

Investment lags far behind the potential for return and is far below investments in health in the first five years and in primary education after age 5 years. Table 1.1 compares our recommendations for additional spending with current spending on education and with spending on health for children under age 5 years.

This bias in investment is paralleled by a similar bias in research. Approximately 99 percent of publications in Google Scholar and 95 percent in PubMed on the first 20 years of life focus on children under age 5 (annex 1A shows the number of publications since 2004 that our search found that include the terms *health*, *mortality*, or *cause of death*). The availability of age-specific publications reflects a lack of research funding for and attention to middle childhood and adolescence, resulting in a lack of data. The analysis for the Global Burden of Disease 2013 came to a similar conclusion, pointing out that most of the unique data sources for risk factors for adolescents ages 15–19 years were from school-based surveys, that children younger than age 5 had the most data available of any age group, and that adolescents ages 10–14 years had the fewest data sources (Mokdad and others 2016). The *World Development Report 2007: Development and the Next Generation* similarly found

severe data shortcomings for these older age groups (World Bank 2006), whereas Hill and others found no empirical studies of mortality rates for the age group 5–14 years in countries without vital statistics, which include the majority of low- and middle-income countries (LIMCs) (Hill, Zimmerman, and Jamison 2017). The estimates, based on Demographic and Health Surveys Program data, reported here result in sharp upward adjustments in estimated numbers of deaths in that age range (Hill, Zimmerman, and Jamison 2017). This strong bias toward early childhood in the health literature may have been helpful in the successful United Nations Millennium Development Goals (MDG) drive to reduce under-five mortality. But it seems to have caused us to lose sight of the fact that the subsequent decades of growth and development in the transition to adulthood involve complex processes and critical periods that are sensitive to intervention.

This volume focuses on the scientific evidence, but local contexts, including culture, beliefs, lifestyles, and health systems, as well as other key determinants such as gender, race, ethnicity, sexuality, geography, socioeconomic status, and disability, are important for developing practical policies (Chandra-Mouli, Lane, and Wong 2015).

Table 1.1 Estimates of Public Sector Investment in Human Development in Low- and Lower-Middle-Income Countries

US$, billions per year

	Low-income countries	Lower-middle-income countries	Total for both low- and lower-middle-income countries
Current spending			
Basic education[a]	19	190	210
First 1,000 days[b]	4.4	24	29
Proposed new package			
School-age children package (excluding school feeding)	0.13	0.38	0.51
School-age children package (including school feeding)[c]	0.47	2.8	3.3
Adolescent package[c]	0.88	2.7	3.6
Total proposed spending on new packages in middle childhood and adolescence (including school feeding)[c]	1.4	5.5	6.9

a. These estimates are from *The Learning Generation* (International Commission on Financing Global Education Opportunity 2016, 37). They estimate current public sector spending on basic (primary-level) education in low- and lower-middle-income countries. The report calls for increases to US$50 billion and US$712 billion, respectively, by 2030.

b. These estimates are from *DCP3*, volume 2 and are for the cost of two packages: (1) maternal and newborn and (2) under-five child health. The editors of volume 2 estimate current spending in low- and lower-middle-income countries. Estimated incremental annual investments of US$7 billion and US$14 billion, respectively, are needed to achieve full coverage.

c. These estimates are summarized in table 1.4. They are the estimated total cost of implementing the school-age and adolescent packages in low- and lower-middle-income countries. There are no formal estimates of current coverage, but it is likely in the range of 20 percent to 50 percent of these figures.

Some groups that tend to be marginalized and overlooked when planning intervention strategies, such as ethnic minorities, LGBT (lesbian, gay, bisexual, or transgender) youth, persons with disabilities, youth in conflict areas, and refugees, are also likely to have the greatest need for health and development support.

A CONCEPTUAL FRAMEWORK FOR UNDERSTANDING CHILD AND ADOLESCENT HEALTH AND DEVELOPMENT

In this volume, we develop a conceptual framework for exploring the processes and inputs that determine physical and cognitive growth from birth to adulthood (Bundy and Horton 2017, chapter 6 in this volume). The framework recognizes the importance of the first 1,000 days. It further notes that during the first two decades of life, there are at least three other critically important development phases: middle childhood (ages 5 to 9 years), the early adolescent growth spurt (ages 10 to 14 years), and the later adolescent phase of growth and consolidation (ages 15 to 19 years) when age-specific interventions are necessary. See figure 1.2.

Rates of physical growth are indeed at their highest at ages below age two, emphasizing the importance of the first 1,000 days. However, at the peak of the adolescent growth spurt, the growth rate for girls is similar to—and for boys exceeds—the rate at age two years and growth begins to occur in quite different ways (Tanner 1990). Furthermore, a review in chapter 8 in this volume (Watkins, Bundy, and others 2017) suggests that human growth remains relatively plastic throughout much of childhood, with potentially important amounts of catch-up growth. We need to be more careful about claiming that early insults are irreversible and recognize that more can be done to help older children catch up, especially in middle childhood. The data signal how unintended research bias and the scarcity of studies of ages 5–19 have had perverse policy consequences.

Evidence from neuroscience over the past 15 years suggests that critical phases of brain development occur beyond the first 1,000 days and in some cases long after. By age six years, the brain has reached approximately 95 percent of its adult volume, but size is not everything; rather, the connections within the brain are of growing importance through middle childhood and adolescence (Grigorenko 2017, chapter 10 in this volume). Different areas of the brain have different functions and develop at different rates. Peak development of the sensorimotor cortex—which is associated with vision, hearing, and motor control—occurs relatively early, and development is limited after puberty. The parietal and temporal association complex, responsible for language skills and numeracy, develops the fastest a little later; thus by about age 14 years, although it is possible to learn new languages, it is more difficult to speak a new language in the same way as a native speaker (Dahl 2004). The prefrontal cortex develops later still; this area is associated with higher brain functions, such as executive control (figure 1.2, panel b).

There is a sequence of brain development, and the kind of growth in middle childhood and adolescence differs from the kind of growth in early life. It is possible to see some of these differential growth rates in brain capabilities by studying the size of the subcortical regions as shown in figure 1.2, panel c (Goddings and others 2014).

The panel shows the pattern for adolescent boys. The patterns are similar for girls but occur at earlier ages because of different patterns of puberty. The panel shows that the regions associated with movement (such as the caudate and globus pallidus) are shrinking in size during early adolescence because these structures become more efficient as the functions become more mature. In contrast, regions associated with memory, decision making, and emotional reactions (amygdala and hippocampus) are still developing and growing in size during adolescence.

Brain development during infancy and early childhood is marked by the development of primary

Figure 1.2 Human Development to Age 20 Years

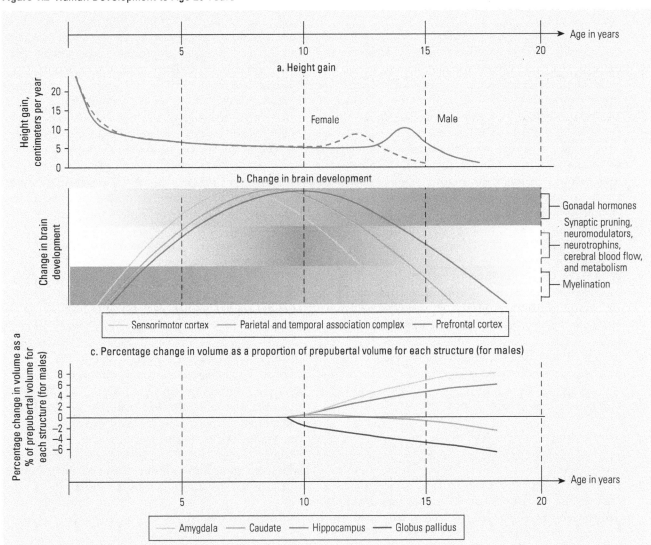

Sources: Adapted from Tanner 1990; Goddings and others 2014; Grigorenko 2017.
Note: Behavioral attributes are paralleled by hormonal and neurobiological changes that target specific brain regions and cell populations (shown in shaded gray to capture the dynamic influences of hormones, various brain processes, and myelination). The vertical axis in panel b shows relative rate of growth of three brain areas from 0 to highest. The progressive shading indicates when the indicated activity is at its most intense (darkest shading).

cognitive and emotional abilities. With the onset of the hormonal changes of puberty in middle childhood, a new phase of brain development commences in which the individual's interactions with the social, cultural, and educational environment shapes the processes of myelination and synaptic pruning of centers involved in emotional processing and higher executive functioning (Viner, Allen, and Patton 2017). Although primary cognitive abilities in stunted children may improve during middle childhood (Crookston and others 2013), brain development during these years and during adolescence is primarily focused on acquiring the higher-level cognitive, emotional, and social skills essential for functioning in complex social systems. As in earlier childhood, nutritional as well as social environments shape brain development (Andersen and Teicher 2008; Blakemore and Mills 2014).

Early intervention is critical for setting human development on an effective trajectory. However, the emphasis on the proposition that harm experienced in early life is irreversible is not only weakly supported by the evidence but also has led to an unfortunate lack of emphasis on exploring interventions later in childhood (Prentice and others 2013). Similarly, the widely cited conceptual framework of continuously declining rates of return with age (Heckmann 2011) is at variance with what is now known about the plasticity of brain development (Black, Gove, and Merseth 2017, chapter 19 in this volume) and of physical growth during much of middle childhood (Watkins, Bundy, and others 2017, chapter 8 in this volume), and it also fails to take into account the intergenerational benefits of actions in later childhood and adolescence. Some interventions make sense only at specific points in development; for example, some famous tennis players attribute their success to learning to play at age eight years, but they recognize that no amount of tennis lessons at age three would have achieved the same outcome. Current evidence suggests that there are substantial returns on investments made throughout the first two decades of life.

THE UNFINISHED AGENDA OF MORTALITY REDUCTION

During middle childhood and adolescence, the major consequences of ill health are related to morbidity rather than mortality. This fact does not mean that mortality is unimportant in older children. A new analysis of mortality was specifically conducted for this volume using Demographic and Health Surveys to estimate death rates for ages 5 to 19 years in the same way that data have been used to estimate rates for children under age 5 (Hill, Zimmerman, and Jamison 2017, chapter 2).

The estimates for 2010 suggest that the total annual mortality in LMICs in the 5 to 19 age group is around 2.3 million. The number of deaths estimated for children ages 5 to 9 years are 935,000, which is higher than the estimates of the United Nations Population Division and the Institute for Health Metrics and Evaluation (IHME) for this age group. Congruence of the new estimates with the UN and IHME data is closer for the 10 to 14 age group and closer yet for the 15 to 19 age group.

These results suggest that we need to do more to understand mortality in older children. A natural conclusion for policy would be to extend major national and international programmatic efforts that assess levels and causes of mortality in children under age 5 years to include the entire age range from birth through age 19 years. The United Nations Inter-agency Group for Child Mortality Estimation (IGME), which provides child mortality estimates through the Child Mortality Estimation (CME) database, and the Child Health Epidemiology Reference have historically focused on children under age 5 years, which helps explain why the data are so poor, and so poorly known, for children in middle childhood and adolescence. At least in part because of the focus in this volume on mortality levels in older children, IGME is expanding its work to cover this age range (Masquelin 2017). Although empirical estimates are still evolving, it is to be expected that IGME's effort will soon provide stable and up-to-date estimates that are country specific.

Morbidity is even more poorly documented than mortality for children over age five years. The volume explores the evidence for geographical and social differences in four key outcome measures—education, anthropometric status, micronutrient deficiency, and adolescent health— and describes major geographic variation in all four development outcomes (Galloway 2017; Wu 2017; Patton and others 2017, chapters 3–5, respectively, in this volume), but there is no systematic collection of morbidity data for this age-group, especially in LMICs. In exploring morbidity, we have begun to see that health and education are strongly linked in this age group; the education analysis shows that individual differences in health between students contribute to differences between educational outcomes and that differences in health are amenable to intervention in the short term.

ESSENTIAL PACKAGES OF INTERVENTIONS FOR SCHOOL-AGE CHILDREN AND ADOLESCENTS

Appropriate health interventions for the first 1,000 days are addressed in detail in volume 2, which describes

Table 1.2 Essential Package of Interventions for School-Age Children (Ages 5–14 Years)

Health area	Population	Community	Primary health center	School	Benefit of delivering interventions in schools
Physical health	—	Deworming	Deworming	Deworming	In endemic areas, regular deworming (following WHO guidelines) can be done inexpensively in schools now that the majority of deworming drugs are donated; there are reported benefits in school attendance as a result.
		Insecticide-treated net promotion	Insecticide-treated net promotion	Insecticide-treated net promotion	Education concerning the use of insecticide-treated nets in endemic areas is important because schoolchildren tend to use nets less often than do mothers and small children.
		Tetanus toxoid and HPV vaccination	Tetanus toxoid and HPV vaccination	Tetanus toxoid and HPV vaccination	Schools can be a good venue for administering tetanus boosters, which benefit not only young people themselves but also babies born to those young women.
		Oral health promotion	Oral health promotion and treatment	Oral health promotion	Education on oral health is important; poor households generally cannot afford dental treatment.
			Vision screening and provision of glasses	Vision screening and treatment	Vision screening and provision of inexpensive ready-made glasses boost school performance.
Nutrition	—	Micronutrient supplementation	—	Micronutrient supplementation	—
		Multifortified foods	—	Multifortified foods	—
				School feeding	School meals promote attendance and education outcomes.

Source: Fernandes and Aurino 2017 (chapter 25 in this volume).
Note: — = not available; HPV = human papillomavirus; WHO = World Health Organization. School-age children do not regularly come in contact with the health system unless they seek treatment. With the remarkable success of the Millennium Development Goals in increasing school enrollment and participation and the continuing focus on universal education with the Sustainable Development Goals, it makes sense to use schools to promote health in this age group and to deliver preventive and curative health interventions. These interventions are affordable and also the highest priority, given their health and educational benefits. Table 1.4 presents the cost of components of the essential package of investments for school-age children.

two essential packages of interventions targeted at young children: one on maternal and newborn health and the other on child health. In volume 8, we complement these packages with an analysis of early childhood development (Alderman and others 2017; Black, Gove, and Merseth 2017; Horton and Black 2017; Horton and others 2017, chapters 7, 19, 24, and 26, respectively, in this volume). Our analysis suggests that there is significant value in adding "responsive stimulation" to these health packages (box 1.3). More detailed analysis of the cost and relative effectiveness of the early child development package is presented in chapter 2 of volume 9 (Watkins, Nugent, and others 2018).

This volume focuses on the three phases of development for those older than age five years: middle childhood growth and consolidation, the adolescent growth spurt, and adolescent growth and consolidation (figure 1.1). We argue that intervention during each of these stages is essential to enhanced survival and to effective development; in addition, each stage provides an opportunity to remedy earlier failures in development, at least to some extent.

First we discuss a package of interventions aimed at school-age children (see table 1.2); this package addresses both middle childhood growth and consolidation (ages 5–9 years) and the adolescent growth spurt (ages 10–14 years). We then discuss a package aimed at later adolescence, which addresses adolescent growth and consolidation (ages 15–19 years) (table 1.3). In practice, there is considerable overlap between the age groups able to benefit from these two packages, and both packages are required to cover the needs of adolescents from ages 10 to 19 years.

As illustrated in maps 1.1 and 1.2, school-age children and adolescents (that is, the age group of 5–19 years) together constitute a substantial proportion of the overall population of all countries, with the proportion greatest in the poorest countries: 17.2 percent of high-income countries and rising to 37.2 percent of low-income countries. The essential health and development

Table 1.3 Essential Package of Investments for Adolescents (Ages 10–19 Years, Approximately)

Health area	Population	Community	Primary health center	School	Benefit of targeting interventions to adolescents
Physical health	Healthy lifestyle messages: tobacco, alcohol, injury, accident avoidance, and safety	Adolescent-friendly health services	Adolescent-friendly health services: provision of condoms to prevent STIs, provision of reversible contraception, treatment of injury in general and abuse in particular, screening and treatment for STIs	Healthy lifestyle education, including accident avoidance and safety	National media messages on healthy life choices in formats designed to appeal to adolescents, combined with national policy efforts to support healthy choices (limiting access of adolescents to products most harmful to their health)
	Sexual health messages	—	—	Sexual health education	Additional health education in schools aimed at issues relevant to older ages, intended to supplement messages for younger children in the school-age package
				Adolescent-friendly health services	Provision of adolescent-friendly health services within schools or within health care facilities in ways that respect adolescent needs
Nutrition	Nutrition education messages	—	—	Nutrition education	—
Mental health	Mental health messages	—	Mental health treatment	Mental health education and counseling	—

Source: Horton and others 2017 (chapter 26 in this volume).
Note: — = not available; STI = sexually transmitted infection. Adolescents are the hardest group to reach because many are no longer in school and feel uncomfortable accessing health services predominantly designed for adults. They may fear lack of confidentiality, and in some cases (such as teen pregnancy) may be stigmatized by health care workers. The total costs of the school-age package are about US$10 per child in the 5–14 years age group and US$9 per adolescent in the 10–19 years age group. Table 1.4 presents the cost of components of the essential package of investments for adolescents.

packages for school-age children and adolescents have particular relevance in low- and lower-middle-income countries where the population that can benefit from these developmental interventions constitutes approximately one-third of the total population.

Essential Package of Interventions for School-Age Children

Health and nutrition programs targeted through schools are among the most ubiquitous for school-age children in LMICs. Since the inclusion of school health programs in the launch of Education for All in 2000, it is difficult to find a country that is not attempting to provide school health services at some level, although the coverage is often limited (Sarr and others 2017). The World Food Programme estimates that more than 360 million school-children receive school meals every day (Drake and others 2017, chapter 12 in this volume), many of whom live in LMICs, and the World Health Organization (WHO) estimates that more than 450 million schoolchildren—more

than half of the target population—are dewormed annually (Bundy, Appleby, and others 2017, chapter 13 in this volume) in nearly all LMICs. These largely public efforts are variable in quality and coverage, but the large scale of existing programs indicates a willingness by governments to invest in health as well as education for this age group.

The school system represents an exceptionally cost-effective platform through which to deliver an essential package of health and nutrition services to this age group, as has been well documented in high-income countries (HICs) (Shackleton and others 2016). It is also increasingly equitable, especially because increases in primary enrollment and attendance rates, and narrowing of gender gaps, are among the greatest achievements of the Millennium Development Goals (Bundy, Schultz, and others 2017, chapter 20 in this volume). In LMICs with weak health systems, the education system is particularly well-situated to promote health among school-going children and adolescents who may not be reached by health services. There are typically more schools than health facilities in all income settings,

Map 1.1 Proportion of Country Population That Comprises Children in Middle Childhood (between Ages 5–9)
Percent

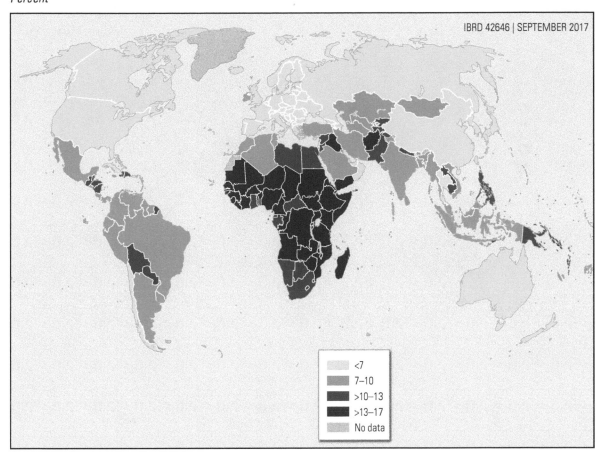

IBRD 42646 | SEPTEMBER 2017

<7
7–10
>10–13
>13–17
No data

Source: United Nations, *World Population Prospects: The 2015 Revision*, July 2015.

and rural and poor areas are significantly more likely to have schools than health centers.

In this section, we examine the investment case for providing an integrated package of essential health services for children attending school in low- and lower-middle-income countries (see table 1.2). "School-age" includes both middle childhood and younger adolescence.

Middle Childhood Growth and Consolidation Phase

An important economic rationale for targeting the health and development of school-age children is to promote learning at an age when they have what may be their only opportunity to attend school. Ill health can be a catalyst for extended absence from or dropping out of school; for example, malaria and worm infections can reduce enrollment, and anemia resulting from malaria or worm infections can affect cognition, attention span, and learning (Benzian and others 2017; Brooker and others 2017; Bundy, Appleby, and others 2017; Drake and others 2017; LaMontagne and others 2017; Lassi, Moin, and Bhutta 2017 [chapters 11–16 in

this volume]). Estimates suggest that in areas where malaria and worm infections are prevalent, poor students could gain the equivalent of 0.5 to 2.5 extra years of schooling if given appropriate health interventions, while sustaining benefits across multiple years of schooling could improve cognitive abilities by 0.25 standard deviation, on average. Extrapolating the benefits of improved accumulation of human capital could translate to roughly a 5 percent increase in earning capacity over the life course (Ahuja and others 2017, chapter 29 in this volume).

Chapter 8 in this volume (Watkins, Bundy, and others 2017) shows that some of these interventions also have important roles to play in maintaining and sustaining the gains of earlier investments, and children who slip through the early safety net can still achieve some catch-up growth with interventions in middle childhood. Furthermore, the new mortality analyses presented in chapter 2 (Hill, Zimmerman, and Jamison 2017) show that, for those ages five to nine years, survival continues to be a significant challenge, largely

Map 1.2 Proportion of Country Population That Comprises Adolescents (between Ages 10–19)
Percent

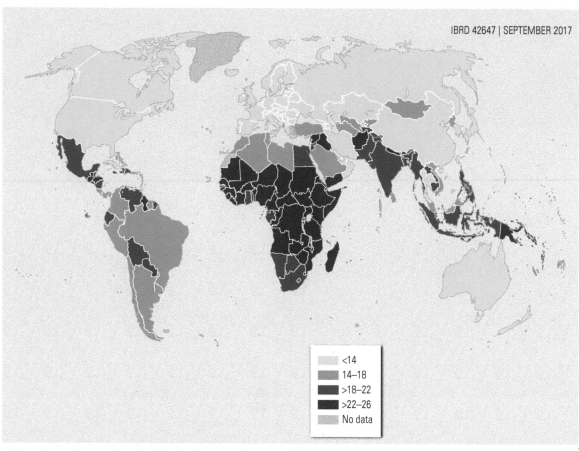

IBRD 42647 | SEPTEMBER 2017

<14
14–18
>18–22
>22–26
No data

Source: United Nations, *World Population Prospects: The 2015 Revision*, July 2015.

because of the persistently high prevalence of infectious diseases, including pneumonia, diarrhea, and malaria. The control of infectious diseases therefore remains a critical element of intervention in this age group.

In many malaria-endemic areas, successful control programs have reduced the level of transmission substantially (Noor and others 2014; O'Meara and others 2008; WHO 2015). However, since the age pattern of clinical malaria is determined by the level of transmission and the consequent level of acquired immunity (Carnerio and others 2010; Snow and others 1997), clinical attacks of malaria are becoming more common in older children. In The Gambia, the peak age of hospital admission for severe malaria increased from 3.9 years in 1999–2003 to 5.6 years in 2005–2007 (Ceesay and others 2008); similar changes have been seen in Kenya (O'Meara and others 2008). This has created a new challenge for intervention, because none of the population-based presumptive treatment approaches are recommended for the school-age group and the current policy of testing and treating with Artemisinin-based combination therapy does not appear cost-effective in this age-group (Brooker and others 2017, chapter 14 in this volume; see also Babigumira, Gelband, and Garrison 2017, chapter 15 in volume 6). Analyses in this volume (Bundy, Appleby, and others 2017, chapter 13) and in volume 6 (Fitzpatrick and others 2017, chapter 16) also show that intestinal worm burdens are often greatest in school-age children, and whereas there is broad consensus on the benefits of treating infected children, there is controversy regarding the most cost-effective approach to school-based delivery. In practice, most countries use school-based mass treatment—that is, treatment of all children at risk, without prior screening. In 2015, more than 450 million children were treated, and India alone claims to have treated 340 million children in 2016.

Adolescent Growth Spurt Phase

The pubertal growth spurt is a watershed feature in the transition from childhood to adolescence, a process that occurs earlier for girls and that can be modified by external factors, including diet. The phase may provide the best opportunity for catch-up growth, with growth velocities reaching equivalence to those of children at age two years.

The growth spurt is a time of rapidly increasing muscle, bone, and organ mass, and of high dietary demand. One way of responding to this—providing meals in schools—is arguably the most prevalent publicly funded resource transfer program worldwide, with some 360 million children being fed every school day. A narrow focus on health outcomes underestimates the benefits of multiple cross-sectoral outcomes, including promoting school participation, especially for girls; providing a productive social safety net in hard-to-reach communities; and stimulating rural economies through the procurement of local produce (Drake and others 2017, chapter 12 in this volume). School feeding should be viewed as an option among other transfer programs with multiple outcomes. From a social perspective—often taken in economic evaluation—the net cost of a transfer is often close to zero, or the 10 percent to 15 percent of the total cost that is required for delivery (see discussion of the costs of cash and other transfer programs from multiple perspectives in chapter 23 in this volume, de Walque and others 2017). School feeding can thus be viewed as conditional (because school attendance triggers the transfer) non-cash transfer programs, and evaluations suggest that offering school meals typically increases attendance rates by 8 percent (Drake and others 2017). From this effect alone, benefit-cost ratios of 2 or more can be inferred.

School-based delivery of vaccination is particularly effective at this age, especially for girls. Tetanus toxoid vaccination lowers the risk of contracting tetanus both for recipients and for the children of adolescent girls, thus providing an intergenerational benefit. In addition, 70 percent coverage of human papillomavirus vaccine that is effective over a lifetime could avert more than 670,000 cases of cervical cancer in Sub-Saharan Africa over consecutive birth cohorts of girls vaccinated as young adolescents (LaMontagne and others 2017, chapter 15 in this volume). There is evidence that school-based vaccination programs can achieve effective coverage.

Early adolescence is the age when the most common vision problems—refractive errors—first emerge, and school-based screening of children in select grades is a cost-effective way to detect and correct refractive errors of vision that could otherwise increase the probability of dropping out of school, perhaps leading to lifelong visual impairment (Graham and others 2017, chapter 17 in this volume). Early adolescence is also a key phase for promoting lifelong healthy behaviors (World Bank 2006), including oral hygiene and good dietary practices. This phase may be particularly sensitive to diet, as it is associated with the emergence of micronutrient deficiency diseases, such as anemia and iodine deficiency.

Essential Package of Interventions for Later Adolescence

A phase of adolescent growth and consolidation begins around 15 years of age, continues into the 20s, and requires a package of age-specific interventions (table 1.3). This period has traditionally been viewed as socially important but has lacked concerted attention as a critical period for health and development. This is an age when self-agency becomes increasingly important, and although the concept of adolescent-friendly health services has been widely adopted, in reality the quality and coverage rarely respond to the need, in particular, ensuring that adolescents are able to make their own decisions about their health. School-based interventions that go beyond the teaching of health education in classrooms and encompass changes to the curriculum and the wider social environment, as well as engagement with families and the community, are more likely to improve sexual health, reduce violence, and decrease substance abuse (Reavley and others 2017, chapter 18 in this volume; Shackleton and others 2016). In the broader population, intersectoral action has been central to public health gains in many countries, including transport sector actions to reduce road traffic injuries and taxes to achieve tobacco control (Elvik and others 2009; Farrelly and others 2013).

With the exception of sexual and reproductive health, available evidence on preventive interventions derives largely from high-income countries and the United States in particular. The social and environmental determinants of adolescent health and well-being act at different levels and across different sectors. The most effective responses are likely to operate at multiple levels of particular settings (Viner and others 2012). The lives of young people are affected by community behavior and norms as well as by the values of adults and other adolescents. Community interventions have commonly involved local government, families, youth-focused and religious organizations, and schools.

Universal health coverage for adolescents requires training health care providers not only to respond to specific health problems beyond a focus on sexual and reproductive health but also to adopt nonjudgmental attitudes, to maintain confidentiality, and to engage with adolescents—while maintaining lines of communication with families. There needs to be a focus on addressing the financial barriers that are especially important for adolescents to overcome, such as making out-of-pocket payments and finding accessible platforms for health delivery that work for this age group. There is growing recognition of the importance of agency for this age group and of the importance of identifying approaches to health that enhance decision making and engagement of adolescents around their health and health care. Lack of adolescent agency is particularly common in LMICs.

Particularly for girls, the expansion of secondary education, which is one of the Sustainable Development Goals (SDGs) targeted for 2030, offers remarkable opportunities to improve health and well-being. Secondary education is effective in increasing the age at marriage and first pregnancy (Verguet and others 2017, chapter 28 in this volume). Participation in quality secondary education enhances cognitive abilities; improves mental, sexual, and reproductive health; lowers risks for later-life noncommunicable diseases; and offers significant intergenerational benefits (Blank and others 2010). Secondary schools also provide a platform for health promotion that can strengthen self-agency around health; provide essential health knowledge, including comprehensive sexuality education; and help to maintain lifestyles that minimize health risks. Equally, achieving the educational and economic benefits that secondary schools offer requires the avoidance of early pregnancy, infectious diseases, mental disorders, injury-related disabilities, and undernutrition.

Media messages have particular salience during the adolescent years and provide an essential platform for health action and have proven effective in HICs. Adolescents are biologically, emotionally, and developmentally primed for engagement beyond their families, and the media, particularly social media, offer that opportunity. Social media may also bring hazards, among the most conspicuous being online grooming, cyberbullying, and a growing preoccupation with body image, and so any intervention has to take these negatives into account (Durlak, Weissberg, and Dymnicki 2011; Farahmand and others 2011; Murray and others 2007).

Economic Analysis of the Essential Packages

Table 1.1 summarizes current levels of public investment in three important areas for child and adolescent health and development in LMICs: basic education (pre-primary, primary, and secondary), health in the first 1,000 days, and the two intervention packages for ages 5–19 years in low- and lower-middle-income countries. Table 1.4 summarizes the costs of the essential packages to promote health of school-age children and adolescents.

Of the three areas, education attracts the largest investment at US$206 billion per year in 2015, much of which is from the public sector and is intended to provide pre-primary, primary, and secondary education free at the point of delivery. The International Commission on Financing Global Education Opportunity (2016) calls for governments to increase domestic public expenditures to support universal provision of primary education in low- and lower-middle-income countries by 2030, requiring an increase from 4.0 to 5.8 percent of gross domestic product (GDP), which is equivalent to an annual rate of growth in public education spending of 7 percent over a 15-year period. In addition to education interventions, the commission identifies 13 nonteaching interventions as "highly effective practices to increase access and learning outcomes," including three health interventions: school feeding, malaria prevention, and micronutrient intervention. The achievement of universal secondary education by 2030 is a specific Sustainable Development Goal and is also cited in the report of the *Lancet* Commission on Adolescent Health and Wellbeing as key to adolescent growth and development.

In contrast to these very large public expenditures for education, the current annual investment for children younger than age five years is an estimated US$28.6 billion, which includes investments in maternal and newborn health, as well as child health for children under age five years. It is estimated, based on current prices, that the cost of increasing coverage to 80 percent would be an additional US$27.3 billion annually (table 1.1). This is based on estimates in volume 2 (Black, Walker, and others 2015) of the cost of the two packages: maternal and newborn health, and health of children under five.

For interventions in the health and development of children in the age range of 5–19 years in low- and lower-middle-income countries, we have no direct estimate of current expenditure. We present here the estimated total and incremental costs of providing a school-age package and an adolescent package to this age group (table 1.1). We estimate the total cost as US$6.9 billion, comprising US$1.4 billion and US$5.5 billion in low- and lower-middle-income countries, respectively (not including HPV vaccination). Assuming that current provision is on the order of 20 percent to 50 percent of need, this implies an incremental need of between US$3.4 billion and US$5.4 billion annually, representing between 0.03 percent and 0.07 percent of GDP, dramatically less

Table 1.4 Cost of Components of Essential Packages to Promote Health of School-Age Children and Adolescents in Low- and Lower-Middle-Income Countries

Intervention	Mode of delivery	Approximate cost per child who benefits (US$) in low- and lower-middle-income countries	Approximate cost per child (US$) in relevant age group	Aggregate cost in low-income countries (US$, millions, per year)	Aggregate cost in lower-middle-income countries (US$, millions, per year)
School-age children					
School feeding programs	Meals (fortified with micronutrients) provided at school	41 (targeted to 20% of population in most food-insecure or poor areas)	8.2 per child ages 6–12 years	340	2,400
Health education (oral health, ITN use)	ITN education delivered only in endemic areas	0.50 per educational message (ITN message delivered only in endemic areas; assumed 50% of children in low- and lower-middle-income countries)	0.75 per child ages 6–12 years	31	110
Vision screening	Prescreening by teachers; vision tests and provision of ready-made glasses on site by eye specialists	3.6 per child to screen and provide glasses to the fraction of the age group needing glasses	0.60 per child ages 6–12 years	25	90
Deworming	Medication for soil-transmitted helminths or schistosomiasis delivered by teachers once a year in endemic areas	0.70 per child; 50% of endemic areas	0.35 per child ages 6–12 years	14	52
Tetanus toxoid booster	Single-dose booster administered to all children in one grade by nurse or similar health care worker	2.4 per child	0.40 per child ages 6–12 years	16	59
HPV vaccine	Part of the cancer essential package	10 per fully vaccinated girl (Gavi-eligible countries)	0.83 per child ages 6–12 years	43	74
Aggregate costs without HPV vaccine		48	10	430	2,700
Aggregate costs without school feeding programs but with HPV vaccine		17	2	130	390
Adolescents					
Media messages on national policy regarding health	Messages concerning use of tobacco, alcohol, and illicit drugs; sexual and reproductive health; mental health; healthy eating or physical activity	1 per adolescent	1 per adolescent ages 10–19 years	—	—
Health education in schools	Education for targeted age group	9 per year per adolescent ages 14–16 years	3 per adolescent ages 10–19 years	90	450
Adolescent-friendly health services	Health services offering respectful and confidential access for adolescents	5 per adolescent	5 per adolescent ages 10–19 years	790	2,300
Aggregate costs		15 per adolescent ages 10–19 years	9 per adolescent ages 10–19 years	880	2,700

Source: Fernandes and Aurino 2017 (chapter 25 in this volume); Horton and others 2017 (chapter 26 in this volume).

Note: — = not available; Gavi = Gavi, the Vaccine Alliance; HPV = human papillomavirus; ITN = insecticide-treated bednet. The total cost of the school-age package is about US$10 per child in the 5–14 years age group and about US$9 per adolescent in the 10–19 years age group. Compared with per capita public expenditures on health in 2013 of about US$31, this does not seem unreasonable, but it is high for low-income countries, which spent only US$14 per capita on health in 2013.

than the increments sought for education or for the health programs for children under five years of age.

The single most costly component is school meals, which account for almost half of the additional investment required. We have argued earlier that this is a special case and is neither paid for by the Ministry of Health nor primarily aimed at improving health. It is standard in *DCP3* to distinguish between interventions within the health sector and those delivered and financed outside the health sector. School meals, although part of the health package, are intersectoral in origin. For this reason, table 1.1 shows the costs with and without school meals. See also volume 9 for further discussion of this issue (chapter 2 [Watkins, Nugent, and others 2018]).

Taken together, these analyses suggest two important conclusions for investing in health in the 5 to 19 age group. It is apparent that education investments dominate all other public investments in human development during the first two decades of life. Using our estimates of current expenditure, the current costs of providing access in low- and lower-middle-income countries to basic education and a health care services package for under-fives (including maternal and newborn health) are US$206 billion and US$28.6 billion, respectively. The cost of the additional essential health and development packages for those ages 5–19 years are between US$1.4 billion and US$3.4 billion, respectively. Given that the latter two health and development investments underpin those in education, it seems difficult to justify investing in education without making the complementary investments in health and human development for this age group, especially given the comparatively low cost of the health and development packages. The modest cost of the two packages suggests that scaling up the health packages for those ages 5–19 is therefore a high return and low-cost investment that addresses the most pressing development needs throughout the first two decades of life.

HEALTH AND EDUCATION: TWO SIDES OF THE SAME COIN

This volume makes a strong case for providing both education and health services during middle childhood and adolescence. The view that education and health are separate silos in human development reflects an administrative and bureaucratic reality but does not best serve the needs of the growing child and adolescent. The common sense view that growing children need both health and education—*mens sana in corpore sano*—is supported by the evidence for strong links between health

outcomes and educational attainment (Bundy, Schultz, and others 2017, chapter 20 in this volume; Plaut and others 2017, chapter 22 in this volume), and between educational attainment and health outcomes (Pradhan and others 2017). Years of schooling and quality of schooling (as measured by standardized test scores) reduce mortality rates in adults and children. Chapter 30 of this volume (Pradhan and others 2017) reports research that has recently incorporated both adult mortality outcomes and education quality into the literature. If rates of return to educational investments are recalculated to take into account reasonable estimates of the value of reducing mortality, the returns to education increase by about one-third. For example, in lower-middle-income countries, the estimated internal rate of return to one additional year of education increases from 7.0 percent to 9.3 percent if the effect of education on mortality is included. In this volume we explore both of these directions of influence.

Health, Education, and Social Outcomes

Exposing young children to drought and social shocks in Zimbabwe was shown to adversely affect height in adolescence, which, in turn, adversely affected schooling (Alderman, Hoddinott, and Kinsey 2006). Effect sizes were large: if individuals had reached median height for age, they would have been 3.4 centimeters taller, started school six months earlier, and have achieved an additional 0.85 years of schooling. There are also some trials in low- and middle-income countries that indicate impact: for example, young children with better diets in the Philippines did better in school than their less-advantaged siblings (Glewwe, Jacoby, and King 2001). Micronutrient deficiencies (particularly of iodine and iron, both known to affect cognition) have adverse effects on grade repetition and scores on cognitive tests (surveyed by Alderman and Bleakley 2013). In contrast, a recent systematic review, largely in LMICs, provides a more ambiguous picture of the impact of school-based interventions (Snilstveit and others 2015). We now recognize that development outcomes are crucially dependent upon the age-specific timing of intervention and upon the duration of follow-up. This is an area where longitudinal studies are particularly important but are currently rare. Chapter 7 of this volume (Alderman and others 2017) uses the lifecycle approach to assess the benefit-cost ratios of interventions in nutrition and child development in LMICs where nutrition is a risk factor, with a focus on the first five years of life. Chapter 12 (Drake and others 2017) summarizes the effects of school feeding programs (which alleviate hunger) on improved school attendance and test scores.

Chapter 27 (Nandi and others 2017) discusses the long-term human capital and economic benefits of early-life interventions.

Chapter 14 in this volume (Brooker and others 2017) reviews the effect of malaria on education. Randomized controlled trials found that treatment of malaria reduced absenteeism and that treatment provided in childhood improved schooling attainment in adolescence; in two countries, schoolchildren receiving malaria prophylaxis had better attention spans. Chapter 13 (Bundy, Appleby, and others 2017) and chapter 29 (Ahuja and others 2017) emphasize the importance of deworming for education.

Uncertainty about the appropriate metrics is one reason the scale of the contribution of ill health to unrealized cognitive attainment, and hence learning, is poorly understood. Both the WHO and IHME estimate the effect of ill health on cognition using a threshold approach, typically the proportion of the affected population that scores below some threshold—for example, an intelligence quotient (IQ) of 75, indicative of severe cognitive disability. A more informative metric would be some population level metric of the extent to which individuals reach their cognitive potential, analogous to the assessment of anthropometric status. There is also a need for an impact model that takes into account the overlapping benefits of multiple interventions. Given the secular trend for IQ scores to drift upward (Flynn 2007), it might be helpful to estimate the extent to which improved health will contribute to the achievement of cognitive potential.

Education and Health Outcomes

An extensive literature documents the correlation between higher levels of education and lower levels of mortality, illness, and health risk. The earliest data showed no association: in the late nineteenth century, mortality levels of individuals with high education were no lower than those of individuals with little education. However, by the early twentieth century, U.S. census data revealed a strong association between health and education. This transition has been attributed to the scientific revolution launched by Koch and Pasteur with the germ theory of disease, which gave households and states practicable means of interrupting the transmission of infectious disease (Preston and Haines 1991). Without such knowledge, an educated person could do little more than could an illiterate compatriot, but the more educated person learned about and adopted the newly available science from Europe much more quickly. This conclusion has close parallels with research on the value of education to economic productivity: in the

presence of access to new markets, new seeds, or new crops, educated farmers quickly surpass illiterate farmers, but in closed, stagnant economies, formal education confers no advantage (Schultz 1993).

Rapidly changing knowledge and greater access to powerful drugs and vaccines should have led education to play an important role in halving the mortality rate for adolescents and adults 15–60 years of age around the world in the half century since 1970. But rates of decline varied markedly from country to country. Why such variation? For child mortality, variation in income growth explained a modest amount of cross-country differences (Jamison, Murphy, and Sandbu 2016). The number of available medical professionals explained more, and the pace at which some countries were able to adopt powerful and low-cost child survival technologies explained even more. About 9 percent of the reduction in child mortality from 1970 to 2000 in LMICs resulted from increased levels of education, as discussed in chapter 30 (Pradhan and others 2017).

Similarly, strong controls for country-specific effects in both the level and the rate of change of child and adult mortality resulted in education effects that were quantitatively and statistically highly significant (Pradhan and others 2017, chapter 30 in this volume). This study suggests that education's effects on adult mortality rates are about the same as the effects on child mortality (around 2–3 percent reduction per additional year of education and per one standard deviation improvement in test scores). If rates of return to educational investments are recalculated to take into account reasonable estimates of the value of mortality reduction, the returns to education increase by about one-third. For example, in lower-middle-income countries, the estimated internal rate of return to one additional year of education increases from 7.0 to 9.3 percent if the effect of education on mortality is included.

RESEARCH AND DEVELOPMENT PRIORITIES

The analyses presented here suggest some priorities for future research, with a focus on longer-term periods of observation that will capture developmental outcomes, assessment of multiple and complementary interventions, and, most important, a greater focus on children in middle childhood and adolescents. Specifically, future research should take into account the following issues.

1. *Collect better data on health and development needs in the 5 to 21 age range.* As shown in annex 1A, there has been a strong research focus on the health and development of children under five and a concomitant

relative absence of research on the needs of children in middle childhood and adolescence. There is a particular lack of information on children five to nine years of age.

2. *Pilot and evaluate packages of interventions for middle childhood and adolescence.* The packages proposed in this volume are based on the published literature for the individual interventions. In many cases, the evidence is partial and overly reliant on experiences in high-income countries. This suggests a need to carefully pilot and evaluate the packages under local circumstances before going to scale.

3. *Conduct more long-term longitudinal studies.* Most of the available analyses are too short term (typically less than a year) to provide useful guidance on development, which is inherently a long-term issue. To be useful, studies need to track outcomes over multiple years. A key question concerns the relative importance to development outcomes of intervention at different phases.

4. *Measure multiple outcomes of interventions.* Studies generally assess a single or a few outcomes, whereas the focus of development is inherently multisectoral and multifactorial. In particular, more studies are needed that simultaneously assess physical growth and cognitive development to assess the mutual benefits for health and education outcomes.

5. *Track mortality beyond age 5.* The new evidence that mortality is higher than recognized in those ages 5–14 indicates a need for more clarity about appropriate survival interventions for this age group. A starting point in middle childhood would be to assess the applicability of interventions that have proved successful in reducing the mortality of children under five; however, the causes of death are likely to be quite different for older adolescents, in particular.

6. *Examine the social dimensions of intervention in childhood and adolescence.* The social ecology of children's lives is poorly understood, especially in low- and lower-middle-income countries. There is a specific need for locally relevant research on the importance of families and teachers and of the gender context.

7. *Understand biological differences as a development issue.* There are sex differences in growth and development. For example, pubertal development differs by sex, so the timing of the growth spurt and the accompanying physiological changes also happen on a different timeline and scale. We now know that large differences are also apparent in brain development, yet we know little of the implications for behavioral intervention.

8. *Estimate the scale of the contribution of disability to development.* Children with disabilities are less able to benefit from prosperity, and disability remains a largely hidden topic. This is particularly true of mental health challenges in low-income countries and LMICs, and even more so of behavioral and social challenges, including autism. IHME estimates suggest that one in six children ages 5–19 years is severely or very severely disabled.

In reviewing these research issues, two short-term responses could be quickly implemented if there is to be a serious effort to understand the health and development needs of middle childhood and adolescence: (1) support existing longitudinal studies to define returns on interventions in middle childhood and adolescence, and (2) extend current mortality surveillance tools to include those ages 5–19 years.

In this volume, we propose intervening during ages that have not traditionally been given policy priority, especially in low-income countries. Developing an appropriate response will require stronger investment in implementation research that addresses the specific needs of middle childhood and adolescence. A potential way to move forward efficiently would be to expand the age range and interventions explored in current research models designed to assess developmental outcomes longitudinally. Examples include the 20-year-old Matlab Health and Socioeconomic Survey in Bangladesh; the 40-year-old Medical Research Council Keneba study in The Gambia; and the 15-year-old Young Lives studies in Ethiopia, India, Peru, and Vietnam, all of which are still ongoing. One of the key questions might be, what intervention is necessary to achieve remediation for children who slipped through the early safety net?

The burden of mortality and serious disease in the 5–19 age group is substantially higher than had been realized. During the Millennium Development Goals era, there was notable success in reducing under-5 mortality, and a key contributor was the creation of two new mechanisms for tracking mortality in children in this age group: the United Nations Inter-agency Group for Child Mortality Estimation, which provides current child mortality estimates through the Child Mortality Estimation database; and the Child Health Epidemiology Reference Group, which develops improved evidence on the causes of child mortality. If the world is to be similarly successful in addressing mortality in older children, there will need to be a similarly strong evidence-based approach to mortality in ages beyond five. This could be achieved if both of these groups extended the age range up to 21 and engaged with the research and public health communities working with these older age groups.

CONCLUSIONS

Although the current investment focus on the first 1,000 days of human development is necessary, it is not enough. The narrow focus on investing in health in the earliest childhood years underserves our children and adolescents by failing to support their development at other critical phases during the first two decades of life and by failing to secure the early gains. This unbalanced approach has not only resulted in a neglect of health service provision after the first 1,000 days but has also deflected research away from middle childhood and adolescence.

The issue is not that the first 1,000 days are less important than previously thought, but rather that the subsequent 7,000 days before the child reaches age 21 have much greater importance than has been recognized. Based largely on cost-effectiveness and benefit-cost analyses, we have identified two essential packages of interventions that together can help address these health and development demands in middle childhood and adolescence. A school-age package, largely built around school-based delivery, can address many of the needs during middle childhood and the adolescent growth spurt. An adolescence package, built both around the school and around access to non-stigmatizing, affordable, and confidential health care, can help further address the needs during the adolescent growth spurt and the very particular needs of later adolescence. The purposes of the two packages overlap, as do the age ranges of the target populations, and so both packages are required to support development through middle childhood and adolescence. It is important to recognize that the school and the education sector are key participants in these processes, both by providing an infrastructure for delivery and, just as important, by providing the learning, understanding, and life skills that have contributed, for example, about 30 percent of the observed decline in maternal mortality since 1990.

There are powerful opportunities for synergy between health and education that are currently underexploited. The school and the education sector should be recognized as key participants in promoting health, both by providing an infrastructure for delivery and, just as important, by providing the learning, understanding, and life skills that, for example, have

contributed about 30 percent of the observed decline in maternal mortality since 1990. However, the health of school-age children and adolescents, especially in low- and lower-middle-income countries, is an important determinant of education outcomes, having consequences for both education access and learning. The analyses presented here for the first 8,000 days indicate that investments in health leverage education outcomes, and investments in education leverage health.

The current world view is that education is a high priority and that the MDGs have helped ensure near-universal access to free primary education that is free at the point of delivery. One of the new Sustainable Development Goals is to achieve the same for secondary education. There is also increasing recognition that the RMNCH (reproductive, maternal, newborn and child health) demands of the 1,000 days should also be viewed as a high priority. Here we argue that, for similar reasons, the incremental costs of addressing health and development needs during middle childhood and adolescence should be viewed in the same way. Our calculations suggest that the proposed essential packages are a practical and affordable investment, even for LMICs. Based on current expenditures world-wide in LMICs, the annual cost of providing access to health care for children under five is US$28.6 billion, and the cost of providing primary education is US$206 billion. For the same countries, the estimated incremental cost of the essential health and development packages for ages 5 to 19 would add between US$1.4 billion and US$3.4 billion. This is a small increment to leverage the existing investments in early childhood and education and to secure the health and development of the next generation. Given the current levels of development assistance and domestic investment in both the first 1,000 days and in education, there would seem to be a strong economic case for leveraging these investments with critical, but more modest, health investments during the next 7,000 days, with benefits for equity, for realizing individual potential, and for maximizing the opportunities for the next generation.

The implication is that public policy needs to align with parental commitments and to the commitment to addressing health, development, and education through the first two decades of life. More countries already emphasize the social and legal importance of the 21st birthday, and our analyses suggest that it is necessary and affordable for all countries to translate that commitment into practical investments in middle childhood and adolescence.

ANNEX

The annex to this chapter is as follows. It is available at http://www.dcp-3.org/CAHD.

- Annex 1A. Analysis of Published Literature Describing Health and Mortality, Ages 0–19 Years

NOTE

World Bank Income Classifications as of July 2014 are as follows, based on estimates of gross national income (GNI) per capita for 2013:

- Low-income countries (LICs) = US$1,045 or less
- Middle-income countries (MICs) are subdivided:
  a) lower-middle-income = US$1,046 to US$4,125
  b) upper-middle-income (UMICs) = US$4,126 to US$12,745
- High-income countries (HICs) = US$12,746 or more.

REFERENCES

Ahuja, A., S. Baird, J. Hamory Hicks, M. Kremer, and E. Miguel. 2017. "Economics of Mass Deworming Programs." In *Disease Control Priorities* (third edition): Volume 8, *Child and Adolescent Health and Development*, edited by D. A. P. Bundy, N. de Silva, S. Horton, D. T. Jamison, and G. C. Patton. Washington, DC: World Bank.

Alderman, H., J. Behrman, P. Glewwe, L. Fernald, and S. Walker. 2017. "Evidence of Impact on Growth and Development of Interventions during Early and Middle Childhood." In *Disease Control Priorities* (third edition): Volume 8, *Child and Adolescent Health and Development*, edited by D. A. P. Bundy, N. de Silva, S. Horton, D. T. Jamison, and G. C. Patton. Washington, DC: World Bank.

Alderman, H., and H. Bleakley. 2013. "Child Health and Educational Outcomes." In *Education Policy in Developing Countries,* edited by P. Glewwe, 107–36. Chicago, IL: University of Chicago Press.

Alderman, H., J. Hoddinott, and B. Kinsey. 2006. "Long Term Consequences of Early Childhood Malnutrition." *Oxford Economic Papers* 58 (3): 450–74.

Andersen, S. L., and M. H. Teicher. 2008. "Stress, Sensitive Periods and Maturational Events in Adolescent Depression." *Trends in Neuroscience* 31 (4): 183–91.

Babigumira, J. B., H. Gelband, and L. P. Garrison Jr. 2017. "Cost-Effectiveness of Strategies for Diagnosis and Treatment of Febrile Illness in Children." In *Disease Control Priorities* (third edition): Volume 6, *Major Infectious Diseases*, edited by K. K. Holmes, S. Bertozzi, B. R. Bloom, and P. Jha. Washington, DC: World Bank.

Benzian, H., B. Varenne, N. Stauf, R. Garg, and B. Monse. 2017. "Promoting Oral Health through Programs in Middle Childhood and Adolescence." In *Disease Control Priorities* (third edition): Volume 8, *Child and Adolescent Health and Development*, edited by D. A. P. Bundy, N. de Silva, S. Horton, D. T. Jamison, and G. C. Patton. Washington, DC: World Bank.

Black, M., A. Gove, and K. A. Merseth. 2017. "Platforms to Reach Children in Early Childhood." In *Disease Control Priorities* (third edition): Volume 8, *Child and Adolescent Health and Development*, edited by D. A. P. Bundy, N. de Silva, S. Horton, D. T. Jamison, and G. C. Patton. Washington, DC: World Bank.

Black, R., R. Laxminarayan, M. Temmerman, and N. Walker, editors. 2015. *Disease Control Priorities* (third edition): Volume 2, *Reproductive, Maternal, Newborn, and Child Health*. Washington, DC: World Bank.

Black, R., N. Walker, R. Laxminarayan, and M. Temmerman. 2015. "Reproductive, Maternal, Newborn, and Child Health: Key Messages of This Volume." In *Disease Control Priorities* (third edition): Volume 2, *Reproductive, Maternal, Newborn, and Child Health*, edited by R. Black, R. Laxminarayan, M. Temmerman, and N. Walker. Washington, DC: World Bank.

Blakemore, S. J., and K. L. Mills. 2014. "Is Adolescence a Sensitive Period for Sociocultural Processing?" *Annual Review of Psychology* 65 (January): 187–207.

Blank, L., S. Baxter, E. Goyder, P. Naylor, L. Guillaume, and others. 2010. "Promoting Well-Being by Changing Behaviour: A Systematic Review and Narrative Synthesis of the Effectiveness of Whole Secondary School Behavioural Interventions." *Mental Health Review Journal* 15 (2): 43–53.

Brooker, S., S. Clarke, D. Fernando, C. Gitonga, J. Nankabirwa, D. Schellenberg, and others. 2017. "Malaria in Middle Childhood and Adolescence." In *Disease Control Priorities* (third edition): Volume 8, *Child and Adolescent Health and Development*, edited by D. A. P. Bundy, N. de Silva, S. Horton, D. T. Jamison, and G. C. Patton. Washington, DC: World Bank.

Brown, D. S., X. Fang, and C. S. Florence. 2011. "Medical Costs Attributable to Child Maltreatment: A Systematic Review of Short- and Long-Term Effects." *American Journal of Preventive Medicine* 41 (6): 627–35.

Bundy, D. A. P., L. Appleby, M. Bradley, K. Croke, D. Hollingsworth, and others. 2017. "Mass Deworming Programs in Middle Childhood and Adolescence." In *Disease Control Priorities* (third edition): Volume 8, *Child and Adolescent Health and Development*, edited by D. A. P. Bundy, N. de Silva, S. Horton, D. T. Jamison, and G. C. Patton. Washington, DC: World Bank.

Bundy, D. A. P., and S. Horton. 2017. "Impact of Interventions on Health and Development during Childhood and Adolescence: A Conceptual Framework." In *Disease Control Priorities* (third edition): Volume 8, *Child and Adolescent Health and Development*, edited by D. A. P. Bundy, N. de Silva, S. Horton, D. T. Jamison, and G. C. Patton. Washington, DC: World Bank.

Bundy, D. A. P., L. Schultz, B. Sarr, L. Banham, P. Colenso, and L. Drake. 2017. "The School as a Platform for Addressing Health in Middle Childhood and Adolescence." In *Disease*

Control Priorities (third edition): Volume 8, *Child and Adolescent Health and Development*, edited by D. A. P. Bundy, N. de Silva, S. Horton, D. T. Jamison, and G. C. Patton. Washington, DC: World Bank.

Carnerio, I., A. Roca-Feltrer, J. T. Griffin, L. Smith, M. Tanner, and others. 2010. "Age-Patterns of Malaria Vary with Severity, Transmission Intensity and Seasonality in Sub-Saharan Africa: A Systematic Review and Pooled Analysis." *PLos One* 5: e8988.

Ceesay, S. J., C. Casals-Pascual, J. Erskine, S. E. Anyam No. O. Duah, and others. 2008. "Changes in Malaria Indices between 1999 and 2007 in The Gambia: A Retrospective Analysis." *The Lancet* 372: 1545–54.

CDC (Centers for Disease Control and Prevention). 2015. *THRIVES: A Global Technical Package to Prevent Violence against Children.* Atlanta, GA: Division of Violence Prevention, National Center for Injury Prevention and Control, CDC. https://stacks.cdc.gov/view/cdc/31482.

Chandra-Mouli, V., C. Lane, and S. Wong. 2015. "What Does Not Work in Adolescent Sexual and Reproductive Health: A Review of Evidence on Interventions Commonly Accepted as Best Practices." *Global Health Science and Practice* 3 (3): 333–40.

Crookston, B. T., W. Schott, S. Cueto, K. A. Dearden, P. Engle, and others. 2013. "Postinfancy Growth, Schooling, and Cognitive Achievement: Young Lives." *American Journal of Clinical Nutrition* 98 (6): 1555–63.

Currie, J., and C. S. Widom. 2010. "Long-Term Consequences of Child Abuse and Neglect on Adult Economic Well-Being." *Child Maltreatment* 15 (2): 111–20.

Dahl, R. E. 2004. "Adolescent Brain Development: A Period of Vulnerabilities and Opportunities." Keynote Address: *Annals of the New York Academy of Sciences* 1021: 1/22.

de Walque, D., L. Fernald, P. Gertler, and M. Hidrobo. 2017. "Cash Transfers and Child and Adolescent Development." In *Disease Control Priorities* (third edition): Volume 8, *Child and Adolescent Health and Development*, edited by D. A. P. Bundy, N. de Silva, S. Horton, D. T. Jamison, and G. C. Patton. Washington, DC: World Bank.

Drake, L., M. Fernandes, E. Aurino, J. Kiamba, B. Giyosa, and others. 2017. "School Feeding Programs in Middle Childhood and Adolescence." In *Disease Control Priorities* (third edition): Volume 8, *Child and Adolescent Health and Development*, edited by D. A. P. Bundy, N. de Silva, S. Horton, D. T. Jamison, and G. C. Patton. Washington, DC: World Bank.

Durlak, J. A., R. P. Weissberg, and A. B. Dymnicki. 2011. "The Impact of Enhancing Students' Social and Emotional Learning: A Meta-Analysis of School-Based Universal Interventions." *Child Development* 82 (1): 405–32.

Elvik, R., A. Hoye, T. Vaa, and M. Sorensen. 2009. *The Handbook of Road Safety Measures* (second edition). Bingley, U.K.: Emerald Group Publishing Limited.

Fang, X., D. A. Fry, K. Ji, D. Finkelhor, J. Chen, and others. 2015. "The Burden of Child Maltreatment in China: A Systematic Review." *Bulletin of the World Health Organization* 93 (3): 176–85c.

Farahmand, F. K., K. E. Grant, A. J. Polo, and S. N. Duffy. 2011. "School-Based Mental Health and Behavioral Programs for Low-Income, Urban Youth: A Systematic and Meta-Analytic Review." *Clinical Psychology* 18 (4): 372–90.

Farrelly, M. C., B. R. Loomis, B. Han, J. Gfroerer, N. Kuiper, and others. 2013. "A Comprehensive Examination of the Influence of State Tobacco Control Programs and Policies on Youth Smoking." *American Journal of Public Health* 103 (3): 549–55.

Fernandes, M., and E. Aurino. 2017. "Identifying an Essential Package for School-Age Child Health: Economic Analysis." In *Disease Control Priorities* (third edition): Volume 8, *Child and Adolescent Health and Development*, edited by D. A. P. Bundy, N. de Silva, S. Horton, D. T. Jamison, and G. C. Patton. Washington, DC: World Bank.

Fitzpatrick, C., U. Nwankwo, E. Lenk, S. J. de Vlas, and D. A. P. Bundy. 2017. "An Investment Case for Ending Neglected Tropical Diseases." In *Disease Control Priorities* (third edition): Volume 6, *Major Infectious Diseases*, edited by K. K. Holmes, S. Bertozzi, B. R. Bloom, and P. Jha. Washington, DC: World Bank.

Flynn, J. R. 2007. *What Is Intelligence?* Cambridge, U.K., and New York: Cambridge University Press.

Galloway, R. 2017. "Global Nutrition Outcomes at Ages 5 to 19." In *Disease Control Priorities* (third edition): Volume 8, *Child and Adolescent Health and Development*, edited by D. A. P. Bundy, N. de Silva, S. Horton, D. T. Jamison, and G. C. Patton. Washington, DC: World Bank.

Gertler, P., J. Heckman, R. Pinto, A. Zanolini, C. Vermeersch, and others. 2014. "Labor Market Returns to an Early Childhood Stimulation Intervention in Jamaica." *Science* 344 (6187): 998–1001.

Glewwe, P., H. Jacoby, and E. King. 2001. "Early Childhood Nutrition and Academic Achievement: A Longitudinal Analysis." *Journal of Public Economics* 81 (3): 345–68.

Goddings, A., K. L. Mills, L. S. Clasen, J. N. Giedd, R. M. Viner, and S. Blakemore. 2014. "The Influence of Puberty on Subcortical Brain Development." *NeuroImage* 88: 242–51.

Graham, N., L. Schultz, S. Mitra, and D. Mont. 2017. "Disability in Middle Childhood and Adolescence." In *Disease Control Priorities* (third edition): Volume 8, *Child and Adolescent Health and Development*, edited by D. A. P. Bundy, N. de Silva, S. Horton, D. T. Jamison, and G. C. Patton. Washington, DC: World Bank.

Grantham-McGregor, S. M., C. A. Powell, S. P. Walker, and J. H. Himes. 1991. "Nutritional Supplementation, Psychosocial Stimulation, and Mental Development of Stunted Children: The Jamaican Study." *The Lancet* 338 (8758): 1–5.

Grigorenko, E. 2017. "Brain Development: The Effect of Interventions on Children and Adolescents." In *Disease Control Priorities* (third edition): Volume 8, *Child and Adolescent Health and Development*, edited by D. A. P. Bundy, N. de Silva, S. Horton, D. T. Jamison, and G. C. Patton. Washington, DC: World Bank.

Heckmann, J. J. 2011. "Effective Child Development Strategies." In *The Pre-K Debates: Current Controversies and Issues,* edited by E. Zigler, W. S. Gilliam, and W. S. Barnett. Baltimore, MD: Paul H. Brookes Publishing.

Hill, K., L. Zimmerman, and D. T. Jamison. 2017. "Mortality at Ages 5 to 19: Levels and Trends, 1990–2010." In *Disease Control Priorities* (third edition): Volume 8, *Child and Adolescent Health and Development*, edited by D. A. P. Bundy, N. de Silva, S. Horton, D. T. Jamison, and G. C. Patton. Washington, DC: World Bank.

Horton, S., and M. Black. 2017. "Identifying an Essential Package for Early Childhood Development: Economic Analysis." In *Disease Control Priorities* (third edition): Volume 8, *Child and Adolescent Health and Development*, edited by D. A. P. Bundy, N. de Silva, S. Horton, D. T. Jamison, and G. C. Patton. Washington, DC: World Bank.

Horton, S., J. Waldfogel, E. De la Cruz Toledo, J. Mahon, and J. Santelli. 2017. "Identifying an Essential Package for Adolescent Health: Economic Analysis." In *Disease Control Priorities* (third edition): Volume 8, *Child and Adolescent Health and Development*, edited by D. A. P. Bundy, N. de Silva, S. Horton, D. T. Jamison, and G. C. Patton. Washington, DC: World Bank.

International Commission on Financing Global Education Opportunity. 2016. *The Learning Generation: Investing in Education for a Changing World*. New York: International Commission on Financing Global Education Opportunity. http://report.educationcommission.org.

Jamison, D. T., J. G. Breman, A. R. Measham, G. Alleyne, M. Claeson, D. B. Evans, P. Jha, A. Mills, and P. Musgrove, editors. 2006. *Disease Control Priorities in Developing Countries* (second edition). Washington, DC: Oxford University Press and World Bank.

Jamison, D. T., W. Mosley, A. R. Measham, and J. Bobadilla, editors. 1993. *Disease Control Priorities in Developing Countries* (first edition). New York: Oxford University Press.

Jamison, D. T., S. M. Murphy, and M. E. Sandbu. 2016. "Why Has Under-5 Mortality Decreased at Such Different Rates in Different Countries?" *Journal of Health Economics* 48 (July): 16–25.

Jukes, M. C. H., L. J. Drake, and D. A. P. Bundy. 2008. *Leveling the Playing Field: School Health Nutrition for All*. Oxfordshire, U.K.: CABI Publishing.

LaMontagne, D. S., T. Cernushi, A. Yabuku, P. Bloem, D. Watson-Jones, and J. Kim. 2017. "School-Based Delivery of Vaccines to 5 to 19 Year Olds." In *Disease Control Priorities* (third edition): Volume 8, *Child and Adolescent Health and Development*, edited by D. A. P. Bundy, N. de Silva, S. Horton, D. T. Jamison, and G. C. Patton. Washington, DC: World Bank.

Lassi, Z., A. Moin, and Z. Bhutta. 2017. "Nutrition in Middle Childhood and Adolescence." In *Disease Control Priorities* (third edition): Volume 8, *Child and Adolescent Health and Development*, edited by D. A. P. Bundy, N. de Silva, S. Horton, D. T. Jamison, and G. C. Patton. Washington, DC: World Bank.

Masquelin, B. 2017. "Global, Regional, and National Levels and Trends in Mortality among Older Children (5–9)

and Young Adolescents (10–14) from 1990–2015." Paper prepared for UN Inter-agency Group for Child Mortality Estimation (IGME), UNICEF, New York.

Mock, C. N., O. Kobusingye, R. Nugent, and K. Smith, editors. 2017. *Disease Control Priorities* (third edition): Volume 7, *Injury Prevention and Environmental Health*. Washington, DC: World Bank.

Mokdad, A., M. H. Forouzanfar, F. Daoud, A. A. Mokdad, C. El Bcheraoui, and others. 2016. "Global Burden of Diseases, Injuries, and Risk Factors for Young People's Health During 1990–2013: A Systematic Analysis for the Global Burden of Disease Study 2013." *The Lancet* 387: 2383–401.

Murray, N. G., B. J. Low, C. Hollis, A. W. Cross, and S. M. Davis. 2007. "Coordinated School Health Programs and Academic Achievement: A Systematic Review of the Literature." *Journal of School Health* 77 (9): 589–600.

Nandi, A., J. R. Behrman, S. Bhalotra, A. B. Deolalikar, and R. Laxminarayan. 2017. "The Human Capital and Productivity Benefits of Early Childhood Nutritional Interventions." In *Disease Control Priorities* (third edition): Volume 8, *Child and Adolescent Health and Development*, edited by D. A. P. Bundy, N. de Silva, S. Horton, D. T. Jamison, and G. C. Patton. Washington, DC: World Bank.

Noor A. M., D. K. Kinyoki, C. W. Mundia, et al. 2014. "The Changing Risk of Plasmodium Falciparum Malaria Infection in Africa: 2000–10: A Spatial and Temporal Analysis of Transmission Intensity." *The Lancet* 383: 1739–47.

Norman, R. E., M. Byambaa, R. De, A. Butchart, J. Scott, and others. 2012. "The Long-Term Health Consequences of Child Physical Abuse, Emotional Abuse, and Neglect: A Systematic Review and Meta-Analysis." *PLoS Medicine* 9 (11): 1–31.

O'Meara, W. P., P. Bejon, T. W. Mwangi, E. A. Okiro, N. Peshu, and others. 2008. "Effect of a Fall in Malaria Transmission on Morbidity and Mortality in Kilifi, Kenya." *The Lancet* 372 (9649): 1555–62.

Patton, G. C., P. Azzopardi, E. Kennedy, C. Coffey, and A. Mokdad. 2017. "Global Measures of Health Risks and Disease Burden in Adolescents." In *Disease Control Priorities* (third edition): Volume 8, *Child and Adolescent Health and Development*, edited by D. A. P. Bundy, N. de Silva, S. Horton, D. T. Jamison, and G. C. Patton. Washington, DC: World Bank.

Patton, G. C., S. M. Sawyer, J. S. Santelli, D. A. Ross, R. Afifi, and others. 2016. "Our Future: A *Lancet* Commission on Adolescent Health and Wellbeing." *The Lancet* 387 (10036): 2423–78.

Plaut, D., T. Hill, M. Thomas, J. Worthington, M. Fernandes, and N. Burnett. 2017. "Getting to Education Outcomes: Reviewing Evidence from Health and Education Interventions." In *Disease Control Priorities* (third edition): Volume 8, *Child and Adolescent Health and Development*, edited by D. A. P. Bundy, N. de Silva, S. Horton, D. T. Jamison, and G. C. Patton. Washington, DC: World Bank.

Pradhan, E., E. M. Suzuki, S. Martínez, M. Schäferhoff, and D. T. Jamison. 2017. "The Effects of Education Quantity and Quality on Mortality." In *Disease Control Priorities* (third edition): Volume 8, *Child and Adolescent Health and Development*, edited by D. A. P. Bundy, N. de Silva, S. Horton, D. T. Jamison, and G. C. Patton. Washington, DC: World Bank.

Prentice, A. M., K. A. Ward, G. R. Goldberg, L. M. Jarjou, S. E. Moore, and others. 2013. "Critical Windows for Nutritional Interventions against Stunting." *American Journal of Clinical Nutrition* 97 (5): 911–18.

Preston, S., and M. Haines. 1991. *Fatal Years: Child Mortality in Late Nineteenth Century America*. Princeton, NJ: Princeton University Press.

Reavley, N., G. C. Patton, S. Sawyer, E. Kennedy, and P. Azzopardi. 2017. "Health and Disease in Adolescence." In *Disease Control Priorities* (third edition): Volume 8, *Child and Adolescent Health and Development*, edited by D. A. P. Bundy, N. de Silva, S. Horton, D. T. Jamison, and G. C. Patton. Washington, DC: World Bank.

Sarr, B., B. McMahon, F. Peel, M. Fernandes, D. A. P. Bundy, and others. 2017. "The Evolution of School Health and Nutrition in the Education Sector 2000–2015." *Frontiers in Public Health*. https://doi.org/10.3389/fpubh.2016.00271.

Schultz, T. W. 1993. *Origins of Increasing Returns*. Oxford, U.K.: Blackwell.

Shackelton, N., F. Jamal, R. M. Viner, K. Dickson, G. C. Patton, and C. Bonell. 2016. "School-Level Interventions to Promote Adolescent Health: Systematic Review of Reviews." *Journal of Adolescent Health* 58 (4): 382–96.

Snilstveit, B., J. Stevenson, D. Phillips, M. Vojtkova, E. Gallagher, and others. 2015. "Interventions for Improving Learning Outcomes and Access to Education in Low- and Middle-Income Countries: A Systematic Review," Final Review. London: International Initiative for Impact Evaluation (3ie).

Snow, R. W., J. A. Omumbo, B. Lowe, C. S. Molyneaux, J. O. Obiero, and others. 1997. "Relation between Severe Malaria Morbidity in Children and Level of Plasmodium Falciparum Transmission in Africa." *The Lancet* 349 (9006): 1650–54.

Tanner, J. L. 1990. *Fetus into Man: Physical Growth from Conception to Maturity*. Cambridge, MA: Harvard University Press.

United Nations. 2015. *Transforming Our World: The 2030 Agenda for Sustainable Development*. New York: United Nations.

United Nations General Assembly. 1989. "Convention on the Rights of the Child." United Nations Treaty Series, volume 1577, United Nations, New York.

Verguet, S., A. K. Nandi, V. Filippi, and D. A. P. Bundy. 2017. "Postponing Adolescent Parity in Developing Countries through Education: An Extended Cost-Effective Analysis." In *Disease Control Priorities* (third edition): Volume 8, *Child and Adolescent Health and Development*, edited by D. A. P. Bundy, N. de Silva, S. Horton, D. T. Jamison, and G. C. Patton. Washington, DC: World Bank.

Viner, R. M., A. B. Allen, and G. C. Patton. 2017. "Puberty, Developmental Processes, and Health Interventions." In *Disease Control Priorities* (third edition): Volume 8, *Child and Adolescent Health and Development*, edited by D. A. P. Bundy, N. de Silva, S. Horton, D. T. Jamison, and G. C. Patton. Washington, DC: World Bank.

Viner, R. M., E. M. Ozer, S. Denny, M. Marmot, M. Resnick, and others. 2012. "Adolescence and the Social Determinants of Health." *The Lancet* 379 (9826): 1641–52.

Watkins, K., D. A. P. Bundy, D. T. Jamison, F. Guenther, and A. Georgiadis. 2017. "Evidence of Impact on Health and Development of Intervention during Middle Childhood and School Age." In *Disease Control Priorities* (third edition): Volume 8, *Child and Adolescent Health and Development*, edited by D. A. P. Bundy, N. de Silva, S. Horton, D. T. Jamison, and G. C. Patton. Washington, DC: World Bank.

Watkins, D., R. Nugent, G. Yamey, H. Saxenian, C. N. Mock, and others. 2018. "Intersectoral Policies for Health." In *Disease Control Policies* (third edition): Volume 9, *Disease Control Priorities: Improving Health and Reducing Poverty*, edited by D. T. Jamison, R. Nugent, H. Gelbrand, S. Horton, P. Jha, R. Laxminarayan, and C. N. Mock. Washington, DC: World Bank.

World Bank. 1993. *World Development Report 1993: Investing in Health*. New York: Oxford University Press.

———. 2006. *World Development Report 2007: Development and the Next Generation*. Washington, DC: World Bank.

WHO (World Health Organization). 2015. *Guidelines for the Treatment of Malaria*. 3rd ed. Geneva: WHO.

Wu, K. B. 2017. "Global Variation in Education Outcomes at Ages 5 to 19." In *Disease Control Priorities* (third edition): Volume 8, *Child and Adolescent Health and Development*, edited by D. A. P. Bundy, N. de Silva, S. Horton, D. T. Jamison, and G. C. Patton. Washington, DC: World Bank.

Zielinski, D. S. 2009. "Child Maltreatment and Adult Socioeconomic Well-Being." *Child Abuse and Neglect* 33 (10): 666–78.

Chapter 2

Mortality at Ages 5 to 19: Levels and Trends, 1990–2010

Kenneth Hill, Linnea Zimmerman, and Dean T. Jamison

INTRODUCTION

During the past 15 years, the attention of the international community, as reflected in the Millennium Declaration and its associated Development Goals (UN 2000), has focused on the health of children under age five years and of adults. Adolescents and children older than age five years have been relatively neglected. However, publication of the report of a *Lancet* Commission on Adolescent Health and Wellbeing (Patton and others 2016), as well as the essays in this volume, suggest the beginning of serious concern for this neglected age group.

Mortality rates provide the most significant single indicator of health, but two publications (UN 2014; Wang and others 2012) have arrived at different estimates of numbers of deaths in the age 5–19 years range. Both the UN and Wang studies use models to generate mortality estimates. This chapter reviews and expands on a third set of estimates of mortality rates and numbers of deaths in those ages 5–19 years in low- and middle-income countries (LMICs) for 1990 and 2010 (Hill, Zimmerman, and Jamison 2015). The purpose of the Hill, Zimmerman, and Jamison (2015) study was to generate empirical estimates of mortality rates to check against the modeled numbers from UN (2014) and Wang and others (2012). It compares and contrasts the empirical estimates with those from the two previous modeling exercises. More specifically, the chapter summarizes the findings in Hill, Zimmerman, and Jamison (2015) on gender-specific mortality risks and numbers of deaths by World Bank geographical region for ages 5–9 years and 10–14 years for 1990 and 2010, and on the rates of change in these risks and numbers during the two decades. It then extends these findings to ages 15–19 years. The chapter concludes by reporting the World Health Organization's (WHO) estimates of percentage of deaths by broad cause of death category. We do not discuss risk factors or potential interventions. Definitions of age groupings and age-specific terminology used in this volume can be found in chapter 1 (Bundy and others 2017).

The age range of 5–19 years encompasses the inflection point of human mortality risks, with infectious disease mortality declining from the high risks of early childhood before noncommunicable disease risks start their exponential increase in adulthood. Despite being a healthy age range relative to all others, the number of deaths exceeded an estimated 2 million in 2010. This age range is also crucial for human development. In most societies, it covers the large majority of educational attainment; in many societies, it also covers the start of family formation (Sawyer and others 2012; UNICEF 2012). This chapter attempts to ground this volume's discussion of these larger issues with a reminder that the mortality reduction agenda remains unfinished and substantial.

Corresponding author: Kenneth Hill, Stanton-Hill Research, Moultonborough, NH, United States; kenneth_hill_1@yahoo.com.

MORTALITY AT AGES 5 TO 19 YEARS

Methods and Data

The methodology used by Hill, Zimmerman, and Jamison (2015) to develop the new estimates is fully described in their paper and summarized here. The empirical basis for their estimates is the full birth histories collected by Demographic and Health Surveys (DHS) (Rutstein and Rojas 2006) in more than 70 LMICs. These full birth histories—which consist of information on dates of birth, survival status, and age at death if relevant for all live births of a representative sample of women of reproductive age—are the primary source of information on mortality under age five years in LMICs, given that most of these countries lack accurate civil registration systems (UN 2014). Because the birth histories collect data on all births, and deaths to those births at all ages, they provide information, albeit increasingly selected by age of mother, about the mortality of older children and adolescents. The method used to estimate mortality risks for ages five years and older is the same as that used for mortality under age five years (Hill 2013). The numbers of deaths are much smaller above age 5 years, and particularly above age 10 years, than below, however, and estimates have been calculated for the 10 calendar years before each survey.

Although the coverage of the DHS program has been wide, not all countries have conducted such surveys; China is the most notable exception. Given the importance of China for global estimates, we adopted a different estimation strategy for that country, using census data from 1990 and 2010, adjusted for coverage. Because the DHS program does not cover all LMICs, and because individual countries are represented in the dataset for some years and not others, we adopted a model-based estimation method. We used the empirical survey-specific dataset to estimate relationships between risks of dying at ages 5–9, 10–14, and 15–19 years to the under-5 mortality rate (U5MR), and then applied those relationships to regional estimates of U5MR in 1990 and 2010, as produced by the Interagency Group on Mortality Estimation (UN 2014).

The empirical dataset is derived from 213 surveys covering 77 countries; the earliest survey is from 1986, and the latest is from 2011. Before turning to modeled estimates, it is of interest to examine the empirical observations themselves. Table 2.1 reports the mean mortality risks for both genders for ages 0–4, 5–9, 10–14, and 15–19 years, as calculated for the 10 calendar years before each survey. Across all observations, which are weighted toward Sub-Saharan Africa because of the geographic distribution of the DHS, the median U5MR is 85.6 per 1,000 live births; the risk of dying for ages 5–9 years is 15.8 per 1,000 survivors to age 5 years; the risk of dying for ages 10–14 years is 9.3 per 1,000 survivors to age 10; and the risk of dying for ages 15–19 years is 11.7 per

Table 2.1 Median Conditional Probabilities of Dying per 1,000 at Ages 0–4, 5–9, 10–14, and 15–19 Years, Estimated from DHS by World Bank Region

		World Bank Low- and Middle-Income Country Regions					
	All	**East Asia and Pacific, excluding China**	**Europe and Central Asia**	**Latin America and the Caribbean**	**Middle East and North Africa**	**South Asia**	**Sub-Saharan Africa**
Number of DHS analyzed	213	17	14	40	17	17	108
Age range (years)							
0–4	80 (50, 113)	42 (39, 72)	39 (19, 49)	53 (35, 74)	44 (34, 75)	69 (53, 81)	110 (85, 138)
5–9	13 (6.6, 23)	9.4 (7.0, 13)	3.2 (1.6, 3.7)	5.6 (3.4, 8.1)	4.3 (3.2, 8.5)	12 (8.5, 18)	23 (15, 30)
10–14	7.5 (4.2, 13)	5.8 (4.5, 6.4)	2.4 (1.8, 3.3)	4.3 (2.9, 5.8)	4.0 (2.5, 5.8)	5.7 (5.2, 7.7)	13 (9.0, 16.2)
15–19	10 (7.1, 15)	8.1 (6.3, 9.5)	5.1 (2.6, 7.3)	8.5 (5.6, 10)	5.6 (4.3, 7.4)	9.0 (7.1, 11)	14 (11, 20)

Note: Numbers in parentheses are the 25th and 75th percentiles. DHS = Demographic and Health Surveys.

1,000 survivors to age 15. The risks are highest in Sub-Saharan Africa in all age ranges; in this region, these risks are also higher relative to the U5MR.

Results: Mortality Risks

Across all regions, the lowest risk is in ages 10–14 years. The increase in risk from 10–14 to 15–19 years is substantially larger in two regions, Latin America and the Caribbean, and Europe and Central Asia. To bring out the relationships between risks in different age groups, figure 2.1 plots the risk of dying, for both genders combined, at ages 10–14 against 5–9 years, and 15–19 against 10–14 years. The risk at 10–14 years is lower than that at 5–9 years in almost all cases; risk at 15–19 years is generally higher than at 10–14 years, although there are numerous exceptions. The risk at 15–19 years relative to that at 10–14 years seems to increase at lower mortality levels and thus presumably at higher levels of economic development.

Figure 2.2 shows empirical relationships by gender for all three age ranges. Patterns are less clear than in figure 2.1, but further analysis through paired *t*-tests of the basic observations indicates that male mortality risks are higher than female risks in each age range, by about 12 percent for ages 5–9 years, 8 percent for 10–14 years, and 6 percent for 15–19 years; the first two differences are significant at 1 percent or higher, but the third misses significance at the 10 percent level. Once again, there is some indication that the pattern changes at low levels of mortality toward larger male disadvantages.

To obtain estimates for regions that include some countries that have not conducted surveys or have not conducted them consistently, we estimated models by regressing survey-specific mortality risks for ages 5–9, 10–14, and 15–19 years on the U5MR, and then estimated regional risks for 1990 and 2010 using regional estimates of U5MR. The models relating mortality at ages 5–9 and 10–14 years are statistically much stronger than the model for mortality at ages 15–19 years. This occurs partly because of smaller numbers of recorded deaths at ages 15–19 years, but also partly because the relationship itself seems to be more variable across countries, so the estimates for ages 15–19 years are substantially more uncertain.

Given its size and importance in any regional or global estimates, we adopted a different approach for China. Following the work of Banister and Hill (2004), we used information on population and deaths by age from the Chinese population censuses of 1990 (National Bureau of Statistics 1993) and 2010 (National Bureau of Statistics 2012), after adjustment for estimated undercoverage of deaths, and calculated mortality risks directly.

Table 2.2 shows the regional mortality risks by gender for ages 5–9, 10–14, and 15–19 years for 1990 and 2010 derived from the regression equations outlined; the table also shows the annual average rates of change between 1990 and 2010. For all LMICs, the probabilities of dying per 1,000 survivors at the beginning of the age intervals 5–9, 10–14, and 15–19 years decline from 16 to 8, from 8.5 to 5.5, and from 11.5 to 8.0, respectively. Overall, and in all geographic areas studied except China, declines have been fastest for ages 5–9 years, and slowest for ages 15–19 years. In China, declines were fastest for ages 5–9 years but slowest for ages 10–14 years, with a notably rapid decline of more than 6 percent per year for females ages 15–19 years. Across all regions and all age ranges, the declines were faster for females than for males.

Figure 2.1 Observed Probabilities of Dying at Ages 10–14 versus Ages 5–9 Years, and at Ages 15–19 versus Ages 10–14 Years, Both Genders

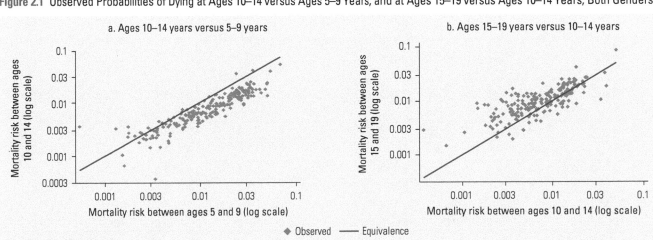

Figure 2.2 Observed Probabilities of Dying by Gender: Ages 5–9, 10–14, and 15–19 Years

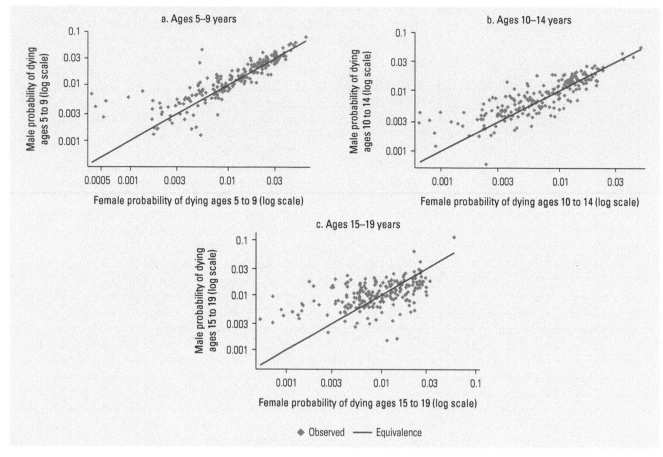

♦ Observed — Equivalence

Table 2.2 Estimated Conditional Probabilities of Dying at Ages 5–9, 10–14, and 15–19 Years, by Gender: World Bank Regions, Annual Average Rates of Change, 1990 and 2010

| World Bank region | Year | Probabilities of Dying per Survivor to Beginning of Age Group | | | | | |
| | | Males | | | Females | | |
		5 to 9	10 to 14	15 to 19	5 to 9	10 to 14	15 to 19
East Asia and Pacific (excluding China)	1990	0.011	0.0068	0.0093	0.0098	0.0061	0.0086
	2010	0.0048	0.0039	0.0059	0.0038	0.0033	0.0051
	Annual rate of change (percent)	−4.3	−2.8	−2.3	−4.7	−3.1	−2.6
China[a]	1990	0.0043	0.0032	0.0056	0.0035	0.0026	0.0051
	2010	0.0020	0.0020	0.0029	0.0014	0.0013	0.0014
	Annual rate of change (percent)	−4.0	−2.3	−3.3	−4.7	−3.6	−6.3
Europe and Central Asia (low and middle income)	1990	0.0085	0.0055	0.0079	0.0069	0.0046	0.0069
	2010	0.0037	0.0032	0.0050	0.0028	0.0025	0.0042
	Annual rate of change (percent)	−4.2	−2.8	−2.3	−4.5	−3.0	−2.5

table continues next page

Table 2.2 Estimated Conditional Probabilities of Dying at Ages 5–9, 10–14, and 15–19 Years, by Gender: World Bank Regions, Annual Average Rates of Change, 1990 and 2010 (continued)

| World Bank region | Year | Probabilities of Dying per Survivor to Beginning of Age Group | | | | | |
| | | Males | | | Females | | |
		5 to 9	10 to 14	15 to 19	5 to 9	10 to 14	15 to 19
Latin America and the Caribbean	1990	0.0085	0.0054	0.0078	0.0068	0.0045	0.0069
	2010	0.0031	0.0028	0.0045	0.0024	0.0023	0.0039
	Annual rate of change (percent)	–5.0	–3.4	–2.8	–5.1	–3.4	–2.8
Middle East and North Africa	1990	0.010	0.0064	0.0088	0.0094	0.0059	0.0084
	2010	0.0038	0.0033	0.0051	0.0032	0.0029	0.0046
	Annual rate of change (percent)	–4.9	–3.3	–2.7	–5.4	–3.7	–3.0
South Asia	1990	0.022	0.012	0.014	0.023	0.012	0.014
	2010	0.0097	0.0068	0.0089	0.010	0.0070	0.0091
	Annual rate of change (percent)	–4.1	–2.8	–2.3	–4.1	–2.8	–2.3
Sub-Saharan Africa	1990	0.037	0.018	0.019	0.032	0.016	0.018
	2010	0.019	0.012	0.013	0.017	0.010	0.012
	Annual rate of change (percent)	–3.2	–2.1	–1.7	–3.2	–2.2	–1.8
Total, low- and middle-income countries	1990	0.017	0.0095	0.012	0.016	0.0074	0.011
	2010	0.0088	0.0063	0.0084	0.0081	0.0049	0.0080
	Annual rate of change (percent)	–3.2	–2.0	–1.7	–3.3	–2.1	–1.8

a. Estimates for China are based on populations and numbers of deaths recorded in the 1990 and 2010 Population Censuses, adjusted as described in the text.

The rates of decline were slowest in Sub-Saharan Africa and generally fastest in Latin America and the Caribbean and the Middle East and North Africa, although China had the fastest declines at ages 15–19 years.

The rates of decline for all LMICs are similar to, or even slower than, the rates of decline for Sub-Saharan Africa, the worst performing region. This statistical oddity arises because Sub-Saharan Africa had the highest risks in both periods, had the slowest rates of decline, and sharply increased its proportional representation among all LMICs because of rapid population growth at these ages.

To confirm that the regional changes in mortality risks by gender and age range were not merely an artifact of the model, reflecting primarily the Interagency Group on Mortality Estimation changes in U5MR, we regressed the (logged) original observations derived directly from DHS data on the year of the survey (the observations are of average mortality risks for the 10 calendar years before each survey), using country fixed effects. These regressions confirmed the broad patterns of the results in table 2.2. The rates of decline were fastest for ages 5–9 years (about 3 percent per year), and slowest for ages 15–19 years (about 1 percent per year), although significantly different from zero for all groups except males ages 15–19 years; in each age range, rates of decline were faster for females than for males. Not surprisingly, the results are not identical to those in table 2.2; there are likely to be unobserved factors determining the selection of countries into the set in which at least two DHS have been conducted. However, the broad support of the basic observations for the results in table 2.2 is reassuring.

The results of an additional analysis drawing on survey data from those 34 countries that conducted two DHS separated by about 10 years (specifically by between 9 and 11 years), the first one in 2000 or earlier, the second in 2001 or later, are shown in figure 2.3, which plots

Figure 2.3 Changes in Probabilities of Dying by Age Group, 1990s and 2000s: Countries with DHS about 10 Years Apart in Each Decade (*N* = 27)

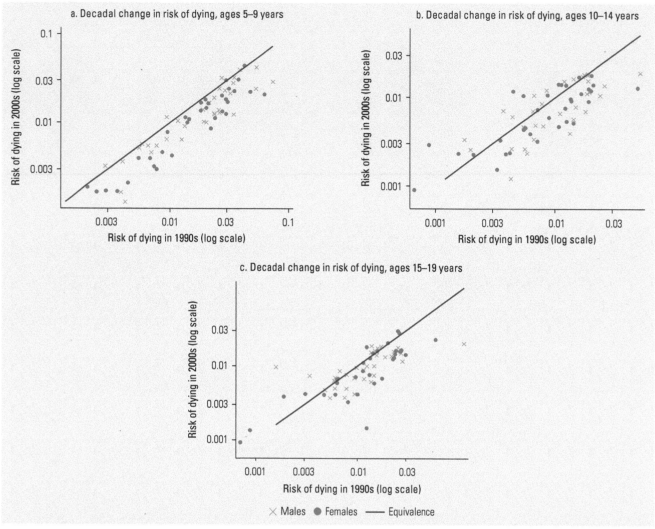

Note: DHS = Demographic and Health Surveys.

mortality risk in the later survey against that in the earlier, for each age range. For ages 5–9 years, the risks from the second survey are almost universally lower than those from the first; for ages 15–19 years, a large majority fits the same pattern. For ages 10–14 years, however, there is more scatter, and the pattern is less clear; before over-interpreting this result, it is important to remember that the number of deaths is lowest in this age group and sampling errors are largest.

Results: Number of Deaths

Table 2.3 repeats the general format of table 2.2 but reports numbers of deaths in 1990 and 2010 and annual rates of change by gender, age range, and region.

The numbers of deaths were estimated by converting the probabilities of dying in table 2.2 into age-specific mortality rates using standard demographic methods (Preston, Heuveline, and Guillot 2001), and then applying those rates to regional populations as estimated by the United Nations Population Division (UN 2013). The resulting numbers are simply the product of population size and risk of dying, and the percentage changes reflect the changes in both of these factors.

The total number of deaths in LMICs between ages 5 and 19 years fell from 3.3 million in 1990 to 2.3 million in 2010; male deaths exceeded female deaths by an estimated 11 percent in 1990 and 15 percent in 2010. The largest number of deaths in both 1990 and 2010 was in

Table 2.3 Estimated Numbers of Deaths at Ages 5–9, 10–14, and 15–19 Years by Gender: World Bank Regions, with Annual Average Rates of Change, 1990 and 2010

World Bank region	Year	Annual Numbers of Deaths (Thousands)					
		Males			Females		
		5 to 9	10 to 14	15 to 19	5 to 9	10 to 14	15 to 19
East Asia and Pacific (excluding China)	1990	69	39	50	58	34	45
	2010	30	24	35	23	19	30
	Annual rate of change (percent)	−4.2	−2.5	−1.7	−4.7	−2.8	−2.0
Chinaª	1990	45	32	69	33	25	59
	2010	15	17	31	9	9	14
	Annual rate of change (percent)	−5.5	−3.3	−4.0	−6.6	−5.0	−7.2
Europe and Central Asia (low and middle income)	1990	31	19	25	24	15	21
	2010	10	8	15	7	6	13
	Annual rate of change (percent)	−5.9	−4.1	−2.5	−6.3	−4.4	−2.7
Latin America and the Caribbean	1990	46	28	36	36	23	31
	2010	18	16	25	13	13	21
	Annual rate of change (percent)	−4.8	−2.8	−1.9	−4.9	−2.9	−2.0
Middle East and North Africa	1990	35	19	22	31	17	20
	2010	13	11	17	10	9	15
	Annual rate of change (percent)	−5.1	−2.8	−1.1	−5.5	−3.1	−1.3
South Asia	1990	340	160	170	330	160	160
	2010	170	120	150	160	110	140
	Annual rate of change (percent)	−3.4	−1.6	−0.65	−3.5	−1.7	−0.68
Sub-Saharan Africa	1990	280	120	100	240	100	94
	2010	250	130	130	210	110	110
	Annual rate of change (percent)	−0.72	0.42	0.97	−0.85	0.32	0.88
Total, low- and middle-income countries	1990	850	410	470	760	370	430
	2010	500	320	400	430	280	350
	Annual rate of change (percent)	−2.6	−1.1	−0.89	−2.8	−1.5	−1.1

a. Numbers of deaths for China are based on numbers of deaths recorded in the 1990 and 2010 Population Censuses, adjusted as described in the text.

ages 5–9 years, although this age group also experienced the fastest rate of decline between those two years; ages 10–14 years recorded the smallest number of deaths, and ages 15–19 years showed the slowest rate of decline from 1990 to 2010. South Asia had the highest number of deaths in 1990, but it was overtaken by Sub-Saharan Africa in 2010 except in ages 15–19 years. These two regions together accounted for almost 70 percent of all deaths in LMICs between ages 5 and 19 years in 1990, and almost 80 percent in 2010.

Comparison with Other Studies

Table 2.4 puts the estimates in this chapter of numbers of deaths in 2010 in the context of global estimates arrived at by the Global Burden of Disease (GBD) exercise (Wang and others 2012) and the United Nations Population Division (UN 2013). We only compared numbers for the world as a whole, for LMICs, and for Sub-Saharan Africa because the three exercises define regions differently. We arrived at the GBD estimates for LMICs by subtracting the sum of deaths in ages 5–9, 10–14, and 15–19 years for high-income Asia and Pacific, Australasia, Central Europe, Western Europe, and high-income North America from global deaths in those age groups; for Sub-Saharan Africa, we summed deaths for Central, Eastern, Southern, and Western Sub-Saharan Africa. The World Population Prospects (WPP) tabulates deaths by age group and five-year period only for 1995–2000, 2000–05, and 2005–10 (UN 2013). We estimated the numbers of deaths for the single year of 2010 by estimating rates of change from 2000–05 to 2005–10, and applying those rates of change to the 2005–10 estimate for 2.5 years, and dividing by 5 to get a single-year figure.

Table 2.4 shows differences between the GBD estimates and those of the other two exercises for ages 5–9 and 10–14 years. At the global level and for LMICs, the GBD numbers are only about 60 percent of the WPP numbers; for Sub-Saharan Africa, they are little more than 35 percent; for ages 15–19 years, the agreement is closer, although the GBD numbers are still 10 percent lower than the WPP numbers globally and for all LMICs, and almost 40 percent lower for Sub-Saharan Africa. In contrast, the Hill, Zimmerman, and Jamison (2015) and WPP (UN 2013) numbers are closer: almost identical for

LMICs for ages 10–14 and 15–19 years, although the Hill, Zimmerman, and Jamison (2015) numbers are higher for LMIC deaths at ages 5–9 years, but lower for Sub-Saharan Africa at ages 10–14 and 15–19 years. The WPP and Hill, Zimmerman, and Jamison (2015) numbers are higher than the GBD estimates for every age-region combination in table 2.4. Hill, Zimmerman, and Jamison (2015) hypothesize that the differences between GBD and the other estimates at ages 5–14 years result from the model life table system used in constructing the GBD estimates.

DEATHS BY CAUSE

We report also in this chapter on deaths by cause. We develop no new estimates but instead rely on the WHO's Global Health Estimates (GHE) for 2012 (WHO 2013). We report only for the age range 5–14 years because the GHE does not provide five-year age breakdowns. A paper (Mokdad and others 2016) prepared in conjunction with *The Lancet* Commission on Adolescent Health and Wellbeing presents recent GBD estimates for the percentage breakdown of deaths by cause for ages 10–24 years.

Table 2.5 shows estimates of the percentage distribution of deaths by cause for LMICs. To provide comparison the table also shows the same results for the age group 1–59 months. Although diarrheal disease, malaria, and respiratory conditions account for an important fraction of mortality in both age groups, these conditions are substantially more important at younger ages. Injury, in contrast, is reported to be more important at older ages.

Table 2.6 shows the GHE estimates of death by cause by World Bank region.

Table 2.4 Comparison of Numbers of Deaths between Ages 5 and 19 Years, 2010, thousands

Geography	GBD[a]			WPP[b]			Hill, Zimmerman, and Jamison (2015)[c]		
	5–9	10–14	15–19	5–9	10–14	15–19	5–9	10–14	15–19
World	450	360	710	710	630	790	n.a.	n.a.	n.a.
Less developed regions	450	360	680	710	620	750	940	600	740
Sub-Saharan Africa	170	110	190	430	330	310	450	240	240

Note: GBD = Global Burden of Disease; WPP = World Population Prospects; n.a. = not applicable.
a. Wang and others 2012.
b. Calculated from UN 2013.
c. See table 2.3.

Table 2.5 Distribution of Deaths by Cause in Low- and Middle-Income Countries, Ages 1–59 Months and 5–14 Years, 2012

	Age Group	
Cause	1–59 months	5–14 years
All causes (thousands)[a]	3,701	1,446
1. Communicable disease		
1.1 Tuberculosis	1.5	0.98
1.2 HIV/AIDS	2.7	6.7
1.3 Diarrheal disease	16	9.8
1.4 Malaria	13	2.2
1.5 Respiratory conditions	23	8.5
2. Noncommunicable disease		
2.1 Malignant neoplasms	0.81	3.4
2.2 Cardiovascular diseases	0.88	3.1
2.3 Congenital anomalies	4.8	2.3
2.4 Epilepsy	0.52	2.2
2.5 Neonatal conditions	5.9	0.01
3. Injuries		
3.1 Unintentional	8.6	22
3.2 Intentional	0.42	3.4
Percentage of deaths in above categories	78	65

Note: HIV/AIDS = human immunodeficiency virus/acquired immune deficiency syndrome.
a. Global Health Estimates, "Estimates for 2000–2012: Causes of Death," WHO 2013. This chapter's estimates of deaths for ages 5–14 years in 2010 is higher at 1.53 million. Deaths by cause are given in percentages.

Table 2.6 Deaths by Cause in Low- and Middle-Income Countries, by World Regional Groups, Ages 5–14, 2012

	Regional Groups							
Causes	High income	Low and middle income	East Asia and Pacific	Europe and Central Asia	Latin America and the Caribbean	Middle East and North Africa	South Asia	Sub-Saharan Africa
All causes (in thousands)	23	1,424	120	18	44	42	342	858
1. Communicable disease								
1.1 Tuberculosis	0.10	1.0	0.50	0.05	0.25	0.36	0.42	1.4
1.2 HIV/AIDS	0.70	6.8	0.85	0.70	2.5	0.40	1.4	10
1.3 Diarrheal disease	1.0	10	2.8	1.1	2.8	1.0	12	11
1.4 Malaria	0.10	2.3	1.5	0	0.23	0.34	0.65	3.4
1.5 Respiratory conditions	4.9	8.5	4.9	6.8	6.7	11	9.9	8.5
2. Noncommunicable disease								
2.1 Malignant neoplasms	17	3.2	11	13	11	12	3.3	1.2
2.2 Cardiovascular diseases	6.2	3.1	6.6	12	6.1	8.8	2.5	2.2

table continues next page

Table 2.6 Deaths by Cause in Low- and Middle-Income Countries, by World Regional Groups, Ages 5–14, 2012 (continued)

Causes	Regional Groups							
	High-income	Low- and middle-income	East Asia and Pacific	Europe and Central Asia	Latin America and the Caribbean	Middle East and North Africa	South Asia	Sub-Saharan Africa
2.3 Congenital anomalies	5.8	2.2	5.1	5.8	4.3	3.2	2.5	1.5
2.4 Epilepsy	1.9	2.2	2.5	3.0	1.6	0.89	1.9	2.4
3. Injuries								
3.1 Unintentional	32	22	33	26	26	23	28	18
3.2 Intentional	7.0	3.3	2.4	5.4	8.5	20	3.5	2.2
Percentage of deaths in above categories	76	65	71	73	70	81	66	62

Note: HIV/AIDS = human immunodeficiency virus/acquired immune deficiency syndrome. Deaths by cause are given in percentages and are from Global Health Estimates, "Estimates for 2000–2012: Causes of Death" (WHO 2013).

CONCLUSIONS

The principle conclusion from this analysis is that, although mortality reaches its minimum in ages 5–19 years, the number of deaths in this age group in LMICs still represents a substantial burden, approximately 2.3 million in 2010. The data show that in most LMICs, mortality risks are lowest in ages 10–14 years; this finding is in contrast to low-mortality, high-income countries, where the risks are lowest in ages 5–9 years. This difference suggests that much of the LMIC burden of mortality at ages 5–9 years is residual mortality from infectious childhood diseases.

In other respects, mortality at ages 5–19 years has behaved largely as has mortality under age 5 years. Males have generally higher risks than females; the risks have fallen since 1990, although not quite as rapidly as for those under age 5 years.

Global estimates of mortality in this age group have shown a discrepancy between the numbers estimated by the United Nations Population Division and the numbers estimated as part of the GBD exercise. This study provides empirical support for the numbers estimated by the United Nations and arrives at numbers that are generally slightly higher still. The discrepancies are not the result of different estimates of U5MR, which are very similar on average, or of very different numbers of population, but of differences in estimated risks of dying.

The full birth histories collected by the DHS and by UNICEF's Multiple Indicator Cluster Surveys program (see http://www.mics.unicef.org) provide estimates of mortality for this age range. However, in many surveys the numbers are small, and the estimates have high uncertainty; as a result, we only estimated rates for periods of 10 years before each survey. The deaths reported at older ages of childhood are also increasingly selected for the young age of mother at the time of the relevant births, because the histories are only collected from women under age 50 years. In countries lacking complete and accurate civil registration systems, these limitations will adversely affect the ability to monitor changes or identify differentials in the mortality of older children and younger adolescents.

A final concern is that we have very little information about the cause-of-death structure for this age range. Verbal autopsy methods applied to deaths of children under age five years occurring shortly before a DHS have improved the data availability for cause of death of younger children (see, for example, Liu and others 2015), but no such efforts have been applied to deaths of older children; in general, sample sizes are probably too small for such an exercise to produce stable results. Nevertheless, our tables 2.5 and 2.6 reproduce current best estimates from WHO. However, some larger surveys in high-mortality settings would provide an adequate basis for such an exercise, which ought to be undertaken; the cost would be relatively modest since the survey identifies the target deaths at virtually zero marginal cost.

NOTE

World Bank Income Classifications as of July 2014 are as follows, based on estimates of gross national income (GNI) per capita for 2013:

- Low-income countries (LICs) = US$1,045 or less
- Middle-income countries (MICs) are subdivided:
  a) lower-middle-income = US$1,046 to US$4,125
  b) upper-middle-income (UMICs) = US$4,126 to US$12,745
- High-income countries (HICs) = US$12,746 or more.

REFERENCES

Banister, J., and K. Hill. 2004. "Mortality in China 1964–2000." *Population Studies* 58 (1): 55–75.

Bundy, D. A. P., N. de Silva, S. Horton, G. C. Patton, L. Schultz, and D. T. Jamison. 2017. "Child and Adolescent Health and Development: Realizing Neglected Potential." In *Disease Control Priorities* (third edition): Volume 8, *Child and Adolescent Health and Development*, edited by D. A. P. Bundy, N. de Silva, S. Horton, D. T. Jamison, and G. C. Patton. Washington, DC: World Bank.

Hill, K. 2013. "Direct Estimation of Child Mortality from Birth Histories." In *Tools for Demographic Estimation*, edited by T. Moultrie, R. Dorrington, A. Hill, K. Hill, I. Timæus, and B. Zaba. Paris: International Union for the Scientific Study of Population. http://www.demographicestimation.iussp.org.

Hill, K., L. Zimmerman, and D. T. Jamison. 2015. "Mortality Risks in Children Aged 5–14 Years in Low-Income and Middle-Income Countries: A Systematic Empirical Analysis." *The Lancet Global Health* 3 (10): 609–16.

Liu, L., S. Oza, D. Hogan, J. Perin, I. Rudan, and others. 2015. "Global, Regional, and National Causes of Child Mortality in 2000–13, with Projections to Inform Post-2015 Priorities: An Updated Systematic Analysis." *The Lancet* 385 (9966): 430–40. doi:10.1016/S0140-6736(14)61698-6.

Mokdad, A. H., M. H. Forouzanfar, F. Daoud, A. A. Mokdad, C. El Bcheraoui, and others. 2016. "Global Burden of Diseases, Injuries, and Risk Factors for Young People's Health During 1990–2013: A Systematic Analysis for the Global Burden of Disease Study 2013." *The Lancet* 387 (10036): 2383–401. http://dx.doi.org/10.1016/S0140-6736(16)00648-6.

National Bureau of Statistics. 1993. *Tabulation on the 1990 Population Census of the People's Republic of China*. 4 vols. Beijing: China Statistics Press.

———. 2012. *Tabulation on the 2010 Population Census of the People's Republic of China*. 3 vols. Beijing: China Statistics Press.

Patton, G. C., S. M. Sawyer, J. S. Santelli, D. A. Ross, R. Afifi, and others. 2016. "Our Future: A *Lancet* Commission on Adolescent Health and Wellbeing." *The Lancet* 387 (10036): 2423–78.

Preston, S. H., P. Heuveline, and M. Guillot. 2001. *Demography: Measuring and Modelling Population Processes*. Oxford, U.K.: Blackwell.

Rutstein, S. O., and G. Rojas. 2006. *Guide to DHS Statistics*. Calverton, MD: Demographic and Health Surveys, ORC-Macro.

Sawyer, S. M., R. A. Afifi, L. H. Bearinger, S. J. Blakemore, B. Dick, and others. 2012. "Adolescence: A Foundation for Future Health." *The Lancet* 379 (9826): 1630–40. doi:101016/so140-6736(12)60072-5.

UN (United Nations). 2000. "United Nations Millennium Declaration." Resolution adopted by the General Assembly, 55th Session of the United Nations General Assembly, New York, September 18.

———. 2013. "World Population Prospects: The 2012 Revision." Demographic Profiles, Department of Economic and Social Affairs, Population Division. http://esa.un.org/wpp/Documentation/pdf/WPP2012_Volume-II-Demographic-Profiles.pdf.

———. 2014. *Levels and Trends in Child Mortality: Report 2014*. United Nations Inter-Agency Group for Mortality Estimation. New York: UNICEF.

UNICEF (United Nations Children's Fund). 2012. *Progress for Children: A Report Card on Adolescents*. New York: UNICEF.

Wang, H., L. Dwyer-Lindgren, K. T. Lofgren, J. K. Rajaratnam, J. R. Marcus, and others. 2012. "Age-Specific and Sex-Specific Mortality in 187 Countries, 1970–2010: A Systematic Analysis for the Global Burden of Disease Study 2010." *The Lancet* 380 (9859): 2071–94.

WHO (World Health Organization). 2013. *Global Health Estimates*. Geneva: WHO.

Chapter 3

Global Nutrition Outcomes at Ages 5 to 19

Rae Galloway

INTRODUCTION

Globally, there are 1.8 billion children and adolescents ages 5–19 years; nearly 90 percent live in low- and middle-income countries (LMICs) (World Bank 2015). The prevalence and consequences of malnutrition and inadequate intake of nutrients leading to increased risk of morbidity and mortality are well studied for children in their first 1,000 days (Black and others 2013). Little information about the prevalence and consequences of malnutrition is available for children and adolescents ages 5–19 years, although they constitute 27 percent of the population in LMICs (World Bank 2015).

This paucity of data makes it difficult to develop policies and strategies on why, if, and how to improve the nutritional situation of children and adolescents in LMICs. Available evidence from smaller studies for selected age groups within this cohort suggests that children ages 5–15 years suffer from high prevalence of nutritional deprivation and its consequences. Malnutrition is manifested as underweight (measured by low weight-for-age or body mass index [BMI]), overweight/obesity (measured by high weight-for-age or BMI), and micronutrient deficiencies (essential fatty acids, vitamins, and minerals). Overweight and obesity are caused by excessive intake of energy and, in most cases, suboptimal intakes of essential fatty acids, vitamins, and minerals because of a poor-quality diet.

The objective of this chapter is to use available national surveys, which provide information on the nutritional status at the beginning and end of the entire age range of 5–19 years, to obtain proxy indicators of malnutrition for school-age children. These indicators are compared with those for the larger age groups—for example, all children younger than age five years and all women of reproductive age (WRA)—collected in these studies. The chapter also discusses what is known about dietary intake and the consequences of malnutrition for this age group, as well as what actions are needed globally to address nutritional needs in these age groups. Chapter 11 of this volume (Lassi, Moin, and Bhutta 2017) also looks at nutrition in middle childhood and adolescence. Definitions of age groupings and age-specific terminology used in this volume can be found in chapter 1 (Bundy and others 2017).

PREVALENCE OF MALNUTRITION IN CHILDREN AND ADOLESCENTS AGES 5–19 YEARS

To obtain information on malnutrition during middle childhood and adolescence, the author reviewed the most recent Demographic and Health Surveys (DHS) from 2000 to 2014. DHS are nationally representative household surveys in LMICs that routinely collect height and weight measurements and anemia prevalence for children ages 0–5 years and WRA ages 15–49 years. These data were disaggregated by age group to obtain information on the nutritional status of boys and girls ages 4–5 years (the age group is 4.00 years to 4.99 years or 48–59 months, or before the child's fifth birthday, which is the approximate age

Corresponding author: Rae Galloway, Independent Consultant, Alexandria, Virginia, United States; rae.galloway2@gmail.com.

when children enter school) and a subset of girls ages 15–19 years.[1] Nutritional status information, including anemia caused primarily by iron deficiency and parasitic infections, was available for girls and boys ages 15–19 years in a smaller number of countries.

Underweight and Anemia in Children Younger than Age Five Years in LMICs

Figure 3.1 shows the prevalence of underweight for children ages 48–59 months, compared with children ages 0–59 months.[2] The figure also shows the prevalence of anemia in children ages 48–59 months, compared with those ages 6–59 months.[3] These data are organized by DHS region.[4]

Underweight

In all regions, children ages 48–59 months are as vulnerable to being underweight as all children ages 0–59 months. In West, Central, and Eastern Africa, approximately 20 percent of children ages 48–59 months are underweight; the prevalence is highest in South and South-East Asia, where 43 percent of children in this age group are underweight. The prevalence of overweight

and obesity in children younger than age five years is not shown here because, based on the available DHS, the prevalence is less than 5 percent in all regions.

Anemia

To determine the level of public health significance for anemia, the World Health Organization (WHO) provides guidance on the severity of anemia by prevalence at the population level (table 3.1).

The prevalence of anemia is higher in children ages 6–59 months than in children ages 48–59 months; but anemia prevalence in children ages 48–59 months is still high (20 percent to more than 50 percent of

Table 3.1 Anemia Prevalence and Public Health Significance

Prevalence of anemia at the population level (percent)	Level of public health significance
<5.0	None
5.0–19.9	Mild
20.0–39.9	Moderate
≥40.0	Severe

Source: WHO 2015.

Figure 3.1 Prevalence of Underweight (Low Weight-for-Age) and Anemia (Hb <11 g/dl) in Children Ages 48–59 Months and Children Ages 6–59 Months

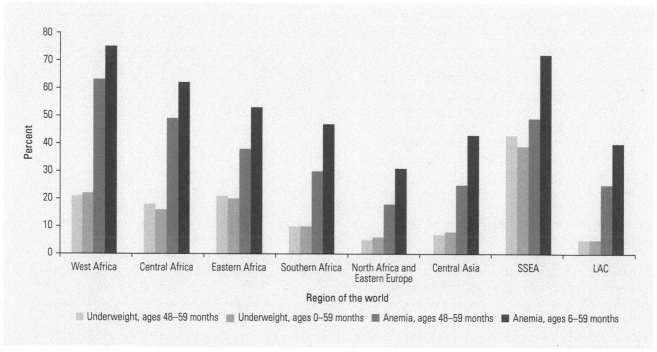

Sources: Statcompiler; Demographic and Health Surveys 2000–14.

Note: g/dl = grams per deciliter; Hb = hemoglobin; LAC = Latin America and the Caribbean; SSEA = South and South-East Asia. If there were two surveys in the country during this period, the most recent survey was used.

children in this age group are anemic in all regions). The highest prevalence of anemia is in children ages 48–59 months in West Africa (63 percent) and South and South-East Asia (49 percent). Based on the WHO definition, anemia is a severe public health problem in children ages 48–59 months in these regions.

Underweight and Overweight/Obesity in Adolescents Ages 15–19 Years

The DHS provide prevalence data on underweight (BMI ≤ 18.5 of body weight in kilograms per square of body height in meters [kg/m²]) and overweight (BMI ≥ 25 kg/m²) for girls and boys in late adolescence, that is, ages 15–19 years, in 17 countries (figures 3.2 and 3.3).

Underweight

The prevalence of underweight in late adolescent girls ages 15–19 years varies from 0.3 percent in the Arab Republic of Egypt (shown as 0 percent in figure 3.2) to 47 percent in India. In boys ages 15–19 years, the prevalence of underweight ranges from 1 percent in Egypt to 66 percent in Ethiopia. In most of the Sub-Saharan African countries shown, the prevalence of underweight in boys is significantly higher than underweight in girls. Data on the prevalence of underweight in males ages 15–49 years were collected in 15 countries.[5] In every country, the prevalence of underweight in late adolescent boys is at least two times higher than the prevalence of underweight in all males ages 15–49 years (data not shown).

Overweight/Obesity

At least 10 percent of either late adolescent boys or girls are overweight or obese in 13 of 17 countries. Overweight/obesity is higher in girls than boys in 13 out of 17 countries; the prevalence in girls is greater than 10 percent in 10 countries, while the prevalence in boys is greater than 10 percent in just 3 countries (figure 3.3). The differential between boys and girls is high in Lesotho, Swaziland, Egypt, and the Dominican Republic. The prevalence of overweight/obesity in girls

Figure 3.2 Prevalence of Underweight (BMI <18.5 kg/m²) in Adolescents Ages 15–19 Years

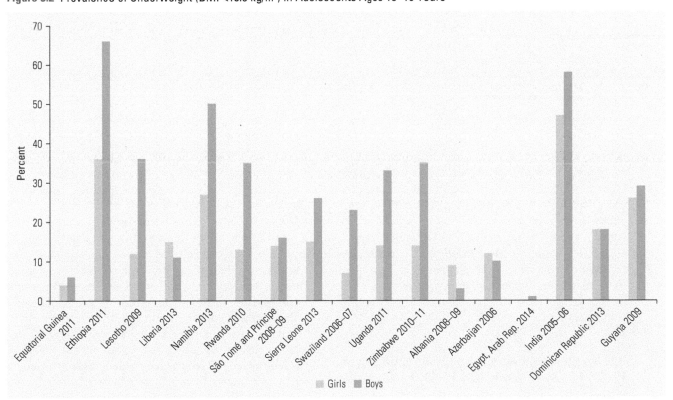

Source: Statcompiler; Demographic and Health Surveys (DHS) 2000–14.

Note: BMI = body mass index. If there were two surveys in the country during this period, the most recent country survey was used. Except in the Arab Republic of Egypt where girls ages 15–19 years are unmarried, girls in late adolescence are included in the DHS sample for women of reproductive age in all countries, with most already having a live birth. Cutoffs for underweight in Egypt use <–2 standard deviations.

Figure 3.3 Prevalence of Overweight/Obesity (BMI ≥25 kg/m²) in Adolescents Ages 15–19 Years

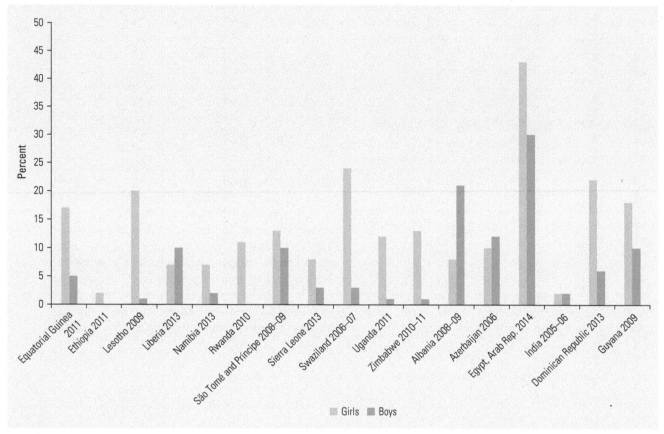

Source: Statcompiler; Demographic and Health Surveys (DHS) 2000–14.
Note: BMI = body mass index. If there were two surveys in the country during this period, the most recent country survey was used. Except in the Arab Republic of Egypt where late adolescent girls ages 15–19 years are unmarried, late adolescent girls are included in the DHS sample for women of reproductive age in all countries, with most already having a live birth. Cutoffs for overweight/obesity in Egypt use >+1 standard deviation.[6]

is lower than in all WRA. For the countries represented in figures 3.2 and 3.3, except Egypt and Equatorial Guinea, where the nutritional status in men ages 15–49 years was not collected, overweight/obesity was significantly higher in men than in late adolescent boys (data not shown). In six countries (Albania, Azerbaijan, Guyana, Namibia, São Tomé and Príncipe, and Swaziland), overweight/obesity in men was greater than 10 percent (data not shown); the prevalence in boys is greater than 10 percent in only three countries (figure 3.3).

Underweight and Overweight/Obesity in Girls Ages 15–19 Years and Women Ages 15–49 Years

Figure 3.4 reviews the prevalence of underweight (BMI < 18.5 kg/m²) in girls ages 15–19 years, compared with all WRA by region; 36 countries in Sub-Saharan Africa, 7 in North Africa and Eastern Europe,[7] 3 in

Central Asia, 7 in South and South-East Asia, and 11 in Latin America and the Caribbean are represented.

In every region except Central Asia, late adolescent girls are more vulnerable to being underweight than all WRA ages 15–49 years. These differences are high in Central Africa, North Africa and Eastern Europe, South and South-East Asia, and Latin America and the Caribbean, although the prevalence is low in some of these regions. In South and South-East Asia, 43 percent of adolescent girls are underweight, compared with slightly more than 33 percent of all WRA.

Overweight and obesity are increasing in late adolescent girls in some regions; based on the available data, however, the prevalence is much lower than in all WRA. An analysis found that overweight/obesity in boys and girls ages 2–19 years in most LMICs was about half of the overweight/obesity in adult men and women. The study also reported that while overweight has been increasing in boys and girls ages 2–19 years in

Figure 3.4 Prevalence of Underweight (BMI <18.5 kg/m^2) in Adolescent Girls Ages 15–19 Years and WRA Ages 15–49 Years

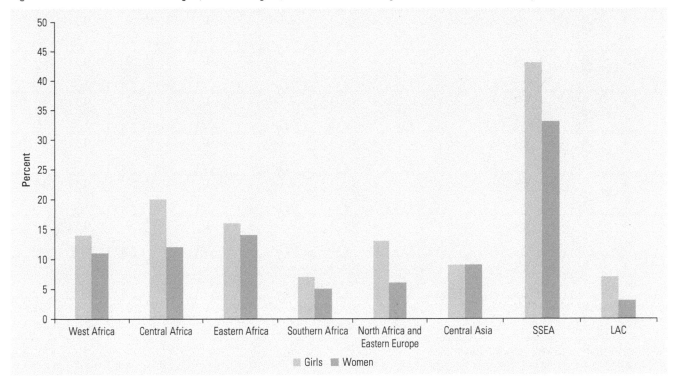

Source: Statcompiler; Demographic and Health Surveys (DHS) 2000–14.
Note: BMI = body mass index; LAC = Latin America and the Caribbean; SSEA = South and South-East Asia; WRA = women of reproductive age. If there were two surveys in the country during this period, the most recent country survey was used. Late adolescent girls ages 15–19 years are included in the DHS sample for WRA in all countries, with most already having a live birth.

LMICs, obesity has not increased significantly (Ng and others 2014).

Anemia in Girls Ages 15–19 Years and Women Ages 15–49 Years

Figure 3.5 compares the prevalence of anemia in girls ages 15–19 years and WRA ages 15–49 years in 28 countries in Sub-Saharan Africa, 6 in North Africa and Eastern Europe,[8] 2 in Central Asia, 5 in South and South-East Asia, and 5 in Latin America and the Caribbean.

Within regions, the prevalence of anemia in late adolescent girls is similar to the prevalence of anemia in all WRA. Nearly 50 percent of women in both groups are anemic in West and Central Asia and South and South-East Asia. In other regions, 25 percent to 40 percent of women are anemic. According to the WHO definition, anemia is a severe public health problem for late adolescent girls and all WRA ages 15–49 years in West Africa, Central Africa, and South and South-East Asia, with prevalence of at least 40 percent (see table 3.1 for cutoff definitions). Anemia is also a severe public health problem for WRA in Central Asia.

Anemia in Boys Ages 15–19 Years and Men Ages 15–49 Years, Selected Countries

Figure 3.6 presents available data on the prevalence of anemia in boys and men in selected countries.

Compared with men ages 15–49 years, anemia is higher in late adolescent boys. However, anemia prevalence is high in all men and late adolescent boys, affecting more than 20 percent of both age groups in 15 of 22 countries. The prevalence of anemia in late adolescent boys (40 percent or higher) is a severe public health problem in eight Sub-Saharan African countries. Anemia in late adolescent boys is generally lower than in girls in the same age range in the same countries (data not shown).

DIETARY INTAKE OF GIRLS AGES 15–19 YEARS

An analysis reviews the available studies, most with small sample sizes, on dietary intake in nonpregnant adolescent girls. These studies are not nationally representative surveys, but they provide information on

Figure 3.5 Prevalence of Anemia (Hb <12 g/dl) in Adolescent Girls Ages 15–19 Years and WRA Ages 15–49 Years

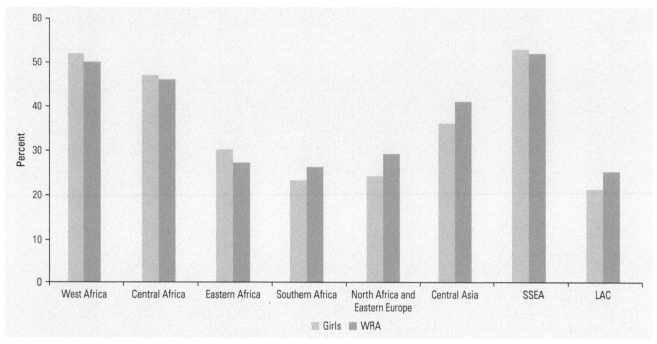

Source: Statcompiler; Demographic and Health Surveys (DHS) 2000–14.
Note: g/dl = grams per deciliter; Hb = hemoglobin; LAC = Latin America and the Caribbean; SSEA = South and South-East Asia; WRA = women of reproductive age. If there were two surveys in the country during this period, the most recent country survey was used. Late adolescent girls ages 15–19 years are included in the DHS sample for WRA in all countries, with most already having a live birth.

Figure 3.6 Prevalence of Anemia (Hb <13 g/dl) in Adolescent Boys Ages 15–19 Years and Men Ages 15–49 Years

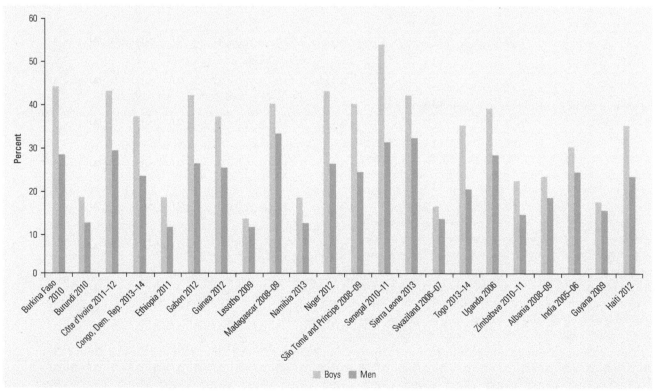

Source: Statcompiler; Demographic and Health Surveys 2000–14.
Note: g/dl = grams per deciliter; Hb = hemoglobin. If there were two surveys in the country during this period, the most recent country survey was used.

more vulnerable girls within the entire cohort of adolescent girls. Energy intake was inadequate and did not meet recommended levels in these girls; intakes were lowest in the Western Pacific and South-East Asia (Caulfield and Elliot 2015). Micronutrient intake was inadequate for iron, calcium, zinc, folate, and vitamin D; fewer than 50 percent of girls have adequate intake (Caulfield and Elliot 2015). Intake of energy-dense, micronutrient-poor, and sugary foods by girls is increasing in urban areas in LMICs.

More information is needed on energy and micronutrient intakes during middle childhood and adolescence, given the relatively high prevalence of underweight and anemia in both genders in this group compared with other age groups, and the increasing prevalence of overweight/obesity, particularly in girls, in some countries.

CONSEQUENCES OF MALNUTRITION

Consequences in Children Younger than Age Five Years

Malnutrition inflicts considerable damage on children in their first 1,000 days and increases the risk of short stature, ill health, cognitive impairment, and reduced productivity and income throughout life (Hoddinott and others 2013). As seen from the available data on prevalence, malnutrition is significant for children when they enter school. The ability of children to recover from a period of compromised growth later in life—catch-up growth—has been deemed unlikely (Martorell, Rivera, and Kaplowitz 1990). The inability to reverse stunting may be the result of changes in genetic expression in early life caused by inadequate food intake and infections that determine growth in stature later in life (Golden 1994).

Emerging evidence, however, suggests that a proportion of stunting may be reversible after age two years in Brazil, Ethiopia, India, Peru, and Vietnam (Lundeen, Behrman, and others 2014), Guatemala, India, the Philippines (Adair 1999), and South Africa (Lundeen, Stein, and others 2014). Chapter 8 in this volume (Watkins and others 2017) provides additional information on catch-up growth attributable to immigration, adoption, and other changes. However, in Lundeen, Stein, and others (2014), height deficits related to the reference median also increased, making the interpretation of recovery more complicated. In addition, little is known about how growth and its timing in school-age children in LMICs compares with the growth of children in high-income countries (HICs)—for example, are growth spurts comparable, and is the timing of puberty experiencing the same secular changes as in children in HICs?

Consequences in Children Ages 5–19 Years

Even if stunting in early childhood is not reversible, further damage to nutritional status and cognitive function needs to be prevented. For children ages five to nine years, malnutrition caused by inadequate food intake and helminth infections increases the risk of underweight, anemia, and illness; these conditions decrease attendance, performance, and years in primary school (Bundy and others 2009). In HICs, 15 percent of adult height and 50 percent of adult weight are attained in adolescence (Heald and Gong 1999). In the United States, the period comprising ages 10–14 years is marked by rapid growth and, for girls, the onset of menses (Sawyer and others 2012). By ages 15–19 years, girls attain their adult height, although their pelvis continues to grow, putting girls at risk of obstructed labor later in life if they are undernourished during pelvic development. Boys continue to gain height and muscle mass through age 24 years. Requirements for iron are high for girls after the onset of menarche and in boys because of muscle mass accretion, increasing their risk of anemia and poor performance in school (Halterman and others 2001). Both iron and iodine deficiencies compromise IQ by 8–15 percentage points at the population level (World Bank 2006). Increasing overweight and poor dietary intake put children at risk for nutrition-related chronic diseases that are on the rise in adolescents in LMICs; 20 percent to 30 percent of adolescents live with chronic illnesses, particularly diabetes (Save the Children 2015).

Adolescent girls are at higher risk of poor birth outcomes (prematurity, stillbirths, and neonatal deaths) and of dying than older WRA (Kozuki and others 2013). One study in the United States found that girls younger than age 15 years were at higher risk of maternal anemia, preterm delivery, postpartum hemorrhage, and preeclampsia, but they were less likely to have a cesarean delivery (Kawakita and others 2015). Becoming pregnant is the main reason why girls drop out of school in LMICs (Save the Children 2015), which results in a loss of income of 1 percent to 30 percent of annual GDP (Chaaban and Cunningham 2011). Adolescent pregnancies also may cause higher prevalence of stunting in children younger than age two years (Dewey and Huffman 2009).

CONCLUSIONS

Few nationally representative surveys are available on the nutritional status of boys and girls ages 5–19 years, and this group continues to be understudied for both prevalence of malnutrition and related outcomes from malnutrition. The dearth of information on nutritional status during middle childhood and early adolescence is particularly striking. Mining DHS data for what has been collected on children ages 48–59 months and boys and girls in late adolescence suggests the prevalence of underweight and anemia are high and, for the most part, are on par with or higher than the prevalence in children ages zero to five years, WRA, and men. Overweight is an emerging problem, particularly in girls during late adolescence, but overweight is lower in girls compared with women and in boys compared with men.

Malnutrition in children ages 5–19 years has profound consequences on education and health outcomes, although more studies and analyses could determine the extent of this impact on national development.

Global resources need to be made available to study all children during middle childhood and adolescence (ages 5–19 years), disaggregating the prevalence of malnutrition to children in middle childhood (5–9 years), early adolescence (10–14 years), and late adolescence (15–19 years). Such disaggregated data would assist in developing policies and introducing programs to address the known and suspected nutrition problems of the entire cohort of middle childhood and adolescence to monitor their impact on the nutritional status in this group.

A better understanding of how to measure malnutrition in this age group also would be useful, although not a prerequisite for action. Knowing more about what indicators reflect and mean, the timing of growth spurts in children, and the timing of puberty could help efforts better target interventions by age group. We know that underweight in children younger than age five years is a composite of chronic malnutrition (stunting) and acute malnutrition (wasting). Can we assume this indicator reflects the same composite of stunting and wasting in children ages 5–15 years? Information is emerging about puberty trends in HICs. For example, Sandhu and others (2006) found the onset of puberty in the United Kingdom to be earlier in boys with higher BMI, while height was higher in boys with later puberty. Studies of this kind are needed in LMICs, where it is unclear how important secular changes in adolescent growth are for long-term health and nutritional status (Karlberg 2002).

Finally, more information is needed about nutrition behaviors and how to influence healthy food choices of school-age children. As they grow older, children can make choices about what they eat based on their own food preferences and peer and media influences. However, all children remain dependent on the food that is available in their environment: collected foods, markets, schools, and household. In addition, age and gender differences may influence how food is distributed within the family; older children may influence, in positive or negative ways, what younger children have available to eat.

NOTES

World Bank Income Classifications as of July 2014 are as follows, based on estimates of gross national income (GNI) per capita for 2013:

- Low-income countries (LICs) = US$1,045 or less
- Middle-income countries (MICs) are subdivided:
  a) lower-middle-income = US$1,046 to US$4,125
  b) upper-middle-income (UMICs) = US$4,126 to US$12,745
- High-income countries (HICs) = US$12,746 or more.

1. The girls in the sample are considered WRA by DHS because they have had at least one live birth and do not represent all girls ages 15–19 years.
2. Indicators are available for low height-for-age (stunting or chronic malnutrition) and low weight-for-height (wasting or acute malnutrition), but because prevalence for these indicators peaks at different times in children ages zero to five years, low weight-for-age, often considered a composite of stunting and wasting, was chosen.
3. DHS collects hemoglobin samples from children ages 6–59 months and does not include children ages 0–5.99 months in the sample.
4. The number of countries for underweight: West Africa (13); Central Africa (5); Eastern Africa (13); Southern Africa (3); North Africa and Eastern Europe (7); Central Asia (2); South and South-East Asia (7); and Latin America and the Caribbean (8). The number of countries for anemia: West Africa (11); Central Africa (6—one study is a Malaria Indicators Survey); Eastern Africa (9); Southern Africa (3); North Africa and Eastern Europe (6); Central Asia (1); South and South-East Asia (5); Latin America and the Caribbean (5).
5. Albania 2008–09, Azerbaijan 2006, Bangladesh 2011, Ethiopia 2011, Guyana 2009, India 2005–06, Lesotho 2009, Namibia 2013, Rwanda 2010, São Tomé and Príncipe 2008–09, Senegal 2010–11, Sierra Leone 2013, Swaziland 2006–07, Uganda 2011, and Zimbabwe 2010–11.
6. Overweight is between +1 standard deviation and ≤+2 standard deviations; obesity is >+2 standard deviations.
7. The Republic of Yemen DHS for 2013 was excluded from the calculations because it was not available on the DHS Statcompiler at the time.
8. The Republic of Yemen was excluded.

REFERENCES

Adair, L. S. 1999. "Filipino Children Exhibit Catch-Up Growth from Age 2 to 12 Years." *Journal of Nutrition* 129 (6): 1140–48.

Black, R. E., C. G. Victora, S. P. Walker, Z. A. Bhutta, P. Christian, and others. 2013. "Maternal and Child Undernutrition and Overweight in Low-Income and Middle-Income Countries." *The Lancet* 382 (9890): 427–51. http://dx.doi.org/10.1016/S0140-6736(13)60937-X.

Bundy, D. A. P., C. Burbano, M. Grosh, A. Gelli, M. Jukes, and others. 2009. *Rethinking School Feeding: Social Safety Nets, Child Development, and the Education Section.* Washington, DC: World Bank.

Bundy, D. A. P., N. de Silva, S. Horton, G. C. Patton, L. Schultz, and D. T. Jamison. 2017. "Child and Adolescent Health and Development: Realizing Neglected Potential." In *Disease Control Priorities* (third edition): Volume 8, *Child and Adolescent Health and Development,* edited by D. A. P. Bundy, N. de Silva, S. Horton, D. T. Jamison, and G. C. Patton. Washington, DC: World Bank.

Caulfield, L. E., and V. Elliot. 2015. *Nutrition of Adolescent Girls and Women of Reproductive Age in Low and Middle Income Countries: Current Context and Scientific Basis for Moving Forward.* Arlington, VA: USAID/Strengthening Partnerships, Results, and Innovations in Nutrition Globally (SPRING) Project.

Chaaban, J., and W. Cunningham. 2011. "Measuring the Economic Gain of Investing in Girls: The Girl Effect Dividend." Policy Research Working Paper 5753, World Bank, Washington, DC.

Dewey, K. G., and S. L. Huffman. 2009. "Maternal, Infant, and Young Child Nutrition: Combining Efforts to Maximize Impacts on Child Growth and Micronutrient Status." *Food and Nutrition Bulletin* 30 (2): S187–89.

Golden, M. H. N. 1994. "Is Complete Catch-Up Growth Possible for Stunted Malnourished Children?" *European Journal of Nutrition* 48 (Suppl 1): 558–71.

Halterman, J. S., J. M. Kaczorowski, C. A. Aligne, P. Auinger, and P. G. Szilagyi. 2001. "Iron Deficiency and Cognitive Achievement among School-Aged Children and Adolescents in the United States." *Pediatrics* 107 (6): 1381–86.

Heald, F. P., and E. J. Gong. 1999. "Diet, Nutrition, and Adolescence." In *Modern Nutrition in Health and Disease,* ninth edition, edited by M. E. Shils, J. A. Olson, M. Shike, and A. C. Ross. Baltimore, MD: Williams and Wilkins.

Hoddinott, J., H. Alderman, J. R. Behrman, L. Haddad, and S. Horton. 2013. "The Economic Rationale for Investing in Stunting Reduction." *Maternal and Child Nutrition* 9 (Suppl 2): 69–82.

Karlberg, J. A. 2002. "Secular Trends in Pubertal Growth Development." *Hormone Research* 57 (Suppl 2): 19–30.

Kawakita, T., K. Wilson, K. L. Grantz, H. J. Landy, C.-C. Huang, and others. 2015. "Adverse Maternal and Neonatal Outcomes in Adolescent Pregnancy." *Journal of Pediatric and Adolescent Gynecology* 29 (2): 1130–36. doi:10.1016/j.jpag.2015.08.006.

Kozuki, N., A. C. Lee, M. F. Silveira, A. Sania, J. P. Vogel, and others. 2013. "The Association of Parity and Maternal Age with Small-for-Gestational Age, Preterm, and Neonatal Infant Mortality: A Meta-Analysis." *BMC Public Health* 13 (Suppl 3). doi:10.1186/1471-2458-13-S3-S2.

Lassi Z., A. Moin, and Z. Bhutta. 2017. "Nutrition in Middle Childhood and Adolescence." In *Disease Control Priorities* (third edition): Volume 8, *Child and Adolescent Health and Development,* edited by D. A. P. Bundy, N. de Silva, S. Horton, D. T. Jamison, and G. C. Patton. Washington, DC: World Bank.

Lundeen, E. A., J. R. Behrman, B. T. Crookston, K. A. Dearden, P. Engle, and others. 2014. "Growth Faltering and Recovery in Children Aged 1–8 Years in Four Low- and Middle-Income Countries: Young Lives." *Public Health Nutrition* 17 (9): 2131–37. doi:10.1017/S1368980013003017.

Lundeen, E. A., A. D. Stein, L. S. Adair, J. R. Behrman, S. K. Bhargava, and others. 2014. "Height-for-Age Z Scores Increase Despite Increasing Height Deficits among Children in 5 Developing Countries." *American Journal of Clinical Nutrition* 100 (3): 821–25.

Martorell, R., J. Rivera, and H. Kaplowitz. 1990. "Consequences of Stunting in Early Childhood for Adult Body Size in Rural Guatemala." *Annals of Nestlé* 48: 85–92.

Ng, M., T. Fleming, M. Robinson, B. Thomson, N. Graetz, and others. 2014. "Global, Regional, and National Prevalence of Overweight and Obesity in Children and Adults during 1980–2013: A Systematic Analysis for the Global Burden of Disease Study 2013." *The Lancet* 384 (9945): 766–81. http://dx.doi.org/10.1016/S0140-6736(14)60460-8.

Sandhu, J., Y. Ben-Shlomo, T. J. Cole, J. Holly, and G. Davey Smith. 2006. "The Impact of Childhood Body Mass Index on Timing of Puberty, Adult Stature and Obesity: A Follow-Up Study Based on Adolescent Anthropometry Recorded at Christ's Hospital (1936–1964)." *International Journal of Obesity* 30 (1): 14–22. doi:10.1038/sj.ijo.0803156.

Save the Children. 2015. *Adolescent Nutrition: Policy and Programming in SUN+ Countries.* London: Save the Children.

Sawyer, S. M., R. A. Afifi, L. H. Bearinger, S. J. Blakemore, B. Dick, and others. 2012. "Adolescence: A Foundation for Future Health." *The Lancet* 379 (9826): 1630–40.

Watkins, K. L., D. A. P. Bundy, D. T. Jamison, G. Fink, and A. Georgiadis. 2017. "Evidence of Impact of Interventions on Health and Development during Middle Childhood and School Age." In *Disease Control Priorities* (third edition): Volume 8, *Child and Adolescent Health and Development,* edited by D. A. P. Bundy, N. de Silva, S. Horton, D. T. Jamison, and G. C. Patton. Washington, DC: World Bank.

WHO (World Health Organization). 2015. *Global Prevalence of Anaemia 2011.* Geneva: WHO.

World Bank. 2006. *Repositioning Nutrition as Central to Development. A Strategy for Large-Scale Action.* Directions in Development Series. Washington, DC: World Bank.

———. 2015. "Population Estimates and Projections." World Bank, Washington, DC. http://data.worldbank.org/data-catalog/population-projection-tables.

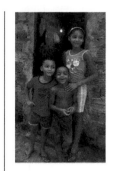

Chapter 4

Global Variation in Education Outcomes at Ages 5 to 19

Kin Bing Wu

INTRODUCTION

Education produces far-reaching benefits to populations by improving health, increasing individual productivity and earnings, enhancing civic engagement, and facilitating economic and social intergenerational mobility (Hannum and Xie 2016; Montenegro and Patrinos 2014; OECD 2013c; Schultz 1961). In the aggregate, it enhances economic growth by contributing to technological change and innovation (Becker 1964; Mankiw, Romer, and Weil 1992; Mincer 1974; Solow 1956; Pradham and others 2016, chapter 30 of this volume).

Education outcomes are affected by a number of factors. At the child or student level, nutrition, health, and interactions with parents and other adults affect brain development, emotional and psychological well-being, and the capacity to learn (Crookston and others 2013). At the school level, education quality is enhanced by school leadership, an orderly and safe environment, high expectations, positive reinforcement, regular assessment, constructive school-home relations, and opportunity to learn (OTL) (Sammons, Hillman, and Mortimore 1995). Education, health, and social policies can create an enabling environment and equalize opportunities for all students through resource allocation, monitoring and supervision, curriculum improvement, teacher management, policy toward the language of instruction, and interventions targeted to disadvantaged groups. Chudgar and Luschei's (2009) study of 25 participating systems in international studies found that although family background affects

outcomes more, schools are an important source of variation in student achievement in poor countries and can bridge the achievement gap. Definitions of age groupings and age-specific terminology used in the volume can be found in chapter 1 (Bundy and others 2017).

INTERNATIONAL ASSESSMENT OF STUDENT ACHIEVEMENT

Cross-national studies confirm the positive relationship between educational attainment, as measured by average years of schooling, and economic growth (Barro 1991, 1997). However, student achievement can vary widely across countries, even across countries with the same average years of schooling. Education quality is the most critical component because the capability to use technology and to innovate is contingent on the improvement of cognitive skills. Hanushek and Woessmann (2015) found a strong positive relationship between student achievement and gross domestic product (GDP) per capita growth between 1964 and 2003; they also found that cognitive skills explained differences in growth rates between regions. For example, 10 East Asia and Pacific countries in their sample experienced growth that was at least 2.5 percentage points per year faster than the typical country in the world, attributable to their knowledge capital. Although other qualities, such as resilience, collaboration, and entrepreneurship, are very important, cognitive skills lend themselves more easily to international comparison.

Corresponding author: Kin Bing Wu, Lead Education Specialist, World Bank (Retired), Menlo Park, California, United States; kbwu_2000@yahoo.com.

The International Association for the Evaluation of Educational Achievement (IEA) and the Organisation for Economic Co-operation and Development's (OECD's) Programme for International Student Assessment (PISA) conducted 21 cross-country studies of student achievement in mathematics, science, and reading between 1964 and 2015 (see annex 4A and table 4.1 for the history of international student assessments).

The IEA organized the first, second, and third mathematics, science, and reading tests from the 1960s to the 1990s, about once every decade, to study the differences between education systems and outcomes. The IEA subsequently conducted the Trends in International Mathematics and Science Study (TIMSS) once every four years and the Progress in International Reading Literacy Study (PIRLS) once every five years. Participating

Table 4.1 History of International Assessments of Student Achievement and Adult Skills

Studies conducted by the International Association for the Evaluation of Educational Achievement	Year	Age (years) and grade	Participating education systems
FIMS	1964	13 and final year	11
FISS	1970–71	10, 14, and final year	14, 16, 16
FIRS	1970–72	13	12
SIMS	1980–82	13 and final year	17, 12
SISS	1983–84	10, 13, and final year	15, 17, 13
SIRS	1990–91	9, 13	26, 30
TIMSS	1994–95	9 (grade 3 or 4), 13 (grade 7 or 8), final year	29, 46, 21
TIMSS-R	1999	13 (grade 8)	38
PIRLS	2001	9 (grade 4)	36
TIMSS	2003	9 (grade 4), 13 (grade 8)	26, 47
PIRLS	2006	9.5 (grade 4)	45
TIMSS	2007	9.5 (grade 4), 13.5 (grade 8)	37, 50
PIRLS	2011	9 (grade 4)	57
TIMSS	2011	9 (grade 4), 13 (grade 8)	50, 42
TIMSS	2015	9 (grade 4), 13 (grade 8)	48, 40
PISA, conducted by the OECD	**Year**	**Age (years)**	**Participating education systems**
PISA	2000, 2002	15	31, 10
PISA	2003	15	40
PISA	2006	15	57
PISA	2009	15	65
PISA	2012	15	65
PISA (to be published in late 2016)	2015	15	74
PIAAC, conducted by the OECD	**Year**	**Age (years)**	**Countries**
PIAAC	2011	16–65	24
PIAAC	2014	16–65	33

Sources: Hanushek and Woessmann 2015; NCES (National Center for Education Statistics) Trends in International Mathematics and Science Study (TIMSS), http://www.nces.ed .gov/TIMSS//countries.asp; NCES Progress in International Reading Literacy Study (PIRLS), http://www.nces.ed.gov/surveys/pirls/countries.asp; NCES Programme for International Student Assessment (PISA), http://www.nces.ed.gov/surveys/pisa/countries.asp.
Note: FIMS = First International Mathematics Study; FIRS = First International Reading Study; FISS = First International Science Study; OECD = Organisation for Economic Co-operation and Development; PIAAC = Programme for the International Assessment of Adult Competencies; PIRLS = Progress in International Reading Literacy Study; PISA = Programme for International Student Assessment; SIMS = Second International Mathematics Study; SIRS = Second International Reading Study; SISS = Second International Science Study; TIMSS = Trends in International Mathematics and Science Study; TIMMS-R = Trends in International Mathematics and Science Study-Repeat.

educational systems increased from the original 11 in 1964 to more than 50 in recent years; they include systems from Europe, East Asia, the Middle East and North Africa, Latin America and the Caribbean, South Asia, and Sub-Saharan Africa.

The IEA has historically assessed three student populations: upper primary (third or fourth grade), lower secondary (seventh or eighth grade), and the final year of upper secondary school. Participating educational systems agree on the content to ensure that the test covers topics in their curricula. The IEA enforces strict sampling rules and protocols to ensure that an educational system under study is representative, whether of a country or of a region of a country. A properly drawn sample of several hundred schools and several thousand students could yield results representative of an education system.

In 2000, PISA began testing the mathematics, science, and reading competency of 15-year-olds every three years, irrespective of the grade of enrollment. PISA assesses students' acquisition of the knowledge and skills that are essential for full participation in modern societies, with the goal of identifying ways in which students can learn better, teachers can teach better, and schools can operate more effectively (OECD 2010).

Both IEA and PISA provide training to participating education systems in sampling, test administration, and data cleaning and analysis. They also validate the results to ensure comparability across countries. The IEA and PISA scores are highly correlated at the national level (Hanushek and Woessmann 2015). Over 100 countries or regions of a country have participated in at least one of the IEA or OECD tests (annex 4A).[1] Financial constraints and consideration of the results' political impact often are the main deterrents to participation.

LESSONS FROM INTERNATIONAL ASSESSMENTS

Education system performance varies tremendously, and country rankings in the international league table often generate headlines. However, in addition to the previously mentioned student-level and school-level factors, student achievement at the system level is affected by size of the rural population, diversity of terrain, adult literacy rates, income distribution, ethnicity and languages, attitudes toward gender equality, and history of conflict. It is important to put the results in a broader context when interpreting them.

Changes in Student Performance and Adult Skills

Education system performance can improve or decline over time. For example, in TIMSS 1995, six education systems scored at the top of the international league table in eighth-grade mathematics: Singapore; Japan; the Republic of Korea; Hong Kong SAR, China; Belgium (Flemish); and the Czech Republic. In TIMSS 2011, the Republic of Korea's score increased by 32 points, rising to the top spot; Hong Kong SAR, China, increased by 17 points; and Singapore increased by 2 points. Over this period, Japan's score decreased by 11 points, Belgium's (Flemish) by 13 points, and the Czech Republic's by 42 points (Loveless 2013). Between PISA 2000 and PISA 2012, Peru made the greatest gains among all participating systems (increasing by 76 points in mathematics), albeit from a very low base, while Brazil and Chile were among the top 10 countries with the greatest gains during this period (Patrinos 2013). In PISA 2009 and 2012, Shanghai, China, overtook Finland as the top performer (annex 4B). Vietnam, a lower-middle-income economy, scored higher than the OECD average (OECD 2013a). These changes in performance demonstrate that cognitive skills are not fixed but can be developed. The relationship between education quality and economic development is not linear; relatively low income countries can make great strides, thereby changing the trajectory of their development.

The reasons for changes in student achievement are complex and country specific, and they may be attributable to a combination of interventions at the student, school, and policy levels and broader social trends. Where girls' performance in mathematics and science lagged behind boys', programs to improve girls' proficiency in these subjects increased the overall national average, as in the Republic of Korea (Chiu, personal communication 2016).[2] Countries that had previously divided their educational systems into general and vocational education saw improved academic achievement by postponing tracking and exposing more students to general education, as in Poland (OECD 2011). Germany increased its scores and ranking from 2003 to 2012 after it adopted a national educational standard in all federal states and put significant effort into teacher training and assessment (Chiu, personal communication 2016). Teaching math through strong visual presentation and improving student engagement improved test scores, as in Singapore (Cavendish 2015). Curriculum change that unintentionally reduced coherence led to a decline in test scores, as in Taiwan, China (Chiu, personal communication 2016). Linking strong schools with weak schools raised teachers' competency in weaker schools, as in Shanghai (Liang, Kidwai, and Zhang 2016). Using international assessment to guide educational interventions has substantially improved student outcomes, as in Germany and Peru (Anderson, Chiu, and Yore 2010; Patrinos 2013). The opening up, particularly to women, of more nonteaching professions with better remuneration and expanded migration opportunities with open borders made it harder for the education sector to retain capable teachers and recruit new talent, thereby affecting education quality (Chui, personal communication, 2016).

Findings from the OECD's first survey of adult skills, the Programme for the International Assessment of Adult Competencies (PIAAC), launched in 2011, confirmed that educational systems could shape people's skill profiles (OECD 2013b). The Republic of Korea was among the three lowest-performing countries when comparing the performance of adults ages 55–65 years with other countries, but it followed Japan in skill proficiency among the younger generation of workers ages 16–24 years. The United Kingdom was among the three highest-performing countries in literacy proficiency among adults ages 55–65 years, but it was among the bottom three in literacy proficiency among those ages 16–24 years. High school–educated adults ages 25–34 years in Japan and the Netherlands outperformed Italian and Spanish university graduates of the same age (annex 4C).

The PIAAC found that skills have a major impact on each person's life chances. The median hourly wage of workers scoring at the highest two levels in literacy (levels 4 and 5) is more than 60 percent higher than that for workers scoring at or below level 1. Those with lower skills also tend to report poorer health and lower civic engagement, and they are less likely to be employed (OECD 2013b). Countries would benefit from using mixed-method case studies to examine how decadal changes in education policy affect generational changes in skill profiles.

Characteristics of High-Performing Systems

Examining the distribution of student achievement at different levels of proficiency is important for assessing the depth of skills. For example, PISA has five levels of proficiency in ascending order, from level 1 to level 5. In PISA 2012, 55 percent of students in Shanghai, 40 percent in Singapore, and 37 percent in Taiwan, China, scored at level 5 in mathematics, compared with 13 percent of OECD students. Only 4 percent of students in Shanghai, 8 percent in Singapore, and 13 percent in Taiwan, China, performed below level 2, compared with 23 percent in OECD countries (annex 4B; OECD 2013a).

High-performing education systems tend to have standards-based external examinations and allocate resources more equitably across all types of schools. Systems that create more competitive environments in which schools vie for students do not systematically perform better. High teacher salaries relative to national income are associated with better student performance.

School autonomy has a positive relationship with student performance when public accountability measures are in place, when school principals and teachers collaborate in school management, or when both occur. Schools with better disciplinary climates, more collaboration among teachers, and more positive teacher-student relationships tend to perform better. Stratification in school systems into general and vocational streams and grade repetition are negatively related to equity and student achievement. School systems with higher percentages of students having attended preprimary education tend to produce better results (OECD 2010, 2013b).

Variance in Achievement between Schools and between Students

International comparisons of the percentage of variance in achievement attributable to between-school differences and between-student (within-school) differences can provide direction for policy intervention. Variance in achievement attributable to between-school differences results from education policies, school resources, teacher characteristics, and instructional strategies. The smaller the between-school variance, the more equitable the school system. In Finland, less than 10 percent of the variance in PISA 2009 was attributable to between-school differences, suggesting that student achievement was less likely to be affected by which school they attended. In Hong Kong SAR, China; the Republic of Korea; Shanghai; and Taiwan, China, the variance in between-school achievement ranged from 30 percent to 35 percent, indicating relatively inequitable schools. In low-performing countries, such as Argentina and Trinidad and Tobago, the variance in student achievement between schools in PISA 2009 was 90 percent and more (OECD 2010). Where between-school variance is large, policy interventions could be directed to improving school-related factors to equalize the OTL.

Variance in achievement attributable to differences between students (within-school) results from students' family characteristics, innate ability, nutrition and health status, early childhood education, and learning strategies. PISA found that students whose parents read to them in their early years and who had attended preprimary school performed better than those without these types of support. Policy interventions directed at students and families could improve achievement. However, international student assessments focus on collecting the characteristics of education systems, schools, teachers, and students; they do not collect data on nutrition and health, which could be very important determinants of education outcomes, particularly in low-income countries and disadvantaged communities.

STUDENT ACHIEVEMENT IN POOR REGIONS OF INDIA AND CHINA

The high-performing education systems in TIMSS, PIRLS, PISA, and PIAAC are relatively small in size and population. Managing an educational system well is much more challenging in countries with more than a billion people and with highly variable geography and income. For example, top-performing Shanghai is a municipality of 23 million people and has the highest per capita income in China. The key question is how students in the poor regions of populous countries fare, relative to the more advanced regions of the same country and to international averages. This section addresses this question by reporting the findings of two surveys conducted in poor regions of India and China, using selected TIMSS mathematics items.

The India survey was part of the World Bank's study on secondary education in India. It was conducted in 2005, involving 3,418 students in 114 schools in Rajasthan (in the west) and 2,856 students in 109 schools in Orissa (in the east) (Wu, Sankar, and Azam 2006). These states have a significantly lower per capita GDP than the national average. The eighth grade was part of elementary education in Rajasthan but was part of secondary education in Orissa. The differences in the education structure in these two states led to selection of the ninth grade for testing because it was part of secondary education in both states. Thirty-six test items designed for the eighth grade internationally were selected from published items from the TIMSS 1999 (TIMSS-R) and administered to the sampled ninth-graders in both states (annex 4D). The survey also administered questionnaires to the sampled students, teachers, and schools to assess factors affecting student performance (annex 4E).

The China survey was part of a 2006 World Bank study on compulsory education (Wu, Boscardin, and Goldschmidt 2011). The same test items from TIMSS-R used in India were used to test a sample of 4,103 eighth-graders in 138 schools in Gansu province in China. Located in arid northwest China, Gansu is the second poorest province in the country. As in India, the survey administered questionnaires to the sampled students, teachers, and schools to assess factors affecting student performance, but a question on breakfast and measurement of weight and height were added to the student questionnaire (annex 4F).

Major differences existed between the two countries. India's per capita GDP was less than one-fourth of China's. Infrastructure and the telecommunication systems were relatively well developed, even in China's poor western regions, but much less so in India in 2006. India lagged far behind China in health indicators (WHO 2010). India did not have a national curriculum; each state determined its own education structure, curriculum, and language of instruction. China has a national curriculum that applies to all public schools irrespective of location. Chinese schools were far better resourced than Indian schools. In both countries, local educational authorities were consulted on the appropriateness of applying the test to their students. Stratified random sampling was used in both countries, but the sampling frames were different (and they were different from that of TIMSS-R). As such, the findings are only suggestive, not representative or definitive, of student achievement in the hinterland of these two large countries and its potential link with TIMSS performance. The results should be treated as a test case for further investigation.

Gansu's eighth-graders' average of 72 percent correct of the 36 items was above the international average of 52 percent; Rajasthan's and Orissa's ninth-graders scored 34 percent and 37 percent correct on average, respectively. Item by item, the Gansu students scored above the international average on 34 of 36 items, while Orissa students had lower scores on 35 of 36 items, and Rajasthan students performed below on all items. Given that students in Rajasthan and Orissa had the benefit of an additional year of education, their low scores should be a concern for policy makers. Figure 4.1 illustrates the differences in percentage correct for each item. These results to some extent foreshadow the relatively weak performance of two of the better-performing Indian states (Tamil Nadu and Himachal Pradesh) on PISA 2009 and the stellar performance of Shanghai, China, on the same test. Yet, a significant achievement gap between Gansu and Shanghai could be inferred given the latter's top position in PISA 2009 and 2012.

A multilevel analysis was performed to explore the determinants of achievement in Rajasthan, Orissa, and Gansu (Wu, Boscardin, and Goldschmidt 2011; Wu, Sankar, and Azam 2006). The unconditional analytical models found that school quality was highly variable in the poor regions of both large countries—46 percent of the variance in achievement in Rajasthan and 50 percent of the variance in Orissa was attributable to differences between schools; in Gansu, 55 percent of the variance was attributable to between-school differences (annex 4E). The paragraphs that follow and annexes 4F and 4G report only those variables with statistical significance and could inform policy.

India

Student Level

At the student level in Rajasthan and Orissa, the analysis found a statistically significant association between good

Figure 4.1 Average Percentage Correct by Item in Gansu, China, and Rajasthan and Orissa, India, Compared with International Average

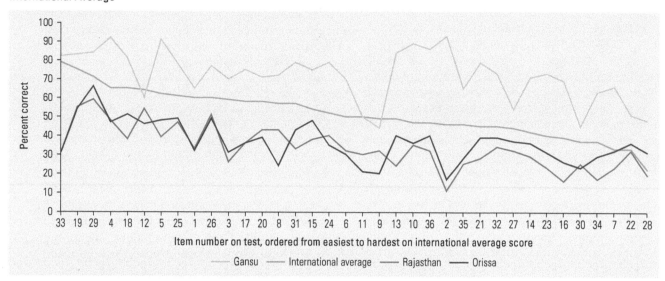

Source: Wu, Boscardin, and Goldschmidt 2011.

performance on the one hand, and being male, higher education levels of mothers, higher parental expectations, advanced resources at home, and OTL on the other hand. Boys outperformed girls, on average, in both states. In Rajasthan, students who belonged to Scheduled Tribes[3] performed below nontribal students. In Orissa, Scheduled Caste students performed lower than the general students, on average. The OTL through homework and examination had positive effects on student achievement (annex 4F).

School Level

When students' family resources were aggregated at the school level, a significant effect on student achievement in both states was found. School types made a difference in Rajasthan: students enrolled in government-aided schools and unaided (private) schools performed better than government schools (annex 4F).

In the full model, student-level variables explained only 8 percent of the variance in achievement and school-level variables explained 33 percent in Rajasthan. Student-level variables explained only 4 percent of the variance in achievement between students, and school-level variables explained 19 percent in Orissa (annex 4E).

China

Student Level

In Gansu, significant factors at the student level were as follows: gender, age, students' prior achievement,

parental expectations, and having had breakfast. On average, girls performed lower than boys. Increase in age and grade repetition were associated with lower performance. Students with parents who expected them to complete tertiary education performed better. Students who rarely had breakfast before school performed lower than students who had breakfast. The last variable is particularly important because 43 percent of students rarely had breakfast. However, there was insufficient variation in weight and height at the ninth-grade level to link those measures with student performance (annex 4G).

School Level

At the school level, teacher qualification, teacher preparation, and teaching strategy were positively associated with student achievement. Students with teachers who had higher levels of education performed much higher. An increase of an additional hour of lesson preparation by the teacher was associated with a small but significant increase in student performance. Additional teacher time spent during class time discussing questioning strategies was positively associated with student performance. Schools with more resources and facilities, ranging from drinking water and electricity to computers, student dormitories, and televisions, were positively associated with student performance. Schools with a high percentage of minority students were negatively associated with student performance, although at the individual student level, minority status was not associated with student outcome (annex 4G).

In the full model, the student-level variables only explained 7 percent of the variance in achievement between students, and the school-level variables only explained 12 percent of variance between schools (annex 4E).

Discussion

In both the India and China studies, the collected data explained a much smaller portion of the variance in achievement between students than the variance between schools. This outcome suggests that a singular focus on education policy without simultaneous interventions at the student level is unlikely to improve achievement on a large and sustained scale. Although it is difficult to change family characteristics, socioeconomic backgrounds, and innate abilities, it is entirely possible to improve students' nutrition and health, and to provide opportunity for early child development.

Longitudinal studies in a number of countries have found significant long-term impacts of nutrition and health on educational outcome (Crookston and others 2013; Hannum, Liu, and Frongillo 2014; Lundeen and others 2014). Several randomized controlled trials in elementary schools in western China that took blood samples from elementary students to use as independent variables to predict their test scores confirmed that giving the treatment group multivitamins, including iron, raised hemoglobin and increased mathematics test scores by 0.2–0.4 standard deviation compared with those of a control group (Kleiman-Weiner and others 2013; Luo and others 2012). These studies suggest that directly measuring nutrition and health through blood tests can help target interventions at the student level to increase their educational outcomes.

CONCLUSIONS

The evidence from international student assessments supports the overall relationship between knowledge capital and economic growth, although it is not linear. The PIAAC findings on adult skills suggest that countries with low skill levels are at a competitive disadvantage in the global knowledge economy. Yet TIMSS and PISA have shown that education systems can improve student achievement on a large scale. Future international assessments could consider including a more detailed questionnaire on nutrition and health and collection of biomarkers through blood tests, at least in a subsample. Availability of such integrated information on education, nutrition, and health on an international scale could explain in greater depth the differences in achievement across countries and between students, help countries prioritize their

interventions, and enable international donors to target their resources more effectively.

ANNEXES

The annexes to this chapter are as follows. They are available at http://www.dcp-3.org/CAHD.

- Annex 4A. Participating Educational Systems in International Assessment of Student Achievement, 1995–2015
- Annex 4B. Performance of 15-Year-Old Students in 10 Top-Performing Educational Systems in PISA, 2012
- Annex 4C. Comparison of Skill Proficiency among Adults, 2011
- Annex 4D. Average Percentage Correct, by Item, in Gansu, China, and Rajasthan and Orissa, India, Compared with International Average
- Annex 4E. Percentage of Variance in Achievement Explained by Differences between Schools and between Students in Rajasthan, Orissa, and Gansu
- Annex 4F. Factors Associated with Student Achievement in Grade 9 in Rajasthan and Orissa, India
- Annex 4G. Factors Associated with Student Achievement in Grade 8 in Gansu

NOTES

World Bank Income Classifications as of July 2014 are as follows, based on estimates of gross national income (GNI) per capita for 2013:

- Low-income countries (LICs) = US$1,045 or less
- Middle-income countries (MICs) are subdivided:
  a) lower-middle-income = US$1,046 to US$4,125
  b) upper-middle-income (UMICs) = US$4,126 to US$12,745
- High-income countries (HICs) = US$12,746 or more.

1. Other regional student assessment programs focus on Latin America and the Caribbean, as well as on English-speaking and French-speaking countries in Sub-Saharan Africa. However, this chapter only focuses on the IEA and PISA assessments because of their international scope and long history.
2. M. H. Chiu was interviewed by the author in Taiwan, China, on June 23, 2016. Dr. Chiu is Professor at the Graduate Institute of Science Education, National Taiwan Normal University and President, National Association for Research in Science Teaching (NARST), United States.
3. Scheduled Tribes are indigenous peoples and Scheduled Castes are the most disadvantaged social groups in India. They are recognized in India's constitution as eligible for support.

REFERENCES

Anderson, J. O., M. H. Chiu, and L. D. Yore. 2010. "First Cycle of Pisa (2000–2006)—International Perspectives on Successes and Challenges: Research and Policy Directions." *International Journal of Science and Mathematics Education* 8 (3): 373–88.

Barro, R. J. 1991. "Economic Growth in a Cross Section of Countries." *Quarterly Journal of Economics* 106 (2): 407–43.

———. 1997. *Determinants of Economic Growth: A Cross-Country Empirical Study.* Cambridge, MA: MIT Press.

Becker, G. S. 1964. *Human Capital: A Theoretical and Empirical Analysis, with Special Reference to Education.* Cambridge, MA: National Bureau of Economic Research.

Bundy, D. A. P., N. de Silva, S. Horton, G. C. Patton, L. Schultz, and D. T. Jamison. 2017. "Child and Adolescent Health and Development: Realizing Neglected Potential." In *Disease Control Priorities* (third edition): Volume 8, *Child and Adolescent Health and Development,* edited by Bundy, D. A. P., N. de Silva, S. Horton, D. T. Jamison, and G. C. Patton. Washington, DC: World Bank.

Chudgar, A., and T. F. Luschei. 2009. "National Income, Income Inequality, and the Importance of Schools: A Hierarchical Cross-National Comparison." *American Educational Research Journal* 46 (3): 626–58.

Crookston, B., W. Schott, S. Cueto, K. A. Dearden, P. L. Eagle, and others. 2013. "Post-Infancy Growth, Schooling, and Cognitive Achievement: Young Lives." *American Journal of Clinical Nutrition* 98 (6): 1555–63.

Hannum, E., J. Liu, and A. Frongillo. 2014. "Poverty, Food Insecurity, and Nutritional Deprivation in Rural China: Implication for Children's Literacy Achievement." *International Journal of Educational Development* 34: 90–97.

Hannum, E., and Y. Xie. 2016. "Education." In *The Oxford Handbook of the Social Science of Poverty,* edited by D. Brady and L. Burton, chapter 20. New York: Oxford University Press.

Hanushek, E. A., and L. Woessmann. 2015. *The Knowledge Capital of Nations: Education and the Economics of Growth.* Cambridge, MA: MIT Press.

Kleiman-Weiner, M., R. Luo, L. Zhang, Y. Shi, A. Medina, and S. Rozelle. 2013. "Eggs versus Chewable Vitamins: Which Intervention Can Increase Nutrition and Test Scores in Rural China?" *China Economic Review* 24: 165–76.

Liang, X., H. Kidwai, and M. Zhang. 2016. *How Shanghai Does It: Insights and Lessons from the Highest Ranking Education System in the World.* Directions in Development. Washington, DC: World Bank.

Loveless, T. 2013. "The Latest TIMSS and PIRLS Scores." Brown Center Report on American Education, Part I. Brookings Institution, Washington, DC.

Lundeen E. A., J. R. Behrman, B. T. Crookston, K. A. Dearden, P. Engle, and others. 2014. "Growth Faltering and Recovery in Children Aged 1–8 Years in Four Low- and Middle-Income Countries: Young Lives." *Public Health Nutrition* 9: 2131–37.

Luo, R., Y. Shi, L. Zhang, C. Liu, S. Rozelle, and others. 2012. "Nutrition and Educational Performance in Rural China's Elementary Schools: Results of a Randomized Control Trial in Shaanxi Province." *Economic Development and Cultural Change* 60 (4): 735–72.

Mankiw, G., D. Romer, and D. Weil. 1992. "A Contribution to the Empirics of Economic Growth." *Quarterly Journal of Economics* 107 (2): 407–37.

Marshall Cavendish. 2015. *Math in Focus: Singapore Math.* Singapore: Marshall Cavendish Education, distributed by Houghton Mifflin Harcourt.

Mincer, J. 1974. *Schooling, Experience, and Earnings.* New York: National Bureau of Economic Research.

Montenegro, C. E. and H. A. Patrinos. 2014. "Comparable Estimates of Return to Schooling around the World." Policy Research Working Paper WP57020, World Bank, Washington, DC.

NCES (National Center for Education Statistics). Various years a. "Trends in International Mathematics and Science Study (TIMSS)." NCES, US Department of Education. http://www.nces.ed.gov/TIMSS//countries.asp.

———. Various years b. "Progress in International Reading Literacy Study (PIRLS)." NCES, US Department of Education. http://www.nces.ed.gov/surveys/pirls/countries.asp.

———. Various years c. "Programme for International Student Assessment (PISA)." NCES, US Department of Education. http://www.nces.ed.gov/surveys/pisa/countries.asp.

OECD (Organisation for Economic Co-operation and Development). 2010. *PISA 2009 Results: What Makes a School Successful? Resources, Policies and Practices.* Vol. IV. Paris: OECD Publishing. http://dx.doi.org/10.1787/9789264091559-en.

———. 2011. "The Impact of the 1999 Education Reform in Poland." OECD Education Working Paper No. 49, OECD Publishing, Paris. http://dx.doi.org/10.1787/5kmbjgkm1m9x-en.

———. 2013a. *PISA 2012 Results in Focus: What 15-Year-Olds Know and What They Can Do with What They Know.* Paris: OECD. http://www.oecd.org/pisa/keyfindings/pisa-2012-resultsoverview.pdf.

———. 2013b. *PISA 2012 Results: What Makes a School Successful? Resources, Policies and Practices.* Vol. IV. Paris: OECD Publishing. http://dx.doi.org/10.1787/9789264201156-en.

———. 2013c. *OECD Skills Outlook 2013: First Results from the Survey of Adult Skills.* OECD Publishing. http://dx.doi.org/10.1787/9789264204256-en.

Patrinos, H. 2013. "PISA Results: Which Countries Improved Most?" Education for Global Development: A blog about the power of investing in people. http://blogs.worldbank.org/education/pisa-results-which-countries-improve-most.

Sammons, P., J. Hillman, and P. Mortimore. 1995. *Key Characteristics of Effective Schools: A Review of School Effectiveness Research.* London: International School Effectiveness and Improvement Center, Institute of Education, University of London for the Office of Standards in Education.

Schultz, T. W. 1961. "Investment in Human Capital." *American Economic Review* 51 (1): 1–17.

Solow, R. M. 1956. "A Contribution to the Theory of Economic Growth." *Quarterly Journal of Economics* 70 (1): 65–94.

WHO (World Health Organization). 2010. *World Health Statistics 2010.* Geneva: WHO. http://www.who.int/whosis /whostat/2010/en.

Wu, K. B., D. Sankar, and M. Azam. 2006. "Secondary Education in India." Technical Notes. Unpublished. World Bank, Washington, DC.

Wu, K. B., C. K. Boscardin, and P. Goldschmidt. 2011. "A Retrospective on Educational Outcomes in China: From Shanghai's 2009 PISA Results to Factors that Affected Student Performance in Gansu in 2007." Unpublished. Background paper for *China 2030: Building a Modern, Harmonious, and Creative Society.* 2013. Washington, DC: World Bank and Development Research Center of the State Council, the People's Republic of China.

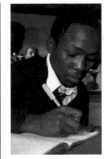

Global Measures of Health Risks and Disease Burden in Adolescents

George C. Patton, Peter Azzopardi, Elissa Kennedy,
Carolyn Coffey, and Ali Mokdad

INTRODUCTION

Adolescents are commonly viewed as healthy in comparison with other age groups (Sawyer and others 2012). Adolescence is an age at which many positive attributes of health peak, and these positive attributes predict health in later life. Physical fitness peaks about age 20 years; it remains high until the early 30s, when it declines steadily to old age (Rockwood, Song, and Mitnitski 2011). Those with the highest fitness levels in their 20s are more likely to stay physically healthy throughout life, using less health service as they age (Rockwood, Song, and Mitnitski 2011). Adolescent cardiorespiratory fitness, muscular strength, and body composition are also predictive of lower all-cause mortality and cardiovascular disease in later life (Ruiz and others 2009). Adolescence is similarly central in skeletal health. Bone mineral density, a primary determinant of later-life osteoporosis and its complications, peaks in the late teens to early 20s (Baxter-Jones and others 2011). In the two years of peak skeletal growth, adolescents accumulate more than 25 percent of adult bone mass; patterns of physical activity and adolescent nutrition are important modifiable influences (Julián-Almárcegui and others 2015; Whiting and others 2004).

Increasingly, adolescence is recognized as a time of changing trajectories and health across the life course (Patton and Viner 2007; Sawyer and others 2012). This is evident in mortality shifts showing a rise in deaths that are largely preventable: deaths from intentional and nonintentional injuries; deaths due to human immunodeficiency virus/acquired immune deficiency syndrome (HIV/AIDS), tuberculosis, and other infectious diseases; and deaths due to maternal causes (Patton and others 2009). Patterns of nonfatal disease burden also shift across these years. The prevalence of mental disorders rises sharply across adolescence (Gore and others 2011). Many risk processes leading to chronic noncommunicable diseases (NCDs) in later life, including tobacco use, alcohol and illicit substance use, unsafe sex, obesity, and lack of physical activity, typically emerge in these years (Gore and others 2011). Definitions of age groupings and age-specific terminology used in this volume can be found in chapter 1 (Bundy and others 2017).

HEALTH INFORMATION SYSTEMS AND ADOLESCENCE

Sound information is essential for selecting priorities in health and social policy and monitoring the effects of subsequent actions (AbouZahr, Adjei, and Kanchanachitra 2007). Global and national health information systems have paid little attention to the

Corresponding author: George C. Patton, Department of Paediatrics, University of Melbourne; and Murdoch Children's Research Institute, Melbourne, Australia; george.patton@rch.org.au.

adolescent age group, in part because of the prevailing view of young people as healthy. Very few attempts to systematically measure their health have been made. Initiatives in adolescent health metrics have more commonly arisen from interest in particular aspects of health, such as sexual and reproductive health or adolescent-onset risks for NCDs in later life. The Millennium Development Goals (MDGs), for example, proposed indicators on the development of young people in low- and middle-income countries (LMICs) but with a health focus predominantly on sexual and reproductive health (Beaglehole and Bonita 2008).

Broad conceptual frameworks for reporting adolescent health have been used in only a small number of high-income countries (HICs) that undertake regular reports on the health status of young people (AIHW 2003; Kolbe and others 1997; Office of the Minister for Children and Youth Affairs 2008; Ministry of Social Development 2008). In these countries reporting has moved from a focus on age-disaggregation of routinely collected health and demographic statistics to reporting behavioral and risk factor data collected directly from young people (UNICEF 2007).

Current Data Surveys and Databases for Adolescent Health

Planning responses to adolescent health requires data that are timely, developmentally relevant, age- and gender-disaggregated, and defined to a local level. Ideally, these data would allow comparisons over time and tracking of inequalities within and between countries. In reality existing global data systems for adolescents are uncoordinated, inconsistent in coverage and timing, inadequately disaggregated, and missing large groups of adolescents, and they fail to deal with the spectrum of health problems and their determinants. This situation matters because LMICs are, to a large extent, dependent on global surveys, such as Demographic and Health Surveys (DHS), for data for health policy and programming.

Map 5.1 and annex table 5A outline the available surveys and databases that provide data on adolescent health problems, health risks, and social determinants of health. Adolescent health and well-being is currently assessed in a patchwork of surveys that include school- and household-based surveys.

Health Behaviour in School-Aged Children (HBSC) is the oldest of the school-based surveys. It is supported by an academic network and has, over the past three decades, collected data on younger adolescents in schools in many HICs and middle-income countries, with intermittent, ad hoc support from some national governments. The Global Youth Tobacco Survey and the Global School-Based Student Health Survey (GSHS) were both established in the past two decades, primarily to gain greater information on NCD risks that emerge in adolescence. They are both administered by the World Health Organization (WHO), with support from the U.S. Centers for Disease Control and Prevention, and focus on younger adolescents ages 13–15 years in schools in LMICs. Although broadly focused on risks for NCDs, the GSHS also covers other aspects of adolescent health.

The DHS are the most well established of the global household surveys. It is supported by the U.S. Agency for International Development and operates in LMICs. It has provided some health information for ages 15–25 years over the past three decades, predominantly around sexual and reproductive health. It has more recently been complemented by the Multiple Indicator Cluster Surveys (MICS), administered by the United Nations Children's Fund. MICS use methodologies similar to those of DHS, with a predominant focus on the sexual and reproductive health of married women and girls.

HEALTH INDICATORS AND COVERAGE FOR ADOLESCENTS

Health indicators are summary measures chosen to describe particular aspects of health, health risk, or health system performance. They are generally developed in the context of a specific policy initiative and conceptual framework. Indicators are commonly defined within the context of specific disease-related initiatives, a process that has led to rapid inflation in numbers of indicators, presenting a major challenge for global health information systems (Murray 2007). Many indicators remain poorly measured, leading to calls to define smaller numbers of core health indicators focused on mortality, morbidity, service coverage, and risk factors (Bchir and others 2006).

The MDGs brought a focus to indicators for HIV/AIDS and maternal health in adolescents. There have been a number of subsequent calls to expand indicators and data collection systems beyond this focus on sexual and reproductive health to take into account rapid transitions in adolescent health in many countries (Boerma and Stansfield 2007). More comprehensive approaches would consider relevant social determinants of health, as well as the contribution of adolescent-onset risk factors to future disease burden (Walker, Bryce, and Black 2007).

Growing evidence suggests the importance of sound information to promote effective responses to the

Map 5.1 Global Coverage of Adolescent Health by International Data Collections, 2000–12

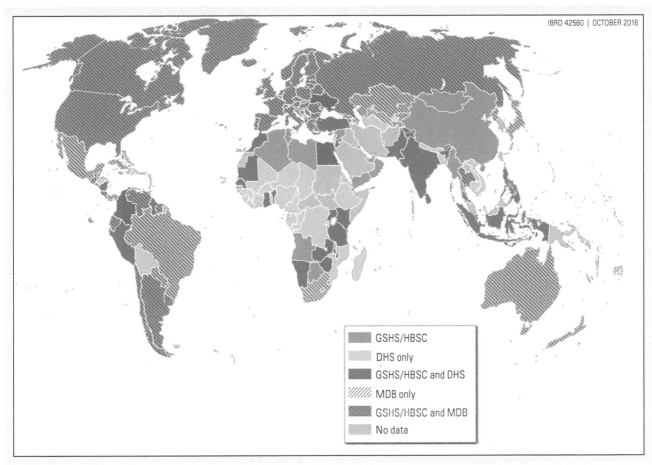

IBRD 42560 | OCTOBER 2016

GSHS/HBSC

DHS only

GSHS/HBSC and DHS

MDB only

GSHS/HBSC and MDB

No data

Source: Reprinted from *The Lancet* 379 (9826): Patton, G. C., C. Coffey, C. Cappa, D. Currie, L. Riley, and others, "Health of the World's Adolescents: A Synthesis of Internationally Comparable Data," 1665–75, © 2012, with permission from Elsevier.
Note: DHS = Demographic and Health Surveys; GSHS = Global School-Based Student Health Survey; HBSC = Health Behaviour in School-Aged Children; MDB = World Health Organization Global Mortality Database.

health problems of young people, including prevention of traffic injury (Shope and others 2001); reducing adolescent alcohol abuse (Wagenaar 2003); responding to underweight and malnutrition; and promoting the social, neighborhood, and school engagement background for healthy development (Hawkins and others 2009; Patton and others 2006). Despite this growing recognition of the importance of good information for adolescent health, there is as yet no current internationally agreed-upon set of indicators. The *2012 Lancet Adolescent Health Series* conceptual framework was adopted for the purpose of defining indicators relevant to adolescent health (figure 5.1). It incorporates elements from earlier national reports, including measures of health and well-being (AIHW 2007), social role transitions (Department for Children, Schools, and Families 2010), risk and protective factors (Bronfenbrenner 1979), and health service system

Figure 5.1 Conceptual Framework on Adolescent Health

Social, educational, and economic policies and interventions

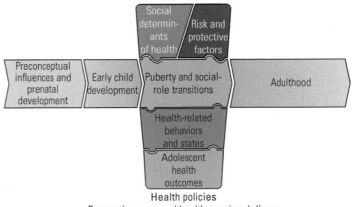

Health policies
Preventive care and health-service delivery

Source: Reprinted from *The Lancet* 379 (9826): Sawyer, S. M., R. A. Afifi, L. H. Bearinger, S. J. Blakemore, B. Dick, and others, "Adolescence: A Foundation for Future Health," 1630–40, © 2012, with permission from Elsevier.

responses (Rosen and Levine 2010). The series selected indicators across five areas:

- Health outcomes reflecting major causes of death and incident disability in ages 10–24 years
- Health-related behaviors and states that carry risks for current or later-life disease and typically emerge in adolescence and young adulthood
- Risk and protective factors derived from the immediate social contexts affecting emerging health risks
- Markers of social role transitions that are associated with altered patterns of health risk
- Health service policy interventions provided to adolescents that have the potential to influence current or later health status.

The indicators drew on the four categories of data outlined in annex 5A including the global mortality database, international household surveys, international school-based surveys, and other United Nations (UN) sources. The indicators included the most recent data available, collected since 2000, even if the data were not available for the entire age spectrum or were available only at a subnational level. Regional subgroups were defined according to the 2010 Global Burden of Disease study (Murray and others 2012).

The Lancet series used indicator definitions with the best comparable data to optimize global coverage. Where available, the series used well-accepted and consistent definitions, although definitions varied considerably for many indicators. In these instances, the series examined currently available data sources (annex 5A) to derive definitions that allowed comparisons to be made across a maximum possible number of countries.

Global Coverage of Adolescent Health

Given the widespread perception of adolescence as a healthy life phase, it is not surprising that this picture of young people's health is patchy, with a range of data gaps. Global coverage of the 25 indicators selected for the 2012 *Lancet* series on adolescent health are outlined in annex 5B. Comparable data coverage was higher for indicators that have been the focus of the MDGs. However, only a few indicators had global coverage greater than 50 percent; coverage was very low for some indicators, particularly around mental health, substance use, and health service delivery. Accurate population data on the major causes of nonfatal health-related disability in this age group, even for HIV/AIDS, is telling for its absence. This lack of good health information reflects a number of gaps that can be classified into four categories.

Indicators Needing Better Measures

Much work needs to be done on indicator development and measurement. Sexual and reproductive health in adolescents has had the greatest policy and programmatic attention, leading to a greater degree of consensus on definitions of indicators and, in turn, the production of data. In other areas, there are difficulties in defining and measuring indicators. The lack of investment in, and agreement around, mental health indicators is one striking gap that is relevant for an age group in which the peak onset for mental disorders occurs (Gore and others 2011). This void reflects a lack of clarity about the definition of an indicator and a lack of agreement about which standardized and practical measures might be used widely in health surveys. Potentially useful measures exist, however, in that the K-6 (Kessler-6), PHQ-2 (Patient Health Questionnaire), and PHQ-9 seem brief enough to be useful in the major surveys (Green and others 2010; Richardson and others 2010).

Indicators of health service delivery to young people were poorly measured other than an MDG-related focus on HIV/AIDS. In some instances, such as human papillomavirus (HPV) vaccination, this gap is likely to reflect the comparatively recent introduction and as yet absence of wide-scale implementation (Goldie and others 2008). In other instances, such as health care responses to major mental disorders, it reflects both lack of agreement about the indicator and measurement problems. In delineating indicators of intervention coverage, there is scant evidence about the effectiveness of interventions such as youth-friendly primary health care and longer-term outcomes of treatment for mental disorders (Tylee and others 2007). Such evidence is needed to define indicators of health service coverage and quality. Current international surveys, such as those conducted by the Commonwealth Fund, provide data on unmet health care needs but focus on a small number of HICs and lack scope for disaggregation by age group. Given that the delivery of high-quality interventions is likely to be the main way in which health systems may effect change in adolescent health, this gap is concerning.

One area that few national or international reports have addressed well is measurement of risk and protective factors related to the social contexts of child and adolescent development. In addition to being important determinants of adolescent health, these factors are commonly the areas for which good evidence around prevention exists (Catalano and others 2012). Positive family, school, and community connections are measured in school health surveys, but much more work needs to be done to clarify cross-culturally valid indicators in these areas (McNeely and Barber 2010).

Indicators Needing Agreed-Upon Definitions

Sometimes which indicator and definition is most valid, and whether a single indicator is sufficient, is unclear, for example, maternal mortality rate and ratio. Both the choice and definition of indicators in earlier national and international reports have varied greatly, in part reflecting the available data. Many HICs have used the HBSC; this practice has led not only to comparable measures but also to the adoption of similar definitions (UNICEF 2007). Even so, in areas such as tobacco and substance use, and physical activity, measurement is not a major problem; however, these areas do have substantial differences in the definitions used that limit comparisons between countries and over time.

International comparability can be optimized where similar methods of sampling and measurement are used across surveys (Pirkis and others 2003). Such harmonization of data collection is evident in the major household surveys (MICS, DHS, Reproductive Health Surveys, AIDS Indicator Surveys), but it is not yet optimal for the major international school-based surveys, even though some comparisons are possible. The GSHS complements the more established HBSC in providing new data on adolescents in LMICs. Despite the difficulties inherent in international comparisons, there appear to be sufficient similarities between these two international surveys to suggest that aggregated analyses might be feasible in the future (Pirkis and others 2003). This comparability could be strengthened even further with alignment of sampling and measurement strategies.

Indicators Needing Extended or Different Data Collection

Some of the difficulties in capturing a complete picture of young people's health lie in the limits of international data collection. Mortality indicators are one example. Although arguably a poorer guide to health status of adolescents than for other age groups with higher death rates, these estimates depend on good national registers of death. Those countries with the highest mortality rates, and therefore where mortality is a more important indicator, tend to be those without national registers.

The capacity to measure and respond to the health risk behaviors that emerge in adolescence and young adulthood will be central in prevention efforts for NCDs (Strong and others 2008; WHO 2000). Investment has increased since the 2000 World Health Assembly call for surveillance to track the major risks for chronic NCDs (WHO 2000). Yet many adolescent estimates in LMICs are based on only one data point, with little certainty about whether and when serial measurements

of indicators will be feasible. Recently introduced surveys, such as the GSHS, are also limited to younger adolescents in school rather than being population based. School-based surveys provide no information on those outside of school, almost certainly a higher-risk population for many health problems (Bovet and others 2006). Additionally, because retention rates drop with progression through secondary school, the predominant focus of school surveys has been early adolescence, arguably too young an age group in which to track important risk processes related to alcohol abuse and illicit drug use that tend to emerge at a later age (Patrick and Schulenberg 2011).

To what extent the measurement of young people's health best takes place in adolescent school-based surveys or augmentation of existing household surveys that include older age groups is an important question. School-based surveys are efficient where a high proportion of adolescents are in school; for those countries and regions where school retention rates are low or absenteeism high, however, it is unlikely to be a sufficient strategy without data collection on the higher-risk groups outside of school. This situation will be particularly true for girls in countries with lower enrollment rates because girls are less likely to be in school than boys. Furthermore, because of lower school retention in later secondary school, school-based surveys, even in HICs, are likely to provide a better measure of the health of younger rather than older adolescents. Yet it is in older adolescence that many health risk behaviors, such as tobacco, alcohol, and other substance use; obesity; and physical activity, and health states become established. The younger adolescent age group with the greatest coverage is arguably too young for the extent of these problems to be adequately assessed.

Although some programs do capture risk behaviors and states in older groups (for example, the European School Survey Project on Alcohol and Other Drugs, the WHO's STEPwise approach to Surveillance), the range of country coverage globally is limited and depends on high retention rates in upper secondary schools. For this reason, the extension of household surveys with a broader range of measures is likely to be important. These surveys collect fewer data from men and remain largely restricted to sexual and reproductive health, even though the MICS have taken recent steps to extend to other areas of health. There are challenges beyond survey design, respondent burden, and cost. Questions may also arise about whether an adolescent or a parent is the better informant, who can provide consent, and whether confidentiality can be maintained.

Strategies relevant to socially marginalized young people, including those out of school, out of home, and in juvenile detention, are needed. These young people are unlikely to be included in current data collections and health profiles, and their access to health services is often very poor. Strategies for health surveillance are needed in these groups, such as focused institutional surveys or respondent-driven sampling, methods that have been used to track HIV prevalence and risk behaviors at a local level (Chopra and others 2009).

Digital technologies potentially offer an alternative path, either in the context of existing surveys or development of new surveys. In countries with conspicuous acute adolescent health problems—such as intentional and nonintentional injuries, HIV/AIDS, and mental disorders—it may be possible to use these technologies to tap into data from existing facilities where young people are seeking care. Web-based sampling and assessment methods, the use of mobile phones and hand-held devices for data collection, and new data-sharing strategies also have great potential to increase the range and use of data (Lang 2011). So, too, digital technologies offer scope for collection of data on health service encounters, the weakest aspect in current adolescent health data systems (Simmons, Fajans, and Ghiron 2007). Combined with the use of logic models, these technologies might also generate data that are useful at local levels to guide practice responses and secure support for data collection by decision makers.

Indicators for which Data Are Not Fully Utilized

No clear inclusive forum exists for the collection and collation of global data on young people's health. As a result, countries such as Australia, Brazil, and New Zealand, despite having sophisticated survey and health information systems, do not have data that are easily internationally comparable (AIHW 2007). A simple solution of incorporating at least some elements of the HBSC into national surveys in these countries, as well as adopting an agreed-upon international core set of indicators, would do much to ensure international comparability.

However, more systematic approaches will be needed. A range of UN agencies and other groups contribute elements to current surveillance, but they do so without any clear coordinating mechanism (Murray and Lopez 2010). In more targeted areas of global health, the development of mechanisms for the coordination of strategic information has underpinned many advances. In HIV/AIDS, malaria control, vaccine-preventable diseases, and diarrheal diseases monitoring and evaluation groups have been organized and may extend across UN agencies (Stein and others 2007). The Child Health Epidemiology Reference Group (CHERG) was established in 2001 in response to the need for better information on infant and child mortality in pursuit of MDG 4. CHERG subsequently extended its work to examine the relationship between infant and maternal mortality; CHERG has produced reports that have shaped global policy responses and information systems around early childhood mortality and disease. A coordinating entity for the measurement of young people's health might have a work plan that includes conducting research that would lead to better measures of important and neglected indicators, refining indicator definitions with optimal validity, determining the best methods of capturing data in this adolescent age group, and ensuring the full use of available data. Ultimately, this effort could lead to harmonization across the different data sources, establishment of a consensus set of global indicators, development of a global index of adolescent health, and better use of data in policy formation.

Outside of HICs, with a few notable exceptions, relatively few countries have compiled status reports on the health and development of young people. The absence of data on intervention coverage suggests that even in the development of policy within the health sector, the data currently collected may receive little attention and have little capacity to drive health program delivery at a country level. Without such bottom-up data collection capacity that can specify local priorities and document health intervention coverage, securing either political or donor engagement may be difficult (Boerma and AbouZahr 2005).

GLOBAL PATTERNS OF ADOLESCENT DISEASE AND HEALTH RISK

The 2012 *Lancet* series illustrated wide international variations in almost all areas of young people's health. These differences existed both between and within regions, such as those defined by the WHO. The poorest regional health profiles were generally for young people in Sub-Saharan Africa, where mortality, rates of HIV/AIDS infection, and role transitions such as early childbirth linked to health risk were high. There were striking regional differences that included death rates from violence in Latin American countries and wide variations in rates of suicide and traffic injury deaths. With regard to risks for later NCDs, the available data suggest that HICs had some of the poorest profiles relating to patterns of alcohol abuse, mental disorders, and overweight.

Adolescent Health Outcomes

HIV seroprevalence based on household surveys was available from 29 countries representing 29 percent of the global population. Data were predominantly from Sub-Saharan Africa and to a lesser extent from central and southern Asia. We have not included estimates from sentinel surveillance sites or women attending antenatal clinics because these generally overestimate prevalence (Wilson and others 2010). In areas where HIV/AIDS is endemic, rates are substantially higher in females ages 15–24 years than in males. Swaziland had the highest estimated rates of HIV/AIDS infection. Countries with higher rates of HIV/AIDS that have not had country-wide surveys include Angola, Botswana, Eritrea, The Gambia, Guinea-Bissau, Namibia, Nigeria, South Africa, Somalia, and Sudan. Countries outside of Africa without seroprevalence data include Pakistan, Papua New Guinea, the Russian Federation, Thailand, and Ukraine.

Axis 1 psychiatric disorder in the past 12 months in those ages 18–24 years was only available from 23 countries representing 37 percent of the global population. In a number of countries with smaller sample sizes (less than 4,000 for all age groups, for example, Belgium, France, Germany, and Lebanon) or with subregional samples (for example, Japan), confidence intervals around the estimates for those ages 18–24 years were greater than 5 percent. No comparable data are available for those younger than age 18 years. Rates of disorder tended to be higher in females than males in most countries. There was a threefold difference in rates across countries, with low rates in Bulgaria, India, Italy, and the Netherlands, and high rates in Brazil, France, New Zealand, Spain, and the United States. Erskine and others (2016) estimated the coverage of prevalence data for mental disorder in children ages 5–17 years. The overall global coverage was very poor; 124 out of 187 countries have no data at all on the prevalence of mental disorders. The mean global coverage for mental disorders in this age group was 6.7 percent (Erskine and others 2016).

Health Risk Behaviors and States

Coverage for health risk behaviors ranged between 40 and 85 countries. In general, there was good to excellent coverage of health risk behaviors and states in North America, the European Region, and southern Latin America.

Tobacco Use

Tobacco use in the past 30 days was available in 62 countries representing 45 percent of the global population of young people. Rates of tobacco use were high in a number of Western European countries, Chile, Jamaica, Namibia, Tonga, and in males in Indonesia. In the European Region, North America, Latin America, and many Sub-Saharan African countries, rates of tobacco use appeared similar in males and females. In most Asian regions and the Caribbean, rates were higher in males.

Binge Drinking

Data on binge drinking in the past month were available for 51 countries and 17 percent of the global population. Definitions are not strictly comparable between the GSHS and HBSC. The former defines binge drinking as the consumption of at least five units of alcohol on any day in the past month; the latter defines it as getting drunk at least once in the past month. Rates are substantially higher for age 15 years than for age 13 years. In general, estimates for binge drinking from HICs were substantially higher than derived from LMICs, with the exception of some Latin American countries. Austria, Ireland, and the United States had the highest rates, with close to one-third of 15-year-olds reporting binge drinking in the past month.

Illicit Substance Use

Data on illicit substance use in the past 30 days were available in 41 countries representing 12 percent of the global population. The best data available were for the European Region and North America. There were substantial variations in the rates of use; the highest were in Canada, France, Spain, the Netherlands, and the United States.

Underweight

Underweight in those ages 13–15 years could be defined in 72 countries representing 48 percent of the global population. The greatest availability of body mass index (BMI) data was in the European Region. Limited data were available for Sub-Saharan Africa and Central Asia, regions where the prevalence of underweight might be expected to be highest. Rates of underweight were generally less than 10 percent in the European regions and North America. In regions with higher rates of underweight, males tended to fall into this category more than females. South-East Asia had high rates of underweight with Indonesia, Myanmar, and Sri Lanka particularly high. Limited data exist for other regions; Djibouti, Fiji, and the Republic of Yemen stood out for their high rates, particularly in males.

Overweight

Overweight in those ages 13–15 years was available for a similar range of countries as underweight. In HICs, rates of overweight were substantially higher in males than females. Canada, Greece, Italy, Malta, and the United States stand out for their high rates, particularly in young males where more than one-third were overweight. LMICs demonstrated substantial variation in rates of overweight; the lowest rates were in Malawi,

Mongolia, Myanmar, Pakistan, and Sri Lanka. It is striking that many LMICs had substantial rates of overweight; between one-fifth and one-third of young males are overweight in Latin American countries, Oceania, China, Thailand, and Mauritania. Tonga had the highest rates of overweight, with approximately 60 percent of those ages 13–15 years fulfilling the criteria.

Physical Activity

Physical activity data were available for 86 countries representing more than 50 percent of the global population. Boys were generally more likely than girls to fulfill the recommended level of activity. HICs displayed some tendency to have higher rates of reported activity than LMICs. In most HICs, a majority of those ages 13 and 15 years meet the guidelines of at least 60 minutes of moderate physical activity on most days of the week; the rates were lower in older females. Among HBSC countries, Bulgaria, Croatia, France, Greece, Israel, Italy, Malta, Romania, and Russia stand out for their low rates

of physical activity. The rates of physical activity are lower in LMICs, particularly for females, in the Middle East and North Africa, many Sub-Saharan African countries, Pakistan, and the Philippines.

Sexual and Reproductive Health

Indicators of sexual and reproductive health were generally more available. Map 5.2 provides an illustration of information on sexual health risks available from household surveys. The surveys do not collect data on those younger than age 15 years.

- **Sexual activity by age 15 years** was relatively well populated if the data sources extended to school-based surveys. Theoretically, data were available for 117 countries and almost 50 percent of the global population. Generally, more information was available for females than males. The household survey data derive from retrospective reports in samples ages 15–24 years, while available school-based survey

Map 5.2 Sexual Health Risks in Adolescents in Countries with Available Household Data

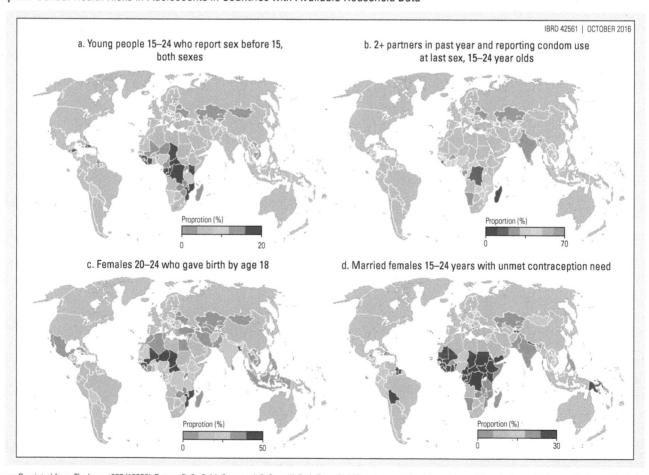

Source: Reprinted from *The Lancet* 387 (10036): Patton, G. C., S. M. Sawyer, J. S. Santelli, D. A. Ross, R. Alifi, and others, "Our Future: A Lancet Commission on Adolescent Health and Wellbeing," 2423–78, © 2016, with permission from Elsevier.

data cover having had sex by the time of report. Rates from retrospective reports appeared to be lower than those from concurrent reports in countries where both sets of data are available. European countries surveyed through HBSC showed an almost fourfold variation in rates for males and females and up to an eightfold variation between countries. Coverage was poorest in the Middle East and North Africa, and coverage was limited in HICs in East Asia and Pacific. Bulgaria, the Central African Republic, Denmark, Iceland, Mauritania, Mozambique, the United States, and Zambia appeared to have higher rates of early sexual activity in females.

- *Female marriage before age 18 years* had good data coverage for much of Sub-Saharan Africa, and mixed coverage in Asia, the Middle East, and Latin America and the Caribbean. Similar data may be available in HICs (Stein and others 2007), but they are not collated according to this definition to allow international comparability. Rates of early marriage were high in Southern Asia; Bangladesh reported the highest rate globally, with two-thirds of women marrying before age 18 years. Very high rates of early marriage were reported for most of Sub-Saharan Africa. Rates in Eastern Europe and Latin America were generally in the intermediate range but with striking variations among countries.

- *Child birth by age 18 years* had relatively good coverage with data available for 57 percent of the world's young women in 96 countries across a wide range of incomes. Rates of early childbirth closely mirrored rates of early marriage, with high rates in Southern Asia, Sub-Saharan Africa, and countries in Latin America and the Caribbean. Namibia, South Africa, and Swaziland stand out for their relatively high early birth rates and lower rates of early marriage.

ALTERNATIVES TO HARMONIZATION IN DATA COLLECTION

The current low rates of coverage do not allow an adequate picture to be developed of health and health risks in adolescents in most countries. Recent attempts have been made to model the use of existing sources of information to provide a more comprehensive picture of global health and health risks (Murray and others 2012). Multiple definitions from different data sources are modeled in Murray and others (2012) using ordinary least-squares regression to generate estimates of frequency within particular categories. Maps 5.3–5.8 illustrate global patterns of three health risks that emerge prominently during the adolescent years and the changes over the past two decades.

Map 5.3 Prevalence of Daily Smoking in Ages 10–24 Years, 2012
Percent

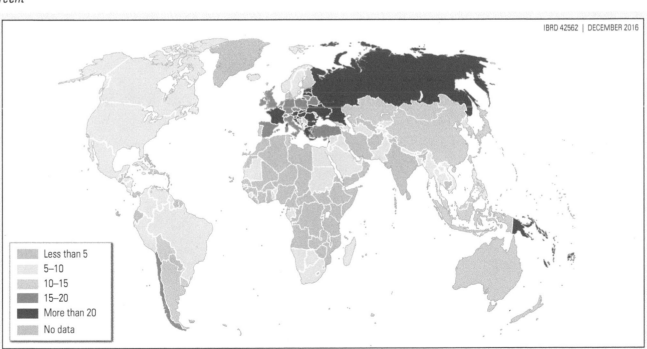

Legend:
- Less than 5
- 5–10
- 10–15
- 15–20
- More than 20
- No data

IBRD 42562 | DECEMBER 2016

Source: Reprinted from *The Lancet* 387 (10036): Patton, G. C., S. M. Sawyer, J. S. Santelli, D. A. Ross, R. Alifi, and others, "Our Future: A Lancet Commission on Adolescent Health and Wellbeing," 2423–78, © 2016, with permission from Elsevier.

Map 5.4 Annual Change in Daily Smoking in Ages 10–24 Years, 1990–2012
Percent

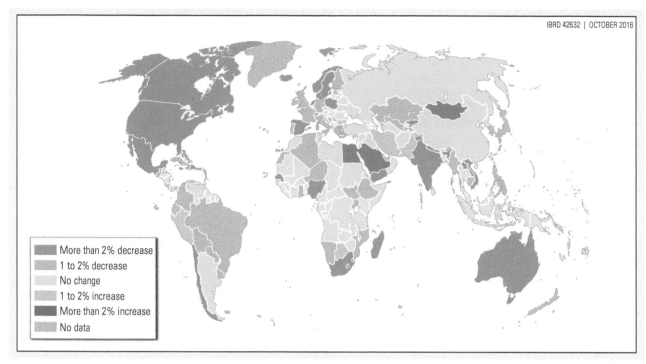

IBRD 42632 | OCTOBER 2016

- More than 2% decrease
- 1 to 2% decrease
- No change
- 1 to 2% increase
- More than 2% increase
- No data

Source: Reprinted from *The Lancet* 387 (10036): Patton, G. C., S. M. Sawyer, J. S. Santelli, D. A. Ross, R. Alifi, and others, "Our Future: A Lancet Commission on Adolescent Health and Wellbeing," 2423–78, © 2016, with permission from Elsevier.

Map 5.5 Ages 15–24 Years Reporting Binge Drinking in the Past 12 Months, Both Genders, 2013
Percent

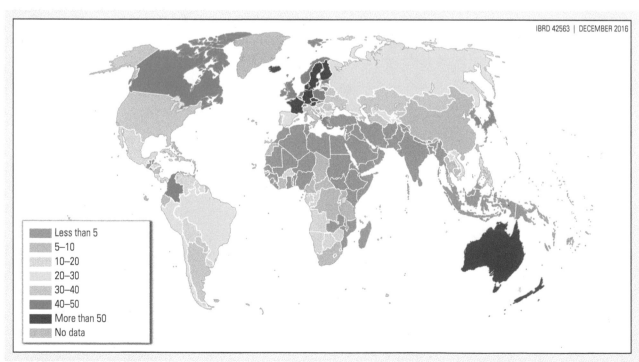

IBRD 42563 | DECEMBER 2016

- Less than 5
- 5–10
- 10–20
- 20–30
- 30–40
- 40–50
- More than 50
- No data

Source: Reprinted from *The Lancet* 387 (10036): Patton, G. C., S. M. Sawyer, J. S. Santelli, D. A. Ross, R. Alifi, and others, "Our Future: A Lancet Commission on Adolescent Health and Wellbeing," 2423–78, © 2016, with permission from Elsevier.

Map 5.6 Annual Change in Ages 15–24 Years Reporting Binge Drinking in the Past 12 Months, Both Genders, 1990–2013
Percent

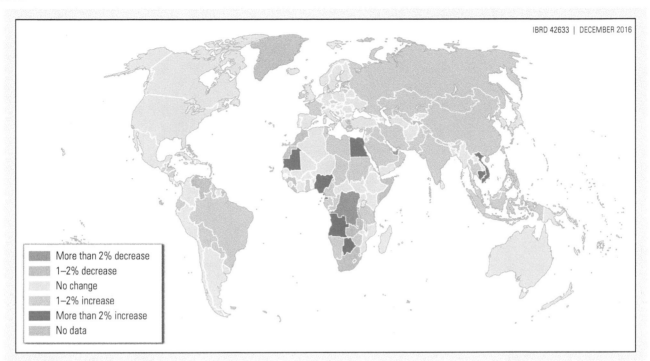

IBRD 42633 | DECEMBER 2016

More than 2% decrease
1–2% decrease
No change
1–2% increase
More than 2% increase
No data

Source: Reprinted from *The Lancet* 387 (10036): Patton, G. C., S. M. Sawyer, J. S. Santelli, D. A. Ross, R. Afifi, and others, "Our Future: A Lancet Commission on Adolescent Health and Wellbeing," 2423–78, © 2016, with permission from Elsevier.

Map 5.7 Prevalence of Overweight and Obesity in Ages 10–24 Years, 2013

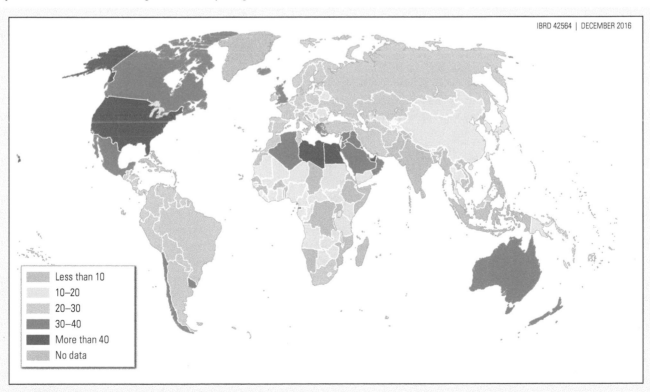

IBRD 42564 | DECEMBER 2016

Less than 10
10–20
20–30
30–40
More than 40
No data

Source: Reprinted from *The Lancet* 387 (10036): Patton, G. C., S. M. Sawyer, J. S. Santelli, D. A. Ross, R. Afifi, and others, "Our Future: A Lancet Commission on Adolescent Health and Wellbeing," 2423–78, © 2016, with permission from Elsevier.

Map 5.8 Annual Change in Overweight and Obesity in Ages 10–24 Years, 1990–2013
Percent

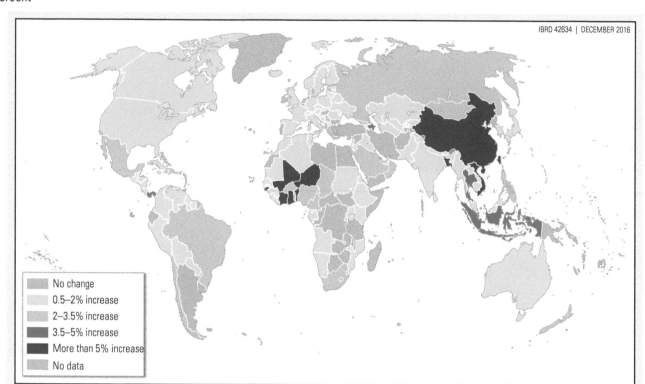

IBRD 42634 | DECEMBER 2016

No change
0.5–2% increase
2–3.5% increase
3.5–5% increase
More than 5% increase
No data

Source: Reprinted from *The Lancet* 387 (10036): Patton, G. C., S. M. Sawyer, J. S. Santelli, D. A. Ross, R. Alifi, and others, "Our Future: A Lancet Commission on Adolescent Health and Wellbeing," 2423–78, © 2016, with permission from Elsevier.

The prevalence of smoking was defined as tobacco smoking at least once per day. Smoking prevalence data were available for 186 countries for ages 10–14, 15–19, and 20–24 years, and for males and females.

Tobacco use is a major risk factor for NCDs later in life and overwhelmingly has its onset in adolescence. Maternal smoking during pregnancy is also a well-established risk factor for poor fetal growth as well as for later-life illness in offspring (Bruin, Gerstein, and Holloway 2010). Overall, tobacco use has declined since 1990, but progress has been mixed. Rates of daily smoking remain greater than 15 percent in ages 10–24 years across most European countries. In Russia, one in four people ages 10–24 years smokes daily. Across all groups of countries, daily smoking is more common in males than females. A number of countries in Sub-Saharan Africa, Eastern Europe, and the Middle East have seen increases. Many nonsignatories to the Framework Convention on Tobacco Control have not seen any decline in adolescent and young adult tobacco use.

Alcohol use disorders typically begin during the young adult years. As with nicotine addiction, younger age of drinking is a particular risk factor (Bonomo, Patton, and Bowes 2006; Viner and Taylor 2007). Alcohol consumption in adulthood is linked to eight different cancers, hypertension, hemorrhagic stroke, atrial fibrillation, and various forms of liver disease and pancreatitis (Parry, Patra, and Rehm 2011). Greater use of alcohol in pregnancy has prominent intergenerational harms in the form of fetal alcohol syndrome (Riley and McGee 2005).

Binge drinking was defined as consuming 48 grams of alcohol in a single occasion for females and 60 grams for males in the past year, per Global Burden of Disease definitions. Alcohol prevalence data were available for 188 countries for a combined 15–24 age group, and for males, females, and both genders combined. The modeled estimates were for a 15–24 year age band that assumed constant prevalence across all ages in this group. Data were available for 1990, 1995, 2000, 2005, 2010, and 2013.

Binge drinking was considerably more prevalent in males than in females in every country grouping. Little progress has been made in reducing adolescent and young adult binge drinking since 1990. An increasing trend for binge drinking is clear; both males and females in LMICs are likely to overtake HICs in binge drinking in the coming years.

Overweight and obesity increase markedly across adolescence and young adulthood with very high persistence, particularly for obesity (Patton and others 2011). The risks in later life include premature mortality, chronic disability, type 2 diabetes, ischemic heart disease, hypertension, and cerebrovascular disease (Reilly and Kelly 2011). Preconception maternal obesity increases risks for miscarriage, gestational diabetes, operative delivery, preeclampsia, infant perinatal mortality, and macrosomia (Yu, Teoh, and Robinson 2006).

For those ages 19–24 years, overweight was defined as BMI ≥ 25 to < 30 kilograms per square meter (kg/m²) and obesity as BMI ≥ 30 kg/m². For those ages 10–18 years, classification was based on percentiles using the International Obesity Task Force definition. Overweight and obesity prevalence data were available for 188 countries for age groups 10–14, 15–19, and 20–24 years, and for males, females, and both sexes combined. Data were available for all years from 1990 to 2013.

Adolescent overweight and obesity have increased in prevalence across almost all countries since 1990, as shown in map 5.8. Notable exceptions are Argentina, Bulgaria, the Islamic Republic of Iran, Turkey, and countries in central Sub-Saharan Africa. The annual increase has been about 10 percent in China and Vietnam; there have also been marked increases in other countries across South-East Asia, as well as in Sub-Saharan Africa. If their recent increases in obesity continue, middle-income countries will soon outstrip HICs in rates of overweight and obesity.

CONCLUSIONS

Current knowledge of adolescent health reflects many of the broader gaps in global health information systems. Adolescents are further disadvantaged on a number of counts.

- Younger adolescents are poorly covered, especially in LMICs, with no coverage for those out of school in any survey.
- Fewer data are available on males and unmarried young women.
- Beyond sexual and reproductive health, most aspects of adolescent health and health risks are not included in household surveys.

- The capacity to understand health trends has been limited by funding constraints resulting in lack of investment in repeat surveys in many countries.

Moving forward will require responses in multiple areas, including the following:

- *Improving the harmonization of assessments across surveys based on standardized indicators and measures.* Where harmonization is not possible, studies are needed to understand how different survey approaches might be complementary.
- *Extending the coverage of current surveys to new and emerging problems and health risks, including mental disorders and emotional well-being, substance use, and injury risks.* Doing so is likely to require the development of new indicators and measures.
- *Extending existing surveys to provide adequate coverage of younger adolescents, as well as developing systems for assessing structural and social determinants of health.*

Digital technologies will offer great opportunities for more affordable and more effective data collection systems, training, and support of in-country expertise in data analysis.

ANNEXES

The annexes to this chapter are as follows. They are available at http://www.dcp-3.org/CAHD.

- Annex 5A. Characteristics of Important International Data Sources Used in Adolescent Health Indicators
- Annex 5B. Availability of Information from International Data Collections to Populate Indicators of Adolescent Health, 2000–12

NOTE

World Bank Income Classifications as of July 2014 are as follows, based on estimates of gross national income (GNI) per capita for 2013:

- Low-income countries (LICs) = US$1,045 or less
- Middle-income countries (MICs) are subdivided:
  a) lower-middle-income = US$1,046 to US$4,125
  b) upper-middle-income (UMICs) = US$4,126 to US$12,745
- High-income countries (HICs) = US$12,746 or more.

REFERENCES

AbouZahr, C., S. Adjei, and C. Kanchanachitra. 2007. "From Data to Policy: Good Practices and Cautionary Tales." *The Lancet* 369 (9566): 1039–46.

AIHW (Australian Institute of Health and Welfare). 2003. *Australia's Young People: Their Health and Well-Being 2003.* Canberra: AIHW.

———. 2007. Young Australians: Their Health and Wellbeing. Canberra: AIHW.

Baxter-Jones, A. D., R. A. Faulkner, M. R. Forwood, R. L. Mirwald, and D. A. Bailey. 2011. "Bone Mineral Accrual from 8 to 30 Years of Age: An Estimation of Peak Bone Mass." *Journal of Bone and Mineral Research* 26 (8): 1729–39.

Beaglehole, R., and R. Bonita. 2008. "Global Public Health: A Scorecard." *The Lancet* 372 (9654): 1988–96.

Bchir, A., Z. Bhutta, F. Binka, R. Black, D. Bradshaw, and others. 2006. "Better Health Statistics Are Possible." *The Lancet* 367 (9506): 190–3.

Boerma, J. T., and C. AbouZahr. 2005. "Monitoring Global Health: Bottom Up Approach Is More Likely to Be Successful." *BMJ* 330 (7484): 195–96.

Boerma, J. T., and S. K. Stansfield. 2007. "Health Statistics Now: Are We Making the Right Investments?" *The Lancet* 369 (9563): 779–86.

Bonomo, Y. A., G. C. Patton, and G. Bowes. 2006. "What Are the Longer Term Outcomes of Adolescent Alcohol Consumption in Young Adulthood? Results from a 10-Year Cohort Study." *Alcoholism: Clinical and Experimental Research* 30 (9): 117A.

Bovet, P., B. Viswanathan, D. Faeh, and W. Warren. 2006. "Comparison of Smoking, Drinking, and Marijuana Use between Students Present or Absent on the Day of a School-Based Survey." *Journal of School Health* 76 (4): 133–37.

Bronfenbrenner, U. 1979. *The Ecology of Human Development: Experiments by Nature and Design.* Cambridge, MA: Harvard University Press.

Bruin, J. E., H. C. Gerstein, and A. C. Holloway. 2010. "Long-Term Consequences of Fetal and Neonatal Nicotine Exposure: A Critical Review." *Toxicological Sciences* 116 (2): 364–74.

Bundy, D. A. P., N. de Silva, S. Horton, G. C. Patton, L. Schultz, and D. T. Jamison. 2017. "Child and Adolescent Health and Development: Realizing Neglected Potential." In *Disease Control Priorities* (third edition): Volume 8, *Child and Adolescent Health and Development,* edited by D. A. P. Bundy, N. de Silva, S. Horton, D. T. Jamison, and G. C. Patton. Washington, DC: World Bank.

Catalano, R. F., A. A. Fagan, L. E. Gavin, M. T. Greenberg, C. E. Irwin Jr., and others. 2012. "Worldwide Application of Prevention Science in Adolescent Health." *The Lancet* 379 (9826): 1653–64.

Chopra, M., L. Townsend, L. Johnston, C. Mathews, M. Tomlison, and others. 2009. "Estimating HIV Prevalence and Risk Behaviors among High-Risk Heterosexual Men with Multiple Sex Partners: Use of Respondent-Driven Sampling." *Journal of Acquired Immune Deficiency Syndromes* 51 (1): 72.

Department for Children, Schools, and Families. 2010. *Every Child Matters: Outcome Framework.* London: Department for Children, Schools, and Families.

Erskine H., A. Baxter, G. C. Patton, T. E. Moffatt, V. Patel, and others. 2016. "The Global Coverage of Prevalence Data for Mental Disorders in Children and Adolescents." *Epidemiology and Psychiatric Sciences*: 1–8. Epub ahead of print January 20.

Goldie, S. J., M. O'Shea, M. Diaz, and S. Y. Kim. 2008. "Benefits, Cost Requirements and Cost-Effectiveness of the HPV16,18 Vaccine for Cervical Cancer Prevention in Developing Countries: Policy Implications." *Reproductive Health Matters* 16 (32): 86–96.

Gore, F. M., P. Bloem, G. C. Patton, J. Ferguson, J. V. Coffey, and others. 2011. "Global Burden of Disease in Young People Aged 10–24 Years: A Systematic Analysis." *The Lancet* 377 (9783): 2093–102.

Green, J. G., M. J. Gruber, N. A. Sampson, A. M. Zaslavsky, and R. C. Kessler. 2010. "Improving the K6 Short Scale to Predict Serious Emotional Disturbance in Adolescents in the USA." *International Journal of Methods in Psychiatric Research* 19 (Suppl 1): 23–35.

Hawkins, J. D., S. Oesterle, E. C. Brown, M. W. Arthur, R. D. Abbott, and others. 2009. "Results of a Type 2 Translational Research Trial to Prevent Adolescent Drug Use and Delinquency: A Test of Communities That Care." *Archives of Pediatrics and Adolescent Medicine* 163 (9): 789–98.

Julián-Almárcegui, C., A. Gómez-Cabello, I. Huybrechts, A. González-Aqüero, J. M. Kaufman, and others. 2015. "Combined Effects of Interaction between Physical Activity and Nutrition on Bone Health in Children and Adolescents: A Systematic Review." *Nutrition Reviews* 73 (3): 127–39.

Kolbe, L., L. Kann, S. Everett, and C. Hannan. 1997. "Frameworks to Inform the Development of U.S. Adolescent Health Indicators for the 21st Century." *Global Health Promotion* 4 (4): 32–6.

Lang, T. 2011. "Advancing Global Health Research through Digital Technology and Sharing Data." *Science* 331 (6018): 714–17.

McNeely, C., and B. K. Barber. 2010. "How Do Parents Make Adolescents Feel Loved? Perspectives on Supportive Parenting from Adolescents in 12 Cultures." *Journal of Adolescent Research* 25 (4): 601–31.

Ministry of Social Development. 2008. *Children and Young People: Indicators of Wellbeing in New Zealand 2008.* Wellington, New Zealand: Ministry of Social Development.

Murray, C. J. L. 2007. "Towards Good Practice for Health Statistics: Lessons from the Millennium Development Goal Health Indicators." *The Lancet* 369 (9564): 862–73.

Murray, C. J. L., M. Ezzati, A. D. Flaxman, S. Lim, R. Lozano, and others. 2012. "GBD 2010: Design, Definitions, and Metrics." *The Lancet* 380 (9859): 2063–66.

Murray, C. J. L., and A. D. Lopez. 2010. "Production and Analysis of Health Indicators: The Role of Academia." *PLoS Medicine* 7. doi:10.1371/journal.pmed.1001004.

Office of the Minister for Children and Youth Affairs. 2008. *State of the Nation's Children.* Dublin: Office of the Minister for Children and Youth Affairs.

Parry, C. D., J. Patra, and J. Rehm. 2011. "Alcohol Consumption and Non-Communicable Diseases: Epidemiology and Policy Implications." *Addiction* 106 (10): 1718–24.

Patrick, M. E., and J. E. Schulenberg. 2011. "How Trajectories of Reasons for Alcohol Use Relate to Trajectories of Binge Drinking: National Panel Data Spanning Late Adolescence to Early Adulthood." *Developmental Psychology* 47 (2): 311–17.

Patton, G. C., L. Bond, J. B. Carlin, L. Thomas, H. Butler, and others. 2006. "Promoting Social Inclusion in Secondary Schools: A Cluster Randomised Trial." *American Journal of Public Health* 96 (9): 1582–89.

Patton, G. C., C. Coffey, C. Cappa, D. Currie, L. Riley, and others. 2012. "Health of the World's Adolescents: A Synthesis of Internationally Comparable Data." *The Lancet* 379 (9826): 1665–75.

Patton, G. C., C. Coffey, J. B. Carlin, S. M. Sawyer, J. Williams, and others. 2011. "Overweight and Obesity between Adolescence and Young Adulthood: A 10-Year Prospective Cohort Study." *Journal of Adolescent Health* 48 (3): 275–80.

Patton, G. C., C. Coffey, S. M. Sawyer, R. M. Viner, D. M. Haller, and others. 2009. "Global Patterns of Mortality in Young People: A Systematic Analysis of Population Health Data." *The Lancet* 374 (9693): 881–92.

Patton, G. C., S. M. Sawyer, J. S. Santelli, D. A. Ross, R. Alifi, and others. 2016. "Our Future: A *Lancet* Commission on Adolescent Health and Wellbeing." *The Lancet* 387 (10036): 2423–78.

Patton, G. C., and R. Viner. 2007. "Pubertal Transitions in Health." *The Lancet* 369 (9567): 1130–9.

Pirkis, J. E., C. E. Irwin, C. Brindis, G. C. Patton, and M. G. Sawyer. 2003. "Adolescent Substance Use: Beware of International Comparisons." *Journal of Adolescent Health* 33 (4): 279–86.

Reilly, J., and J. Kelly. 2011. "Long-Term Impact of Overweight and Obesity in Childhood and Adolescence on Morbidity and Premature Mortality in Adulthood: Systematic Review." *International Journal of Obesity* 35 (7): 891–98.

Richardson, L. P., C. Rockhill, J. E. Russo, D. C. Grossman, J. Richards, and others. 2010. "Evaluation of the PHQ-2 as a Brief Screen for Detecting Major Depression among Adolescents." *Pediatrics* 125 (5): E1097–103.

Riley, E. P., and C. L. McGee. 2005. "Fetal Alcohol Spectrum Disorders: An Overview with Emphasis on Changes in Brain and Behavior." *Experimental Biology and Medicine* 230 (6): 357–65.

Rockwood, K., X. Song, and A. Mitnitski. 2011. "Changes in Relative Fitness and Frailty across the Adult Lifespan: Evidence from the Canadian National Population Health Survey." *Canadian Medical Association Journal* 183 (8): E487–94.

Rosen, J. E., and R. Levine. 2010. *Mainstreaming Adolescent Girls into Indicators of Health Systems Strengthening*. Washington, DC: Center for Global Development.

Ruiz, J. R., J. Castro-Piñero, E. G. Artero, F. B. Ortega, M. Siostrom, and others. 2009. "Predictive Validity of Health-Related Fitness on Youth: A Systematic Review." *British Journal of Sports Medicine* 43 (912): 909–23.

Sawyer, S. M., R. A. Afifi, L. H. Bearinger, S. J. Blakemore, B. Dick, and others. 2012. "Adolescence: A Foundation for Future Health." *The Lancet* 379 (9826): 1630–40.

Shope, J. T., L. J. Molnar, M. R. Elliott, and P. F. Waller. 2001. "Graduated Driver Licensing in Michigan." *Journal of the American Medical Association* 286 (13): 1593.

Simmons, R., P. Fajans, and L. Ghiron. 2007. *Scaling Up Health Service Delivery: From Pilot Innovations to Policies and Programmes*. Geneva: WHO.

Stein, C., T. Kuchenmuller, S. Hendrickx, A. Prüss-Ustün, L. Wolfson, and others. 2007. "The Global Burden of Disease Assessments: WHO Is Responsible?" *PLoS Neglected Tropical Diseases* 1 (3): e161.

Strong, K., C. Mathers, J. Epping-Jordan, S. Resnikoff, and A. Ullrich. 2008. "Preventing Cancer through Tobacco and Infection Control: How Many Lives Can We Save in the Next 10 Years?" *European Journal of Cancer Prevention* 17 (2): 153–61.

Tylee, A., D. M. Haller, T. Graham, R. Churchill, and L. A. Sanci. 2007. "Youth-Friendly Primary-Care Services: How Are We Doing and What More Needs to Be Done?" *The Lancet* 369 (9572): 1565–73.

UN (United Nations). 2011. *World Population Prospects: The 2010 Revision, CD-ROM Edition*. Department of Economic and Social Affairs, Population Division. New York: UN.

UNICEF (United Nations Children's Fund). 2007. *An Overview of Child Well-Being in Rich Countries. Report Card 7*. Florence, Italy: UNICEF Innocenti Research Centre.

Viner, R. M., and B. Taylor. 2007. "Adult Outcomes of Binge Drinking in Adolescence: Findings from a UK National Birth Cohort." *Journal of Epidemiology and Community Health* 61 (10): 902–7.

Wagenaar, A. C. 2003. "Research Affects Public Policy: The Case of the Legal Drinking Age in the US." *Addiction* 88 (s1): 75S–81S.

Walker, N., J. Bryce, and R. E. Black. 2007. "Interpreting Health Statistics for Policymaking: The Story behind the Headlines." *The Lancet* 369 (9565): 956–63.

Whiting, S. J., H. Vatanparast, A. Baxter-Jones, R. A. Faulkner, R. Mirwald, and others. 2004. "Factors That Affect Bone Mineral Accrual in the Adolescent Growth Spurt." *Journal of Nutrition* 134 (3): 696S–700S.

WHO (World Health Organization). 2000. "Global Strategy for the Prevention and Control of Noncommunicable Disease." (WHAA53/14). WHO, Geneva.

Wilson C. M., P. F. Wright, J. T. Safrit, and B. Rudy. 2010. "Epidemiology of HIV Infection and Risk in Adolescents and Youth." *Journal of Acquired Immune Deficiency Syndromes* 54 (Suppl 1): S5.

Yu, C., T. Teoh, and S. Robinson. 2006. "Obesity in Pregnancy." [Review Article.] *British Journal of Obstetrics and Gynaecology* 113 (10): 1117–25.

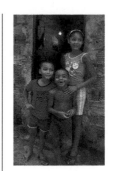

Chapter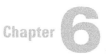

Impact of Interventions on Health and Development during Childhood and Adolescence: A Conceptual Framework

Donald A. P. Bundy and Susan Horton

This chapter provides a conceptual framework for exploring the processes and inputs that determine the physical, cognitive, and intellectual growth of human beings from birth to adulthood. This task is made particularly difficult by the absence of a holistic academic discipline that provides an overview of this critical phase in the human life course. It is also complicated by the curiously partial approach to studies in this area; much of the literature on child health ends when a child reaches age two years, while much of the literature on child education does not begin until a child reaches age five years. This significant mismatch in the literature reflects a similar lack of connection between the scale of public investment in primary education—one of the few public goods that attracts near-universal support—and the scale of investments in health and nutrition during middle childhood and adolescence.

Development during adolescence (ages 10–19 years) has received greater attention than the middle childhood years (ages 5–9 years; see, for example, Patton and others 2016). The unfortunate tendency to treat adolescence as separate from childhood has impeded efforts to enhance the understanding of the interrelationships between adolescence and earlier development and of the contribution of health and nutrition to the development of the next generation. Definitions of age groupings and age-specific terminology used in this volume can be found in chapter 1 (Bundy and others 2017).

The focus on the first 1,000 days—from the first day of pregnancy until age two years—has caused us to lose sight of the fact that child and adolescent growth and development are complex processes with multiple periods of sensitivity to intervention. Early intervention is undoubtedly critical to human development. However, the emphasis on the proposition that harm experienced in early life is irreversible not only is weakly supported by the evidence, but also has led to an unfortunate lack of emphasis on exploring important and relevant interventions later in childhood. Similarly, the declining rate of return on educational investments posited by Heckmann (2011) may need to be reconsidered following recent neurobiological research on brain development and a broader recognition of the complexity of intellectual skills, which extend well beyond numeracy and literacy.

INTERVENTIONS DURING MIDDLE CHILDHOOD AND ADOLESCENCE

Volume 2 of the third edition of *Disease Control Priorities, Reproductive, Maternal, Newborn, and Child Health* (Black and others 2016), explores evidence of the importance of maternal and young child health for subsequent child development. This chapter complements those findings by exploring evidence of the consequences of intervention at later points throughout the life course. This chapter places

Corresponding author: Donald A. P. Bundy, Bill & Melinda Gates Foundation, Seattle, Washington, United States; Donald.bundy@gatesfoundation.org.

particular emphasis on giving equivalent weight to the understanding of the role of interventions at all stages, from early childhood through middle years and adolescence. To provide a conceptual scaffolding, we developed figure 6.1 to assemble evidence of effects along the same age-specified life course.

Figure 6.1 illustrates the value of a perspective that extends beyond the first 1,000 days. Rates of physical growth are indeed the highest at younger than age two years, when nutrition is critical. However, the rates at the peak of the adolescent growth spurt for girls are similar to—and for boys exceed—the rates at age two years (figure 6.1, panel a). It has long been recognized

that stunting before age three years can be partially reversed by delayed maturation and a longer period of catch-up (Martorell, Khan, and Schroeder 1994), given the right circumstances. A review in chapter 8 in this volume (Watkins and others 2017) presents evidence for smaller, but potentially important, amounts of catch-up growth in older children before the onset of puberty. These data may mean that we need to be more careful about assuming that early insults are irreversible and pay more attention to what can be done for children in middle childhood. The scarcity of studies in this age group also may show the influence of unintended research bias on policy.

Figure 6.1 Human Development to Age 20 Years

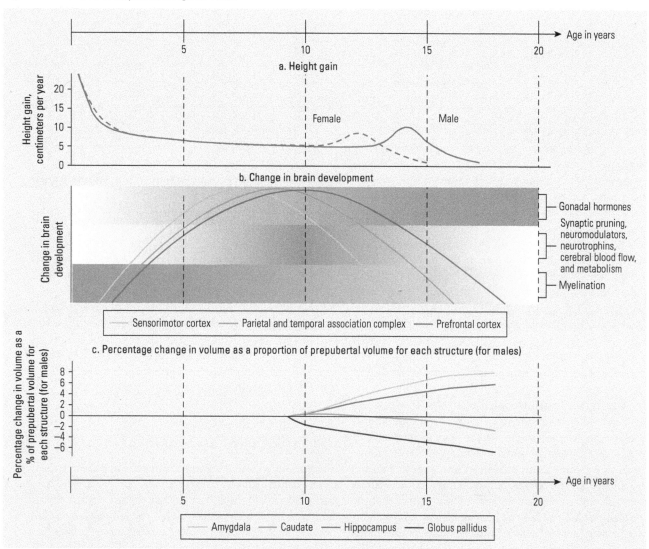

Sources: Panel a adapted from Tanner 1990; panel b adapted from Grigorenko 2017; panel c adapted from Goddings and others 2014.
Note: The vertical axis in panel b shows relative rate of growth of three brain areas from 0 to highest. The progressive shading indicates when the indicated activity is at its most intense (darkest shading). Behavioral attributes are paralleled by hormonal and neurobiological changes that target specific brain regions and cell populations (shown in shaded gray to capture the dynamic influences of hormones, various brain processes, and myelination).

Although the first 1,000 days are clearly a key period for brain development, evidence from neuroscience from the past 15 years has given us greater insight into the complexities of brain development. By age 6 years, the brain has reached approximately 95 percent of its adult volume; the volume of gray matter peaks about age 12 years in boys (figure 6.1, panel c) (Goddings and others 2014). For the brain, however, size is not everything. Connections within the brain are of greater importance to functioning than size. The process of myelination speeds up the processing of signals, and the process of synaptic pruning leads to strengthening of particular pathways. White matter in the brain, which reflects increased myelin, peaks in early adulthood. These processes of brain development also depend on individuals' interactions with their environments, which in turn stimulate their learning.

Different areas of the brain have different functions and develop at different rates. Peak development of the sensorimotor cortex, which is associated with vision, hearing, and motor control, occurs relatively early, and development is limited after puberty. The parietal and temporal association complex, responsible for language skills and numeracy, develops the fastest a little later; hence, the observation that by about age 14 years, although it is possible to learn new languages, it is more difficult to speak a new language in the same way as a native speaker (Dahl 2004). The prefrontal cortex develops later still; this is the area associated with higher brain functions, such as executive control (figure 6.1, panel b) (Grigorenko 2017).

It is possible to see some of these differential growth rates in brain capabilities in the relationship between the size of subcortical regions in figure 6.1, panel c. The figure plots size as a function of stage of puberty using Tanner's well-known five stages, which can be categorized as pre-, early, mid-, late, and postpuberty. The panel shows the pattern for adolescent boys; the patterns are similar for girls but occur at earlier ages because of different patterns of puberty. The panel shows that the size of those regions associated with movement (such as the caudate and globus pallidus) is shrinking during early adolescence because these functions are more mature. In contrast, regions associated with memory, decision making, and emotional reactions (amygdala and hippocampus) are still growing in adolescence.

The development of behaviors and social skills has long been recognized as age dependent, and it is now recognized that this development is closely related to neurological development. The subcortical regions are not fully developed at the point at which they reach maximum size; they require additional time to establish rapid processing and transmission of signals to other parts of the brain. The prefrontal cortex develops later still with maturation continuing into the third decade. This prolonged process helps explain why adolescence is a time of strong passions (Dahl 2004), impulsiveness (Casey, Jones, and Hare 2008), and risk taking (Casey, Jones, and Hare 2008; Steinberg 2007). The earlier development of brain regions associated with these behaviors outstrips the slower development of brain areas associated with control of impulses, delay of gratification, and regulation of emotions (Steinberg 2007). Accordingly, a focus on readily measurable cognitive function, as in much of the educational literature, ignores the more complex and later-developing brain functions that have important consequences for creativity, social functioning, and strategic thinking.

Figure 6.2 was developed to guide human development strategic policy and suggests how key health, nutritional, and educational interventions might be timed according to the different sensitivities at different ages. The figure also indicates the likely levels of school participation at different ages for low- and middle-income populations, showing how important the education sector can be for reaching children in middle childhood and adolescence, and presaging the discussion of delivery platforms in section 4 of this volume, which in turn underpins the discussion of various age- and stage-specific intervention packages discussed in section 5 of this volume.

IMPLICATIONS FOR PHASES OF DEVELOPMENT

Our current understanding of human development during the first two decades of life suggests that there is a series of phases, each of which is critical to development and each of which requires a different set of interventions to support development and sustain the gains of the previous phases. Table 6.1 attempts to represent this process by dividing the first 20 years of life into five phases of physical, behavioral, and emotional development.

The age ranges selected are indicative and simplified; at the population level the phases will each cover a broader range and they will overlap. Middle childhood arguably begins before age five years, but beginning at age five years helps alignment with formal education practice. Middle childhood is also not entirely separable from adolescence, and for many children incorporates an initial period of juvenility followed by the early beginnings of pubertal processes. Similarly, many of the health risks of middle childhood—especially around infectious disease—persist into early adolescence, so that during the adolescent growth spurt phase the school age and the adolescent packages are both relevant. Finally, the end point at age 20 years is a widely accepted marker of the transition from adolescence to adulthood, hence the social and legal importance of the

Figure 6.2 Indicative Rate of School Enrollment in Low- and Middle-Income Countries

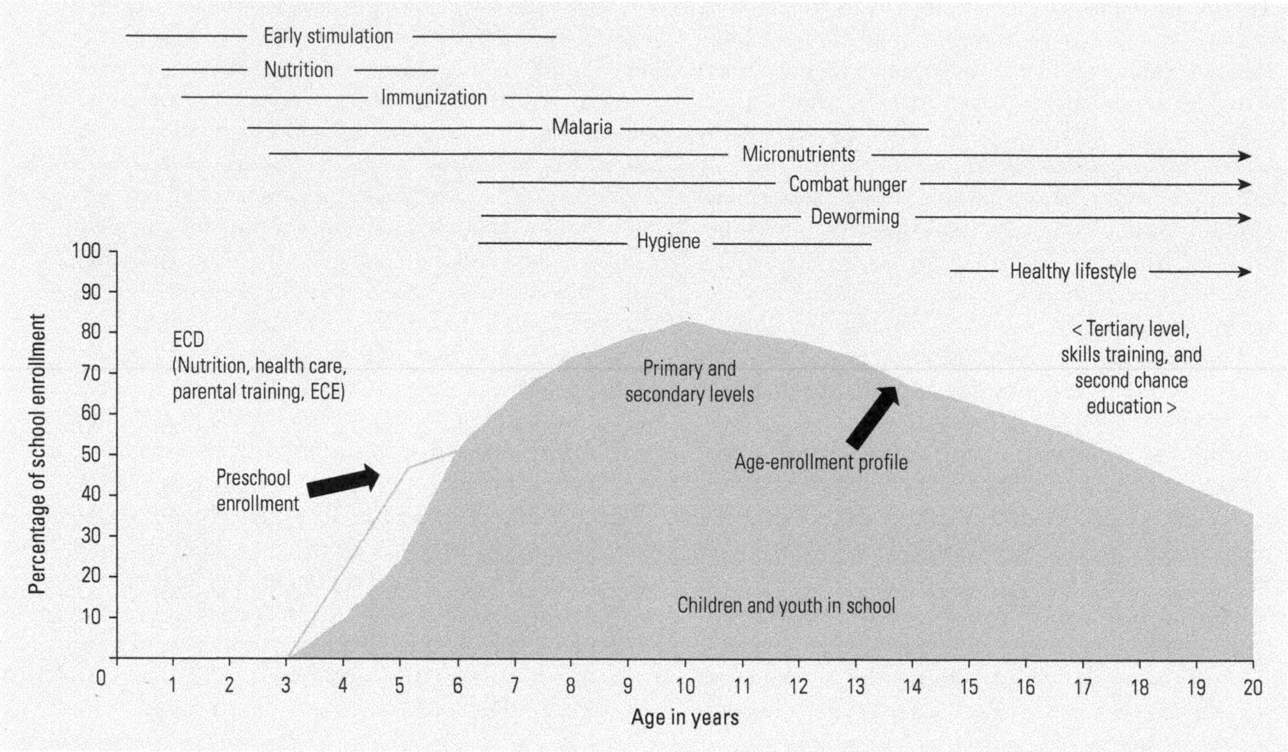

Source: Adapted from World Bank 2011.
Note: ECD = early childhood development; ECE = early childhood education.

Table 6.1 Key Phases of Child and Adolescent Health and Development

Phase	Period	Developmental importance	Examples of interventions	Packages
The First 1,000 Days	Ages 9 months to 2 years	The most rapid growth of body and brain; underpins all subsequent development; highest risk of mortality	Maternal, reproductive, newborn, child health (see volume 2); responsive stimulation	RMNCH (volume 2): Packages on maternal and newborn health and on child health
Middle Childhood Growth and Consolidation	Ages 5 to 9 years	Steady physical growth of body while sensorimotor brain function develops; nontrivial risk of death; some catch-up growth possible	Infection control, diet quality, and promotion of healthy behaviors and well-being	The school-age package
Adolescent Growth Spurt	Ages 10 to 14 years	Rapid physical growth, attaining growth velocities not seen since age 2 years, and rapid growth of centers for emotional development; main phase for remedial catch-up growth	Age-appropriate variants on above, plus vaccination, structured physical exercise, and promotion of healthy emotional development	The school-age and adolescent packages
Adolescent Growth and Consolidation	Ages 15 to 19 years	Consolidation of physical growth and especially of links in the brain; risk-taking behavior associated with socioemotional development; last chance for remedial growth in height	More focus on reproductive health, incentives to stay in school, protection from excessive risk taking, and early identification of mental health issues	The adolescent package

Note: RMNCH = Reproductive, Maternal, Newborn, and Child Health.

twenty-first birthday, but it is now recognized that significant late-stage adolescent changes continue through to the mid-twenties.

Table 6.1 also indicates the packages of interventions that can be developed to respond to the specific needs of each phase of development.

OVERVIEW OF SECTION 2 OF THIS VOLUME

The following chapters in this section expand on the this discussion of intervention and the life course and are based on the conceptual framework illustrated in figure 6.1.

- Chapter 7 in this volume (Alderman and others 2017) examines in more detail the timing of investments and provides equity arguments for investment in those children who were disadvantaged in the investments received before age five years.
- Chapter 8 in this volume (Watkins and others 2017) explores the issue of the irreversibility of early insult by asking whether catch-up is possible for children whose physical or cognitive growth has been limited in the first 1,000 days.
- Chapter 9 in this volume (Viner, Allen, and Patton 2017) explores age-specific adolescent development.
- Chapter 10 in this volume (Grigorenko 2017) provides a more detailed explication regarding brain development.

REFERENCES

Alderman, H., J. R. Behrman, P. Glewwe, L. Fernald, and S. Walker. 2017. "Evidence of Impact of Interventions on Growth and Development during Early and Middle Childhood." In *Disease Control Priorities* (third edition): Volume 8, *Child and Adolescent Health and Development*, edited by D. A. P. Bundy, N. de Silva, S. Horton, D. T. Jamison, and G. C. Patton. Washington, DC: World Bank.

Black, R., R. Laxminarayan, M. Temmerman, and N. Walker. 2016. *Reproductive, Maternal, Newborn, and Child Health*, volume 2 in *Disease Control Priorities* (third edition), edited by D. T. Jamison, R. Nugent, H. Gelband, S. Horton, P. Jha, R. Laxminarayan, and C. N. Mock. Washington, DC: World Bank.

Bundy, D. A. P., N. de Silva, S. Horton, G. C. Patton, L. Schultz, and D. T. Jamison. 2017. "Child and Adolescent Health and Development: Realizing Neglected Potential." In *Disease Control Priorities* (third edition): Volume 8, *Child and Adolescent Health and Development*, edited by D. A. P. Bundy, N. de Silva, S. Horton, D. T. Jamison, and G. C. Patton. Washington, DC: World Bank.

Casey, B. J., R. M. Jones, and T. A. Hare. 2008. "The Adolescent Brain." *Annals of the New York Academy of Sciences* 1124: 111–26.

Dahl, R. E. 2004. "Adolescent Brain Development: A Period of Vulnerabilities and Opportunities." Keynote Address. *Annals of the New York Academy of Sciences* 1021: 1–22.

Goddings, A.-L., K. L. Mills, L. S. Clasen, J. N. Giedd, R. M. Viner, and others. 2014. "The Influence of Puberty on Subcortical Brain Development." *NeuroImage* 88: 242–51.

Grigorenko, E. L. 2017. "Evidence on Brain Development and Interventions." In *Disease Control Priorities* (third edition): Volume 8, *Child and Adolescent Health and Development*, edited by D. A. P. Bundy, N. de Silva, S. Horton, D. T. Jamison, and G. C. Patton. Washington, DC: World Bank.

Heckmann, J. J. 2011. "Effective Child Development Strategies." In *The Pre-K Debates: Current Controversies and Issues*, edited by E. Zigler, W. S. Gilliam, and W. S. Barnett. Baltimore, MD: Paul H. Brookes Publishing.

Martorell, R., L. K. Khan, and D. G. Schroeder. 1994. "Reversibility of Stunting: Epidemiological Findings in Children from Developing Countries." *European Journal of Clinical Nutrition* 48: S45–57.

Patton, G. C., S. M. Sawyer, J. S. Santelli, D. A. Ross, R. Afifi, and others. 2016. "Our Future: A *Lancet* Commission on Adolescent Health and Well Being." *The Lancet* 387 (10036): 2423–78.

Steinberg, L. 2007. "Risk Taking in Adolescence: New Perspective from Brain and Behavioral Science." *Current Directions in Psychological Science* 16: 55–59.

Tanner, J. L. 1990. *Fetus into Man: Physical Growth from Conception to Maturity*. Cambridge, MA: Harvard University Press.

Viner, R. M., N. B. Allen, and G. C. Patton. 2017. "Puberty, Developmental Processes, and Health Interventions." In *Disease Control Priorities* (third edition): Volume 8, *Child and Adolescent Health and Development*, edited by D. A. P. Bundy, N. de Silva, S. Horton, D. T. Jamison, and G. C. Patton. Washington, DC: World Bank.

Watkins, K., D. A. P. Bundy, D. T. Jamison, G. Fink, and A. Georgiadis. 2017. "Evidence of Impact of Interventions on Health and Development during Middle Childhood and School Age." In *Disease Control Priorities* (third edition): Volume 8, *Child and Adolescent Health and Development*, edited by D. A. P. Bundy, N. de Silva, S. Horton, D. T. Jamison, and G. C. Patton. Washington, DC: World Bank.

World Bank. 2011. *World Bank Group Education Strategy 2020*. Washington, DC: World Bank.

Evidence of Impact of Interventions on Growth and Development during Early and Middle Childhood

Harold Alderman, Jere R. Behrman, Paul Glewwe, Lia Fernald, and Susan Walker

INTRODUCTION

Worldwide patterns of linear growth faltering, based on data from many low- and middle-income countries (LMICs) (Victora and others 2010), indicate deterioration of child nutritional status, on average, from age 0 to 24 months; after this period, nutritional status levels off or slightly reverses (for example, Prentice and others 2013; Stein and others 2010). Analyses of the five countries in the Consortium of Health-Orientated Research in Transitioning Societies (COHORTS) study found that low birth weight or undernutrition at age two years (or both) were associated with shorter adult height, less schooling, and lower economic productivity (Victora and others 2008). The 2008 *Lancet* series on nutrition argued that height-for-age is the best nutritional predictor of adult human capital (Victora and others 2008).

These results influenced prioritization of global efforts to combat undernutrition in the first 1,000 days, from conception to age 24 months. More broadly, these 1,000 days are seen as a critical period for establishing the physical, cognitive, and socioemotional foundation for later life (Walker, Wachs, and others 2011) and are viewed as the period of greatest plasticity (Gluckman and others 2009). As reviewed by Halfon and others (2014), new approaches to life course development have integrated biological systems, drawing from genetics as well as epigenetics, with social and behavioral models. The approach in this chapter unites economic theory with health science.

We use the lifecycle approach to assess the benefit-cost ratios of interventions in nutrition and child development in LMICs, where undernutrition is a risk factor, with a focus on the first five years of life. Definitions of age groupings and age-specific terminology used in this volume can be found in chapter 1 (Bundy and others 2017).

Birth weight and linear growth in the first two years are associated with many beneficial outcomes later in life (Adair and others 2013). The 2013 *Lancet* nutrition series also acknowledged the need to address both undernutrition and increased obesity in LMICs (Black and others 2013), recognizing that there is a high prevalence of both conditions and that the conditions often are linked. The 2013 series connected the importance of prenatal nutrition and adolescent girls' nutrition (Bhutta and others 2013). Women's height affects risks for pregnancy complications (Toh-Adam, Srisupundit, and Tongsong 2012) and low birth weight (Black and others 2013); given associations of birth weight with subsequent undernutrition (Christian and others 2013), these findings bring the discussion full circle. Thus, the 1,000-day window could be made much longer—even going back to mothers' childhoods.

Corresponding author: Harold Alderman, International Food Policy Research Institute, Washington, DC, United States; h.alderman@cgiar.org.

Children's early years are critically important for cognitive, language, and socioemotional development, and strong evidence indicates that the window of influence extends well beyond the first 1,000 days. Protective and risk factors for undernutrition are often similar to the factors influencing cognitive and socioemotional development (Walker, Wachs, and others 2011). For example, shared risk factors include intrauterine growth retardation, nutrient deficiencies, and social and economic conditions. Risks specific to poor cognitive development include inadequate learning opportunities and inadequate quality of caregiver-child interactions. Shared protective factors include breastfeeding and maternal education.

The overlapping risk factors, timing of peak vulnerabilities, and the possibility that early deficits have long-lasting impacts have motivated interest in interventions that integrate nutritional and other approaches to promote overall child development (Alderman and others 2014). Ideally, policies and programs must move from a focus on single issues to a wider-reaching, more integrated approach across the life course, which would allow for each child to develop as well as possible and mitigate the impact of constraints under which their development may be occurring (Fine and Kotelchuck 2010). Such integration, however, requires clearer understanding of individuals' developmental timing and age-dependent responses to external factors (Wachs and others 2014). Cognitive functions, receptive and expressive language, and socioemotional skills develop at different ages (Grantham-McGregor and others 2007). Development in brain structure and function supporting acquisition of cognitive, language, and socioemotional skills is most rapid during early childhood, with continued development in later years for many skills.

The early years, beginning in utero and extending to age 36 months, are the best stage in which to prevent stunting. The debate continues as to whether children who become stunted before age 24 months can catch up later in their lives. Population averages from cross-sectional data show some limited catch-up in height-for-age z scores, though average height deficits widen beyond age two years into adulthood (Leroy and others 2014; Lundeen and others 2014). Longitudinal studies report considerable individual movements in both directions between stunted and nonstunted status after age 24 months that are associated with family and community characteristics, suggesting potential for catch-up or prevention of faltering (Crookston and others 2013; Lundeen and others 2013; Mani 2012; Prentice and others 2013; Schott and others 2013). Catch-up may, however, have some risks; for example, weight gain on small frames has been associated with subsequent obesity and adult chronic diseases (Monteiro and Victora 2005; Yajnik 2004, 2009).

As with malnutrition, cognitive delays can occur throughout infancy, childhood, and adolescence, understood in this volume as birth through age 19 years. Measurable differences in receptive language by socioeconomic groups are apparent in preschool children ages three to five years (Paxson and Schady 2007; Schady and others 2015); differences in cognitive ability have been observed even in the first two years (Fernald and others 2012). Early life stress—often toxic if extreme—can also have difficult-to-reverse lifetime consequences (Shonkoff and Garner 2012). Individual responsiveness to interventions implemented after initial developmental insults are widely debated (see chapter 8 in this volume, Watkins and others 2017).

More than 3 million children younger than age five years died in 2011; half of these deaths were associated with fetal growth restriction, suboptimal breastfeeding, stunting, wasting, and vitamin A and zinc deficiencies (Black and others 2013). Given that about 75 percent of child deaths before age five years occur in the first year, addressing catch-up growth beyond the 1,000-day window is driven less by concern for mortality risk and more by concerns relating to later-life consequences for survivors.

Some evidence indicates that skill accumulation is more plastic than physical growth; skills such as executive function—a component of cognitive function—and socioemotional development have time paths different from those of conventional cognitive abilities (Borghans and others 2008). Still, very little is known about time paths of effective interventions for addressing nutritional, cognitive, and socioemotional development, particularly in LMICs. Maximum gains relative to costs, particularly for cognitive and socioemotional developmental outcomes, are likely to require early investment, followed by appropriate nutritional and educational investments and continued support for effective parent-child interaction over childhood and adolescence. Determining which later-life interventions cost-effectively reduce consequences of early malnutrition or cognitive delay is important if efforts at prevention fall short, as they already have for hundreds of millions of children.

LIFECYCLE FRAMEWORK FOR ASSESSMENT OF BENEFITS AND COSTS OF INTERVENTIONS TO SUPPORT CHILD DEVELOPMENT

The lifecycle framework highlights the age dimension for both outcomes and determinants of child and adolescent development. Figure 7.1 presents such a

Figure 7.1 Physical Growth and Other Developmental Outcomes within a Lifecycle Framework

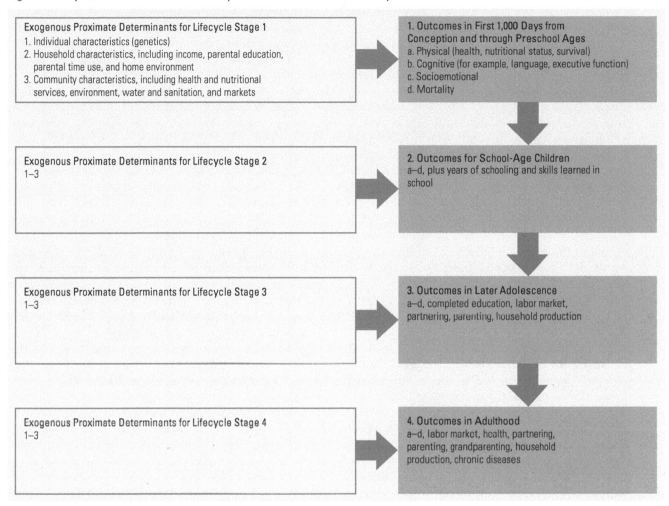

framework, with three formative stages extending from conception through childhood and adolescence, continuing to an adult stage.[1]

- Lifecycle Stage 1 from conception through preschool age
- Lifecycle Stage 2 primary and early secondary school ages
- Lifecycle Stage 3 late adolescence
- Lifecycle Stage 4 adulthood.

Individuals who survive each stage continue on to the next stage, as indicated by the green arrows in the figure (see also Nandi and others 2017, chapter 27 in this volume). The sections in this chapter and in chapter 8 (Watkins and others 2017) present evidence of opportunities for interventions in the first three lifecycle stages—preschool, school-age, and late adolescence—including evidence on costs, returns to investments, and implications for tradeoffs.

The lifecycle could be divided into fewer or more stages, but the pattern by which actions in one stage influence both outcomes in that period and in subsequent stages, either directly or indirectly, is generalizable. Moreover, the timing of exit from one stage and entry into the subsequent one is itself partially dependent on earlier outcomes and concurrent decisions; for example, entry into school depends in part on nutritional status (Alderman and others 2001; Glewwe, Jacoby, and King 2001); entry into the labor force depends on both physical stature and schooling achievement (Pitt, Rosenzweig, and Hasan 2012; Yamauchi 2008). Even transitions that are biological, such as menarche and the beginning and duration of the adolescent growth spurt, are partially dependent on earlier health outcomes and on behavioral and hormonal responses to cultural and environmental contexts.

Broadly speaking, the outcomes in each lifecycle stage can be classified into three categories: physical growth, cognitive development (including language, executive function, mathematics, and reasoning), and socioemotional development. The relevant outcomes of these categories vary at the different stages. The risk of early mortality is particularly relevant in the first stage; school attainment is most relevant in the second and third stages; and employment is most relevant in the third and fourth stages. Establishing priorities for investment or integrating mortality with other outcomes, such as improved development for survivors, is particularly challenging without a common metric. Most other outcomes can be assessed by measuring their financial value relative to their cost, but there is no consensus on how to make such an assessment for mortality. A wide range of estimates of the value of averted mortality have been proposed. These, however, range from the cost of the cheapest alternative for averting mortality to what compensating differentials individuals require to assume more risk, for example, based on wage tradeoffs (Summers 1992; Viscusi and Aldy 2003).

Usefulness of the Lifecycle Framework

A particular conceptual value of a lifecycle model is that it can illustrate how inputs in one stage influence outcomes in later stages. For example, higher stocks of health (or health skills) in one stage may create even higher health later. Cunha and Heckman (2007) term this process *self-productivity*. Similarly, the model can highlight cross-productivities in which better health in one stage increases cognitive skills in the same or subsequent stages. Cross-productivities may also occur if cognitive skills in one period enhance socioemotional skills in another (Helmers and Patnam 2011), or if dimensions of health in one period influence other developmental dimensions subsequently. The model also describes what Cunha and Heckman (2007) call *dynamic complementarities,* by which higher health or skills in one stage lead to greater returns to investments in subsequent stages.

Dynamic complementarities have important implications from an economic efficiency perspective: more investments should be targeted to those with better initial health and greater skills, although doing so would widen disparities as children age. This is not only a possible outcome of decisions by governments, but may also pertain to households' investments in siblings. Given dynamic complementarities, do households invest more in their children who have higher potential, or do they seek more equity and compensate by investing more in "less productive" children? However, whether dynamic complementarities predominate is an empirical issue—there may be dynamic substitution if investments in one period have a greater return when provided to children

with worse outcomes in the earlier period. Whether governments or households prefer strategies that reinforce earlier differentials, or whether they prefer to invest to compensate for disparities, is also an empirical question.

This framework also helps deepen our understanding of how short-term health shocks may affect future outcomes. If dynamic complementarities are strong, then moderate shocks to children's health in early life may lead to major differences in schooling and other later outcomes if nothing is done to compensate for these shocks. Similarly, self-productivity is consistent with long-term impacts of early-life nutritional deficits, morbidity, inadequate stimulation, and toxic stress (National Scientific Council on the Developing Child 2014).

To quantify the links in the framework illustrated in figure 7.1, the challenge imposed by the multiple proximate determinants of the outcomes of interest in each lifecycle stage must be addressed. With the rare exception of randomized controlled trials or transitory natural experiments that alter one of them, these determinants are likely to be highly correlated across different lifecycle stages. Accordingly, the causal effects of growth in one period on outcomes in subsequent stages may be overstated because this approach attributes to the previous stage the effect not only of growth in that stage on subsequent growth (the green arrow) but also the effects of correlated determinants across stages (the blue arrows).

Additionally, it is difficult to separate the physical, cognitive, and socioemotional dimensions of growth over the lifecycle. For example, to examine the impact of an investment in physical growth, either the investment has to affect only physical growth, or else other dimensions of child development need to be controlled. Randomized controlled trials or natural experiments directed only at physical growth with impacts measured over multiple lifecycle phases might permit such an assessment to be made, but such studies are rare. If observational data are used, and channels for the impacts of investment other than physical growth are not controlled for in the analysis, the impacts of physical growth are likely to be misrepresented because physical growth will almost certainly be positively correlated with impacts of the investment through other channels. Since one of those channels is cognitive development, for example, identifying the impacts of physical growth as distinct from the impacts of cognitive development is challenging.

Prioritization of Interventions

Prioritization of interventions involves an understanding of these causal impacts, as well as the costs of these interventions, in the context of LMICs. The costs of interventions include the total resource costs of changes in the boxes on the left-hand side of figure 7.1, where resource costs mean the use of resources for this intervention that have value in other uses. Many interventions have resource costs for both public sector providers and private individuals. If parents have to take their children to health clinics to receive interventions, resource costs are incurred in the form of transportation costs and the costs of the parents' time, in addition to the public resource costs of the clinic. In addition, there are likely to be distortion costs from raising funds to finance public expenditures; these distortion costs have been estimated to be approximately 25 percent of public expenditures (Devarajan, Squire, and Suthiwart-Narueput 1997). If only service provider costs are incorporated into the analyses, total resource costs are likely to be understated.

A further consideration related to costs may be the budget envelope, that is, the short-term constraint on available revenue or line item for a sector. Policy makers may perceive that the budget envelope constrains their choices so that, for example, increases to public sector expenditures on one item, such as preschool programs, must come at the expense of other items, such as primary school teacher salaries, even if the benefit-cost ratios of both options are considerably greater than one. The budgetary process imposes a constraint on their choices that, from their perspective, is an additional cost component. The impact of the budget envelope is particularly likely to affect new initiatives because endowment effects and vested interests may make it difficult to reduce public sector expenditures on items purchased in the past even if their benefit-cost ratios are smaller than those of proposed new interventions. Although the budget envelope does not represent real resource costs, it may be a real constraint on public sector choices, especially for new initiatives.

Policy makers who think they are constrained by budget envelopes have incentives to offload real program costs onto private entities, to the extent possible. For example, if new services are provided and a choice is made between expenditure of public sector funds to improve households' access to those services and higher private transportation costs to be borne by those households, the constraint imposed by budget envelopes creates incentives to choose the latter even if those costs are borne by very poor people. This last point is related to a more general distortion present in many policy discussions that wrongly equate public sector expenditures with real resource costs, ignoring the fact that important components of real resource costs may be private sector costs and that components of public sector expenditures such as transfers may not be real resource costs. Considerations such as budget envelopes and endowment effects should not be confused with real resource costs, even though they may have implications for real resource costs.

In addition, because of the interest in longer-term impacts, it is important to recognize that the timing of both impacts and costs matters if there is an advantage to obtaining returns earlier rather than later because the returns can be reinvested to generate further returns. This is particularly important if early-life interventions have impacts decades later through their effects on adult productivity and chronic diseases. In this context, the intertemporal discount rate used may make a considerable difference. Hoddinott, Alderman, and others (2013) provide a scenario in which the benefit-cost ratio for reducing stunting in Bangladesh is 17.9 with a 3 percent discount rate, but this ratio declines to 8.9 with a 5 percent discount rate, and 3.3 with an 8 percent discount rate.

Finally, the framework in figure 7.1 is context dependent. Resources, environments, policies, cultures, and markets are likely to vary considerably, and careful assessment is needed within the particular context for which an intervention is being considered.

QUANTIFYING THE MODEL: ILLUSTRATIONS OF BENEFIT-COST RATIOS AND RELATIVE RATES OF RETURN FOR INTERVENTIONS FOR DIFFERENT AGES IN A LIFECYCLE FRAMEWORK

The benefits and costs or, equivalently, internal rates of return from interventions are needed to guide decisions about choices among different interventions to mitigate inadequate child development versus other possible interventions. We illustrate some dimensions of benefit-cost ratios with an example of interventions to prevent or reduce inadequate physical growth early in the preschool stage of the lifecycle, and then we discuss a well-known stylized characterization of relative rates of return to investments over the lifecycle.

Benefits over the Lifecycle: An Illustration

On the benefit side, including all the important impacts is critical—which means that different types of benefits need to be expressed in the same terms—as is accountng for the fact that some impacts may be realized only years after the intervention and need to be discounted to the present to obtain present discounted values (PDVs). Table 7.1 illustrates moving one child out of low–birth weight (LBW) status in a low-income country, based on the best estimates of causal links over the lifecycle. The major impacts include three from the

Table 7.1 Estimates of Present Discounted Values of Seven Major Impacts of Moving One Infant Out of Low–Birth Weight Status in a Low-Income Country

Impacts	Present Discounted Value (2004 US$)		
	3% annual discount rate	5% annual discount rate	10% annual discount rate
Reduced infant mortality	95	99	89
Reduced neonatal care	42	42	42
Reduced costs of infant and child illness	36	35	34
Productivity gain directly from increased adult height	152	85	25
Productivity gain from increased schooling and cognitive ability	367	205	60
Reduced costs of chronic diseases	49	15	1
Intergenerational effects	92	35	6
Total benefits	832	516	257

Source: Based on Alderman and Behrman 2006.

preschool lifecycle stage and four from the adult lifecycle stage. The adult stage includes the productivity impacts that encompass intermediate effects through channels such as schooling without double-counting; for example, the productivity gains from increasing adult height must be additional to those from increasing cognitive skills (Alderman and Sahn 2016). All of the impacts have been put into the same terms (U.S. dollars), with the most contestable value being that for averted mortality in the preschool stage, for which case the cost of vaccinations, the cheapest alternative means of averting mortality, was used (Summers 1992). The PDVs of total benefits vary a fair amount with the discount rates because of the gains from being able to reinvest returns that are realized sooner rather than later and are half as large using a 10 percent discount rate than when using a 5 percent rate, and are 39 percent smaller using a 5 percent discount rate than when using a 3 percent rate.

The estimated impacts shown in the table are primarily from productivity gains with 3 percent and 5 percent discount rates (62 percent and 57 percent of the total benefits, respectively). Productivity gains remain a substantial part of the total (33 percent), even with the 10 percent discount rate, because these gains are realized each year during the working lives of surviving adults. If these economic productivity gains were ignored by focusing only on direct health impacts, overall benefits would be substantially underestimated.

Finally, even though the early-life origins of chronic diseases have received increasing attention in recent decades, the estimated PDV of gains from this source are relatively small—5.9 percent of the total benefits with a 3 percent discount rate, 2.9 percent with a 5 percent

discount rate, and 0.4 percent with a 10 percent discount rate—because the impacts (assumed equal to a decade of income) are obtained late in the lifecycle and so are discounted considerably to obtain their present values.

The relevant costs include the intervention-provider resource costs, the private resource costs, and the distortion costs of using taxes to fund public expenditures on the program. The total resource costs are not the same as public budget expenditures, which ignore private and distortion costs and tend to underestimate the resource costs; they also can include considerable transfers, such as in-kind transfer or conditional cash transfer programs and so might overstate resource costs.

Benefit-cost ratios are the PDV of benefits divided by the PDV of costs. If the ratio exceeds 1.0, then the expected PDV of benefits exceeds the PDV of costs, and the intervention is warranted. Because both the benefits and the costs tend to vary substantially by context, the benefit-cost ratios related to the impacts in table 7.1 are likely to vary greatly across LMICs. An alternative means of summarizing such information is the internal rate of return, which is defined as the discount rate that makes the benefit-cost ratio exactly equal to one.

Relative Rates of Return to Human Capital Investments over the Lifecycle

A well-known example of relative rates of return to investments in skills formation over the lifecycle is described by Cunha, Lochner, and Masterov (2006), who found declining rates of return to age-specific investments in human capital as a child's age increases. Accordingly, investments before birth appear to have higher returns than investments in the first two years of life, which appear to have higher returns than preschool programs directed toward children ages three to five years. These, in turn, appear to have higher returns than additional years of schooling, which also have higher returns than postschooling job training. A key implication is that interventions should be concentrated early in life, when the highest overall returns are obtained, until reaching a point at which diminishing marginal rates of return make investments later in life relatively more productive. Current human capital investment levels may yield declining rates of return, but optimal investments would yield equal rates of return for all age levels.

The stylized returns of Cunha, Lochner, and Masterov (2006) and the myriad discussions the returns have engendered raise the question, why do the rates of return differ so much by age? If private rates of return are so high for early-life investments, why do families not take immediate advantage of such high-return opportunities? Is it because of lack of knowledge or credit market constraints? Perhaps private rates of return are not as high as social rates of return because of positive externalities. If so, then another set of questions arises: Why does public investment not follow? Is it lack of knowledge, high discount rates for policy makers because of political cycles, the combination of the budget envelope and endowment effects, or a concern that the evidence is too thin or is based on studies from distant countries? Again, understanding why the age pattern of rates of return exists, as well as clarifying the extent to which they differ from private and social perspectives, would be very useful for developing effective policy responses, such as whether emphasis should be placed on enhancing information, improving capital markets, subsidizing providers of services relevant to early-life development, increasing the direct public provision of services relevant to early-childhood development, empowering mothers, or other possibilities.

Many presume that such age patterns of rates of return to investments in human skills prevail in many LMICs. There does seem to be some support for relatively high rates of return on investing in nutrition and stimulation during the first 1,000 days of life (Gertler and others 2014; Hoddinott and others 2008; Hoddinott, Alderman, and others 2013; Hoddinott, Behrman, and others 2013), as well as for investing in preschool programs across a number of countries for children ages three to five years (Engle and others 2011) in some settings. Nevertheless, the age pattern of rates of return is much less well documented for most LMICs than for the United States. For example, it would be desirable to be able to base policy recommendations for other LMICs on more extensive information than on the available

very careful analysis of a few small special samples from Guatemala, Jamaica, and the United States, or on analyses of cross-country data such as in Engle and others (2011). The available evidence is insufficient to indicate a wide range of possible heterogeneous investments. This concern pertains to average returns across subpopulations as well as any complementarities of inputs and the possibility that the return to an investment in one stage depends on investments in previous stages.

Benefit-Cost Ratios for Investments in Nutrition

We document the recent prevalence of nutritional deficits to establish that they are major problems and turn to estimated benefit-cost ratios of interventions designed to reduce some of these deficits.

Table 7.2 gives the prevalence, by world region, of key indicators of preschool-age malnutrition based on the most recent data available from the United Nations Children's Fund before the February 2014 conference for the third edition of *Disease Control Priorities*: low birth weight; whether exclusively breastfed for the first six months of life; and, for children younger than age five years, moderate and severe underweight, severe underweight, wasting defined as weight-for-height, overweight or obese, and stunting. Although availability of data on these indicators has improved considerably in recent decades, substantial data problems remain that are discussed in the original sources. For example, China is not included in the East Asia and Pacific and World aggregates for the last five indicators (although we have included values for China for other indicators when available), and coverage in some cases is otherwise limited. Table 7.3 gives further estimates and projections, from 1990 to 2020 and by major region, of the prevalence—and number of children affected (in millions)—of overweight/obesity and stunting among children younger than age five years.

Low Birth Weight

Low–birth weight (LBW) babies (less than 2,500 grams) face a greater risk of dying in their early months and years compared with normal birth weight babies; if LBW babies survive, they have greater risks of cognitive disabilities, impaired immune function, diabetes, and heart disease later in life (UNICEF 2006b, n.d.; UNICEF and WHO 2004). The prevalence of LBW varies considerably across regions: South Asia's rate of 27 percent is almost twice the rate in Sub-Saharan Africa (15 percent), which is the region with the second-highest rate. Approximately 19.5 million LBW babies are born annually, half of whom are born in only three countries: India (38.0 percent), Pakistan (7.7 percent), and

Table 7.2 Children's Nutritional Status in Major World Regions, Most Recent Available Data

Region or subregion	Low birth weight (< 2,500 grams, %)	Exclusive breastfeeding of children for first 6 months (%)	Children Younger than Age Five Years				
			Underweight (moderate and severe, %)[a]	Underweight (severe, %)	Wasting (moderate and severe, %)[a]	Overweight/ obese (%)[a]	Stunting (moderate and severe, %)[a]
Sub-Saharan Africa	15	—	21	7	9	7	40
East and Southern Africa	14	41	18	5	7	5	40
West and Central Africa	15	20	23	8	12	9	39
Middle East and North Africa	12	29	8	—	9	12	20
South Asia	27	38	33	14	16	3	39
East Asia and Pacific[b]	6	43	6	4	4	5	12
China	3	—	4	—	2	7	10
Latin America and the Caribbean	9	—	3	—	2	7	12
Central and Eastern Europe/Commonwealth of Independent States	6	22	2	—	1	16	12
High-income countries	7	—	2	—	2	15	7
Least developed countries	17	—	23	7	10	4	38
World[b]	14	—	16	10	8	7	26

Sources: For low birth weight, http://www.childinfo.org/low_birthweight_profiles.php; for exclusive breastfeeding, http://www.unicef.org/progressforchildren/2006n4/index_breastfeeding.html; all others, http://www.childinfo.org/malnutrition_nutritional_status.php A1. (All accessed January 11, 2014; all last updated February 2013.)

Note: — = not available.

a. Regional averages for underweight (moderate and severe), wasting (moderate and severe), overweight/obese, and stunting (moderate and severe) are estimated using statistical modeling of data from the UNICEF and WHO Joint Global Nutrition Database, 2011 revision (completed July 2012). The severe underweight indicator was not included in this exercise; regional averages for this indicator are based on population-weighted averages calculated by UNICEF. "Moderate" ("severe") is defined as more than 2 (3) standard deviations from the age-gender-specific reference median (below the medians except for overweight/obese).

b. Data exclude China for last five columns (children younger than age five years).

Nigeria (3.9 percent) (UNICEF 2013). Trend analysis is complicated by the lack of comparable estimates over time, both within and among countries. A population-weighted average for available surveys shows that the incidence of LBW remained unchanged from the 1990s to 2010 for both Sub-Saharan Africa and Asia (UNICEF 2013).

Breastfeeding

Exclusive breastfeeding in the first six months of life stimulates babies' immune systems, protects them from diarrhea and acute respiratory infections—two of the major causes of infant mortality in LMICs—and improves their responses to vaccination (UNICEF 2006a). Particularly in unhygienic conditions, breast milk substitutes carry high risks of infection that can be fatal for infants. Yet only slightly more than one-third of all infants in LMICs are exclusively breastfed for the first

six months of life. There is a fair amount of variation in the prevalence of breastfeeding, from 20 percent and 22 percent, respectively, in West and Central Africa and Central and Eastern Europe to 38 percent to 43 percent in South Asia, East and Southern Africa, and East Asia and Pacific.

Underweight

Globally, 16 percent of children younger than age five years are moderately or severely underweight. The high prevalence of moderate and severe underweight of 33 percent (14 percent for severe) in South Asia stands out in comparison with other regions; Sub-Saharan Africa (with West and Central Africa a little higher) is next, with 21 percent. All other regions have prevalence of less than 10 percent; the lowest is 2 percent to 3 percent for Central and Eastern Europe/Commonwealth of Independent States and Latin America and the Caribbean.

Table 7.3 Estimated Prevalence and Number of Children (Millions) Younger than Age Five Years Who Are Overweight/Obese or Stunted in Major Regions, 1990–2020

	Overweight/Obese				Stunted			
	1990	2000	2010	2020	1990	2000	2010	2020
Prevalence (%)								
Africa	4.0	5.7	8.5	12.7	40.3	39.3	38.2	37.1
Asia	3.2	3.7	4.9	6.8	48.6	37.7	27.6	19.0
Southern and Central Asia	2.3	2.9	3.5	4.3	60.7	48.4	36.4	25.9
LAC	6.8	6.8	6.9	7.2	23.7	18.1	13.5	10.0
All developing countries	3.7	4.5	6.1	8.6	44.4	36.1	29.2	23.7
Global	4.2	5.1	6.7	9.1	39.7	32.9	26.7	21.6
Children younger than age five years (millions)								
Africa	4.5	7.4	13.3	22.0	44.9	51.3	60.0	64.1
Asia	12.4	13.7	17.7	24.3	189.9	138.0	99.5	68.4
Southern and Central Asia	4.2	5.4	6.6	8.0	110.1	90.9	69.0	48.4
LAC	3.8	3.8	3.7	3.5	13.2	10.2	7.2	4.9
All developing countries	20.7	25.0	34.7	49.9	248.4	199.9	167.2	137.9
Global	26.9	31.4	42.8	59.4	253.0	203.8	171.4	142.0

Sources: de Onis, Blössner, and Borghi 2010, 2011.
Note: LAC = Latin America and the Caribbean. Overweight/obese is defined as > 2 standard deviations from weight-for-height median. Stunting is defined as more than two standard deviations below the height-for-age median.

Wasting

Children who suffer from wasting are at substantially increased risk of severe acute malnutrition and death. Globally, 8 percent of children suffer from wasting. South Asia has the highest prevalence of wasting (16 percent), and the highest prevalence of underweight (33 percent). Sub-Saharan Africa has 9 percent prevalence of wasting, the second-highest rate.

Obesity

Increasing trends in child overweight/obesity have occurred in the past two decades in most regions. Globally, an estimated 42.8 million (7 percent) of children younger than age five years were overweight or obese in 2010, a 59 percent increase from an estimated 26.9 million in 1990. Projections are for a further increase of 39 percent from 2010 to 59.4 million in 2020, of which 49.9 million are projected to be in LMICs. Latin America and the Caribbean had the highest prevalence in 1990, at 6.8 percent, which increased slowly to 6.9 percent in 2010 and is projected to be 7.2 percent in 2020. Other LMIC regions had much more rapid increases in the past two decades; Sub-Saharan Africa was notable because of the increase from 4.0 percent in 1990 to 8.5 percent in 2010, projected to be 12.7 percent in 2020. Throughout the period 1990–2020, Southern and Central Asia has the lowest prevalence, but still has substantial increases from 4.2 million in 1990 to 8.0 million projected for 2020.

Stunting

Globally, 26.7 percent of children younger than age five years were stunted in 2010, an estimated 171.4 million children. Southern and Central Asia and Sub-Saharan Africa have particularly high prevalence rates of between 36 percent and 38 percent. However, although prevalence in these two regions is similar for 2010, the trends are different. For Sub-Saharan Africa, the prevalence of 40.3 percent in 1990 (44.9 million children) declined very slowly to 38.2 percent in 2010, and it is projected to be 37.1 percent by 2020 (64.1 million). In contrast, in Southern and Central Asia, the prevalence in 1990 was much higher at 60.7 percent, an estimated 110.1 million stunted children, yet the rate dropped to 36.4 percent (69 million) in 2010; it is projected to be 25.9 percent (48.4 million) in 2020.

Benefit-Cost Estimates for Nutritional Interventions

Some consensus exists on the benefits of specific nutritional interventions. Often using meta-analyses of controlled trials, reviews such as Bhutta and others (2013) indicate the expected changes in outcomes of stunting or anemia for a given intervention. A body of evidence exists on the costs for achieving such outcomes (Horton and others 2010). These costs, as well as the expected outcomes, can be combined to calculate the relative cost-effectiveness of approaches to achieving a desired improvement in nutrition. However, to estimate a benefit-cost ratio, one needs to convert the multiple relevant outcomes into the same metric as the costs. As indicated in the example in table 7.1, doing so usually involves summing over different outcomes. Some of these, such as a reduction in resources used to care for illness, can be directly assessed in monetary terms. Others, such as increased labor productivity, require estimates of the degree to which the change in nutritional status leads to an increase in earnings, as well as assumptions about the productivity of those not in wage jobs. Most such estimates are based on indirect inference—the changes in schooling or learning attributable to improved nutrition combined with the impact that such increases in learning will have on earnings, often derived from separate studies.

One study, however, has been able to track individuals from the time they participated in a community-randomized program of supplemental feeding when they were infants and toddlers to their adult years about 35 years later (Hoddinott and others 2008; Hoddinott, Behrman, and others 2013). This study found that men who had received better (protein-enriched, higher energy) supplements before age three years earned, on average, 44 percent higher wage rates later in life; this

finding confirms that the body of indirect estimates of returns to nutrition programs based on changes in schooling or cognitive ability discussed in the following sections is in keeping with direct longitudinal evidence.

Table 7.4 lists some estimated benefit-cost ratios for nutritional interventions for preschool children based on Behrman, Alderman, and Hoddinott (2004). The benefits are calculated along the lines of those in table 7.1. Details, including the cost assumptions, are given in the original source, as are some sensitivity analyses (including varying the discount rate between 3 percent and 5 percent) that result in a range of estimates. These interventions can be divided into three groups according to the aim:

- Reduce LBW
- Directly improve infant and child nutrition
- Reduce micronutrient deficiencies.

For each group, estimates are provided for three interventions. Some points to note concerning this table are the following: the benefit-cost ratios are sensitive to the underlying assumptions, so some of the ranges are large; the benefit-cost ratios vary a fair amount within each group, for example, 0.58–35.20 for reducing LBW; and many of these benefit-cost estimates are substantially greater than 1.0, suggesting that even if there is some further discounting to account for uncertainty in such estimates, a number of these interventions merit serious consideration in contexts in which the nutritional deficiencies they are intended to address are prevalent. Table 7.5 provides similar results using different discount rates.

Table 7.4 Benefit-Cost Estimates for Nutritional Interventions for Preschool Children with Discount Rates of 3 Percent to 5 Percent

	Benefit-cost ratio
1. Reducing LBW for pregnancies with high probabilities of LBW	
1a. Treatments for women with asymptomatic bacterial infections	0.6–5.0
1b. Treatment for women with presumptive STD	1.3–10.7
1c. Drugs for pregnant women with poor obstetric history	4.1–35.2
2. Improving infant and child nutrition in populations with high prevalence of child malnutrition	
2a. Breastfeeding promotion in hospitals in which norm has been promotion of use of infant formula	5.6–67.1
2b. Integrated child care programs	9.4–16.2
2c. Intensive preschool program with considerable nutrition for poor families	1.4–2.9
3. Reducing micronutrient deficiencies	
3a. Iodine (per woman of childbearing age)	15.0–520.0
3b. Vitamin A (per child younger than age six years)	4.3–43.0
3c. Iron (pregnant women)	6.1–14.0

Source: Based on Behrman, Alderman, and Hoddinott 2004.
Note: LBW = low birth weight; STD = sexually transmitted disease.

Table 7.5 Sensitivity of Nutritional Intervention Benefit-Cost Ratios to Different Discount Rates and Values of Disability-Adjusted Life Years

Intervention	Discount rate 3%; DALY value of US$1,000	Discount rate 6%; DALY value of US$1,000	Discount rate 3%; DALY value of US$5,000	Discount rate 6%; DALY value of US$5,000
Community nutrition education and promotion	12.5	7.5	62.5	37.5
Vitamin A and zinc supplementation	17.3	10.0	86.5	52.0
Salt iodization	30.0	12.0	30.0	12.0
Iron fortification	8.0	7.0	8.0	7.0
Anthelmintics at preschool	6.0	2.4	6.0	2.4

Source: Based on Horton, Alderman, and Rivera 2009.
Note: DALY = disability-adjusted life year.

Additional estimates of benefit-cost ratios for nutrition interventions in the first 1,000 days that increase preschool linear growth (height) are provided in table 7.6. These ratios are based on recent estimates by Hoddinott, Alderman, and others (2013). On the cost side, Hoddinott, Alderman, and others (2013) provide two sets of estimates of budgetary costs per child—as opposed to costs compiled from ingredients or inputs—to provide 10 evidence-based interventions to reduce stunting and micronutrient deficiencies in children in their first two years of life. On the benefit side, Hoddinott, Alderman, and others (2013) first multiplied the point estimate of the increase in per capita permanent income (consumption) from reducing stunting by 0.20 in recognition of the estimate by Bhutta and others (2013) that this package of interventions will reduce stunting by 20 percent and then assumed that only 90 percent of these income gains are realized.

The first data column in the table reproduces the resulting benefit-to-budgetary-costs ratios using the generally higher cost estimates based on Bhutta and others (2013). However, the procedures in this particular approach underestimate benefits because they include only income or consumption benefits (and not, for example, benefits from averting mortality and resource costs saved as a result of reduced morbidity), and they underestimate resource costs because they do not include private costs and market distortion costs, in particular, the cost of raising revenue to finance the intervention. They also do not exclude the transfer component of public expenditures and so may overstate public sector resource costs; however, for the interventions considered, these transfer components probably are relatively small. Therefore, the second data column includes adjustments to benefits—an increase of 20 percent to represent social benefits beyond increases in income—as well as an increase in costs of 50 percent

to represent private costs and another 25 percent to represent distortion costs. The resulting benefit-cost ratios make interventions to reduce stunting still appear to be an attractive investment given that all the estimates are greater than 1.0, and all except the Democratic Republic of Congo are greater than 6.0, with a median of 12.4 (the estimate for the median country, Bangladesh). The range of estimates also is considerable, from 2.4 for the Democratic Republic of Congo to 33.1 for Indonesia, suggesting that context is important for evaluating such interventions.

A generic concern for these estimates is that the underlying data are often from small-scale studies. Both benefits and costs are likely to change as programs scale up (Alderman, Behrman, and Puett 2017; Menon and others 2014); benefits for hard-to-reach subpopulations may be higher or lower than for the general population, but costs are more likely to increase as programs expand coverage. This is a generic concern, but it is more likely to affect more personnel-intensive programs, such as counseling, relative to micronutrient fortification or supplementation. This is also a concern for most, although not all, estimates of returns to stimulation and preschool.

Benefit-Cost Ratios for Investment in Early Childhood Cognitive and Socioemotional Development

Overview of Programs and Interventions

Disparities in children's development emerge early and are driven by risks associated with poverty that include inadequate nutrition, low maternal education, lack of stimulation, and low levels of maternal well-being. As exposure to risks increases, both in number and duration, low-income children fall further behind more advantaged groups. Without appropriate investments from both their families and the state, children do not

Table 7.6 Benefit-Cost Ratios for Moving Child from Stunting at 24 Months to Not Stunted, in 17 Selected Heavily Burdened Countries

Region	Country	Ratio of income benefit to budgetary cost (Hoddinott, Alderman, and others 2013)	Adjusted benefit-cost ratio[a]
Sub-Saharan Africa	Congo, Dem. Rep.	3.5	2.4
	Madagascar	9.8	6.8
	Ethiopia	10.6	7.3
	Uganda	13.0	9.0
	Tanzania	14.6	10.1
	Kenya	15.2	10.5
	Sudan	23.0	15.9
	Nigeria	24.4	16.9
Middle East and North Africa	Yemen, Rep.	28.6	19.8
South Asia	Nepal	12.9	8.9
	Myanmar	17.2	11.9
	Bangladesh	17.9	12.4
	Pakistan	28.9	20.0
	India	38.6	26.8
East Asia	Vietnam	35.3	24.5
	Philippines	43.8	30.4
	Indonesia	47.7	33.1

Sources: Based on estimates from Hoddinott, Alderman, and others (2013), with cost and intervention data from Bhutta and others (2013).

a. Adjustments include increasing benefits by 20 percent to represent nonincome consumption benefits and increasing costs by 50 percent to represent private costs and by 25 percent to represent distortion costs.

acquire the skills needed to benefit fully from formal education when they enter primary school. Lower ability at school entry is associated with lower achievement and increased drop out (Grantham-McGregor and others 2007), leading to continuing and, in some cases, widening inequality, as well as forgone productivity.

The range of programs to improve child cognitive development in LMICs during the period between birth and the initiation of primary schooling is reviewed in Engle and others (2007) and in Engle and others (2011) and includes programs to promote better parenting and mother-child interaction through home visits by community health workers or by means of group sessions with mothers. Consistent evidence from several countries indicates that interventions that improve parent-child interaction and stimulation benefit children's development; the most current evidence is from interventions delivered through home visits by trained community health workers (Attanasio and others 2014; Hamadani and others 2006; Powell and others 2004; Yousafzai and others 2014). Some evidence indicates that these early interventions have sustained benefits for cognitive ability and behavior

around the age of school entry (Grantham-McGregor and others 1997; Walker and others 2010) and adulthood (Gertler and others 2014; Walker, Chang, and others 2011). Evidence for benefits from other approaches to delivering parenting support, such as through community groups, is also emerging (Singla, Kumbakumba, and Aboud 2015). Center-based approaches, for example, community day care, have been implemented, particularly in Latin America and the Caribbean, with variable benefits depending on program quality (Grantham-McGregor and others 2014). There is, however, a lack of information to guide successful scale-up, including resources required, and more analysis of the implementation process as promising programs are expanded is particularly urgent.

A subset of interventions that enhance child stimulation also provides nutritional supplements, often targeted to children who were born with low birth weights or were stunted. These interventions generally led to improvements in cognitive outcomes and socioemotional development, and sometimes in nutritional outcomes. There is, however, little evidence of synergy between stimulation and nutrition interventions in their outcomes (Grantham-McGregor and others 2014) in the small-scale programs that have been extensively studied, but combining these two types of interventions does not reduce the expected impact of either intervention when delivered independently. There may be synergies in costs if there are economies of scope because some common infrastructure can support both interventions.

Attendance at preschool for children ages three to six years increases development and readiness for formal schooling (Engle and others 2011). The proportions of children in the appropriate age range enrolled vary widely, with an average of 17 percent of children enrolled in low-income countries and 54 percent in middle-income countries (UNESCO 2014). Within regions and countries, lower-income children are less likely to be enrolled (Engle and others 2011). In addition to the need for increased access is a need for investment in improving quality, with improvements in structure (for example, infrastructure, class size) and process (for example, quality of caregiver-child interaction, developmentally appropriate activities); evidence suggests that improvement in process is more critical (Berlinski and Schady 2015).

Rates of Return to Preschool and Early Child Development Programs

Jamaica. An important and influential longitudinal study from Kingston, Jamaica, tracked a cohort of 129 stunted children since they were ages 9–24 months for more than 20 years; the children were initially randomly assigned to four different groups, three of which involved interventions that lasted two years.

- The first group received weekly one-hour home visits from community health workers, who taught parenting skills and encouraged mothers to interact and play with their children in ways that would develop their children's cognitive and socioemotional skills.
- The second group received weekly nutritional supplements of 1 kilogram of a milk-based formula.
- The third group received both home visits and nutritional supplements.
- The fourth group (the control group) received neither.

Gertler and others (2014) directly assessed the impact of these interventions on young adult earnings. Although the children in the home visit stimulation treatment arms were stunted at the time of recruitment into the study, they were able to close the wage gap with a matched nonstunted comparison group. More specifically, the analysis attributed a 25 percent increase in earnings to the stimulation interventions; in contrast, the nutritional arm of the intervention did not close the earnings gap. The authors contend that this increase due

to stimulation was larger than that reported in the few similar interventions from the United States. Although the research design was not set up to assess the relative value of cognitive and socioemotional gains, measures on both of these dimensions of development were improved in the intervention. In addition to the earnings benefit, the intervention also reduced violent behavior (Walker, Chang, and others 2011) and so provided a social benefit, which is not often measured in rates of return.

Turkey. Another long-term panel following an early child development intervention in Turkey looked at the beneficiaries of an intervention in which parents were provided training to improve the home learning environment for their children (Kaytaz 2005). The benefit-cost estimates reported in this study when parental training was center based were 4.3 and 6.4, using plausible discount rates of 10 percent and 6 percent, respectively. The benefit-cost estimates for the home-based parental training using the same discount rates of 10 percent and 6 percent were 5.9 and 8.7, respectively. These benefits are based on the increase in schooling and reduced dropout rates and the expected increase of earnings that can be inferred from these changes in levels of schooling; the earnings of the beneficiaries were not collected. These estimates do not include any increased learning per year of school, and, as Kaytaz (2005) indicates, the benefits are lower-bound estimates.

Bolivia. Behrman, Cheng, and Todd (2004) analyze the impacts of Bolivia's Proyecto Integral de Desarrollo Infantil. The program, which provided feeding as well as day care to groups of up to 15 children in the homes of women in low-income neighborhoods, achieved improvements in measures of language and auditory development, psychosocial skills, gross motor development, and fine motor development, but not in height or weight. Using estimates of the expected increase of schooling that these improvements are assumed to translate into, as well as estimates of the returns to schooling of children in the country, the benefit-cost ratio ranges between 2.0 and 2.9 for children for whom the increase of schooling would be at the intermediate level through grade 8 for discount rates of 5 percent and 3 percent, respectively, and somewhat lower for children for whom the increase in schooling would be at the secondary level that goes until grade 11. The costs in this estimate include the direct program costs, the private opportunity costs of the time devoted to increased schooling, and the expected deadweight cost to the economy from raising the revenue to finance the program.

Colombia. Colombia has been running a similar publicly funded day-care program, Hogares Comunitarios de Bienestar (in fact, Proyecto Integral de Desarrollo Infantil was modeled after this program). Bernal and

Fernández (2013) reported that children ages three years and older who spent at least 15 months in the program showed improvements in both cognitive development and socioemotional skills, although no gains in nutritional status were observed. The benefit-cost ratio was estimated to be between 1.0 and 2.7, using discount rates of 8 percent and 5 percent, respectively.

Both of these studies of day-care centers in Latin America reach children up to age six years, but the centers are not structured preschool programs. Engle and others (2011) provided an order of magnitude estimate of the benefit-cost ratio for such structured preschool programs at scale. This assessment was based on an estimate of the gap between the completed level of schooling for the wealthiest quintile in a given country and that of the poorest as a function of preschool enrollment in the previous 8–12 years. This estimate provided the basis for projecting the expected increase in schooling, and the concomitant increase in earnings, due to an increase in preschool participation, controlling for country effects. Using a discount rate of 3 percent, the assessment indicated that bringing the preschool enrollment rate in all LMICs to 25 percent, starting from each country's base level, would have a benefit-cost ratio of 14.3; bringing the enrollment rate to 50 percent would have a benefit-cost ratio of 17.6. Discounting future returns at a higher rate of 6 percent would lead to benefit-cost ratios of 6.4 and 7.8, respectively.

These estimates have wide ranges and are also sensitive to assumptions about the impact of schooling on wages as well as estimates of the cost of providing this schooling, but these results are similar to program-specific estimates in the literature. For example, Berlinski, Galiani, and Manacorda (2008) presented evidence on schooling outcomes measured a decade after the expansion of preschool enrollment in Uruguay. Their data indicated that as the supply of preschool services increased between 1989 and 2000, participation in preschools increased by 12 percentage points so that well more than 90 percent of all children attended preschool by the end of the period. From their results on the influence of preschool enrollment on school achievement, as well as the cost of construction of classrooms along with local salaries for teachers, they estimated a benefit-cost ratio of 3.2 using a discount rate of 10 percent. If the discount of future earnings is 3 percent, the estimated benefit-cost ratio is 19.1.

Returns to Investments in Schooling

Most estimates of the returns to investments in schooling in LMICs are based on estimates of the association between grades of schooling attainment and the earnings of wage workers. More specifically, if one assumes that the only cost of schooling is forgone wages and that the logarithm of wages is a linear function of schooling and other variables, then the coefficient on schooling from a regression of the log of wages on schooling and those other variables can be interpreted as the private return to time spent in school (see Mincer 1974).

There are at least two problems with such estimates. The first is that they estimate only the private returns to schooling that result from increased wages, and they exclude both other private returns, such as improved health accruing to that person and his or her children, and social returns that accrue to other members of society. These omissions imply that private returns may underestimate total returns. Second, overestimation is also possible because there are other private costs beyond the time spent in school; there are also social costs, in particular, the costs that governments incur by providing schooling opportunities at little or no cost to students and their families. The second problem is that these regressions yield private rates of return to investments in schooling only if the coefficient on schooling measures the causal impact of schooling on wages, and there are several reasons why such estimates may not reflect a causal relationship.

First, regressions of wages on schooling and other variables may not lead to accurate estimates of the causal impact of schooling on wage income because random measurement error in schooling could lead to underestimates of that impact; such measurement errors are particularly likely to be a problem in data from LMICs. Moreover, unobserved factors such as ability, motivation, and family connections could determine both schooling and earnings, even after controlling for wealth and parental schooling, and lead to overestimates in rates of return to schooling. In addition, such estimates from LMICs are almost always for wage earners only, not for the self-employed. Substantial evidence suggests that the return to education among the self-employed is lower than the return to wage earners,[2] which implies that estimates based only on wage earners are likely to be overestimates in countries with large numbers of self-employed workers. Finally, even among wage earners, estimates should, in general, exclude government workers if they are to be interpreted as reflecting productivity as opposed to private returns; yet in most cases, such workers are included. The pay received by government workers with different levels of education mainly reflects government salary policies rather than the productivity of different types of workers.

Given these problems, it is not surprising that compilations of estimates often yield very different results.

Psacharopoulos and Patrinos (2004) presented compilations indicating that the rate of return to an additional year of primary education in Sub-Saharan Africa is 37.6 percent, but Montenegro and Patrinos (2012) reported a much smaller rate of return of 13.4 percent.

Two of these problems can be resolved if valid instrumental variables can be found to predict schooling. A few studies have attempted to use instrumental variable methods to obtain more accurate estimates of the impact of schooling on wages in LMICs. Duflo (2001) used a sharp increase in the construction of primary schools to estimate the impact of schooling on wages in Indonesia. Her estimates indicate that an additional grade of schooling increases wages in that country by 7 percent to 11 percent. She also noted that the instrumented results do not differ appreciably from the uninstrumented estimation. Behrman and others (2013) estimated that an additional grade of schooling increases wages by 9.8 percent in Guatemala; the main identifying instruments were student-teacher ratios, mother's height, and mother's and father's schooling. While more studies would be useful, these two studies suggest that private returns to education are approximately 10 percent in LMICs.

Whatever the impact of additional schooling on adult earnings, there remains the question of what investments may lead to an increase in schooling. School enrollment or grades of schooling completed can be increased by demand-side interventions, such as transfer programs, or by increases in the supply and quality of schooling. The former category includes conditional transfers (Behrman, Parker, and Todd 2011) and school feeding programs (Adelman, Gilligan, and Lehrer 2008). The latter category was reviewed by Glewwe and others (2013), who reported that there are few unambiguous results regarding investments and schooling outcomes. A more comprehensive review can be found in Glewwe and Muralidharan (2016). Although that literature goes far beyond the issues central to disease control priorities, a few salient points are worth discussing here.

- First, although ability affects both schooling attainment and what is learned in school, the latter is the stronger determinant of earnings (Hanushek and Woessmann 2008).
- Second, despite the regular pattern of increased earnings with increased schooling, the quality of education in many settings is discouraging. For example, 52.7 percent of standard 5 (grade 5) students in India could not read a standard 2– (grade 2–) level text (ASER Centre 2014). Similar patterns are found in many Demographic and Health Surveys across the globe. Although many reasons for this waste of resources call for reforms and improvements in school systems, it may be the case that students, or a subset of them, come to school with huge disadvantages that could be offset through interventions in early childhood.
- Third, the impact of specific investments depends, in part, on the ability of students. For example, Glewwe, Kremer, and Moulin (2009) found that an increased supply of books in Kenya benefited the stronger students but had no measurable impact on the others. A different view of complementarity of inputs comes from Grantham-McGregor, Chang, and Walker (1998). This study found that feeding schoolchildren improved attention, but the impact on learning depended on the classroom structure, with stronger results found where the classes were more effectively organized.
- Finally, education responds to health, not only with respect to early-life nutrition, but also with respect to health investments for school-age children. For example, Miguel and Kremer (2004) found deworming in Kenya to be more cost-effective at increasing school participation[3] than supply-side interventions such as the provision of textbooks. Bleakley (2007) noted that hookworm infections in the American South in the early 1900s reduced the income in adulthood of infected children by 43 percent and that this negative outcome was effectively eliminated by a concerted program of hookworm control. Bleakley (2010) estimated a similar impact of malaria-control campaigns on incomes in the United States (circa 1920) and in Brazil, Colombia, and Mexico (circa 1955).

The possibility that healthier children will respond more to schooling inputs is an example of dynamic complementarity and is a major component of the returns to nutrition (Glewwe, Jacoby, and King 2001). However, the interaction of health and schooling may show some dynamic substitution rather than complementarity; there may be educational interventions with higher impacts the lower the initial health conditions. For example, Bobonis, Miguel, and Sharma (2006) studied the provision of iron supplementation and deworming medicine to preschool children in India. Overall, children in the treatment group had less absenteeism, but children who were initially anemic at baseline had a larger response to the intervention. Similarly, iron supplementation costing less than US$5 per child in primary schools in China over a seven-month period led to an improvement in hemoglobin as well as a significant improvement in math test scores (Luo and others 2012), and the academic improvement was found only for children who were anemic before the program.

CONCLUSIONS

Interventions to improve nutrition as well as to enhance cognitive and socioemotional development in each of the early lifecycle stages—preschool ages, schooling ages, and later adolescence—can achieve returns in later stages that greatly exceed their costs. Yet an empirical question remains: at what lifecycle stage, and in what context, are the benefit-cost ratios high enough to warrant investments? The benefit-cost estimates from nutritional interventions in the first 1,000 days are based on extensive data and have been accumulated on a global basis, albeit mostly for small, special samples; there is less evidence on benefits and costs for stimulation and early child development for programs at appreciable scale. Moreover, a review of the cost of programs at scale in Latin America and the Caribbean indicates a wide—and not fully understood—heterogeneity of costs (Araujo and López-Boo 2013). This knowledge gap hinders any definitive generalizations.

Even if estimates of costs were confined to a narrow range over various environments, there is also a general dearth of results on the heterogeneity of impacts. A few studies show that programs may have greater impacts for children who enter these programs at an initial disadvantage (Engle and others 2011). Berlinski, Galiani, and Manacorda (2008) found that the impact of preschool attendance was largest for those children from households with parents who have less schooling, and Jung and Hasan (2014) found that block grants for preschool groups in Indonesia narrowed gaps in language and cognitive development. To the degree that such programs reduce gaps in children's development, they have an additional social value in reducing the intergenerational transmission of poverty with possible gains in efficiency if such programs partially offset capital market failures that result in underinvestments in children. Although a reduction in poverty is usually not translated into benefits that can be aggregated into benefit-cost ratios, the benefits are likely to be real and positive and could be incorporated by weighting outcomes for children from poorer families more heavily.

According to widespread evidence, gradients in cognitive ability by socioeconomic status appear early in life (Fernald and others 2012; Naudeau and others 2011; Schady and others 2015); therefore, the potential to prevent or reverse gaps suggests that nutrition programs, the promotion of early stimulation, and preschool education may have social returns that are appreciably larger than commonly reported.

Some perceive that an ounce of prevention is worth a pound of cure, so that the earlier such interventions can be delivered, the better. The evidence does suggest that, given the current distribution of investments over the lifecycle, in many contexts the rates of return to some additional investments are likely to be highest very early in life. However, there are likely to be diminishing marginal rates of return to such interventions; even if under present circumstances the rates of return were highest to interventions to improve nutrition in the womb or very early in a child's life, it does not follow that all resources should be moved from later to earlier in life. As more resources are moved from later to earlier life, most likely diminishing marginal rates of return will mean that the rates of return to the investments in early life will fall and those to investments in later life will increase. Indeed, it would be socially optimal in an economic sense to move resources directed to human development from older to younger ages until the social rates of return to the use of resources at all ages are equalized.

NOTES

Harold Alderman and Jere R. Behrman acknowledge partial support for their time working on this chapter from Grand Challenges Canada (Grant 0072-03 to the Grantee, The Trustees of the University of Pennsylvania). Behrman also acknowledges partial support from the Bill & Melinda Gates Foundation (Global Health Grant OPP1032713) and Eunice Kennedy Shriver National Institute of Child Health and Human Development (Grant R01 HD070993).

World Bank Income Classifications as of July 2014 are as follows, based on estimates of gross national income (GNI) per capita for 2013:

- Low-income countries (LICs) = US$1,045 or less
- Middle-income countries (MICs) are subdivided:
  a) lower-middle-income = US$1,046 to US$4,125
  b) upper-middle-income (UMICs) = US$4,126 to US$12,745
- High-income countries (HICs) = US$12,746 or more.

1. Halfon and others (2014) propose four phases—generative, acquisition of capacity, maintenance of function, and managing decline—that differ from the stages discussed here, although they are related conceptually.
2. For example, compare the estimates of van der Sluis, van Praag, and Vijverberg (2005) on returns to schooling among the self-employed to the estimate of Psacharopoulos and Patrinos (2004) on the returns to schooling among wage earners.
3. School participation combines enrollment with attendance; among two children enrolled in school, the one with higher attendance in a given year has higher participation, and any child not enrolled has a participation rate of zero.

REFERENCES

Adair, L. S., C. H. D. Fall, C. Osmond, A. D. Stein, R. Martorell, and others. 2013. "Associations of Linear Growth and Relative Weight Gain during Early Life with Adult Health and Human Capital in Countries of Low and Middle Income: Findings from Five Birth Cohort Studies." *The Lancet* 382 (9891): 525–34.

Adelman, S., D. O. Gilligan, and K. Lehrer. 2008. "How Effective Are Food for Education Programs? A Critical Assessment of the Evidence from Developing Countries." Food Policy Review No. 8, International Food Policy Research Institute, Washington, DC.

Alderman, H., and J. R. Behrman. 2006. "Reducing the Incidence of Low Birth Weight in Low-Income Countries Has Substantial Economic Benefits." *World Bank Research Observer* 21 (1): 25–48.

Alderman, H., J. R. Behrman, V. Lavy, and R. Menon. 2001. "Child Health and School Enrollment: A Longitudinal Analysis." *Journal of Human Resources* 36 (1): 185–205.

Alderman, H., J. R. Behrman, and C. Puett. 2017. "Big Numbers about Small Children: Estimating the Economic Benefits of Addressing Undernutrition." *World Bank Research Observer* 32 (1).

Alderman, H., S. Grantham-McGregor, F. Lopez-Boo, and S. Urzua. 2014. "Economic Perspectives on Integrating Early Child Stimulation with Nutritional Interventions." *Annals of the New York Academy of Sciences* 1308: 129–38.

Alderman, H., and D. Sahn. 2016. "Public and Private Returns to Investing in Nutrition." In *Oxford Handbook of Economics and Human Biology*, edited by J. Komlos and I. Kelly. Oxford, U.K.: Oxford University Press.

Araujo, M. C., and F. López-Boo. 2013. *Panorama sobre los servicios de desarrollo infantil temprano en América Latina y el Caribe*. Washington, DC: Inter-American Development Bank.

ASER Centre. 2014. *Annual Status of Education Report 2013*. New Delhi: ASER Centre. http://www.asercentre.org.

Attanasio, O. P., C. Fernandez, E. O. Fitzsimons, S. M. Grantham-McGregor, C. Meghir, and others. 2014. "Using the Infrastructure of a Conditional Cash Transfer Program to Deliver a Scalable Integrated Early Child Development Program in Colombia: Cluster Randomized Controlled Trial." *BMJ* 349: g5785.

Behrman, J. R., H. Alderman, and J. Hoddinott. 2004. "Hunger and Malnutrition." In *Global Crises, Global Solutions*, edited by Bjørn Lomborg, 363–420. Cambridge, U.K.: Cambridge University Press.

Behrman, J. R., Y. Cheng, and P. Todd. 2004. "Evaluating Preschool Programs When Length of Exposure to the Program Varies: A Nonparametric Approach." *Review of Economics and Statistics* 86 (1): 108–32.

Behrman, J. R., J. Hoddinott, J. A. Maluccio, and R. Martorell. 2013. "Brains versus Brawn: Labor Market Returns to Intellectual and Health Human Capital in Guatemala." Working Paper, International Food Policy Research Institute, Washington, DC.

Behrman, J. R., S. Parker, and P. Todd. 2011. "Do Conditional Cash Transfers for Schooling Generate Lasting Benefits? A Five-Year Followup of PROGRESA/Oportunidades." *Journal of Human Resources* 46 (1): 93–122.

Berlinski, S., S. Galiani, and M. Manacorda. 2008. "Giving Children a Better Start: Preschool Attendance and School-Age Profiles." *Journal of Public Economics* 92 (5–6): 1416–40.

Berlinski, S., and N. Schady. 2015. *The Early Years: Child Well-Being and the Role of Public Policy*. Development in the Americas series. New York: Macmillan, and Washington, DC: Inter-American Development Bank.

Bernal, R., and C. Fernández. 2013. "Subsidized Childcare and Child Development in Colombia: Effects of Hogares Comunitarios de Bienestar as a Function of Timing and Length of Exposure." *Social Science and Medicine* 97: 241–49.

Bhutta, Z. A., J. K. Das, A. Rizvi, M. F. Gaffey, N. Walker, and others. 2013. "Evidence-Based Interventions for Improvement of Maternal and Child Nutrition: What Can Be Done and at What Cost?" *The Lancet* 382 (9890): 452–77.

Black, R. E., C. G. Victora, S. P. Walker, Z. A. Bhutta, P. Christian, and others. 2013. "Maternal and Child Undernutrition and Overweight in Low-Income and Middle-Income Countries." *The Lancet* 382 (9890): 427–51.

Bleakley, H. 2007. "Disease and Development: Evidence from Hookworm Eradication in the American South." *Quarterly Journal of Economics* 122 (1): 73–117.

———. 2010. "Malaria in the Americas: A Retrospective Analysis of Childhood Exposure." *American Economic Journal: Applied Economics* 2 (2): 1–45.

Bobonis, G. J., E. Miguel, and C. P. Sharma. 2006. "Anemia and School Participation." *Journal of Human Resources* 41 (4): 692–721.

Borghans, L., A. Duckworth, J. Heckman, and B. ter Weel. 2008. "The Economics and Psychology of Personality Traits." *Journal of Human Resources* 43 (4): 972–10.

Bundy, D. A. P., N. de Silva, S. Horton, G. C. Patton, L. Schultz, and D. T. Jamison. 2017. "Child and Adolescent Health and Development: Realizing Neglected Potential." In *Disease Control Priorities* (third edition): Volume 8, *Child and Adolescent Health and Development*, edited by D. A. P. Bundy, N. de Silva, S. Horton, D. T. Jamison, and G. C. Patton. Washington, DC: World Bank.

Christian, P., S. E. Lee, M. D. Angel, L. S Adair, S. E Arifeen, and others. 2013. "Risk of Childhood Undernutrition Related to Small-for-Gestational Age and Preterm Birth in Low- and Middle-Income Countries." *International Journal of Epidemiology* 42 (5): 1340–55.

Crookston, B. T., W. Schott, S. Cueto, K. A. Dearden, P. Engle, and others. 2013. "Postinfancy Growth, Schooling, and Cognitive Achievement: Young Lives." *American Journal of Clinical Nutrition* 98 (6): 1555–63.

Cunha, F., and J. Heckman. 2007. "The Technology of Skills Formation." *American Economic Review* 97 (2): 31–47.

Cunha, F., L. Lochner, and D. Masterov. 2006. "Interpreting the Evidence on Life Cycle Skill Formation." In *Handbook of the Economics of Education, Vol. 1, edited by E. Hanushek and F. Welch, 697–812. Amsterdam: New Holland-Elsevier.

de Onis, M., M. Blössner, and E. Borghi. 2010. "Global Prevalence and Trends of Overweight and Obesity among Preschool Children." American Journal of Clinical Nutrition 92 (5): 1257–64.

———. 2011. "Prevalence and Trends of Stunting among Pre-School Children, 1990–2020." Public Health Nutrition 1 (1): 1–7.

Devarajan, S., L. Squire, and S. Suthiwart-Narueput. 1997. "Beyond Rate of Return: Reorienting Project Appraisal." World Bank Research Observer 12 (1): 35–46.

Duflo, E. 2001. "Schooling and Labor Market Consequences of School Construction in Indonesia: Evidence from an Unusual Policy Experiment." American Economic Review 91 (4): 795–813.

Engle, P. L., M. M. Black, J. R. Behrman, M. Cabral de Mello, P. J. Gertler, and others. 2007. "Strategies to Avoid the Loss of Developmental Potential in More than 200 Million Children in the Developing World." The Lancet 369 (9557): 229–42.

Engle, P. L., L. Fernald, H. Alderman, J. R. Behrman, C. O'Gara, and others. 2011. "Strategies for Reducing Inequalities and Improving Developmental Outcomes for Young Children in Low and Middle Income Countries." The Lancet 378 (9799): 1339–53.

Fernald, L. C. H., P. K. Kariger, M. Hidrobo, and P. J. Gertler. 2012. "Socio-Economic Gradients in Child Development in Very Young Children: Evidence from India, Indonesia, Peru and Senegal." Proceedings of the National Academy of Sciences 109 (Suppl 2): 17273–80.

Fine, A., and M. Kotelchuck. 2010. "Rethinking MCH: The Life Course Model as an Organizing Framework." U. S. Department of Health and Human Services, Health Resources and Services Administration, Maternal and Child Health Bureau, Washington, DC.

Gertler, P., J. Heckman, R. Pinto, A. Zanolini, C. Vermeerch, and others. 2014. "Labor Market Returns to an Early Childhood Stimulation Intervention in Jamaica." Science 344 (6187): 998–1001.

Glewwe, P., E. Hanushek, S. Humpage, and R. Ravina. 2013. "School Resources and Educational Outcomes in Developing Countries: A Review of the Literature from 1990 to 2010." In Education Policy in Developing Countries, edited by P. Glewwe, 13–64. Chicago, IL: University of Chicago Press.

Glewwe, P., H. Jacoby, and E. King. 2001. "Early Childhood Nutrition and Academic Achievement: A Longitudinal Analysis." Journal of Public Economics 81 (3): 345–68.

Glewwe, P., M. Kremer, and S. Moulin. 2009. "Many Children Left Behind? Textbooks and Test Scores in Kenya." American Economic Journal: Applied Economics 1 (1): 112–35.

Glewwe, P., and K. Muralidharan. 2016. "Improving Education Outcomes in Developing Countries: Evidence, Knowledge Gaps and Policy Implications." In Handbook of the Economics of Education, Vol. 5, edited by E. Hanushek, S. Machin, and L. Woessmann. North Holland: Elsevier.

Gluckman, P. D., M. A. Hanson, P. Bateson, A. S. Beedle, C. M. Law, and others. 2009. "Towards a New Development Synthesis: Adaptive Developmental Plasticity and Human Disease." The Lancet 373 (9675): 1654–57.

Grantham-McGregor, S., Y. B. Cheung, S. Cueto, P. Glewwe, L. Richter, and others. 2007. "Developmental Potential in the First 5 Years for Children in Developing Countries." The Lancet 369 (9555): 60–70.

Grantham-McGregor, S. M., S. Chang, and S. P. Walker. 1998. "Evaluation of School Feeding Programs: Some Jamaican Examples." American Journal of Clinical Nutrition 67 (4): 785S–89S.

Grantham-McGregor, S. M., L. C. H. Fernald, R. M. C. Kagawa, and S. Walker. 2014. "Effects of Integrated Child Development and Nutrition Interventions on Child Development and Nutritional Status." Annals of the New York Academy of Sciences 1308: 11–32.

Grantham-McGregor, S. M., S. P. Walker, C. A. Powell, and S. M. Chang. 1997. "The Effects of Early Childhood Supplementation with and without Stimulation on Later Development in Stunted Children." American Journal of Clinical Nutrition 66 (2): 247–53.

Halfon, N., K. Larson, M. Lu, E. Tullis, and S. Russ. 2014. "Lifecourse Health Development: Past, Present and Future." Maternal and Child Health Journal 18 (2): 344–65.

Hamadani, J. D., S. N. Huda, F. Khatun, and S. M. Grantham-McGregor. 2006. "Psychosocial Stimulation Improves the Development of Undernourished Children in Rural Bangladesh." Journal of Nutrition 136 (10): 2645–52.

Hanushek, E., and L. Woessmann. 2008. "The Role of Cognitive Skills in Economic Development." Journal of Economic Literature 46 (3): 607–68.

Helmers, C., and M. Patnam. 2011. "The Formation and Evolution of Childhood Skill Acquisition: Evidence from India." Journal of Development Economics 95 (2): 252–66.

Hoddinott, J., H. Alderman, J. R. Behrman, L. Haddad, and S. Horton. 2013. "The Economic Rationale for Investing in Stunting Reduction." Maternal and Child Nutrition 9 (Suppl 2): 69–82.

Hoddinott, J., J. R. Behrman, J. A. Maluccio, P. Melgar, A. R. Quisumbing, and others. 2013. "Adult Consequences of Growth Failure in Early Childhood." American Journal of Clinical Nutrition 98 (5): 1170–78.

Hoddinott, J., J. Maluccio, J. R. Behrman, R. Flores, and R. Martorell. 2008. "Effect of a Nutrition Intervention during Early Childhood on Economic Productivity in Guatemalan Adults." The Lancet 371 (9610): 411–16.

Horton, S., H. Alderman, and J. Rivera. 2009. "Hunger and Malnutrition." In Global Crises, Global Solutions, 2nd edition, edited by B. Lomborg. Cambridge, U.K.: Cambridge University Press.

Horton, S., M. Shekar, C. McDonald, A. Mahal, and J. Brooks. 2010. Scaling Up Nutrition: What Will It Cost? World Bank: Washington, DC.

Jung, H., and A. Hasan 2014. "The Impact of Early Childhood Education on Early Achievement Gaps: Evidence from the Indonesia Early Childhood Education and Development Project." Policy Research Working Paper 6794, World Bank, Washington, DC.

Kaytaz, M. 2005. "A Cost Benefit Analysis of Preschool Education in Turkey." AÇEV (Mother Child Education Foundation), Istanbul.

Leroy, J. L., M. Ruel, J.-P. Habicht, and E. A. Frongillo. 2014. "Linear Growth Deficit Continues to Accumulate beyond the First 1000 Days in Low- and Middle-Income Countries: Global Evidence from 51 National Surveys." *Journal of Nutrition* 144 (9): 1460–66.

Lundeen, E. A., J. R. Behrman, B. T. Crookston, K. A. Dearden, P. Engle, and others. 2013. "Growth Faltering and Recovery in Children Aged 1–8 Years in Four Low- and Middle-Income Countries: Young Lives." *Public Health Nutrition* 17 (9): 2131–37.

Lundeen, E. A., D. A. Stein, L. A. Adair, J. R. Behrman, S. K. Bhargava, and others. 2014. "Increases in HAZ Co-Exist with Increasing Deficits in Height among Children in Middle-Income Countries." *American Journal of Clinical Nutrition* 100 (3): 821–25.

Luo, R., Y. Shi, L. Zhang, C. Liu, S. Rozelle, and others. 2012. "Nutrition and Educational Performance in Rural China's Elementary Schools: Results of a Randomized Control Trial in Shaanxi Province." *Economic Development and Cultural Change* 60 (4): 735–72.

Mani, S. 2012. "Is There Complete, Partial, or No Recovery from Childhood Malnutrition? Empirical Evidence from Indonesia." *Oxford Bulletin of Economics and Statistics* 74 (5): 691–715.

Menon, P., N. M. Covic, P. B. Harrigan, S. Horton, N. M. Kazi, and others. 2014. "Strengthening Implementation and Utilization of Nutrition Interventions through Research: A Framework and Research Agenda." *Annals of the New York Academy of Sciences* 1332 (1): 39–59.

Miguel, E., and M. Kremer. 2004. "Worms: Identifying Impacts on Education and Health in the Presence of Treatment Externalities." *Econometrica* 72 (1): 159–217.

Mincer, J. B. 1974. "Education, Experience, and the Distribution of Earnings and Employment." In *Education, Income, and Human Behavior*, edited by F. T. Juster. New York: McGraw-Hill.

Monteiro, P., and C. G. Victora. 2005. "Relation of Serial Changes in Childhood Body-Mass Index to Impaired Glucose Tolerance in Young Adulthood." *Obesity Review* 6 (2): 143–54.

Montenegro, C. E., and H. A. Patrinos. 2012. "Returns to Schooling around the World." Background Paper for the World Development Report 2013, Center for Global Development, Washington, DC.

Nandi, A., J. R. Behrman, S. Bhalotra, A. B. Deolalikar, and R. Laxminarayan. 2017. "Human Capital and Productivity Benefits of Early Childhood Nutritional Interventions." In *Disease Control Priorities* (third edition): Volume 8, *Child and Adolescent Health and Development*, edited by D. A. P. Bundy, N. de Silva, S. Horton, D. T. Jamison, and G. C. Patton. Washington, DC: World Bank.

National Scientific Council on the Developing Child. 2014. "Excessive Stress Disrupts the Architecture of the Developing Brain." Working Paper No. 3, Center on the Developing Child, Harvard University, Cambridge, MA.

Naudeau, S., S. Martinez, P. Premand, and D. Filmer. 2011. "Cognitive Development among Young Children in Low-Income Countries." In *No Small Matter: The Interaction of Poverty, Shocks, and Human Capital Investments in Early Childhood Development*, edited by H. Alderman. Washington, DC: World Bank.

Paxson, C., and N. Schady. 2007. "Cognitive Development among Young Children in Ecuador: The Roles of Wealth, Health, and Parenting." *Journal of Human Resources* 42 (1): 49–84.

Pitt, M. M., M. R. Rosenzweig, and M. N. Hassan. 2012. "Human Capital Investment and the Gender Division of Labor in a Brawn-Based Economy." *American Economic Review* 102 (7): 3531–60.

Powell, C., H. Baker-Henningham, S. Walker, and S. M. Grantham-McGregor. 2004. "Feasibility of Integrating Early Stimulation into Primary Care for Undernourished Jamaican Children: Cluster Randomised Controlled Trial." *BMJ* 329 (7457): 89. doi:10.1136/bmj.38132.503472.7C.

Prentice, A. M., K. A. Ward, G. R. Goldberg, L. M. Jarjou, S. E. Moore, and others. 2013. "Critical Windows for Nutritional Interventions against Stunting." *American Journal of Clinical Nutrition* 97 (5): 911–18.

Psacharopoulos, G., and H. A. Patrinos. 2004. "Returns to Investment in Education: A Further Update." *Education Economics* 12 (2): 111–34.

Schady, N., J. R. Behrman, M. C. Araujo, R. Azuero, R. Bernal, and others. 2015. "Wealth Gradients in Early Childhood Cognitive Development in Five Latin American Countries." *Journal of Human Resources* 50 (2): 446–63.

Schott, W., B. T. Crookston, E. A. Lundeen, A. D. Stein, J. R. Behrman, and others. 2013. "Child Growth from Ages 1 to 8 Years in Ethiopia, India, Peru and Vietnam: Key Distal Household and Community Factors." *Social Science and Medicine* 97: 278–87.

Shonkoff, J., and A. S. Garner. 2012. "The Lifelong Effects of Early Childhood Adversity and Toxic Stress." *Pediatrics* 129 (1): 232–46.

Singla, D. R., E. Kumbakumba, and F. E. Aboud. 2015. "Effects of an Integrated Intervention on Child Development and Maternal Depressive Symptoms in Rural Uganda: A Cluster-Randomized Trial." *The Lancet Global Health* 3 (8): 458–69.

Stein, A. D., M. Wang, R. Martorell, S. A. Norris, L. S. Adair, and others. 2010. "Growth Patterns in Early Childhood and Final Attained Stature: Data from Five Birth Cohorts from Low- and Middle-Income Countries." *American Journal of Human Biology* 22 (3): 353–39.

Summers, L. H. 1992. "Investing in All the People." *Pakistan Development Review* 31 (4): 367–406.

Toh-Adam, R., K. Srisupundit, and T. Tongsong. 2012. "Short Stature as an Independent Risk Factor for Cephalopelvic Disproportion in a Country of Relatively

Small-Sized Mothers." *Archives of Gynecology and Obstetrics* 285 (6): 1513–16.

UNESCO (United Nations Educational, Scientific and Cultural Organization). 2014. *Education for All. Global Monitoring Report 2013/4.* Paris: UNESCO.

UNICEF (United Nations Children's Fund). 2006a. "Progress for Children: Exclusive Breastfeeding." http://www.unicef .org/progressforchildren/2006n4/index_breastfeeding.html.

———. 2006b. "Progress for Children: Low Birthweight." http://www.unicef.org/progressforchildren/2006n4/index _lowbirthweight.html.

———. 2013. "Childinfo.org: Statistics by Area—Low birthweight: Status and Trends."

———. n.d. "Low Birthweight." http://www.unicef.org /specialsession/about/sgreport-pdf/15_LowBirthweight _D7341Insert_English.pdf.

UNICEF and WHO (World Health Organization). 2004. *Low Birthweight: Country, Regional and Global Estimates.* New York: UNICEF.

van der Sluis, J., M. van Praag, and W. Vijverberg. 2005. "Entrepreneurship Selection and Performance: A Meta-Analysis of the Impact of Education in Developing Economies." *World Bank Economic Review* 19 (2): 225–61.

Victora, C. G., L. Adair, C. Fall, P. C. Hallal, R. Martorell, and others. 2008. "Maternal and Child Undernutrition: Consequences for Adult Health and Human Capital." *The Lancet* 371 (9609): 340–57.

Victora, C. G., M. de Onis, P. C. Hallal, M. Blössner, and R. Shrimpton. 2010. "Worldwide Timing of Growth Faltering: Revisiting Implications for Interventions." *Pediatrics* 125 (3): 473–80.

Viscusi, W., and J. Aldy. 2003. "The Value of a Statistical Life: A Critical Review of Market Estimates throughout the World." *Journal of Risk and Uncertainty* 27 (1): 15–76.

Wachs, T., M. Georgieff, S. Cusick, and B. McEwan. 2014. "The Timing of Integrated Early Interventions: Contributions from Nutritional Neuroscience, Stress Neuroscience and Psychological Research." *Annals of the New York Academy of Sciences* 1308: 89–106.

Walker, S. P., S. M. Chang, N. Younger, and S. Grantham-McGregor. 2010. "The Effect of Psychosocial Stimulation on Cognition and Behaviour at 6 Years in a Cohort of Term, Low-Birthweight Jamaican Children." *Developmental Medicine and Child Neurology* 52: e148–54.

Walker, S. P., S. M. Chang, M. Vera-Hernández, and S. M. Grantham-McGregor. 2011. "Early Childhood Stimulation Benefits Adult Competence and Reduces Violent Behavior." *Pediatrics* 127 (5): 849–57.

Walker, S. P., T. D. Wachs, S. M. Grantham-McGregor, M. Black, C. Nelson, and others. 2011. "Inequality in Early Childhood: Risk and Protective Factors for Early Child Development." *The Lancet* 378 (9799): 1325–38.

Watkins, K., D. A. P. Bundy, D. T. Jamison, G. Fink, and A. Georgiadis. 2017. "Evidence of Impact of Interventions on Health and Development of Interventions during Middle Childhood and School Age." In *Disease Control Priorities* (third edition): Volume 8, *Child and Adolescent Health and Development*, edited by D. A. P. Bundy, N. de Silva, S. Horton, D. T. Jamison, and G. C. Patton. Washington, DC: World Bank.

Yajnik, C. 2004. "Early Life Origins of Insulin Resistance and Type 2 Diabetes in India and Other Asian Countries." *Journal of Nutrition* 134: 205–10.

———. 2009. "Nutrient-Mediated Teratogenesis and Fuel-Mediated Teratogenesis: Two Pathways of Intrauterine Programming of Diabetes." *International Journal of Gynecology and Obstetrics* 104 (Suppl 1): S27–31.

Yamauchi, F. 2008. "Early Childhood Nutrition, Schooling, and Sibling Inequality in a Dynamic Context: Evidence from South Africa." *Economic Development and Cultural Change* 56 (3): 657–82.

Yousafzai, A. K., M. A. Rasheed, A. Rizvi, R. Armstrong, and Z. A. Bhutta. 2014. "Effect of Integrated Responsive Stimulation and Nutrition Interventions in the Lady Health Worker Programme in Pakistan on Child Development, Growth, and Health Outcomes: A Cluster-Randomised Factorial Effectiveness Trial." *The Lancet* 384 (9950): 1282–93.

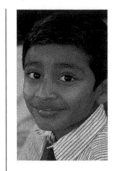

Chapter 8

Evidence of Impact of Interventions on Health and Development during Middle Childhood and School Age

Kristie L. Watkins, Donald A. P. Bundy, Dean T. Jamison,
Günther Fink, and Andreas Georgiadis

INTRODUCTION

A large literature has highlighted the multifaceted and negative long-term consequences of poor health in early life. The large body of evidence linking adversity in the first 1,000 days of life to later life outcomes has created a major policy shift toward the early years, and it has promoted the idea that the consequences of early insults are irreversible. A longitudinal supplementation study in Guatemala of children ages 0–7 years is frequently cited in support of this argument (Martorell, Khan, and Schroeder 1994). The authors concluded that stunting is a condition that results from events in early childhood and that, once present, remains for life. This view was echoed in *The Lancet* series on maternal and child undernutrition: "Poor fetal growth or stunting in the first two years of life leads to irreversible damage, including shorter adult height, lower attained schooling, reduced adult income, and decreased offspring birthweight" (Victora and others 2008, 340).

The available evidence does indeed support the contention that children with a poor start in life are likely to remain on that low trajectory if nothing else changes: indeed, early investment clearly is important. However, this does not mean that children's experiences in later childhood are not important. From a biological perspective, early programming is plausible, but the same obviously also holds for later life gene-environment interactions. Is it possible for children with positive later childhood experiences to catch up with their peers? If yes, to what extent?

This chapter explores evidence regarding whether interventions in school-age children can affect their later development. Definitions of age groupings and age-specific terminology used in this volume can be found in chapter 1 (Bundy, de Silva, and others 2017). The main objective of this chapter is to review the evidence for and against irreversibility: Can interventions after the early years of life help children regain or approach their innate capacity for development? Given that the evidence base for older children is more limited, we do not pursue a systematic review strategy in this chapter, but rather look for specific empirical examples supporting or refuting the idea of lifelong irreversibility; a search for black swans.

CHANGES IN ENVIRONMENT

Changes in environment provide an ideal setting for investigating the irreversibility hypothesis: many children who grow up in poor early life environments move to better environments as a result of migration, adoption, or transfer to different institutional settings. These transitions provide a natural starting point for assessing the potential for catch-up.

Corresponding author: Kristie Lynn Watkins, Imperial College London, London, United Kingdom; kristie.lynn.watkins@gmail.com.

Immigration Studies

One study on immigration found that school-age children who were born in Turkey and then migrated to Sweden were short at first measurement upon immigration but then caught up to achieve heights similar to those of ethnically Turkish children born in Sweden (Mjönes 1987). Similarly, a semilongitudinal study assessed children ages 5–12 years of Chinese, Filipino, Hispanic, and Southeast Asian origins who had migrated to San Francisco (Schumacher, Pawson, and Kretchmer 1987). Upon their arrival, most of the children from the four ethnic groups had mean height and weight between the 5th and 25th percentiles of those of the U.S. population. At follow-up one year later, the median growth rate of most cohorts exceeded that of the U.S. reference, with no differences noted between younger and older children.

Adoption Studies

As Golden (1994) highlighted, immigration studies examine the effect of far-reaching changes to the physical environment of a child, whereas adoption studies examine the effect of a change in the quality of the local or home environment on growth later in life. In general, most adoption studies report anthropometric gains for school-age children—for example, Korean orphans adopted by American families (Lien, Meyer, and Winick 1977; Winick, Meyer, and Harris 1975), Indian girls adopted by Swedish families (Proos, Hofvander, and Tuvemo 1991a, 1991b), and previously abused children taken into foster care or adopted in England (King and Taitz 1985).

Adoption studies offer some of the clearest evidence that improving conditions can reverse the consequences of early childhood deprivation. They also offer evidence that, even if early intervention has been successful, intervention later in life may be necessary to sustain the gains of early intervention. A study in Peru found that children who were treated for severe malnutrition early in life and later adopted were significantly taller at age nine years than were similar children who remained in their original home environments (Graham and Adrianzen 1972). Also in Peru, a unique study (Graham and Adrianzen 1971) admitted children from very poor families to a convalescent unit after birth and maintained them on an optimal diet until an average age of 17.6 months. These children showed initial gains relative to their siblings who did not receive this treatment, but within one year of returning home and through the last measurements at age eight years, there was no significant difference in the heights of the two groups (Adrianzen, Baertl, and Graham 1973; Baertl, Adrianzen, and Graham 1976). These findings suggest that environments promoting growth later in life may be needed to consolidate early gains.

Historical Migration Evidence

Steckel (1987) examined historical data on children brought to the United States as slaves and found that they were initially stunted but grew rapidly through the centiles during adolescence. Similarly, Komlos (1986) examined historical data on students at Hapsburg military schools following the Napoleonic Wars and found that boys who were the sons of poor families and stunted at admission showed sizable catch-up growth, presumably attributable to improved diet and living conditions, once they were admitted to military schools.

SECONDARY STUNTING AND UNDERWEIGHT

Clinical and physiological conditions, such as frequent exposure to diarrhea or worm infections, can be associated with stunting and underweight that are secondary to disease. If the initial effects were irreversible, removing the primary risk factors later in life should not have an impact on growth. However, successful treatment of several conditions has been shown to result in partial or complete catch-up growth for school-age children: celiac disease (Barr, Schmerling, and Prader 1972; Bodé and others 1991; Cacciari and others 1991; Damen and others 1994), growth hormone deficiency (Burns and others 1981; Kemp and others 2005), hypothyroidism (Boersma and others 1996; Pantsiotou and others 1991; Rivkees, Bode, and Crawford 1988), and corticosteroid excess (Davies and others 2005; Prader, Tanner, and von Harnack 1963).

FOOD SUPPLEMENTATION

Studies of food supplementation in school-age children have reported small but significant gains in growth. Kristjansson and others (2007), in a meta-analysis of three randomized controlled trials (RCTs) in low-income countries and lower-middle-income countries (Du and others 2004; Grillenberger and others 2003; Powell and others 1998), reported a small, significant effect of school meals on weight gain (0.39 kilogram), approximately 0.25 kilogram per year factoring in study duration. The review also found a small, nonsignificant effect on height gain (0.38 centimeter).

More recently, the World Food Programme and the World Bank assessed the impact of school feeding programs on anthropometric outcomes in three independent studies in Burkina Faso, the Lao People's Democratic Republic, and Uganda. In Uganda, no significant effects were found on body-mass-index-for-age z-scores or height-for-age z-scores (HAZ) in children ages 6–13 years (Adelman and others 2008). In Burkina Faso, significant gains were reported in weight-for-age (0.21 standard deviation) for children ages 6–10 years, especially boys (Kazianga, de Walque, and Alderman 2014). In Lao PDR, significant improvements were reported in both height-for-age (0.29 standard deviation) and weight-for-age (0.22 standard deviation) among children ages 3–10 years, although the authors suggested that the nutritional findings were inconclusive because of the complications that arise in stratified analyses (Buttenheim, Alderman, and Friedman 2011).

Kristjansson and others (2007) conducted a meta-analysis of three controlled before-and-after studies of school meals in low-income countries and lower-middle-income countries (Agarwal, Agarwal, and Upadhyay 1989; Bailey 1962; Devadas and others 1979). They found greater weight gains of approximately 0.75 kilogram per year, slightly larger than the impacts found in RCTs (0.71 kilogram). In contrast to the RCT evidence, meta-analysis of the three controlled before-and-after studies found a significant effect on height gain (1.43 centimeters), approximately one-third more than in control groups.

MICRONUTRIENT SUPPLEMENTATION

Micronutrient supplementation and fortification have been found to increase growth at school age. A meta-analysis of 33 zinc supplementation studies in prepubertal children conducted by Brown and others (2002) found significant effects for both weight (0.31 kilogram) and height (0.35 centimeter). In seven of the studies, the mean initial age of the children was greater than five years. Ramakrishnan and others (2004), in a meta-analysis of the effects of vitamin A, iron, and multiple-micronutrient interventions on the growth of children younger than age 18 years, found significant improvements in height and weight with multiple-micronutrient interventions, but not with vitamin A or iron alone. Five multiple-micronutrient interventions were included, two of which were in school-age children and reported significant effects on height and weight (Abrams and others 2003; Ash and others 2003). A systematic review focusing on multiple-micronutrient fortification in school-age children reported mixed effects for height and weight gain (Best and others 2011).

DEWORMING

The ability to detect improved growth as a result of anthelmintic treatment of children is controversial. Much of this controversy is about the interpretation of studies of interventions that treat all children in a community irrespective

of their infection status, as discussed in chapters 13 and 29 in this volume (Bundy, Appleby, and others 2017; Ahuja and others 2017, respectively). Here we focus on the observation that effects are generally seen in studies of children who are known to be infected, especially when infection rates are high. For example, deworming of children with intense trichuriasis—which is associated with *Trichuris* dysentery syndrome and severe stunting—results in dramatic catch-up growth (Cooper and others 1995). Similarly, a Cochrane review of the effect of soil-transmitted helminths on growth in children younger than age 16 years found that the three studies that followed up with only those children who had been screened and found to be infected showed a significant mean increase in weight (0.58 kilogram), with no significant difference in height following treatment (Taylor-Robinson and others 2012).

A meta-analysis of 19 RCTs by Hall and others (2008) found that children ages 1–19 years who are treated for intestinal worm infections experience significant improvements in height (9 studies, 0.11 centimeter), weight (11 studies, 0.21 kilogram), HAZ (6 studies, 0.09 standard deviation), weight-for-age z-score (5 studies, 0.06 standard deviation), and weight-for-height z-score (4 studies, 0.38 standard deviation). According to Taylor-Robinson and others (2012), differences in the findings of the two reviews could be due to differences in their protocols.

IMPACT OF INTERVENTIONS AND CATCH-UP GROWTH ON COGNITIVE ACHIEVEMENT AMONG SCHOOL-AGE CHILDREN

Growth- and nutrition-promoting interventions in school-age children have been found to improve learning and cognitive functioning. Although not true for all studies (Gertler and others 2014), several studies on the impact of food supplementation (Cueto, Jacoby, and Pollitt 1998; Muthayya and others 2007), micronutrient supplementation (Soewondo, Husaini, and Pollitt 1989; Zimmermann and others 2006), deworming (Nokes and others 1992), and treatment of growth-hormone deficiencies (Van Pareren and others 2004) on school-age children found that these interventions led to significant improvements in learning and cognitive outcomes.

Evidence from studies using observational data indicates that reversing stunting or achieving catch-up growth among school-age children leads to gains in learning and cognition. Some of these studies used data from the Young Lives child cohort study in Ethiopia, India, Peru, and Vietnam, which follows children from infancy through childhood and adolescence. In particular, the studies by Crookston and others (2013), Crookston and others (2014), Fink and Rockers (2014), and Georgiadis and others (2016) found evidence that children who experienced higher growth, as measured by the change in HAZ, in early primary school years and in adolescence performed better in reading comprehension, vocabulary, and mathematics tests and were less likely to be over-age for their grade than were children with slower growth across the four countries.

Although this evidence is suggestive, it is not conclusive regarding whether catch-up growth among school-age children leads to improvements in learning and cognitive outcomes.

Two studies used observational data to address this issue and to identify the causal effect on cognitive development of growth during school-age years. The first study is by Glewwe and King (2001), who investigated the impact of growth at different periods (from conception to age two years and from ages two to eight years) on the intelligence quotient (IQ) test score of children from the Philippines. The key finding of this study was that only growth in the second year after birth had a significant and positive effect on IQ test scores. The second study is by Georgiadis (2016), who investigated the impact of higher growth during early primary school years, compared with the period from conception to infancy and from infancy through just before starting primary school, on children's achievement in mathematics and vocabulary tests using data from the Young Lives study. In particular, Georgiadis (2016) compared the test scores of children who experienced different growth in these periods as a result of local weather conditions that, in turn, led to differential exposure to pathogens related to parasitic infection. The methodological approach of this study is based on instrumental variables that produce valid results as long as local weather conditions affect cognitive achievement only by influencing child growth. Georgiadis (2016) presents a range of tests that support this key assumption and thereby the validity of his conclusions. His findings suggest that growth in utero and in infancy and its impact on cognitive development can be reversed through parental promotion of nutrition and cognitive development in school-age years.

CONCLUSIONS

The evidence reviewed in this chapter suggests that the effects of early deprivation do not necessarily persist throughout life, especially if environmental circumstances change. Consistent with Golden's (1994) claim that substantial catch-up growth is possible at school age, we find that trajectories of child growth and cognitive development respond rather strongly to growth-promoting interventions after age two years, as summarized by the evidence in table 8.1. Of course, this does not mean that catch-up growth and improvements in cognitive functioning in school-age children always happen; it just means that there is very little evidence to support the notion that early deficits are irreversible, as concluded in the original work by Golden (1994).

Table 8.1 Findings of Studies on the Possibility of Catch-Up Growth

Study	Source of changed conditions	Description	Quantitative findings
Schumacher, Pawson, and Kretchmer 1987	Immigration	Immigrant children ages 5–12 years with low HAZ were studied upon their arrival in the United States and after one year.	On average, 0.1 standard deviation improvement in HAZ occurred after about one year.
Mjönes 1987	Immigration	The growth of school-age children who were born in Turkey and immigrated to Sweden was compared with the growth of Turkish children born in Sweden.	Immigrant children were short on arrival but caught up to heights of ethnically similar children born in Sweden.
Steckel 1987	Improved diet and lower exposure to infection (inference)	Anthropometric data were analyzed from logs of tens of thousands of American slaves between 1820 and 1860.	As children, slaves were about the first or second centile for height; as late adolescents, they exceeded the 25th centile.
Komlos 1986	Move to boarding school	Anthropometric data were analyzed from students who were born between 1775 and 1815 and who attended Hapsburg military schools.	The boys, who were stunted at admission, exhibited sizable catch-up, potentially attributable to improved diet and living conditions.
King and Taitz 1985	Foster care and adoption	Growth of previously abused children was tracked following (1) long-term placement in foster care or adoption or (2) short-term placement in foster care.	The children experienced significant improvements in both HAZ and WAZ, with the long-term foster care group showing the greatest improvement.

table continues next page

Table 8.1 Findings of Studies on the Possibility of Catch-Up Growth (continued)

Study	Source of changed conditions	Description	Quantitative findings
Abrams and others 2003	Micronutrient supplementation	Children ages 6–11 years were administered a beverage fortified with 12 micronutrients for eight weeks.	The treatment group on average gained 0.17 standard deviation in WAZ, significantly different from the 0.08 standard deviation gain in the control group.
Ash and others 2003	Micronutrient supplementation	Children ages 6–11 years were administered a beverage fortified with 10 micronutrients for six months.	The treatment group on average gained 3.2 centimeters in height, significantly different from the 2.6 centimeter gain in the control group.
Cooper and others 1995	Deworming	Children with intense trichuriasis associated with *Trichuris* dysentery syndrome and severe stunting were dewormed.	Six months after deworming, the children exhibited growth in mean height and weight that was two standard deviations greater than the growth of British children their age.
Stephenson and others 1993	Deworming	Primary school boys in a high-prevalence area were given a single dose of deworming treatment and followed up with four months later.	The treatment group exhibited rapid gain in weight, 1.0 kilogram more than the control group, across the four months of the study.

Note: HAZ = height-for-age z-score; WAZ = weight-for-age z-score.

The significant remaining task is to develop and evaluate a range of interventions, including intensive interventions that can be introduced over time into a policy broader than now exists for reaching disadvantaged children throughout their lifecycle. That many of the studies most relevant to understanding catch-up growth and its implication for cognitive development are now decades old points to the need for revitalizing the research and development agenda.

NOTE

World Bank Income Classifications as of July 2014 are as follows, based on estimates of gross national income (GNI) per capita for 2013:

- Low-income countries (LICs) = US$1,045 or less
- Middle-income countries (MICs) are subdivided:
  a) lower-middle-income = US$1,046 to US$4,125
  b) upper-middle-income (UMICs) = US$4,126 to US$12,745
- High-income countries (HICs) = US$12,746 or more.

REFERENCES

Abrams, S. A., A. Mushi, D. C. Hilmers, I. J. Griffin, P. Davila, and others. 2003. "A Multinutrient-Fortified Beverage Enhances the Nutritional Status of Children in Botswana." *Journal of Nutrition* 133 (6): 1834–40.

Adelman, S., H. Alderman, D. O. Gilligan, and J. Konde-Lule. 2008. "The Impact of Alternative Food for Education Programs on Child Nutrition in Northern Uganda." International Food Policy Research Institute, Washington, DC.

Adrianzen, T. B., J. M. Baertl, and G. G. Graham. 1973. "Growth of Children from Extremely Poor Families." *American Journal of Clinical Nutrition* 26: 926–30.

Agarwal, D. K., K. N. Agarwal, and S. K. Upadhyay. 1989. "Effect of Mid-Day Meal Programme on Physical Growth and Mental Function." *Indian Journal of Medical Research* 90: 163–74.

Ahuja, A., S. Baird, J. Hamory Hicks, M. Kremer, and E. Miguel. 2017. "Economics of Mass Deworming Programs." In *Disease Control Priorities* (third edition): Volume 8, *Child and Adolescent Health and Development*, edited by D. A. P. Bundy, N. de Silva, S. Horton, D. T. Jamison, and G. C. Patton. Washington, DC: World Bank.

Ash, D. M., S. R. Tatala, E. A. Frongillo, G. D. Ndossi, and M. C. Latham. 2003. "Randomized Efficacy Trial of a Micronutrient-Fortified Beverage in Primary School Children in Tanzania." *American Journal of Clinical Nutrition* 77 (4): 891–98.

Baertl, J. M., T. B. Adrianzen, and G. G. Graham. 1976. "Growth of Previously Well-Nourished Infants in Poor Homes." *American Journal of the Diseases of Children* 130 (1): 33–36.

Bailey, K. V. 1962. "Rural Nutrition Studies in Indonesia. IX: Feeding Trial on Schoolboys." *Tropical and Geographical Medicine* 14: 129–39.

Barr, D. G., D. H. Schmerling, and A. Prader. 1972. "Catch-Up Growth in Malnutrition Studied in Celiac Disease after Institution of Gluten-Free Diet." *Pediatric Research* 6: 521–27.

Best, C., N. Neufingerl, J. M. Del Rosso, C. Transler, T. van den Briel, and others. 2011. "Can Multi-Micronutrient Food Fortification Improve the Micronutrient Status, Growth, Health, and Cognition of School Children? A Systematic Review." *Nutrition Reviews* 69 (4): 186–204.

Bodé, S. H., E. H. Bachmann, E. Gudmand-Høyer, and G. B. Jensen. 1991. "Stature of Adult Coeliac Patients: No Evidence for Decreased Attained Height." *European Journal of Clinical Nutrition* 45 (3): 145–49.

Boersma, B., B. J. Otten, G. B. A. Stoelinga, and J. M. Wit. 1996. "Catch-Up Growth after Prolonged Hypothyroidism." *European Journal of Pediatrics* 155 (5): 362–67.

Brown, K. H., J. M. Peerson, J. Rivera, and L. H. Allen. 2002. "Effect of Supplemental Zinc on the Growth and Serum Zinc Concentrations of Prepubertal Children: A Meta-Analysis of Randomized Controlled Trials." *American Journal of Clinical Nutrition* 75 (6): 1062–71.

Bundy, D. A. P., N. de Silva, S. Horton, G. C. Patton, L. Schultz, and D. T. Jamison. 2017. "Child and Adolescent Health and Development: Realizing Neglected Potential." In *Disease Control Priorities* (third edition): Volume 8, *Child and Adolescent Health and Development*, edited by D. A. P. Bundy, N. de Silva, S. Horton, D. T. Jamison, and G. C. Patton. Washington, DC: World Bank.

Bundy, D. A. P., L. Appleby, M. Bradley, K. Croke, T. D. Hollingsworth, and others. 2017. "Mass Deworming Programs in Middle Childhood and Adolescence." In *Disease Control Priorities* (third edition): Volume 8, *Child and Adolescent Health and Development*, edited by D. A. P. Bundy, N. de Silva, S. Horton, D. T. Jamison, and G. C. Patton. Washington, DC: World Bank.

Burns, E. C., J. M. Tanner, M. A. Preece, and N. Cameron. 1981. "Final Height and Pubertal Development in 55 Children with Idiopathic Growth Hormone Deficiency, Treated for between 2 and 15 Years with Human Growth Hormone." *European Journal of Pediatrics* 137: 155–64.

Buttenheim, A., H. Alderman, and J. Friedman. 2011. "Impact Evaluation of School Feeding Programs in Lao PDR." Policy Research Working Paper 5518, Development Research Group, World Bank, Washington, DC.

Cacciari, E., G. R. Corazza, S. Salardi, M. G. Pascucci, M. Tacconi, and others. 1991. "What Will Be the Adult Height of Coeliac Patients?" *European Journal of Pediatrics* 150 (6): 407–9.

Cooper, E. S., E. M. Duff, S. Howell, and D. A. P. Bundy. 1995. "'Catch-Up' Growth Velocities after Treatment for *Trichuris* Dysentery Syndrome." *Transactions of the Royal Society of Tropical Medicine and Hygiene* 89 (6): 653.

Crookston, B. T., R. Forste, C. McClellan, A. Georgiadis, and T. Heaton. 2014. "Factors Associated with Cognitive Achievement in Late Childhood and Adolescence: The Young Lives Cohort Study of Children in Ethiopia, India, Peru, and Vietnam." *BMC Pediatrics* 14 (253): 1–9.

Crookston, B. T., W. Schott, S. Cueto, K. A. Dearden, P. Engle, and others. 2013. "Postinfancy Growth, Schooling, and Cognitive Achievement: Young Lives." *American Journal of Clinical Nutrition* 98: 1555–63.

Cueto, S., E. Jacoby, and E. Pollitt. 1998. "Breakfast Prevents Delays of Attention and Memory Functions among Nutritionally At-Risk Boys." *Journal of Applied Developmental Psychology* 19: 219–34.

Damen, G. M., B. Boersma, J. M. Wit, and H. S. A. Heymans. 1994. "Catch-Up Growth in 60 Children with Celiac Disease." *Journal of Pediatric Gastroenterology and Nutrition* 19 (4): 394–400.

Davies, J. H., H. L. Storr, K. Davies, J. P. Monson, G. M. Besser, and others. 2005. "Final Adult Height and Body Mass Index after Cure of Paediatric Cushing's Disease." *Clinical Endocrinology* 62 (4): 466–72.

Devadas, R. P., S. Jamala, V. A. Surabhi, and N. K. Murthy. 1979. "Evaluation of a Food Supplement to School Children." *Indian Journal of Nutrition and Dietetics* 16: 335–41.

Du, X., K. Zhu, A. Trube, Q. Zhang, G. Ma, and others. 2004. "School-Milk Intervention Trial Enhances Growth and Bone Mineral Accretion in Chinese Girls Aged 10–12 Years in Beijing." *British Journal of Nutrition* 92 (1): 159–68.

Fink, G., and P. C. Rockers. 2014. "Childhood Growth, Schooling, and Cognitive Development: Further Evidence from the Young Lives Study." *American Journal of Clinical Nutrition* 100: 182–88.

Georgiadis, A. 2016. "The Sooner the Better, but It's Never Too Late: The Impact of Nutrition at Different Stages of Childhood on Cognitive Achievement." Young Lives Working Paper 159.

Georgiadis, A., L. Benny, B. T. Crookston, L. T. Duc, P. Hermida, and others. 2016. "Growth Trajectories from Conception through Middle Childhood and Cognitive Achievement at Age 8 Years: Evidence from Four Low- and Middle-Income Countries." *Social Science and Medicine Population Health* 2: 43–54. doi.org/10.1016/j.ssmph.2016.01.003.

Gertler, P, J. Heckman, R. Pinto, A. Zanolini, C. Vermeersch, and others. 2014. "Labor Market Returns to an Early Childhood Stimulation Intervention in Jamaica." *Science* 344: 998–1001.

Glewwe, P., and E. King. 2001. "The Impact of Early Childhood Nutritional Status on Cognitive Development: Does the Timing of Malnutrition Matter?" *World Bank Economic Review* 15: 81–113.

Golden, M. H. N. 1994. "Is Complete Catch-Up Possible for Stunted Malnourished Children?" *European Journal of Clinical Nutrition* 48 (Suppl 1): S58–70.

Graham, G. G., and T. B. Adrianzen. 1971. "Growth, Inheritance, and Environment." *Pediatrics Research* 5: 691–97.

———. 1972. "Late 'Catch-Up' Growth after Severe Infantile Malnutrition." *Johns Hopkins Medical Journal* 131 (3): 204–11.

Grillenberger, M., C. G. Neumann, S. P. Murphy, N. O. Bwibo, P. van't Veer, and others. 2003. "Food Supplements Have a Positive Impact on Weight Gain and the Addition of Animal Source Foods Increases Lean Body Mass of Kenyan Schoolchildren." *Journal of Nutrition* 133 (11): S3957–64.

Hall, A., G. Hewitt, V. Tuffrey, and N. de Silva. 2008. "A Review and Meta-Analysis of the Impact of Intestinal Worms on Child Growth and Nutrition." *Maternal and Child Nutrition* 4: 118–236.

Kazianga, H., D. de Walque, and H. Alderman. 2014. "School Feeding Programs, Intrahousehold Allocation, and the Nutrition of Siblings: Evidence from a Randomized Trial in Rural Burkina Faso." *Journal of Development Economics* 106: 15–34.

Kemp, S. F., J. Kuntze, K. M. Attie, T. Maneatis, S. Butler, and others. 2005. "Efficacy and Safety Results of Long-Term Growth Hormone Treatment of Idiopathic Short Stature." *Journal of Clinical Endocrinology and Metabolism* 90 (9): 5247–53.

King, J. M., and L. S. Taitz. 1985. "Catch-Up Growth Following Abuse." *Archives of Disease in Childhood* 60: 1152–54.

Komlos, J. 1986. "Patterns of Children's Growth in East-Central Europe in the Eighteenth Century." *Annals of Human Biology* 13: 33–48.

Kristjansson, B., M. Petticrew, B. MacDonald, J. Krasevec, L. Janzen, and others. 2007. "School Feeding for Improving the Physical and Psychosocial Health of Disadvantaged Students." *Cochrane Database of Systematic Reviews* 1 (CD004676).

Lien, N. M., K. K. Meyer, and M. Winick. 1977. "Early Malnutrition and 'Late' Adoption: A Study of Their Effects on the Development of Korean Orphans Adopted into American Families." *American Journal of Clinical Nutrition* 30: 1734–39.

Martorell, R., L. K. Khan, and D. G. Schroeder. 1994. "Reversibility of Stunting: Epidemiological Findings in Children from Developing Countries." *European Journal of Clinical Nutrition* 48 (Suppl 1): S45–57.

Mjönes, S. 1987. "Growth in Turkish Children in Stockholm." *Annals of Human Biology* 14: 337–47.

Muthayya, S., T. Thomas, K. Srinivasan, K. Rao, A. Kurpad, and others. 2007. "Consumption of a Mid-Morning Snack Improves Memory but Not Attention in School Children." *Physiology and Behavior* 90: 142–50.

Nokes, C., S. M. Grantham-McGregor, A. W. Sawyer, E. S. Cooper, B. A. Robinson, and others. 1992. "Moderate to Heavy Infections of *Trichuris trichiura* Affect Cognitive Function in Jamaican School Children." *Parasitology* 104 (3): 539–47.

Pantsiotou, S., R. Stanhope, M. Uruena, M. A. Preece, and D. B. Grant. 1991. "Growth Prognosis and Growth after Menarche in Primary Hypothyroidism." *Archives of Disease in Childhood* 66: 838–40.

Powell, C. A., S. P. Walker, S. M. Chang, and S. M. Grantham-McGregor. 1998. "Nutrition and Education: A Randomized Trial of the Effects of Breakfast in Rural Primary School Children." *American Journal of Clinical Nutrition* 68: 873–79.

Prader, A., J. M. Tanner, and G. A. von Harnack. 1963. "Catch-Up Growth Following Illness or Starvation." *Journal of Pediatrics* 62: 646–59.

Proos, L. A., Y. Hofvander, and T. Tuvemo. 1991a. "Menarcheal Age and Growth Pattern of Indian Girls Adopted in Sweden. II: Catch-Up Growth and Final Height." *Indian Journal of Pediatrics* 58: 105–14.

———. 1991b. "Menarcheal Age and Growth Pattern of Indian Girls Adopted in Sweden. I: Menarcheal Age." *Acta Paediatrica Scandinavica* 80: 852–58.

Ramakrishnan, U., N. Aburto, G. McCabe, and R. Martorell. 2004. "Multimicronutrient Interventions but Not Vitamin A or Iron Interventions Alone Improve Child Growth: Results of 3 Meta-Analyses." *Journal of Nutrition* 134 (10): 2592–602.

Rivkees, S. A., H. H. Bode, and J. D. Crawford. 1988. "Long-Term Growth in Juvenile Acquired Hypothyroidism: The Failure to Achieve Normal Adult Stature." *New England Journal of Medicine* 318 (10): 599–602.

Schumacher, L. B., I. G. Pawson, and N. Kretchmer. 1987. "Growth of Immigrant Children in the Newcomer Schools of San Francisco." *Pediatrics* 80: 861–68.

Soewondo, S., M. Husaini, and E. Pollitt. 1989. "Effects of Iron Deficiency on Attention and Learning Processes in Preschool Children: Bandung, Indonesia." *American Journal of Clinical Nutrition* 50: 667–74.

Steckel, R. H. 1987. "Growth Depression and Recovery: The Remarkable Case of American Slaves." *Annals of Human Biology* 14: 111–32.

Stephenson, L. S., M. C. Latham, E. J. Adams, S. N. Kinoti, and A. Pertet. 1993. "Physical Fitness, Growth, and Appetite of Kenyan School Boys with Hookworm, *Trichuris trichiura*, and *Ascaris lumbricoides* Infections Are Improved Four Months after a Single Dose of Albendazole." *Journal of Nutrition* 123 (6): 1036–46.

Taylor-Robinson, D. C., N. Maayan, K. Soares-Weiser, S. Donegan, and P. Garner. 2012. "Deworming Drugs for Soil-Transmitted Intestinal Worms in Children: Effects on Nutritional Indicators, Haemoglobin, and School Performance." *Cochrane Database of Systematic Reviews* 11 (CD000371). doi:10.1002/14651858.CD000371.pub5.

Van Pareren, Y., H. Duivenvoorden, F. Slijper, H. Koot, and A. Hokken-Koelega. 2004. "Intelligence and Psychosocial Functioning during Long-Term Growth Hormone Therapy in Children Born Small for Gestational Age." *Journal of Clinical Endocrinology and Metabolism* 89 (11): 5295–302.

Victora, C. G., L. Adair, C. Fall, P. C. Hallal, R. Martorell, and others. 2008. "Maternal and Child Undernutrition: Consequences for Adult Health and Human Capital." *The Lancet* 371 (9609): 340–57.

Winick, M., K. K. Meyer, and R. C. Harris. 1975. "Malnutrition and Environmental Enrichment by Early Adoption." *Science* 190: 1173–75.

Zimmermann, M., K. Connolly, M. Bozo, J. Bridson, F. Rohner, and others. 2006. "Iodine Supplementation Improves Cognition in Iodine-Deficient Schoolchildren in Albania: A Randomized, Controlled, Double-Blind Study." *American Journal of Clinical Nutrition* 83 (1): 108–14.

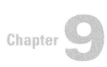

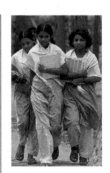

Puberty, Developmental Processes, and Health Interventions

Russell M. Viner, Nicholas B. Allen, and George C. Patton

INTRODUCTION

Adolescence is increasingly recognized as a critical period in the life course, a time when rapid development of the brain, body, and behaviors opens a window of opportunity for interventions that may affect health throughout life.

Puberty results in very rapid somatic growth, brain development, sexual maturation, and attainment of reproductive capacity. It is accompanied by final maturation of multiple organ systems and major changes in the central nervous system and in psychosocial behavior (Patton and Viner 2007). The discovery of continued brain development through adolescence is one of the great advances of neuroscience in the past 20 years. A dramatic spurt in brain development begins during adolescence and continues until the mid-20s, with marked development of both cortical and subcortical structures (Goddings and others 2012).

This rapid development in the body and brain interacts with social changes, including increasing individuation and new peer groups, to facilitate transitions important for individuals to function as productive adults (World Bank 2006). A range of social determinants of health arise in adolescence, with peers, schools, and eventually the workplace becoming strong determinants of health and well-being as the influence of the family wanes (Viner and others 2012). These social changes are apparent even in traditional or more sociocentric cultures. More than half of the top 10 risk factors identified in the Global Burden of Disease study (GBD 2013 Risk Factors Collaborators 2015) are largely determined during adolescence.

Adolescence is also a time when young people may modify or alter the pathways to adult health or illness (Viner and others 2012). Early life experiences may reinforce both good and poor trajectories. Similarly, resilience during adolescence may improve outcomes for young people born into adversity. The transfer from primary to secondary school, sexual debut, and entry into the labor market may be critical points for preventing the accumulation of health risk (Viner and others 2012).

This chapter outlines the key dynamics of adolescent development and examines how they provide opportunities for intervention. Definitions of age groups and age specific terminology used in this volume can be found in chapter 1 (Bundy and others 2017).

PUBERTY AND DEVELOPMENTAL PROCESSES

Puberty is a time of rapid growth in all body systems and changes in brain function and cognitive development (Patton and Viner 2007).

Stages of Puberty

The process of puberty begins earlier than most recognize, that is, between the ages of six and eight years with the early phase of adrenarche, the turning on of the

Corresponding author: Russell M. Viner, UCL Institute of Child Health, University College London, London, United Kingdom; r.viner@ucl.ac.uk.

adrenal glands. Adrenarche has few phenotypic signs in most children, but increasing evidence indicates that adrenal androgens may contribute to the structural and functional development of the brain and associated behaviors in adolescence (Whittle and others 2015). The timing of adrenarche affects the risks for mental health problems (Mundy and others 2015) and a range of cardiometabolic issues. Body mass index (BMI) is associated with adrenal androgens (Corvalan, Uauy, and Mericq 2013); children exhibiting premature adrenarche have been found to have higher levels of insulin and insulin resistance and a predisposition to higher BMI (Ibáñez and others 2008).

The second phase of puberty is gonadarche, the process of sexual maturation and achievement of reproductive capacity (Marshall and Tanner 1968). The production of gonadal steroids stimulates the growth and development of secondary sexual characteristics; it also kindles development across all organ systems, including the central nervous system. Other endocrine systems mature during puberty, including the growth hormone/insulin-like growth factor and thyroid axes.

Marshall and Tanner (1968) developed a system for identifying stages in the external signs of puberty. The earliest external changes—breast buds in girls and testicular enlargement in boys—typically appear about age 11 years, but vary among individuals. Despite a similar age of gonadarche in boys, these early changes are more visible in girls. Menarche, the onset of menstrual periods (menses), typically occurs in late puberty, approximately two years after breast budding. While menses appears to signal reproductive maturity for girls, it largely signals maturity of the uterus because early menstrual periods are irregular and girls are rarely fertile immediately after menarche (Hochberg and Belsky 2013).

Puberty is generally complete within two to four years following gonadarche, but other changes including fat and muscle patterning continue through adolescence. The timing of puberty is partly genetic (Day and others 2016), but intrauterine events, nutrition, family factors, stress, and socioeconomic conditions also play roles (Hochberg and Belsky 2013).

Puberty is increasingly recognized as a time of distinct transitional physiology (Rosenfeld and Nicodemus 2003). The most dramatic change is the pubertal growth spurt, with boys typically growing 30 centimeters and girls growing 25–27 centimeters due to synergy between the sex steroids and growth hormone (Abbassi 1998). For girls, the growth spurt occurs early, with peak growth typically occurring about the time of the start of breast development. For boys, it occurs later. Girls typically stop growing by the end of puberty, adding only about 2.5 centimeters after the

beginning of menses. Boys continue growing slowly after the end of puberty, achieving final height at about age 18 years.

The bone, renal, immune, and cardiovascular systems are also developing, and liver enzymes and blood lipids are maturing. Bone mineral accretion accelerates during puberty under the influence of gonadal steroids, with peak bone mass achieved by the early 20s (Loud and Gordon 2006). Cardiovascular and renal development means that blood pressure and heart rate make a transition to adult values, in parallel with growth in height and mass. The cardiovascular risk profile differs between the genders, with more adverse lipid patterns among boys than girls. Other blood markers, such as hemoglobin levels, similarly change to a sexually dimorphic pattern.

Timing of Puberty

The sequence of pubertal events is remarkably consistent across countries and ethnic groups, although timing varies by country. The timing of puberty is influenced partly by genetics, but largely by nutrition and economic development (Hochberg and Belsky 2013). The mean age at menarche is now 12–13 years in most high-income countries (HICs); it is usually later in low-income countries, even in affluent populations (Parent and others 2003).

The mean age of menarche stopped falling in most HICs after the 1960s, but it is still falling in low-income countries. However, data from the United States (Herman-Giddens and others 1997) and, more recently, Europe (Parent and others 2016) suggest that early pubertal events are occurring at younger ages but that late pubertal events are not. The reasons for this broadening of puberty are unclear, although exposure to endocrine disrupter chemicals and psychosocial stress are possible mechanisms (Parent and others 2016). Recent studies have suggested that earlier pubertal development is likely a response to changing environmental circumstances (Gluckman and Hanson 2006; Hochberg and Belsky 2013). By contrast, the timing of adrenarche appears to be relatively constant across populations (Hochberg 2009).

Effects on Health and Disease

In addition to puberty's direct influences on physiology and growth, the timing of puberty appears to program changes in lifelong health. In particular, strong evidence indicates that higher BMI accelerates the onset of puberty (Burt Solorzano and McCartney 2010; Frisch 1984; Hochberg and Belsky 2013), but early puberty also programs individuals for greater fat accumulation over the life course (Power, Lake, and Cole 1997; Prentice and Viner 2013).

Early puberty is associated with cardiometabolic risk, increasing the risk of cardiovascular events and mortality, type 2 diabetes (Prentice and Viner 2013), and high blood pressure (Hardy and others 2006). These associations appear to be at least partly independent of childhood obesity (Prentice and Viner 2013). Mechanisms likely relate to stress reactivity, the growth hormone/insulin-like growth factor axis (Sandhu and others 2006), and glucose insulin homeostasis (Burt Solorzano and McCartney 2010).

Early puberty is linked to cancer in later life through several mechanisms. Longer exposure to gonadal steroids may increase the risk of steroid-dependent cancers such as breast and ovarian cancer in females (Ahlgren and others 2004; Jordan, Webb, and Green 2005) and possibly prostate cancer in males (Giles and others 2003). Mechanisms may include longer exposure to sex hormones, increased oxidative stress (Vincent and Taylor 2006), or hyperinsulinemia (Frezza, Wachtel, and Chiriva-Internati 2006) related to obesity in early developers or to behavioral risk factors such as substance use (Patton and Viner 2007).

Evolutionary Implications

The relationship of the timing of puberty to environment and nutrition has its origins in evolutionary biology. Severe environmental stress and malnutrition may result in delayed puberty, prioritizing the survival of the individual given that reproduction is not possible. Similarly, ideal environmental conditions may result in delayed puberty, maximizing the individual's later reproductive success. However, environmental stress that is not sufficient to threaten survival may accelerate pubertal development, increasing the likelihood of reproduction before death (Hochberg and Belsky 2013).

In this schema, adrenarche represents a point at which the environment can reprogram reproductive strategies (Del Giudice 2009). It may also allow children time to test their social status in a peer environment free from reproductive imperatives.

Accelerated puberty also increases health risk behaviors, such as early sexual activity and violence. Associations have been found between early pubertal development in girls and sexual abuse, severe psychosocial stress, and even absence of the father. For example, migrant children arriving in HICs frequently experience onset of puberty earlier than would be expected in either their home or host country. Their transition from a threatening to an ideal nutritional environment may accelerate their pubertal development (Hochberg and Belsky 2013).

In an evolutionary context, neurodevelopment during puberty is likely to optimize reproductive success by realigning emotional, social, and metabolic strategies to the external environment (Hochberg and Belsky 2013).

Brain Development

In adolescence, brain development involves two key processes: significant growth and change in regions of the prefrontal cortex (Paus, Keshavan, and Giedd 2008; Steinberg 2005) and improved connectivity between regions of the prefrontal cortex and regions of the limbic system (Casey 2015; Steinberg 2005). These changes are thought to underpin higher-order cognitive functions, such as reasoning, interpersonal interactions, the perception of both short- and long-term risk and reward, and the regulation of behavior and emotion (Paus, Keshavan, and Giedd 2008; Steinberg 2005).

Normative neurodevelopmental processes prepare the brain for responding to the demands of both adolescence and adult life, but may also make adolescents vulnerable to risk behavior and psychopathology (Paus, Keshavan, and Giedd 2008). Dual-system and imbalance models posit that adolescence is a particularly vulnerable period because of the imbalance between early maturation of the limbic motivational and emotional systems and slower, or later, development of the regulatory regions of the prefrontal cortex (Casey 2015). The dual-systems model emphasizes a developmentally normal mismatch between intense affective and behavioral reactions and motivations and limited capacity to regulate them (Steinberg 2005).

Recent studies, however, suggest a more complex picture (Mills and others 2014; Pfeifer and Allen 2012). For example, brain-imaging studies in adolescents do not provide consistent support for the association between immaturity in the frontal cortex and the emergence of risk behavior and psychopathology (Crone and Dahl 2012).

Recent attempts to quantify brain maturation have used measures of the whole brain, such as network-based measurements of resting-state brain function that are independent of specific tasks (Dosenbach and others 2010) or structural data from magnetic resonance imaging (Vértes and Bullmore 2015). Some of these measures may be related to both the emergence of more integrated self-regulatory abilities and plasticity in response to new learning experiences (Crone and Dahl 2012; Dosenbach and others 2010). However, the relationship between these neurodevelopmental patterns and cognitive, affective, and behavioral changes in adolescence is not fully understood.

Cognitive Development

Cognitive domains, including learning, reasoning, information processing, and memory, improve as adolescents develop. Executive functioning capabilities, which facilitate self-regulation of thoughts, actions, and emotions, continue to develop in parallel with changes in the prefrontal cortex (Kesek, Zelazo, and Lewis 2008). These increases in self-regulatory control are thought to support deductive reasoning; information processing; efficiency; and the capacity for abstract, planned, hypothetical, and multidimensional thinking (Steinberg 2005).

Cognitive and Affective Processing

Recent research has focused on both cognitive and affective processing, particularly regarding how these processes interact and influence each other in the context of decision making. First, cognitive skills allow improved self-regulation of affect—the capacity to initiate new or alter ongoing emotional responses—to achieve a goal (Ochsner and Gross 2005). Second, affective influences on cognitive processing, including decision making, risk taking, and judgment, change significantly during adolescence (Hartley and Somerville 2015; Steinberg 2005).

The social and emotional context for cognitive processing during adolescence may include factors such as the presence of peers or the value of performing a task, which are hypothesized to influence the motivational salience of specific contexts and the extent to which cognitive processing is recruited (Johnson, Grossmann, and Kadosh 2009). Moreover, some of these changes in cognitive and affective processing are linked to the onset of puberty (Crone and Dahl 2012), with flexibility of the frontal cortical network greater in adolescence than in adulthood (Jolles and others 2012).

Temporal Discounting

Temporal discounting refers to the inclination to discount the value of future rewards as compared with immediate ones (Christakou, Brammer, and Rubia 2011). This tendency declines sharply between ages 15 and 16 years (de Water, Cillessen, and Scheres 2014). Moreover, the neurobiological basis for temporal discounting is related to developmental changes in dopamine activity (Pine and others 2010). Specifically, increases are evident in both dopaminergic connectivity to the prefrontal cortex (Kalsbeek and others 1988; Verney and others 1982) and the density of dopamine transporters (Spear 2000). Dopamine receptors are overproduced in early adolescence, followed by pruning that is more evident in subcortical than in prefrontal regions (Spear 2000). The net effect is to shift the relative balance between subcortical and cortical dopaminergic systems, with increasing dominance across adolescence of the system responsible for valuing future rewards.

The impact of temporal discounting is consistent with the observed association between adolescence and risk-taking behaviors, despite adequate knowledge of risks (Steinberg 2005). It also suggests that affective valuation of immediate versus long-term outcomes (as opposed to conceptual understanding of them) is likely to be the main way in which adolescent decision making deviates from mature (adult-like) decision making.

Sensitivity to Peer Influence

Adolescents assign greater weight than adults to social outcomes such as peer acceptance. During the transition from childhood to adolescence, the amount of time spent with peers increases dramatically (Brown 2004) and peer and family values increasingly diverge (Gardner and Steinberg 2005; Steinberg 2008). These changes suggest that teenagers are less resistant to peer pressure than either children or adults, although susceptibility to peer influence per se declines over the course of adolescence (Steinberg and Monahan 2007).

Neuroscientific research has begun to explore this resistance to peer influence. Grosbras and others (2007) studied children age 10 years with high or low resistance to peer influence and found that, while viewing angry hand gestures and facial expressions, those with high resistance to peer influence showed more coordinated brain responses across parts of the brain associated with processing nonverbal behavior and with planning and executing movement. The better the brain is at coordinating its response to other people's nonverbal emotional expressions across the emotional and self-regulation networks of the brain, the better the person is at resisting peer influence. Consistent with this, Pfeifer and others (2011) found that adolescents who are better at resisting peer influence have greater activity in a region of the brain involved in reward, positive affect, and emotional regulation.

Executive Control

The literature on the structural and functional changes associated with brain maturation suggests a model in which some regions are tightly integrated into long-range networks, while other regions are segregated into short-range networks. Fjell and others (2012) demonstrated that developmental changes in cognitive control were associated with both the surface area of the anterior cingulate cortex and the properties of large fiber connections. Crone and Dahl (2012) proposed that because these patterns of long-range connectivity are still maturing, some aspects of executive control may be less automatic and more flexible during adolescence, resulting in greater vulnerability when performing attentional and decision-making tasks under high demands (because the ability to integrate control is less automatic) and enabling adolescents to respond in novel and adaptive ways. Thus, specific learning or training experiences during adolescence may guide the final connectivity patterns in some of these long-range cognitive control networks.

ADOLESCENCE AS A TIME OF RISK

The developmental changes that occur in adolescence create greater vulnerability to emotional and behavioral dysregulation (Steinberg 2005).

Although adolescents are relatively physically healthy compared with other age groups, adolescence is a key phase of life for the establishment of risk factors for several highly burdensome diseases. The transition into early adolescence is marked by dramatic increases in morbidity and mortality, often associated with mental health disorders, substance use, and the consequences of risk taking and poor decision making (Blum and Nelson-Mmari 2004; Williams, Holmbeck, and Greenley 2002). The majority of mental health and substance use problems begin before age 21 years (Jones 2013), and poor health outcomes during adolescence may have ongoing and negative impacts on adult life (Sawyer and others 2012). For example, major non-communicable diseases, such as heart disease and cancer, are acutely sensitive to lifestyle and behavioral risk factors that are often established during adolescence, such as nutrition, physical activity, sleep, obesity, stress, and substance use (Lowry and others 1996). The dramatic changes occurring in the brain during adolescence also make this a time of significant neuroplasticity, suggesting that behavioral patterns can become strongly encoded in the brain during this time (Crone and Dahl 2012).

Aggression and Violence

Aggression, including bullying and violence, increases dramatically and peaks in middle adolescence (Krug and others 2002; Patton and Viner 2007). Given the known effects of testosterone on aggression in animals and humans (Archer 1991), researchers focused on the relationship between puberty and aggression in males (Olweus and others 1988). More recently, large-scale studies have found good evidence that the risk of violence and aggression increases with pubertal stage in boys (Hemphill and others 2010).

Depression

Considerable evidence demonstrates that early puberty increases the risk of depression in girls (Hayward and others 1997; Kaltiala-Heino, Kosunen, and Rimpelä 2003; Kaltiala-Heino and others 2003; Mendle, Turkheimer, and Emery 2007). Angold, Costello, and Worthman (1998) found that pubertal stage predicts the risk of major depression in adolescents better than age. Rates of depression are higher in boys than in girls before puberty, but are higher in adult women than in adult men. Girls begin to surpass boys in depression at stage-3 puberty. Puberty may even reduce the prevalence of depression in males (Angold, Costello, and Worthman 1998).

Anxiety

Anxiety disorders increase markedly in both sexes during adolescence. However, the evidence for an association with pubertal timing is much less clear for anxiety than for depression. A recent review of more than 45 empirical studies found only moderate-quality evidence that both earlier timing and more advanced pubertal stage increase anxiety or symptoms in girls after adjusting for age. Findings for boys are even less robust (Reardon, Leen-Feldner, and Hayward 2009).

There is little evidence regarding anxiety disorders. Hayward and others (1992) found an association between panic attacks and pubertal stage, but Graber and others (1997) found no association between anxiety disorders and pubertal timing in boys or girls.

Deliberate Self-Harm

Deliberate self-harm, a major risk factor for suicide, rises sharply in early adolescence. In young women, it peaks about age 15–16 years and falls thereafter (Hawton and others 2002; Madge and others 2008). The literature on puberty and deliberate self-harm is much smaller than that on depression or anxiety. In a large population-based study, strong associations between deliberate self-harm and pubertal stage (adjusted for age) were attenuated when models were adjusted for depressive symptoms, showing that this association was largely or entirely mediated by depression (Patton and others 2007).

Eating Disorders

There is a strong association between puberty and eating disorders, at least in girls. A recent systematic review identified advanced pubertal status or early pubertal timing as a risk factor for eating disorders or disordered eating in more than 40 studies in girls and more than 20 studies in boys. Early-maturing girls and boys have higher risk of a range of eating disorders, including anorexia nervosa and bulimia nervosa, as well as symptoms of eating disorders, including dissatisfaction with body, weight, or shape (Klump 2013). However, some studies found no association between eating disorders and puberty, particularly in boys, and others reported an association between early or advanced puberty and improved body image (McCabe, Ricciardelli, and Banfield 2001).

Physical Health

Less recognized are associations between puberty and physical illnesses. Puberty coincides with a rise in prevalence of many autoimmune conditions and a marked shift in gender ratio toward females (Beeson 1994). In both genders, type 1 diabetes begins in early puberty, although the peak age of onset occurs approximately two years earlier in girls than in boys, reflecting differences in pubertal timing (Pundziute-Lycka and others 2002). Early puberty is an independent risk factor for the persistence of asthma into adolescence and severity of asthma in adulthood (Varraso and others 2005). Seizures often become more frequent and new types of epilepsy emerge during adolescence (Klein, van Passel-Clark, and Pezzullo 2003). The pubertal growth spurt results in new musculoskeletal problems, and puberty is linked with various pain syndromes. The increase in back, facial, and stomach pains in early adolescence is associated with pubertal status in both sexes (LeResche and others 2005). Adult women have higher rates of migraine and tension headaches than adult men; this pattern is evident about age 11 years and is linked with puberty (Wedderkopp and others 2005).

ADOLESCENCE AS A TIME OF OPPORTUNITY

Adolescence is a key time for interventions to improve health. The benefits of intervention in early childhood are well described, and nations have made significant investments in maternal and child health and primary education (Commission on Social Determinants of Health 2008; Conti and Heckman 2012). Adolescence presents an opportunity to preserve investments made in childhood and to switch trajectories (Romeo 2010), while the emergence of new social determinants of health, such as peers, and connection with school, neighborhood, and workplace, offer new vehicles and venues for intervention.

Young people make five key transitions on the pathway to adulthood (World Bank 2006):

- Learning: Transition from primary to secondary schooling and from secondary to higher education
- Work: Transition from education into workforce
- Health: Transition to responsibility for own health
- Family: Transition from family living to autonomy, marriage, and parenthood
- Citizenship: Transition to responsible citizenship.

Transitions are accompanied by new behaviors, including the initiation of many health-related behaviors that track strongly into adult life. They are a time of great opportunity to tread new paths and embark on new trajectories toward health and well-being.

Secondary Education as a Health Intervention

Evidence is emerging that secondary education is efficacious against a range of health outcomes in adolescents and young adults, from sexually transmitted infections to adolescent fertility, mortality, and mental health (Patton and others 2016). Education is one of the strongest determinants of health and human capital (Commission on Social Determinants of Health 2008), and universal primary education is one of the key United Nations Millennium Development Goals. In both rich and poor countries, persons with more education live longer lives with less disability and ill health, and the relationship is likely to be causal (Baker and others 2011; Miyamoto and Chevalier 2010; Pradhan and others 2017, chapter 30 in this volume). The United Nations Sustainable Development Goals include a target for countries to provide every child with access to free primary and secondary education by 2030 (Barro 2013).[1]

Yet the health gains from secondary education have been studied less than those from primary education, despite a dramatic global expansion in the length of education in the past 30 years, with most gains in the late primary and early secondary years (IHME 2015). Among adults in HICs, upper-secondary education is most strongly associated with better health and mental health (Miyamoto and Chevalier 2010), although tertiary education confers additional benefits in U.S. studies (Case and Deaton 2015). Secondary education is known to promote better pregnancy and child health outcomes among adult women internationally (Grépin and Bharadwaj 2015; UNESCO 2010), and a small literature from Sub-Saharan African countries suggests that secondary schooling may have a stronger and more consistent effect on teenage fertility than primary education (Mahy and Gupta 2002).

Nutritional Interventions

Adolescence presents an opportunity to reverse earlier deficits from stunting or wasting in childhood (GBD 2013 Risk Factors Collaborators 2015). Nutritional sufficiency in adolescence is particularly important for pregnancy. Childbearing during adolescence places an additional nutritional burden on the mother and may explain some of the additional risk that pregnancy in adolescence poses to the 16 million teenagers who give birth annually and their offspring (Mundy and others 2015; Whittle and others 2015). Adolescent growth and development therefore provides an opportunity for preconception interventions to ensure adequate nutrition in adolescent girls. These issues are discussed in greater detail in chapter 11 in this volume (Lassi, Moin, and Bhutta 2017).

Psychosocial Interventions

Exposure to an enriching environment during adolescence may offset many of the negative neurobehavioral and physiological consequences of early life adversity (Romeo 2010). The onset of puberty marks the beginning of dramatic changes in the processing of rewards and emotional stimuli and social-cognitive reasoning (Crone and Dahl 2012). Efforts to sensitize young people to their social environment and push them to explore and engage provide opportunities to promote prosocial motivation and goals in early adolescence.

Furthermore, neurodevelopment likely affects a young person's ability to engage with or benefit from interventions, particularly those that target decision making and risk behaviors in peer and affective contexts. In particular, immaturity in cognitive processes, such as temporal discounting, may necessitate a different approach to intervention in early adolescents than in middle to late adolescents. Furthermore, adolescents are uniquely vulnerable to peer influences, both antisocial and prosocial, and this vulnerability can be used to enhance health outcomes. Indeed, resisting negative peer influences is important for self-regulation. Finally, specific experiences may affect neurodevelopment—psychosocial interventions may enhance self-regulation and can have benefits not only during adolescence but also later in life.

Research to date has yielded some efficacious early intervention and prevention approaches to mental disorders during adolescence. For example, both psychosocial and pharmacological treatments with established efficacy are available for treating depression (Kazdin 2003). In particular, research on interpersonal and cognitive behavioral therapy as well as on the use of fluoxetine found that 60 percent to 75 percent of adolescents will recover by the time of posttreatment assessment (Asarnow, Jaycox, and Tompson 2001; March and others 2004). Despite these favorable results, the long-term outcomes of current treatment approaches are unclear. One meta-analysis of psychotherapy for depression in youth found no lasting effects one year following treatment (Weisz, McCarty, and Valeri 2006).

Mental disorders, once established, are difficult to ameliorate fully, highlighting the importance of evidence-based strategies to prevent or slow the onset of disorders in vulnerable individuals. To achieve this goal, it is necessary to identify developmentally significant, modifiable risk factors and to target change in them.

In recent decades, numerous controlled studies have evaluated the effect of programs to prevent mental illness (Durlak and Wells 1997, 1998) and substance use (Tobler and others 2000); problems at school and depression (Gillham, Shatté, and Freres 2000); and aggression and behavior problems, especially in children (Tremblay, LeMarquand, and Vitaro 1999); along with many other conditions. These studies have shown that some programs may strengthen protective factors, such as social and problem-solving skills, stress management skills, prosocial behavior, and social support, and reduce the consequences of risk factors, symptoms, and substance use.

However, few studies have examined how to prevent the onset of case-level mental and substance use disorders, mainly because of the challenges associated with designing and funding studies with enough statistical power to detect such effects (Cuijpers 2003). Such programs have had modest effects (Horowitz and Garber 2006), and there is a need to ascertain which individuals are most likely to benefit from specific interventions. In sum, while prevention and intervention approaches delivered early in life are promising, there is a clear need to understand how to match interventions with individuals to increase their impact and cost-effectiveness.

CONCLUSIONS

Adolescence is a time of great developmental plasticity and risk for the onset of a range of disorders that can carry a high burden of disease throughout the lifespan. It offers a critical developmental window of opportunity for intervention and prevention. Puberty and brain development during adolescence are responsible for dramatic shifts in burden of disease, away from childhood conditions toward injuries and emerging noncommunicable diseases. Knowledge of the unique developmental processes that characterize adolescence and the role they play in both risk and opportunity during this phase of life is expanding rapidly. What remains is the task of translating this knowledge into intervention and prevention methods that target modifiable, developmentally sensitive mechanisms to maximize the effectiveness of intervention approaches during this phase of life.

NOTES

World Bank Income Classifications as of July 2014 are as follows, based on estimates of gross national income (GNI) per capita for 2013:

- Low-income countries (LICs) = US$1,045 or less
- Middle-income countries (MICs) are subdivided:
  a) lower-middle-income = US$1,046 to US$4,125
  b) upper-middle-income (UMICs) = US$4,126 to US$12,745
- High-income countries (HICs) = US$12,746 or more.

1. See the Sustainable Development Knowledge Platform, http://sustainabledevelopment.un.org/.

REFERENCES

Abbassi, V. 1998. "Growth and Normal Puberty." *Pediatrics* 102 (2, Pt 3): 507–11.

Ahlgren, M., M. Melbye, J. Wohlfahrt, and T. I. A. Sørensen. 2004. "Growth Patterns and the Risk of Breast Cancer in Women." *New England Journal of Medicine* 351 (16): 1619–26.

Angold, A., E. J. Costello, and C. M. Worthman. 1998. "Puberty and Depression: The Roles of Age, Pubertal Status, and Pubertal Timing." *Psychological Medicine* 28 (1): 51–61.

Archer, J. 1991. "The Influence of Testosterone on Human Aggression." *British Journal of Psychology* 82 (Pt 1): 1–28.

Asarnow, J. R., L. H. Jaycox, and M. C. Tompson. 2001. "Depression in Youth: Psychosocial Interventions." *Journal of Clinical Child Psychology* 30 (1): 33–47.

Baker, D. P., J. Leon, E. G. Smith Greenaway, J. Collins, and M. Movit. 2011. "The Education Effect on Population Health: A Reassessment." *Population and Development Review* 37 (2): 307–32.

Barro, R. J. 2013. "Education and Economic Growth." *Annals of Economics and Finance* 14 (2): 301–28.

Beeson, P. B. 1994. "Age and Sex Associations of 40 Autoimmune Diseases." *American Journal of Medicine* 96 (5): 457–62.

Blum, R. W., and K. Nelson-Mmari. 2004. "The Health of Young People in a Global Context." *Journal of Adolescent Health* 35 (5): 402–18.

Brown, B. B. 2004. "Adolescents' Relationships with Peers." In *Handbook of Adolescent Psychology*, edited by R. M. Lerner and L. D. Steinberg, 363–94. 2nd ed. Hoboken, NJ: John Wiley and Sons.

Bundy, D. A. P., N. de Silva, S. Horton, G. C. Patton, L. Schultz, and D. T. Jamison. 2017. "Child and Adolescent Health and Development: Realizing Neglected Potential." In *Disease Control Priorities* (third edition): Volume 8, *Child and Adolescent Health and Development*, edited by D. A. P. Bundy, N. de Silva, S. Horton, D. T. Jamison, and G. C. Patton. Washington, DC: World Bank.

Burt Solorzano, C. M., and C. R. McCartney. 2010. "Obesity and the Pubertal Transition in Girls and Boys." *Reproduction* 140 (3): 399–410.

Case, A., and A. Deaton. 2015. "Rising Morbidity and Mortality in Midlife among White Non-Hispanic Americans in the 21st Century." *Proceedings of the National Academy of Sciences* 112 (49): 15078–83.

Casey, B. J. 2015. "Beyond Simple Models of Self-Control to Circuit-Based Accounts of Adolescent Behavior." *Annual Review of Psychology* 66 (1): 295–319.

Christakou, A., M. Brammer, and K. Rubia. 2011. "Maturation of Limbic Corticostriatal Activation and Connectivity Associated with Developmental Changes in Temporal Discounting." *NeuroImage* 54 (2): 1344–54.

Commission on Social Determinants of Health. 2008. *Closing the Gap in a Generation: Health Equity through Action on the Social Determinants of Health.* Geneva: WHO.

Conti, G., and J. J. Heckman. 2012. "The Economics of Child Well-Being." NBER Working Paper No. 18466, National Bureau of Economic Research, Cambridge, MA.

Corvalan, C., R. Uauy, and V. Mericq. 2013. "Obesity Is Positively Associated with Dehydroepiandrosterone Sulfate Concentrations at 7 Y in Chilean Children of Normal Birth Weight." *American Journal of Clinical Nutrition* 97 (2): 318–25.

Crone, E. A., and R. E. Dahl. 2012. "Understanding Adolescence as a Period of Social-Affective Engagement and Goal Flexibility." *Nature Reviews Neuroscience* 13 (9): 636–50.

Cuijpers, P. 2003. "Examining the Effects of Prevention Programs on the Incidence of New Cases of Mental Disorders: The Lack of Statistical Power." *American Journal of Psychiatry* 160 (8): 1385–91.

Day, F. R., B. Bulik-Sullivan, D. A. Hinds, H. K. Finucane, J. M. Murabito, and others. 2016. "Shared Genetic Aetiology of Puberty Timing between Sexes and with Health-Related Outcomes." *Nature Communications* 6: 8842.

Del Giudice, M. 2009. "Sex, Attachment, and the Development of Reproductive Strategies." *Behavioral and Brain Sciences* 32 (1): 1–21; discussion 21–67.

de Water, E., A. H. Cillessen, and A. Scheres. 2014. "Distinct Developmental Pubertal Trajectories of Risk-Taking and Temporal Discounting in Adolescents and Young Adults." *Child Development* 85 (5): 1881–97.

Dosenbach, N. U. F., B. Nardos, A. L. Cohen, D. A. Fair, J. D. Power, and others. 2010. "Prediction of Individual Brain Maturity Using fMRI." *Science* 329 (5997): 1358–61.

Durlak, J. A., and A. M. Wells. 1997. "Primary Prevention Mental Health Programs for Children and Adolescents: A Meta-Analytic Review." *American Journal of Community Psychology* 25 (2): 115–52.

———. 1998. "Evaluation of Indicated Preventive Intervention (Secondary Prevention) Mental Health Programs for Children and Adolescents." *American Journal of Community Psychology* 26 (5): 775–802.

Fjell, A. M., K. B. Walhovd, T. T. Brown, J. M. Kuperman, Y. Chung, and others. 2012. "Multimodal Imaging of the Self-Regulating Developing Brain." *Proceedings of the National Academy of Sciences* 109 (48): 19620–25.

Frezza, E. E., M. S. Wachtel, and M. Chiriva-Internati. 2006. "Influence of Obesity on the Risk of Developing Colon Cancer." *Gut* 55 (2): 285–91.

Frisch, R. E. 1984. "Body Fat, Puberty, and Fertility." *Biological Reviews* 59 (2): 161–81.

Gardner, M., and L. Steinberg. 2005. "Peer Influence on Risk Taking, Risk Preference, and Risky Decision Making in Adolescence and Adulthood: An Experimental Study." *Developmental Psychology* 41 (4): 625.

GBD (Global Burden of Disease) 2013 Risk Factors Collaborators. 2015. "Global, Regional, and National Comparative Risk Assessment of 79 Behavioural, Environmental and Occupational, and Metabolic Risks or Clusters of Risks in 188 Countries, 1990–2013: A Systematic Analysis for the Global Burden of Disease Study 2013." *The Lancet* 386 (10010): 2287–323.

Giles, G. G., G. Severi, D. R. English, M. McRedie, R. MacInnis, and others. 2003. "Early Growth, Adult Body Size, and Prostate Cancer Risk." *International Journal of Cancer* 103 (2): 241–45.

Gillham, J. E., A. J. Shatté, and D. R. Freres. 2000. "Preventing Depression: A Review of Cognitive-Behavioral and Family Interventions." *Applied and Preventive Psychology* 9 (2): 63–88.

Gluckman, P. D., and M. A. Hanson. 2006. "Evolution, Development, and Timing of Puberty." *Trends in Endocrinology and Metabolism* 17 (1): 7–12.

Goddings, A.-L., S. Burnett Heyes, G. Bird, R. M. Viner, and S.-J. Blakemore. 2012. "The Relationship between Puberty and Social Emotion Processing." *Developmental Science* 15 (6): 801–11.

Graber, J. A., P. M. Lewinsohn, J. R. Seeley, and J. Brooks-Gunn. 1997. "Is Psychopathology Associated with the Timing of Pubertal Development?" *Journal of the American Academy of Child and Adolescent Psychiatry* 36 (12): 1768–76.

Grépin, K. A., and P. Bharadwaj. 2015. "Maternal Education and Child Mortality in Zimbabwe." *Journal of Health Economics* 44 (December): 97–117.

Grosbras, M. H., M. Jansen, G. Leonard, A. McIntosh, K. Osswald, and others. 2007. "Neural Mechanisms of Resistance to Peer Influence in Early Adolescence." *Journal of Neuroscience* 27 (30): 8040–45.

Hardy, R., D. Kuh, P. H. Whincup, and M. E. Wadsworth. 2006. "Age at Puberty and Adult Blood Pressure and Body Size in a British Birth Cohort Study." *Journal of Hypertension* 24 (1): 59–66.

Hartley, C. A., and L. H. Somerville. 2015. "The Neuroscience of Adolescent Decision-Making." *Current Opinion in Behavioral Sciences* 5 (October): 108–15.

Hawton, K., K. Rodham, E. Evans, and R. Weatherall. 2002. "Deliberate Self-Harm in Adolescents: Self-Report Survey in Schools in England." *BMJ* 325 (7374): 1207–11.

Hayward, C., J. D. Killen, L. D. Hammer, I. F. Litt, D. M. Wilson, and others. 1992. "Pubertal Stage and Panic Attack History in Sixth- and Seventh-Grade Girls." *American Journal of Psychiatry* 149 (9): 1239–43.

Hayward, C., J. D. Killen, D. M. Wilson, L. D. Hammer, I. F. Litt, and others. 1997. "Psychiatric Risk Associated with Early Puberty in Adolescent Girls." *Journal of the American Academy of Child and Adolescent Psychiatry* 36 (2): 255–62.

Hemphill, S. A., A. Kotevski, T. I. Herrenkohl, J. W. Toumbourou, J. B. Carlin, and others. 2010. "Pubertal Stage and the Prevalence of Violence and Social/Relational Aggression." *Pediatrics* 126 (2): e298–305.

Herman-Giddens, M. E., E. J. Slora, R. C. Wasserman, C. J. Bourdony, M. V. Bhapkar, and others. 1997. "Secondary Sexual Characteristics and Menses in Young Girls Seen in Office Practice: A Study from the Pediatric Research in Office Settings Network." *Pediatrics* 99 (4): 505–12.

Hochberg, Z. 2009. "Evo-Devo of Child Growth II: Human Life History and Transition between Its Phases." *European Journal of Endocrinology* 160 (2): 135–41.

Hochberg, Z., and J. Belsky. 2013. "Evo-Devo of Human Adolescence: Beyond Disease Models of Early Puberty." *BMC Medicine* 11: 113.

Horowitz, J. L., and J. Garber. 2006. "The Prevention of Depressive Symptoms in Children and Adolescents: A Meta-Analytic Review." *Journal of Consulting and Clinical Psychology* 74 (3): 401.

Ibáñez, L., A. López-Bermejo, M. Díaz, M. V. Marcos, and F. Zegher. 2008. "Metformin Treatment for Four Years to Reduce Total and Visceral Fat in Low Birth Weight Girls with Precocious Pubarche." *Journal of Clinical Endocrinology and Metabolism* 93 (5): 1841–45.

IHME (Institute for Health Metrics and Evaluation). 2015. *Global Educational Attainment 1970–2015*. Seattle, WA: IHME.

Johnson, M. H., T. Grossmann, and K. C. Kadosh. 2009. "Mapping Functional Brain Development: Building a Social Brain through Interactive Specialization." *Developmental Psychology* 45 (1): 151.

Jolles, D. D., M. A. van Buchem, S. A. Rombouts, and E. A. Crone. 2012. "Practice Effects in the Developing Brain: A Pilot Study." *Developmental Cognitive Neuroscience* 2 (Suppl 1): S180–91.

Jones, P. B. 2013. "Adult Mental Health Disorders and Their Age at Onset." *British Journal of Psychiatry* 202 (Suppl 54): s5–10.

Jordan, S. J., P. M. Webb, and A. C. Green. 2005. "Height, Age at Menarche, and Risk of Epithelial Ovarian Cancer." *Cancer Epidemiology, Biomarkers, and Prevention* 14 (8): 2045–48.

Kalsbeek, A., P. Voorn, R. M. Buijs, C. W. Pool, and H. B. M. Uylings. 1988. "Development of the Dopaminergic Innervation in the Prefrontal Cortex of the Rat." *Journal of Comparative Neurology* 269 (1): 58–72.

Kaltiala-Heino, R., E. Kosunen, and M. Rimpelä. 2003. "Pubertal Timing, Sexual Behaviour, and Self-Reported Depression in Middle Adolescence." *Journal of Adolescence* 26 (5): 531–45.

Kaltiala-Heino, R., M. Marttunen, P. Rantanen, and M. Rimpelä. 2003. "Early Puberty Is Associated with Mental Health Problems in Middle Adolescence." *Social Sciences and Medicine* 57 (6): 1055–64.

Kazdin, A. E. 2003. "Psychotherapy for Children and Adolescents." *Annual Review of Psychology* 54 (1): 253–76.

Kesek, A., P. D. Zelazo, and M. D. Lewis. 2008. "The Development of Executive Function and Emotion Regulation in Adolescence." In *Adolescent Emotional Development and the Emergence of Depressive Disorders*, edited by N. Allen and L. Sheeber. New York: Cambridge University Press.

Klein, P., L. M. van Passel-Clark, and J. C. Pezzullo. 2003. "Onset of Epilepsy at the Time of Menarche." *Neurology* 60 (3): 495–97.

Klump, K. L. 2013. "Puberty as a Critical Risk Period for Eating Disorders: A Review of Human and Animal Studies." *Hormones and Behavior* 64 (2): 399–410.

Krug, E. G., J. A. Mercy, L. L. Dahlberg, and A. B. Zwi. 2002. "The World Report on Violence and Health." *The Lancet* 360 (9339): 1083–88.

Lassi, Z., A. Moin, and Z. Bhutta. 2017. "Nutrition in Middle Childhood and Adolescence." In *Disease Control Priorities* (third edition): Volume 8, *Child and Adolescent Health and Development*, edited by D. A. P. Bundy, N. de Silva, S. Horton, D. T. Jamison, and G. C. Patton. Washington, DC: World Bank.

LeResche, L., L. A. Mancl, M. T. Drangsholt, K. Saunders, and M. Von Korff. 2005. "Relationship of Pain and Symptoms to Pubertal Development in Adolescents." *Pain* 118 (1–2): 201–9.

Loud, K. J., and C. M. Gordon. 2006. "Adolescent Bone Health." *Archives of Pediatrics and Adolescent Medicine* 160 (10): 1026–32.

Lowry, R., L. Kann, J. L. Collins, and L. J. Kolbe. 1996. "The Effect of Socioeconomic Status on Chronic Disease Risk Behaviors among U.S. Adolescents." *Journal of the American Medical Association* 276 (10): 792–97.

Madge, N., A. Hewitt, K. Hawton, E. J. de Wilde, P. Corcoran, and others. 2008. "Deliberate Self-Harm within an International Community Sample of Young People: Comparative Findings from the Child and Adolescent Self-Harm in Europe (CASE) Study." *Journal of Child Psychology and Psychiatry* 49 (6): 667–77.

Mahy, M., and N. Gupta. 2002. "Trends and Differentials in Adolescent Reproductive Behavior in Sub-Saharan Africa." ORC Macro, Calverton, MD.

March, J., S. Silva, S. Petrycki, J. Curry, K. Wells, and others. 2004. "Treatment for Adolescents with Depression Study (TADS) Team: Fluoxetine, Cognitive-Behavioral Therapy, and Their Combination for Adolescents with Depression; Treatment for Adolescents with Depression Study (TADS) Randomized Controlled Trial." *Journal of the American Medical Association* 292 (7): 807–20.

Marshall, W. A., and J. M. Tanner. 1968. "Growth and Physiological Development during Adolescence." *Annual Review of Medicine* 19 (February): 283–300.

McCabe, M. P., L. A. Ricciardelli, and S. Banfield. 2001. "Body Image, Strategies to Change Muscles and Weight, and Puberty: Do They Impact on Positive and Negative Affect among Adolescent Boys and Girls?" *Eating Behaviors* 2 (2): 129–49.

Mendle, J., E. Turkheimer, and R. E. Emery. 2007. "Detrimental Psychological Outcomes Associated with Early Pubertal Timing in Adolescent Girls." *Developmental Review* 27 (2): 151–71.

Mills, K. L., A. L. Goddings, L. S. Clasen, J. N. Giedd, and S. J. Blakemore. 2014. "The Developmental Mismatch in Structural Brain Maturation during Adolescence." *Developmental Neuroscience* 36 (3–4): 147–60.

Miyamoto, K., and A. Chevalier. 2010. *Improving Health and Social Cohesion through Education*. Paris: OECD Publishing.

Mundy, L. K., H. Romaniuk, L. Canterford, S. Hearps, R. M. Viner, and others. 2015. "Adrenarche and the Emotional and Behavioral Problems of Late Childhood." *Journal of Adolescent Health* 57 (6): 608–16.

Ochsner, K. N., and J. J. Gross. 2005. "The Cognitive Control of Emotion." *Trends in Cognitive Sciences* 9 (5): 242–49.

Olweus, D., A. Mattsson, D. Schalling, and H. Löw. 1988. "Circulating Testosterone Levels and Aggression in Adolescent Males: A Causal Analysis." *Psychosomatic Medicine* 50 (3): 261–72.

Parent, A. S., D. Franssen, J. Fudvoye, A. Pinson, and J. P. Bourguignon. 2016. "Current Changes in Pubertal Timing: Revised Vision in Relation with Environmental Factors Including Endocrine Disruptors." *Endocrine Development* 29: 174–84.

Parent, A. S., G. Teilmann, A. Juul, N. E. Skakkebaek, J. Toppari, and others. 2003. "The Timing of Normal Puberty and the Age Limits of Sexual Precocity: Variations around the World, Secular Trends, and Changes after Migration." *Endocrine Reviews* 24 (5): 668–93.

Patton, G. C., S. A. Hemphill, J. M. Beyers, L. Bond, J. W. Toumbourou, and others. 2007. "Pubertal Stage and Deliberate Self-Harm in Adolescents." *Journal of the American Academy of Child and Adolescent Psychiatry* 46 (4): 508–14.

Patton, G. C., S. M. Sawyer, J. S. Santelli, D. A. Ross, R. Afifi, and others. 2016. "Our Future: A *Lancet* Commission on Adolescent Health and Wellbeing." *The Lancet* 367 (10036): 2473–78. pii: S0140-6736(16)00579-1. doi:10.1016/S0140-6736(16)00579-1.

Patton, G. C., and R. Viner. 2007. "Pubertal Transitions in Health." *The Lancet* 369 (9567): 1130–39.

Paus, T., M. Keshavan, and J. N. Giedd. 2008. "Why Do Many Psychiatric Disorders Emerge during Adolescence?" *Nature Reviews Neuroscience* 9 (12): 947–57.

Pfeifer, J. H., and N. B. Allen. 2012. "Arrested Development? Reconsidering Dual-Systems Models of Brain Function in Adolescence and Disorders." *Trends in Cognitive Sciences* 16 (6): 322–29.

Pfeifer, J. H., C. L. Masten, W. E. Moore, T. M. Oswald, J. Mazziotta, and others. 2011. "Entering Adolescence: Resistance to Peer Influence, Risky Behavior, and Neural Changes in Emotion Reactivity." *Neuron* 69 (5): 1029–36.

Pine, A., T. Shiner, B. Seymour, and R. J. Dolan. 2010. "Dopamine, Time, and Impulsivity in Humans." *Journal of Neuroscience* 30 (26): 8888–96.

Power, C., J. K. Lake, and T. J. Cole. 1997. "Body Mass Index and Height from Childhood to Adulthood in the 1958 British

Born Cohort." *American Journal of Clinical Nutrition* 66 (5): 1094–101.

Pradhan, E., E. M. Suzuki, S. Martínez, M. Schaferhöff, and D. T. Jamison. 2017. "The Effects of Education Quantity and Quality on Child and Adult Mortality: Their Magnitude and Their Value." In *Disease Control Priorities* (third edition): Volume 8, *Child and Adolescent Health and Development*, edited by D. A. P. Bundy, N. de Silva, S. Horton, D. T. Jamison, and G. C. Patton. Washington, DC: World Bank.

Prentice, P., and R. M. Viner. 2013. "Pubertal Timing and Adult Obesity and Cardiometabolic Risk in Women and Men: A Systematic Review and Meta-Analysis." *International Journal of Obesity* 37 (8): 1036–43.

Pundziute-Lycka, A., G. Dahlquist, L. Nystrom, H. Arnqvist, E. Björk, and others. 2002. "The Incidence of Type I Diabetes Has Not Increased but Shifted to a Younger Age at Diagnosis in the 0–34 Years Group in Sweden 1983–1998." *Diabetologia* 45 (6): 783–91.

Reardon, L. E., E. W. Leen-Feldner, and C. Hayward. 2009. "A Critical Review of the Empirical Literature on the Relation between Anxiety and Puberty." *Clinical Psychology Review* 29 (1): 1–23.

Romeo, R. D. 2010. "Adolescence: A Central Event in Shaping Stress Reactivity." *Developmental Psychobiology* 52 (3): 244–53.

Rosenfeld, R. G., and B. C. Nicodemus. 2003. "The Transition from Adolescence to Adult Life: Physiology of the 'Transition' Phase and Its Evolutionary Basis." *Hormone Research* 60 (Suppl 1): 74–77.

Sandhu, J., G. Davey Smith, J. Holly, T. J. Cole, and J. Ben-Shlomo. 2006. "Timing of Puberty Determines Serum Insulin-Like Growth Factor-I in Late Adulthood." *Journal of Clinical Endocrinology and Metabolism* 91 (8): 3150–57.

Sawyer, S. M., R. A. Afifi, L. H. Bearinger, S. J. Blakemore, B. Dick, and others. 2012. "Adolescence: A Foundation for Future Health." *The Lancet* 379 (9826): 1630–40.

Spear, L. P. 2000. "The Adolescent Brain and Age-Related Behavioral Manifestations." *Neuroscience and Biobehavioral Reviews* 24 (4): 417–63.

Steinberg, L. 2005. "Cognitive and Affective Development in Adolescence." *Trends in Cognitive Sciences* 9 (2): 69–74.

———. 2008. "A Social Neuroscience Perspective on Adolescent Risk-Taking." *Developmental Review* 28 (1): 78–106.

Steinberg, L., and K. C. Monahan. 2007. "Age Differences in Resistance to Peer Influence." *Developmental Psychology* 43 (6): 1531.

Tobler, N. S., M. R. Roona, P. Ochshorn, D. G. Marshall, A. V. Streke, and others. 2000. "School-Based Adolescent Drug Prevention Programs: 1998 Meta-Analysis." *Journal of Primary Prevention* 20 (4): 275–336.

Tremblay, R. E., D. LeMarquand, and F. Vitaro. 1999. "The Prevention of Oppositional Defiant Disorder and Conduct Disorder." In *Handbook of Disruptive Behavior Disorders*, edited by H. C. Quay and A. E. Hogan, 525–55. New York: Kluwer.

UNESCO (United Nations Educational, Scientific and Cultural Organization). 2010. *EFA Global Monitoring Report: Reaching the Marginalized.* Paris: UNESCO.

Varraso, R., V. Siroux, J. Maccario, I. Pinn, and F. Kauffmann. 2005. "Asthma Severity Is Associated with Body Mass Index and Early Menarche in Women." *American Journal of Respiratory and Critical Care Medicine* 171 (4): 334–39.

Verney, C., B. Berger, J. Adrien, A. Vigny, and M. Gay. 1982. "Development of the Dopaminergic Innervation of the Rat Cerebral Cortex: A Light Microscopic Immunocytochemical Study Using Anti-Tyrosine Hydroxylase Antibodies." *Developmental Brain Research* 5 (1): 41–52.

Vértes, P. E., and E. T. Bullmore. 2015. "Annual Research Review: Growth Connectomics; the Organization and Reorganization of Brain Networks during Normal and Abnormal Development." *Journal of Child Psychology and Psychiatry, and Allied Disciplines* 56 (3): 299–320.

Vincent, H. K., and A. G. Taylor. 2006. "Biomarkers and Potential Mechanisms of Obesity-Induced Oxidant Stress in Humans." *International Journal of Obesity* 30 (3): 400–18.

Viner, R. M., E. M. Ozer, S. Denny, M. Marmot, M. Resnick, and others. 2012. "Adolescent Health 2: Adolescence and the Social Determinants of Health." *The Lancet* 379 (9826): 1641–52.

Wedderkopp, N., L. B. Andersen, K. Froberg, and C. Leboeuf-Yde. 2005. "Back Pain Reporting in Young Girls Appears to Be Puberty-Related." *BMC Musculoskeletal Disorders* 6: 52.

Weisz, J. R., C. A. McCarty, and S. M. Valeri. 2006. "Effects of Psychotherapy for Depression in Children and Adolescents: A Meta-Analysis." *Psychological Bulletin* 132 (1): 132.

Whittle, S., J. G. Simmons, M. L. Byrne, C. Strikwerda-Brown, R. Kerestes, and others. 2015. "Associations between Early Adrenarche, Affective Brain Function, and Mental Health in Children." *Social Cognitive and Affective Neuroscience* 10 (9): 1282–90.

Williams, P. G., G. N. Holmbeck, and R. N. Greenley. 2002. "Adolescent Health Psychology." *Journal of Consulting and Clinical Psychology* 70 (3): 828.

World Bank. 2006. *World Development Report 2007: Development and the Next Generation.* Washington, DC: World Bank.

Chapter 10

Brain Development: The Effect of Interventions on Children and Adolescents

Elena L. Grigorenko

INTRODUCTION

The landscape of the child public health literature in the twenty-first century has been strongly influenced by the Developmental Origins of Health and Disease (DOHaD) hypothesis (Van den Bergh 2011). This hypothesis proposes that human complex diseases and disorders, regardless of age of onset, have their roots in childhood and adolescence and are products of the dynamics of various forces that substantiate human development. Similar developmentally oriented views have been proposed by other theoretical frameworks (for example, Li 2003), but the DOHaD hypothesis has received the most traction in the literature and is a driving force behind studies that connect early development to lifespan health.

The human brain is arguably the most complex biological system, comprising a diversity of functionally distinct regions, structurally distinct neural circuits, and morphologically distinct cell types. Its lifespan is highly dynamic, encompassing continuity and changes at both structural and functional levels. The brain has a unique developmental trajectory compared with the rest of the body. Whereas at birth an infant is approximately 6 percent of its adult body weight, the brain is already 25 percent of its adult weight; by age two years, these proportions are 20 percent and 77 percent, respectively (Dekaban and Sadowsky 1978). This rapid rate of brain growth is accompanied by a slow rate of functional maturation that extends into early adulthood. One of the major premises of the DOHaD is that both structural and functional characteristics of brain development are highly informative predictors of the lifespan ratio of health and disease. As the brain substantiates behavioral change, understanding its development is key in constructing and disseminating interventions that maximize healthy development and minimize the impact of disabilities and disorders.

This chapter briefly outlines aspects of the brain literature that pertain to public health interventions, programs, and policy approaches to protecting, augmenting, and maximizing the healthy development of the brain. First, the essential characteristics of brain development are outlined. Second, a variety of research on brain development changes associated with public health is briefly discussed. The relevance of this research, conducted predominantly in high-income countries (HICs), is considered, with a view to its applicability in low- and middle-income countries (LMICs). Definitions of age groupings and age-specific terminology used in this volume can be found in chapter 1 (Bundy and others 2017).

DEVELOPMENT OF THE HUMAN BRAIN

Anatomical Maturation

The human brain's maturation is remarkably prolonged and characterized by ongoing dynamic changes throughout the lifespan (Giedd and Rapoport 2010).

Corresponding author: Elena L. Grigorenko, University of Houston, Houston, Texas, United States; elena.grigorenko@times.uh.edu.

Postnatally, it follows (figure 10.1) an inverted U-shaped trajectory that peaks about age eight years and then declines monotonically (Ducharme and others 2016). The brain matures along its two dimensions, gray and white matter. Gray matter is composed chiefly of neuronal cell bodies, which determine the color, as well as dendrites, unmyelinated and relatively few myelinated axons, glial cells including astroglia and oligodendrocytes, synapses, and capillaries. White matter is composed chiefly of myelinated axons; the myelin, which determines the color; and relatively few neuronal cell bodies. In general and simplifying terms, the gray matter forms the structures of the brain, and the white matter ensures that these structures are connected; both are essential for all functions substantiated by the brain. The gray and white matter have different developmental trajectories; their relative proportions and rates of accumulation differ at different developmental stages and in healthy and disordered brains.

Figure 10.1 Developmental Trajectories of Brain Morphometry

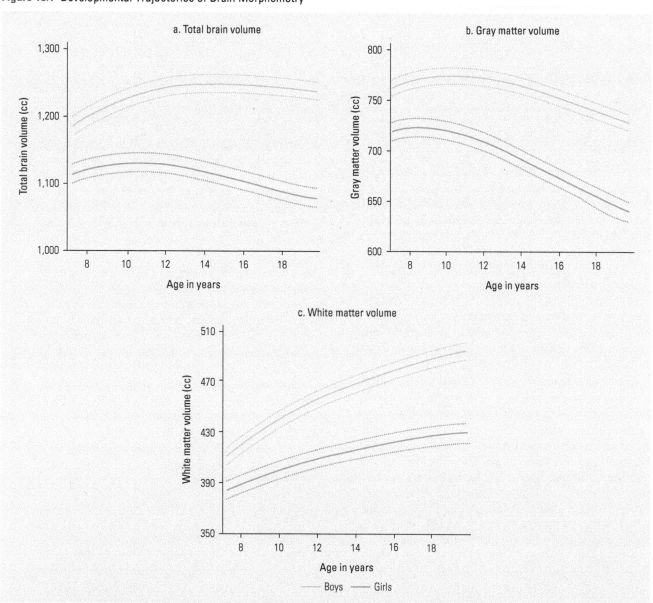

Sources: Adapted from Giedd and Rapoport 2010, adapted from Lenroot and others 2007.
Note: cc = cubic centimeters. The data were collected from a sample of males (*N* = 475 scans) and females (*N* = 354 scans) ages 6–20 years. The middle lines in each set of three lines represent mean values; the upper and lower lines represent upper and lower 95 percent confidence intervals. All curves differ significantly in height and shape.

By age six years, the brain reaches approximately 95 percent of its adult volume. Its size in boys is approximately 10 percent bigger than in girls; this gender difference persists throughout the lifespan, although the bodies of boys do not become larger than bodies of girls until adolescence, suggesting a decoupling of the maturation trajectories of brain and body size (Giedd and Rapoport 2010). The developmental trajectory of gray matter peaks in early childhood, preceding a peak in total brain volume, and then gradually decreases unevenly throughout the brain. The amount of gray matter peaks earliest in the primary sensorimotor areas and latest in the higher-order association areas. The volume of white matter increases gradually into early adulthood. Myelination not only enhances the parameters of signal transmission, it also boosts the connectivity and networking properties of the brain. Some evidence indicates that white matter increases are coupled with the emergence of specific psychological functions, such as language (Paus and others 1999). Recent technological advances resulted in the differentiation of cortical volume into two underlying components, cortical thickness and cortical surface area. Cortical thickness in the majority of brain regions demonstrates linear monotonic decline occurring mostly similarly for boys and girls between the ages of 4.9 and 22 years, with the peak of cortical thickness manifesting no later than age 8 years (Ducharme and others 2016).

Data on the developmental trajectories of the brain in HICs have accumulated rapidly within several initiatives, such as the BRAIN Initiative.[1] Selected findings from these initiatives include the following:

- A remarkable amount of variability of individual brain size occurs, whether across or within groups, making individualized clinical predictions difficult.
- Subtle deviations from normal developmental trajectories of the brain anatomy appear to be at least associated with—if not causal factors of—a number of developmental disorders (Giedd and Rapoport 2010).
- There are different indicators of brain development, and some of them appear to be more clinically informative than others. For example, cortical thickness has a demonstrated association with the manifestation of developmental disorders (Thormodsen and others 2013).
- Cortical thickness appears to correlate with performance on complex cognitive tasks (Karama and others 2011).
- Different areas of the brain have differential maturational dynamics. In general, phylogenetically newer areas mature later than older ones, and higher-order association areas mature after lower-order somatosensory areas (Gogtay and others 2004). For example, the developmental imbalance between the earlier-maturing limbic system networks and later-maturing frontal systems might explain the psychological and behavioral texture of adolescence, which may occur as this imbalance is being resolved (Casey, Duhoux, and Cohen 2010).
- The maturing brain is characterized by the reshaping of its functional properties, particularly its connectivity, which peaks during adolescence and is defined by the physical links between codeveloping brain areas, the co-activational patterns between brain areas engaged in specific tasks, and the etiological connections between brain areas that are co-influenced by the same genetic and environmental factors.

Functional Development

The human brain is commonly represented as a system of tiered networks of highly organized neurons, where spatiotemporal biochemical and bioelectrical activity gives specialized functionality to structural anatomic components of the brain (Power and others 2010). The connection between structure and function is bidirectional, so that specific anatomical characteristics—such as lesions, synaptic development, and myelination—parameterize the functionality of a particular network. The functional dynamics of the network can change physical characteristics of the underlying brain structure. From conception through the lifespan and into senescence, this system's developmental trajectory is shaped by the continuous co-influence of each individual's genome and environome—the immediate system of environmental factors that influence human health and behavior. Understanding the stability and malleability of the system is a fundamental task of modern science and the focus of a number of large-scale projects, such as the Human Connectome Project.[2]

Because the system as a whole and each network emerge developmentally, studies have traditionally engaged research into *where* in the brain a network may be localized and *how* it operates. Such research historically used methods of anatomical localization, for example, through brain surgery or autopsy, but these methods are of limited value in living humans. More recent methods (electroencephalography, positron emission tomography, functional magnetic resonance imaging, and near infrared spectroscopy/optimal imaging) based on various technological advances study the brain in living humans, where the focus, along with anatomical structure, is on functional connectivity. These methods, which at first were technology, skill, cost, and safety demanding, have been evolving to minimize these demands and maximize safety (such as applicability to pediatric populations), transportability (such as use in minimally equipped settings), and utilization (such as usability in low-resource settings).

The current view of the developmental trajectory of the brain's functional networks and their systems converges on the following:

- From infancy into young adulthood, properties of the network change in such a way that initially strong correlations between brain activity in closely located anatomical regions tend to weaken, while initially weak correlations between more distant regions tend to increase (Power and others 2010), allowing, presumably, for the mental and behavioral functional repertoire of an adult to be substituted for that of a newborn.
- This change in the distribution of correlations may be related to anatomical developmental changes in the brain: *synaptic pruning* (Huttenlocher 1979), that is, the process of eliminating synapses connecting different neurons. Synaptic pruning may be the driving factor substantiating the decrease in proximal correlations, whereas myelination (Paus and others 2001)—the process of forming a myelin sheath around a nerve to allow nerve impulses to move more quickly—may be the driving factor for the increase in distal correlations.
- Developmental increases in functional connectivity appear to be, at least in part, due to spontaneous or orchestrated co-occurrences of activity (Lewis and others 2009), namely, the co-activation of different brain structures in the context of, for example, implicit or explicit learning, based on which functional connections within the brain might be established as new skills are acquired.
- Functionally different neural networks are thought to have differential maturational courses.
- Characteristics of functional networks have been associated in adulthood with indicators of intellectual performance (van den Heuvel and others 2009) and executive control (Seeley and others 2007). Although comparable data for children are limited, a careful investigation of the developmental trajectories of brain functional networks in conjunction with other maturing systems—for example, language, cognition, and self-regulation—might enhance the understanding of human development as a systemic transformation of a maturing individual guided by the brain.

GENOME-ENVIRONOME DYNAMICS OF BRAIN DEVELOPMENT

Blueprint of the Genome

The development of the brain is based on the apt expression of integral gene products (the transcriptome) coded by sequences of DNA (the genome), specifically, protein and RNA (Tebbenkamp and others 2014). Recent analyses of the human brain transcriptome[3] have, for the first time, allowed a comprehensive picture of the trajectories of genes associated with specific neurodevelopmental processes to be constructed (figure 10.2). There are strong time-specific correlations between the characteristics of the transcriptome and the morphological and functional specialization of brain regions. Alterations to DNA sequences can result in modifications of gene expression, which can cause changes in the brain and the development of brain-based disorders.

Yet, the brain is a highly open and modifiable system—neuronal circuits, established early in life, undergo remodeling as they develop their adult functional properties in response to both genomic and environmental cues. This room for varying interpretations of a single genotype—that is, when the same genotype can exhibit different phenotypes in variable environments—is referred to as *plasticity*. The capacity of the human brain to respond to the environment and its fluctuations represents an adaptive system that allows individuals to better survive and reproduce. In other words, the brain, metaphorically, is the hub connecting the various information streams from the genome and the environome that allows for the organism's interpretations of and adaptations to genetic and environmental forces.

Nutritional Requirements

As the most metabolically active organ, the brain's adequate balanced nutrition prenatally and postnatally is essential for its development and for the proper maturation of the neural mechanisms substantiating child development (Gómez-Pinilla 2008). Overwhelming evidence demonstrates that malnutrition, especially when severe, has significant and lasting implications for development (Laus and others 2011). Malnutrition slows the brain's development, thinning the cerebral cortex and reducing the numbers of neurons, synapses, dendritic arborization, and myelination—all of which decrease brain size, which, in turn, challenges the brain's functional properties. Specifically, numerous cranial imaging studies of the brains of patients with protein energy malnutrition (for example, Atalabi and others 2010) have demonstrated cerebral atrophy and ventricular dilation, which may lead to inadequate patterns of brain activity. Nutritional rehabilitation during childhood and adolescence can reverse these effects, at least partially.

Similarly, adequate specific microelements are essential for developing brains. For example, both severe lack of iodine and severe exposure to neurotoxins such as lead result in irreversible brain damage (Benton 2010). An adequate concentration of vitamin A is essential for the development of the visual system; levels that are too high or too low prenatally can be teratogenic (Reifen and Ghebremeskel 2001). Moreover, complex dynamics occur among different vitamins; a prenatal imbalance between folate and vitamin B_{12} can increase the risk of postnatal insulin resistance, which is associated with poorer cognitive development (Yajnik and others 2008). The differential developmental trajectories of the brain's features mean there are differential sensitive periods when the violation of nutritional requirements is most detrimental. Because the brain most rapidly develops prenatally and postnatally, these two periods are critical for subsequent outcomes. Yet, because brain development, although not as rapid as at the early stages of development, does not slow down substantially until individuals reach their early 20s, microelement deficiencies and malnutrition are also important in middle childhood and adolescence.

Specific strategies—such as salt iodization to prevent iodine deficiency, home fortification to prevent iron deficiency, and food and specific micronutrient supplementation in food-insecure populations—have been shown to be effective in preventing nutritional deficiencies. Yet, the research literature that qualifies and quantifies the impact of these strategies on brain development is limited (Prado and Dewey 2014).

Environmental Experiences

Substantial evidence indicates that both gray and white matter are susceptible to environmental perturbations (Lupien and others 2009). Although the direction of the causality—from brain to behavior or from behavior to brain—is often unclear, it is indisputable that environment is a critical ingredient of change in the brain's structure and function. For example, children who experienced severe exposure to air pollution in South Mexico City were reported to have prefrontal white matter alterations and the precursors of Alzheimer's disease (Calderon-Garciduenas and Torres-Jardon 2012).

Two environments that contextualize brain development are particularly prominent: socioeconomic status (SES), especially poverty (Hanson and others 2013), and

Figure 10.2 Timeline of Major Human Neurodevelopmental Processes Based on Gene Expression Trajectories

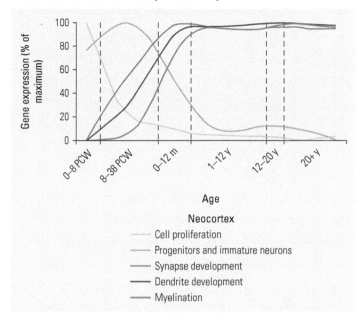

Sources: Adapted from Tebbenkamp and others (2014). The expression levels and trajectories are adapted from Kang and others (2011).
Note: m = months; PCW = postconceptional weeks; y = years. Expression trajectories of genes associated with major neurodevelopmental processes reflect the occurrence and progression of these processes in the human neocortex.

early life experience in general and parenting quality in particular (Kundakovic and Champagne 2015). There is a growing field of studies on socioeconomic neurogradients, defined as neural differences associated with differences in SES (Schibli and D'Angiul 2013). For example, it has been demonstrated that low SES environments in general and poverty in particular influence the rate of human brain development (Hanson and others 2013). Specifically, children from lower SES environments differ in their gray matter accumulation in the frontal and parietal lobes, such that differences widen throughout development as the exposure to impoverished environments continues (figure 10.3). Of note is that volumetric brain differences are associated with the emergence of disruptive behavioral problems (Hanson and others 2013).

Anatomical brain differences have also been associated with characteristics of prenatal and postnatal environments. For example, prenatal maternal stress is associated with decreased dendritic spine density in multiple brain areas (such as the hippocampus and the anterior cingulate and orbitofrontal cortex) substantiating emotional regulation (Murmu and others 2006). Conversely, early maternal support postnatally is strongly

Figure 10.3 Brain Growth Trajectories, by Age and Socioeconomic Status

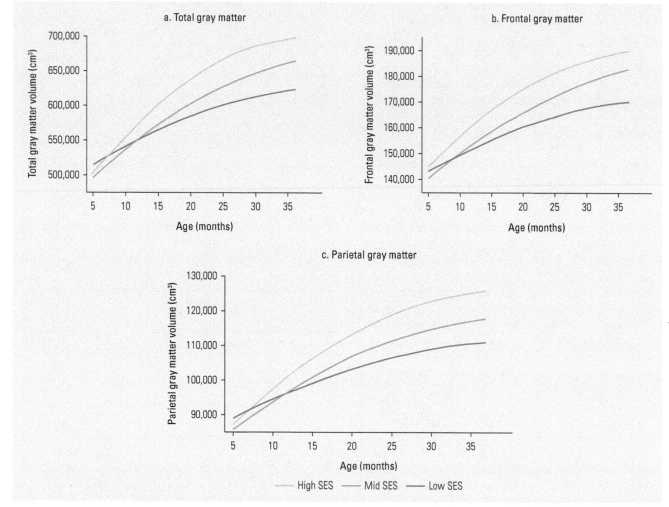

Source: Adapted from Hanson and others 2013.
Note: SES = socioeconomic status; cm³ = cubic centimeters.

predictive at school age of healthy development of the hippocampus, a brain region key to memory and stress modulation (Luby and others 2012).

Neuroplasticity

The overriding principle of neuroplasticity is that behavioral change is associated with a specific gain or loss of synapses within neuronal networks (Caroni, Donato, and Muller 2012). Multiple factors differentiate the types of neuroplasticity in the typically developing brain (Kolb and Gibb 2014).

Neuroplasticity can be characterized as follows:

- *Experience-expectant.* When structural or functional changes in the brain require specific types of

experience, for example, the maturation of binocular vision

- *Experience-independent.* When changes in the brain occur spontaneously and override its initial structure and function, for example, the development of the lateral geniculate nucleus in the maturation of the visual system

- *Experience-dependent.* When changes in the brain allow the acquisition of new behaviors, for example, all types of learning.

Neuroplasticity is related to the relevance, frequency, intensity, and sequences of experiences. It can be adaptive, as in the acquisition of a new skill, or maladaptive, as in the formation of a dependency or disorder. Of note is that changes in the brain that result from the same environmental impact, such as injury, vary remarkably, depending on when in the developmental process the impact occurred. An experience can generate qualitatively different changes in different regions within the same brain. In addition, plastic changes themselves change over time; for example, the overproduction of synapses in the early stages of development is reversed by pruning in adolescence, which continues well into adulthood. One of the most rapidly developing areas of research pertains to the dynamics of infant and toddler neuroplasticity in response to severe negative environmental impacts, such as maltreatment (Graham and others 2015), and remediation, such as training of self-control (Berkman, Graham, and Fisher 2012).

SKILL ACQUISITION AND CHANGES IN THE BRAIN

This section focuses on different behavioral loci associated with brain changes that have been or can become targets for specific public health interventions. Only four selected loci are discussed here—early attachment, language development, acquisition of literacy and numeracy, and self-regulation (SR).

Early Environment and Attachment

Substantial evidence demonstrates that atypical early development in which the presence of the attachment bond between children and significant others—mothers, fathers, or primary caregivers—is disrupted is extremely detrimental for brain and behavior development. One source of such evidence comes from research into orphanhood, when children are raised in institutions, often characterized by nutritional, physical, stimulational (that is, cognitive, linguistic, and emotional), and care deficiencies. Institutionally reared children tend to be characterized by deviations from typical brain development, in particular, a distributed network of alterations in the white matter—limbic and paralimbic pathways, frontostriatal circuitry, and sensory processing pathways (for example, Bick and others 2015). No comparable studies have been completed in LMICs; yet, the frequency of orphaned children in LMICs—given conflict zones, child labor, deadly epidemics, and other maladies—is much higher than in HICs and, therefore, should be a priority for research.

Another source of such evidence comes from studies into the prevalence of childhood maltreatment in LMICs. For example, it has been reported that 25 percent to 50 percent of young South Africans are maltreated by family members (Pieterse 2015). In HICs, maltreatment has been consistently shown to be detrimental to brain development (Painter and Scannapieco 2013). Given the widespread opportunities for maltreatment in LMICs (Tomlinson, Cooper, and Murray 2005) due to early pregnancies, large numbers of children in the same home, high levels of poverty, and low levels of education, it is extremely important to identify programs demonstrated to be effective and efficacious in HICs and transportable, at least potentially, to LMICs. One such program is the Nurse-Family Partnership (Olds and others 1997), which is being introduced to South Africa (Pieterse 2015).

Language Development

Language acquisition occurs during a sensitive period of brain development (Knudsen 2004).

The neural signatures of language acquisition are detectable at very early stages of development (Rivera-Gaxiola, Silvia-Pereyra, and Kuhl 2005). These neural signatures, although themselves dynamically transforming, are highly predictive of numerous other indicators of child development, both linguistic and nonlinguistic.

However, children require several key elements to progress through the language acquisition process:

- First, children need to be immersed in environments in which they have high-frequency exposure to the language because the mechanism thought to be most used is statistical learning, which assumes an ongoing exposure to language data so that linguistic mental representations can be inferred and automatized (Saffran, Aslin, and Newport 1996). Yet, simple exposure to linguistic stimuli, no matter how intense, is not enough.
- Second, the motivation to learn language is social and requires the presence of a social context for language acquisition (Kuhl 2007). The acquisition of language engages and affects the computational and social areas of the brain. To master language, children both capitalize on and enhance systems of cognitive and social skills (Meltzoff and others 2009). Thus, the brain-behavior pathways that underlie and follow language acquisition are highly dynamic and future oriented as their properties predict subsequent steps in child development (Pascoe and Smouse 2012; Prathanee, Lorwatanapongsa, Makarabhirom, and Wattanawongsawang 2010).

These conditions—statistical exposure and social context—form appropriate targets for policies to enhance typical and to remediate atypical brain-behavior development. Such policies, which have been developed in HICs and are being introduced to LMICs, include the following:

- Raising public awareness of atypical development (Mahmoud, Aljazi, and Alkhamra 2014)
- Promoting professional training of specialists able to diagnose, remediate, and support individuals with developmental difficulties (Cheng 2010)
- Facilitating early identification of developmental difficulties (Glumbic and Brojcin 2012; Hamadani and others 2010; Sidhu, Malhi, and Jerath 2010)
- Advocating inclusive preschool education
- Providing additional support to children with developmental language delays (Rakap 2015) and implementing specialized intervention programs (Amato and others 2015; De Cesaro and others 2013; Erasmus and others 2013; Fernandes, De La Higuera Amato, and Molini-Avejonas 2012; Fernandes and others 2014; Kotby, El-Sady, and Hegazi 2010; Pascoe and others 2010; Prathanee, Lorwatanapongsa, Makarabhirom, Suphawatjariyakul, and others 2010).

These systemic changes reflect the emerging emphasis on early child care and education in LMICs in general and language development in particular because all are extremely important for brain development. The relevant research accumulating in LMICs has replicated findings from HICs and reinforces the crucial significance of these systemic changes (Cheng 2010; Günhan 2011; Pascoe and Smouse 2012).

Literacy and Numeracy

Numerous studies have been conducted to isolate and map the specific brain pathways or functional systems that support literacy (Dehaene and Cohen 2007) and numeracy (Butterworth and Walsh 2011). Clearly, the acquisition of these skills is based on the use of existing areas of the brain, which are reorganized structurally and functionally while being recycled and recruited into systems of acquisition (Dehaene and Cohen 2007). Large and growing fields of research are investigating the impact of literacy and numeracy on brain functioning by (1) conducting longitudinal tracking of children as they move from preliteracy and prenumeracy stages into stages of mastery, (2) comparing groups of literate and numerate and illiterate and innumerate adults, and (3) comparing individuals with typical and atypical pathways of acquisition for literacy and numeracy. Each of these approaches is associated with its own methodological challenges, and limitations exist in the interpretations of the relevant data and findings. Yet, there is a

remarkable convergence of multiple studies from different countries, including LMICs, specifying the impact of skill acquisition on brain structure and function.

Literacy

Literacy systems appear to involve brain areas substantiating early vision, script analysis, language analysis, and their mutual associations (Dehaene, Morais, and Kolinsky 2015). Literate individuals have been reported to demonstrate numerous advantages, compared with illiterate individuals, in the speed and accuracy of processing both letter-based and picture-based materials. The specificity of reading as a skill distinguishing literate and illiterate individuals is reflected by the fact that reading recruits a specific brain area located in the left ventral occipito-temporal cortex to become a visual word form area (VWFA)—an area that demonstrates specific, universal, and reproducible responses to script. The patterns of activation in the VWFA are correlated with the degree of mastery of reading.

It is important that adult plasticity in this area underlies the ability to acquire print—the graphic representation of a spoken language—either in a first or in subsequent languages. Also important is that the VWFA is strongly connected, both structurally and functionally, to the brain areas that support spoken language. Because reading assumes a conversion from vision to language, it requires activation of the language network, or at least its component. Indeed, literate, compared with illiterate, individuals demonstrate increased and modified activation of the language-related cortical and subcortical network (in particular, the planum temporale [PT]—an area of the brain that supports, along with surrounding areas, the neuronal representations of the consonants and vowels of spoken language) while engaged in specific language- and reading-related tasks. This means that literacy acquisition not only results in the creation of specific systems supporting reading, but also changes other systems supporting related functions, enhancing and automatizing them. To illustrate (figure 10.4), literacy enhances the connectivity between the ventral temporal lobe (including VWFA) and the inferior parietal and posterior superior temporal regions (including PT) via enhanced myelination. This strengthening may enable the automatization of the grapheme-to-phoneme conversion, crystallization of reading skills, and subsequent development of related higher-order cognitive processes, such as reading comprehension. Moreover, reading mastery has been shown to increase gray-matter density in several regions of the brain that contribute to the establishment and functioning of the brain system that supports literacy.

Numeracy

Although this field is considerably smaller than that of literacy studies, systemic findings include the following (Butterworth, Varma, and Laurillard 2011):

- Groups of multiple-duty neurons that respond to object dimensions such as space, time, object size, and number appear to be located in the intraparietal cortex.
- These neurons are part of an extensive distributed network given that, similar to literacy, numeracy engages multiple processes such as early vision, motor, spatial, and mnemonic functions.
- Neuroimaging studies have converged on the intraparietal sulcus (novel numeric operations) and the angular gyrus (previously learned numeric operations) as the loci of numeric processing.
- The intraparietal sulcus is viewed as the foundational structure in the construction of numeric brain networks; it demonstrates structural abnormalities in individuals with the developmental disorder of mastering numeracy—dyscalculia—and changes in gray-matter density in expert mathematicians.

The evidence that education in general and the acquisition of literacy and numeracy alter the brain structure and function comes primarily from HICs. The relevant research in LMICs is focused predominantly on documenting the manifestation of difficulties in acquiring literacy and numeracy in different languages and societies (Pouretemad and others 2011), frequency of these difficulties (Ashraf and Najam 2014; Hsairi Guidara and others 2013; Jovanovic and others 2013), and the development of relevant intervention approaches (Lee and Wheldall 2011; Obidoa, Eskay, and Onwubolu 2013).

Self-Regulation

One of the ultimate goals of development is to master the skill of SR—goal planning, inhibition, mental flexibility, sustained motivation, executive control, and self-agency. SR is a critical element in the dynamic system of health and disease and the key to productive adulthood and successful aging. SR is supported by a distributed brain system whose main task is to support the adequate appraisal of the system of demands of all relevant factors on individuals and the subsequent formulation of behavior to satisfy these demands. The executive load is developmentally uniquely intensified in adolescence, and corresponding changes occur in the brain (figure 10.5). These changes are related primarily to the maturation of the prefrontal cortex (PFC) and its

Figure 10.4 Impact of Reading Acquisition: Enhanced Connectivity between PT and VWFA

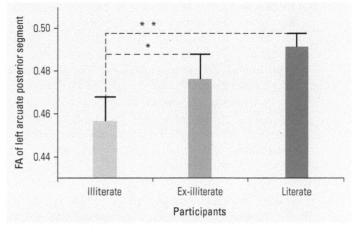

Source: Adapted from Dehaene, Morais, and Kolinsky 2015.
Note: FA = fractional anisotropy; PT = planum temporale; VWFA = visual word form area. The structural link between the visual orthographic (VWFA) and the auditory phonological (PT) systems is enhanced with literacy: there is an increase in the FA in the posterior branch of the left arcuate fasciculus in literate and ex-illiterate (that is, individuals who learned to read in adulthood) relative to illiterate participants. This increase in FA with literacy correlates with activation of the PT in response to spoken sentences. Error bars represent one standard error.
$*p < 0.05$; $**p < 0.001$.

Figure 10.5 Developmental Course of Brain Maturation

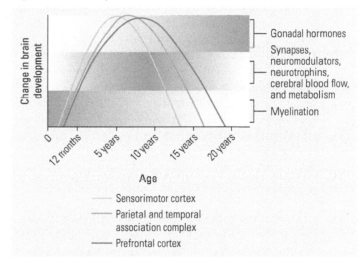

Source: Adapted from Lee and others 2014.
Note: Behavioral attributes are paralleled by hormonal and neurobiological changes that target specific brain regions and cell populations (shown in shaded gray to capture the dynamic influences of hormones, various brain processes, and myelination).

connectivity with other brain areas as it recruits them to substantiate the system of SR.

Specifically, the following changes peak in the adolescent brain (Luciana 2013):

- A general thinning of the cortex and pruning in subcortical structures (gray matter) and an increase in the volume and enhanced organization of brain connections (white matter) crescendo. This results in

increasingly efficient functioning within and across brain networks.
- Heightened distinctions occur in regional brain volumes, and functional brain responses to reward intensify.
- Maturation of the PFC and the SR network requires exposure to key environmental experiences, such as positive incentive and reward. Such exposures are particularly important in adolescence because they are coupled with age-dependent experience-expectant increases in dopaminergic tone (that is, the amount of distribution of the neurotransmitter dopamine) in the brain.

Dopaminergic signaling—the engagement of dopamine-based reward systems, exposure to uncertain and risky environments, behavioral explorations, and independence seeking—contributes to the maturation of the PFC and the related distributed system in general and the cross-talk between subcortical (limbic) and cortical (prefrontal) regions in particular. As consolidation through learning occurs, a brain system emerges whose role is to support decision making based on calculations of the probability and magnitude of risk and reward.

Our current knowledge of the development of the brain systems substantiating SR, although largely empirically based rather than explanatory, suggests several approaches for intervention. These interventions are connected to the nature of reward responsivity, its intersection with social strivings, and socioemotional context and content. Numerous relevant intervention approaches have been developed in HICs (Rothbart and Posner 2015), but their distribution has been limited in LMICs.

CONCLUSIONS

The DOHaD hypothesis assumes continuity between the adult profile of health and disease and the dynamics of child development in general and brain development in particular. The hypothesis also assumes another continuity—that between interventions and sensitive periods given that the presence of such periods is not limited to early childhood. Although the DOHaD hypothesis has been increasingly supported by empirical evidence in HICs, the corresponding evidence in LMICs is limited.

As this empirical evidence is being accumulated, it is becoming clear that the brain helps ensure both types of continuity. The brain is an ever-changing system whose structure and function reflect, at any given time, both the endowment of the genome and the investment

opportunities available in various environmental contexts, including educational systems, public health policies, and specific intervention programs. As knowledge of the brain's developmental trajectories accumulates, the extent of the brain's modifiability, especially in response to targeted interventions, will become clearer. This understanding will help guide the development of intervention approaches suitable for and most effective at the sensitive periods of brain development that occur across the lifespan.

NOTES

Work on this essay was supported by NIH grants R01 HD085836 (Elena L. Grigorenko, PI) and P50 HD052120 (Richard Wagner, PI). Grantees undertaking such projects are encouraged to express freely their professional judgment. This chapter, therefore, does not necessarily reflect the position or policies of the abovementioned agency, and no official endorsement should be inferred. I am grateful to Eileen Luders and Tuong Vi Nguyen for providing helpful comments on the manuscript, to Mei Tan for her editorial assistance, and to Janet Croog for preparing the figures.

World Bank Income Classifications as of July 2014 are as follows, based on estimates of gross national income (GNI) per capita for 2013:

- Low-income countries (LICs) = US$1,045 or less
- Middle-income countries (MICs) are subdivided:
  a) lower-middle-income = US$1,046 to US$4,125
  b) upper-middle-income (UMICs) = US$4,126 to US$12,745
- High-income countries (HICs) = US$12,746 or more.

1. BRAIN Initiative, Washington, DC.
2. The Human Connectome Project: http://www.humanconnectomeproject.org/.
3. BrainSpan: Atlas of the Developing Human Brain: http://www.brainspan.org.

REFERENCES

Amato, C. A. H., T. H. F. Santos, I. Y. I. Sun, L. Segeren, and F. Fernandes. 2015. "Serving the Underserved: Language Intervention to Children with Disorders of the Autism Spectrum in Brazil." *European Psychiatry* 30 (Suppl 1): 438.

Ashraf, F., and N. Najam. 2014. "Validation of Learning Disabilities Checklist in Public Sector Schools of Pakistan." *Pakistan Journal of Psychological Research* 29 (2): 223–44.

Atalabi, O. M., I. A. Lagunju, O. O. Tongo, and O. O. Akinyinka. 2010. "Cranial Magnetic Resonance Imaging Findings in Kwashiorkor." *International Journal of Neuroscience* 120 (1): 23–27. doi:0.3109/00207450903315727.

Benton, D. 2010. "The Influence of Dietary Status on the Cognitive Performance of Children." *Molecular Nutrition and Food Research* 54 (4): 457–70.

Berkman, E. T., A. M. Graham, and P. A. Fisher. 2012. "Training Self-Control: A Domain-General Translational Neuroscience Approach." *Child Development Perspectives* 6 (4): 374–84. doi:10.1111/j.1750-8606.2012.00248.x.

Bick, J., T. Zhu, C. Stamoulis, N. A. Fox, C. Zeanah, and others. 2015. "Effect of Early Institutionalization and Foster Care on Long-Term White Matter Development: A Randomized Clinical Trial." *Journal of the American Medical Association Pediatrics* 169 (3): 211–19. doi:10.1001 /jamapediatrics.2014.3212.

Bundy, D. A. P., N. de Silva, S. Horton, G. C. Patton, L. Schultz, and D. T. Jamison. 2017. "Child and Adolescent Health and Development: Realizing Neglected Potential." In *Disease Control Priorities* (third edition): Volume 8, *Child and Adolescent Health and Development*, edited by D. A. P. Bundy, N. de Silva, S. Horton, D. T. Jamison, and G. C. Patton. Washington, DC: World Bank.

Butterworth, B., S. Varma, and D. Laurillard. 2011. "Dyscalculia: From Brain to Education." *Science* 332 (6057): 1049–53. doi:10.1126/science.1201536.

Butterworth, B., and V. Walsh. 2011. "Neural Basis of Mathematical Cognition." *Current Biology* 21 (16): R618–21. doi:http://dx.doi.org/10.1016/j.cub.2011.07.005.

Calderon-Garciduenas, L., and R. Torres-Jardon. 2012. "Air Pollution, Socioeconomic Status, and Children's Cognition in Megacities: The Mexico City Scenario." *Frontiers in Psychology* 3: 217. doi:10.3389/fpsyg.2012.00217.

Caroni, P., F. Donato, and D. Muller. 2012. "Structural Plasticity upon Learning: Regulation and Functions." *Nature Reviews Neuroscience* 13 (7): 478–90.

Casey, B. J., S. Duhoux, and M. M. Cohen. 2010. "Adolescence: What Do Transmission, Transition, and Translation Have to Do with It?" *Neuron* 67 (5): 749–60.

Cheng, L. R. 2010. "Emerging Issues in Health and Education in Asia-Pacific: A Focus on Speech-Language Pathology." *Folia Phoniatrica et Logopaedica* 62 (5): 238–45. doi:10.1159/000314787.

De Cesaro, B. C., L. G. Gurgel, G. P. Nunes, and C. T. Reppold. 2013. "Child Language Interventions in Public Health: A Systematic Literature Review." *Codas* 25 (6): 588–94. doi:10.1590/s2317-17822014000100012.

Dehaene, S., and L. Cohen. 2007. "Cultural Recycling of Cortical Maps." *Neuron* 56 (2): 384–98.

Dehaene, S., J. Morais, and R. Kolinsky. 2015. "Illiterate to Literate: Behavioural and Cerebral Changes Induced by Reading Acquisition." *Nature Reviews Neuroscience* 16 (4): 234–44.

Dekaban, A. S., and D. Sadowsky. 1978. "Changes in Brain Weights during the Span of Human Life: Relation of Brain Weights to Body Heights and Body Weights." *Annals of Neurology* 4 (4): 345–56.

Ducharme, S., M. D. Albaugh, T.-V. Nguyen, J. J. Hudziak, J. M. Mateos-Pérez, and others. 2016. "Trajectories of Cortical Thickness Maturation in Normal Brain Development—The Importance of Quality Control Procedures." *NeuroImage* 125: 267–79. doi:http://dx.doi .org/10.1016/j.neuroimage.2015.10.010.

Erasmus, D., L. Schutte, M. van der Merwe, and S. Geertsema. 2013. "Speech-Language Therapy for Adolescents with Written-Language Difficulties: The South African Context." *South African Journal of Communication Disorders* 60: 50–58.

Fernandes, F. D. M., C. A. H. Amato, D. A. Defense-Netrval, and D. R. Molini-Avejonas. 2014. "Speech-Language Intervention for Children with Autism Spectrum Disorder in Brazil." *Topics in Language Disorders* 34 (2): 155–67. doi:10.1097/tld.0000000000000011.

Fernandes, F. D. M., C. A. De La Higuera Amato, and D. R. Molini-Avejonas. 2012. "Language Therapy Results with Children of the Autism Spectrum." *Revista de Logopedia, Foniatría y Audiología* 32: 2–6. doi:10.1016/j .rlfa.2011.12.001.

Giedd, J. N., and J. L. Rapoport. 2010. "Structural MRI of Pediatric Brain Development: What Have We Learned and Where Are We Going?" *Neuron* 67 (5): 728–34. doi:http:// dx.doi.org/10.1016/j.neuron.2010.08.040.

Glumbic, N., and B. Brojcin. 2012. "Factor Structure of the Serbian Version of the Children's Communication Checklist-2." *Research in Developmental Disabilities* 33 (5): 1352–59. doi:10.1016/j.ridd.2012.03.010.

Gogtay, N., J. N. Giedd, L. Lusk, K. M. Hayashi, D. Greenstein, and others. 2004. "Dynamic Mapping of Human Cortical Development during Childhood through Early Adulthood." *Proceedings of the National Academy of Sciences of the United States of America* 101 (21): 8174–79. doi:10.1073 /pnas.0402680101.

Gómez-Pinilla, F. 2008. "Brain Foods: The Effects of Nutrients on Brain Function." *Nature Reviews Neuroscience* 9 (7): 568–78. doi:10.1038/nrn2421.

Graham, A. M., J. H. Pfeifer, P. A. Fisher, W. Lin, W. Gao, and others. 2015. "The Potential of Infant fMRI Research and the Study of Early Life Stress as a Promising Exemplar." *Developmental Cognitive Neuroscience* 12: 12–39. doi:http:// dx.doi.org/10.1016/j.dcn.2014.09.005.

Günhan, N. E. 2011. "Review of Communication Disorders in Turkish." *Clinical Linguistics and Phonetics* 25 (4): 335–37.

Hamadani, J. D., H. Baker-Henningham, F. Tofail, F. Mehrin, S. N. Huda, and others. 2010. "Validity and Reliability of Mothers' Reports of Language Development in 1-Year-Old Children in a Large-Scale Survey in Bangladesh." *Food and Nutrition Bulletin* 31 (2 Suppl): S198–206.

Hanson, J. L., N. Hair, D. G. Shen, F. Shi, J. H. Gilmore, and others. 2013. "Family Poverty Affects the Rate of Human Infant Brain Growth." *PLoS One* 8 (12): e80954.

Hsairi Guidara, I., I. Ayadi, E. Ellouz, I. Abid, F. Kamoun, and others. 2013. "Study of a Tunisian Population of Children with Learning Disorders." *Tunisie Medicale* 91 (6): 382–86.

Huttenlocher, P. R. 1979. "Synaptic Density in Human Frontal Cortex: Developmental Changes and Effects of Aging." *Brain Research* 163 (2): 195–205.

Jovanovic, G., Z. Jovanovic, J. Bankovic-Gajic, A. Nikolic, S. Svetozarevic, and others. 2013. "The Frequency of Dyscalculia among Primary School Children." *Psychiatria Danubina* 25 (2): 170–74.

Kang, H. J., Y. I. Kawasawa, F. Cheng, Y. Zhu, X. Xu, and others. 2011. "Spatio-Temporal Transcriptome of the Human Brain." *Nature* 478 (7379): 483–89.

Karama, S., R. Colom, W. Johnson, I. J. Deary, R. Haier, and others. 2011. "Cortical Thickness Correlates of Specific Cognitive Performance Accounted for by the General Factor of Intelligence in Healthy Children Aged 6 to 18." *NeuroImage* 55 (4): 1443–53. doi:http://dx.doi.org/10.1016/j.neuroimage.2011.01.016.

Knudsen, E. I. 2004. "Sensitive Periods in the Development of the Brain and Behavior." *Journal of Cognitive Neuroscience* 16 (8): 1412–25.

Kolb, B., and R. Gibb. 2014. "Searching for the Principles of Brain Plasticity and Behavior." *Cortex* 58: 251–60. doi:http://dx.doi.org/10.1016/j.cortex.2013.11.012.

Kotby, M. N., S. El-Sady, and M. Hegazi. 2010. "Thirty-Five Years of Care of Child Language in Egypt." *Topics in Language Disorders* 30 (1): 84–91.

Kuhl, P. K. 2007. "Is Speech Learning 'Gated' by the Social Brain?" *Developmental Science* 10 (1): 110–20.

Kundakovic, M., and F. A. Champagne. 2015. "Early-Life Experience, Epigenetics, and the Developing Brain." *Neuropsychopharmacology* 40 (1): 141–53. doi:10.1038/npp.2014.140.

Laus, M. F., L. D. M. F. Vales, T. M. B. Costa, and S. S. Almeida. 2011. "Early Postnatal Protein-Calorie Malnutrition and Cognition: A Review of Human and Animal Studies." *International Journal of Environmental Research and Public Health* 8 (2): 590–612. doi:10.3390/ijerph8020590.

Lee, F. S., H. Heimer, J. N. Giedd, E. S. Lein, N. Šestan, and others. 2014. "Adolescent Mental Health—Opportunity and Obligation." *Science* 346 (6209): 547–49. doi:10.1126/science.1260497.

Lee, L. W., and K. Wheldall. 2011. "Acquisition of Malay Word Recognition Skills: Lessons from Low-Progress Early Readers." *Dyslexia* 17 (1): 19–37. doi:10.1002/dys.421.

Lenroot, R. K., N. Gogtay, D. K. Greenstein, E. M. Wells, G. L. Wallace, and others. 2007. "Sexual Dimorphism of Brain Developmental Trajectories during Childhood and Adolescence." *Neuroimage* 36 (4): 1065–73. doi:http://dx.doi.org/10.1016/j.neuroimage.2007.03.053.

Lewis, C. M., A. Baldassarre, G. Committeri, G. L. Romani, and M. Corbetta. 2009. "Learning Sculpts the Spontaneous Activity of the Resting Human Brain." *Proceedings of the National Academy of Sciences* 106 (41): 17558–63.

Li, S.-C. 2003. "Biocultural Orchestration of Developmental Plasticity across Levels: The Interplay of Biology and Culture in Shaping the Mind and Behavior across the Life Span." *Psychological Bulletin* 129 (2): 171–94.

Luby, J. L., D. M. Barch, A. Belden, M. S. Gaffrey, R. Tillman, and others. 2012. "Maternal Support in Early Childhood Predicts Larger Hippocampal Volumes at School Age." *Proceedings of the National Academy of Sciences of the United States of America* 109 (8): 2854–59.

Luciana, M. 2013. "Adolescent Brain Development in Normality and Psychopathology." *Development and Psychopathology* 25 (4 Pt 2): 1325–45. doi:10.1017/S0954579413000643.

Lupien, S. J., B. S. McEwen, M. R. Gunnar, and C. Heim. 2009. "Effects of Stress throughout the Lifespan on the Brain, Behaviour and Cognition." *Nature Review Neuroscience* 10 (6): 434–45.

Mahmoud, H., A. Aljazi, and R. Alkhamra. 2014. "A Study of Public Awareness of Speech-Language Pathology in Amman." *College Student Journal* 48: 495–510.

Meltzoff, A. N., P. K. Kuhl, J. Movellan, and T. J. Sejnowski. 2009. "Foundations for a New Science of Learning." *Science* 325 (5938): 284–88. doi:10.1126/science.1175626.

Murmu, M. S., S. Salomon, Y. Biala, M. Weinstock, K. Braun, and others. 2006. "Changes of Spine Density and Dendritic Complexity in the Prefrontal Cortex in Offspring of Mothers Exposed to Stress during Pregnancy." *European Journal of Neuroscience* 24 (5): 1477–87. doi:10.1111/j.1460-9568.2006.05024.x.

Obidoa, M. A., M. Eskay, and C. O. Onwubolu. 2013. "Remedial Help in Inclusive Classrooms: Gender Differences in the Enhancement of Mathematics Achievement of Students through PAL (Peer-Assisted Learning)." *US-China Education Review* 3 (3): 172–80.

Olds, D. L., J. Eckenrode, C. R. Henderson Jr., H. Kitzman, J. Powers, and others. 1997. "Long-Term Effects of Home Visitation on Maternal Life Course and Child Abuse and Neglect: Fifteen-Year Follow-Up of a Randomized Trial." *Journal of the American Medical Association* 278 (8): 637–43. doi:10.1001/jama.1997.03550080047038.

Painter, K., and M. Scannapieco. 2013. "Child Maltreatment: The Neurobiological Aspects of Posttraumatic Stress Disorder." *Journal of Evidence-Based Social Work* 10 (4): 276–84.

Pascoe, M., Z. Maphalala, A. Ebrahim, D. Hime, B. Mdladla, and others. 2010. "Children with Speech Difficulties: An Exploratory Survey of Clinical Practice in the Western Cape." *South African Journal of Communication Disorders* 57: 66–75.

Pascoe, M., and M. Smouse. 2012. "Masithethe: Speech and Language Development and Difficulties in isiXhosa." *South African Medical Journal* 102 (6): 469–71.

Paus, T., D. L. Collins, A. C. Evans, G. Leonard, B. Pike, and others. 2001. "Maturation of White Matter in the Human Brain: A Review of Magnetic Resonance Studies." *Brain Research Bulletin* 54 (3): 255–66.

Paus, T., A. Zijdenbos, K. Worsley, D. L. Collins, J. Blumenthal, and others. 1999. "Structural Maturation of Neural Pathways in Children and Adolescents: In Vivo Study." *Science* 283 (5409): 1908–11.

Pieterse, D. 2015. "Childhood Maltreatment and Educational Outcomes: Evidence from South Africa." *Health Economics (United Kingdom)* 24 (7): 876–94. doi:http://dx.doi.org/10.1002/hec.3065.

Pouretemad, H. R., A. Khatibi, M. Zarei, and J. Stein. 2011. "Manifestations of Developmental Dyslexia in Monolingual Persian Speaking Students." *Archives of Iranian Medicine* 14 (4): 259–65. doi:0011144/aim.007.

Power, J. D., D. A. Fair, B. L. Schlaggar, and S. E. Petersen. 2010. "The Development of Human Functional Brain Networks."

Neuron 67 (5): 735–48. doi:http://dx.doi.org/10.1016/j.neuron.2010.08.017.

Prado, E. L., and K. G. Dewey. 2014. "Nutrition and Brain Development in Early Life." *Nutrition Reviews* 72 (4): 267–84. doi:10.1111/nure.12102.

Prathanee, B., P. Lorwatanapongsa, K. Makarabhirom, R. Suphawatjariyakul, R. Thinnaithorn, and others. 2010. "Community-Based Model for Speech Therapy in Thailand: Implementation." *Journal of the Medical Association of Thailand* 93 (Suppl 4): S1–6.

Prathanee, B., P. Lorwatanapongsa, K. Makarabhirom, and W. Wattanawongsawang. 2010. "Thai Speech and Language Norms for Children 2 1/2 to 4 Years of Age." *Journal of the Medical Association of Thailand* 93 (Suppl 4): S7–15.

Rakap, S. 2015. "Quality of Individualised Education Programme Goals and Objectives for Preschool Children with Disabilities." *European Journal of Special Needs Education* 30: 173–86. doi:http://dx.doi.org/10.1080/08856257.2014.986909.

Reifen, R., and K. Ghebremeskel. 2001. "Vitamin A during Pregnancy." *Nutrition and Health* 15: 237–43.

Rivera-Gaxiola, M., J. Silvia-Pereyra, and P. K. Kuhl. 2005. "Brain Potentials to Native and Non-Native Speech Contrasts in 7- and 11-Month-Old American Infants." *Developmental Science* 8 (2): 162–72.

Rothbart, M. K., and M. I. Posner. 2015. "The Developing Brain in a Multitasking World." *Developmental Review* 35 (March): 42–63.

Saffran, J., R. Aslin, and E. Newport. 1996. "Statistical Learning by 8-Month-Old Infants." *Science* 274 (5294): 1926–28.

Schibli, K., and A. D'Angiul. 2013. "The Social Emotional Developmental and Cognitive Neuroscience of Socioeconomic Gradients: Laboratory, Population, Cross-Cultural and Community Developmental Approaches." *Frontiers in Human Neuroscience* 7: 788. doi:10.3389/fnhum.2013.00788.

Seeley, W. W., V. Menon, A. F. Schatzberg, J. Keller, G. H. Glover, and others. 2007. "Dissociable Intrinsic Connectivity Networks for Salience Processing and Executive Control." *Journal of Neuroscience* 27 (9): 2349–56.

Sidhu, M., P. Malhi, and J. Jerath. 2010. "Multiple Risks and Early Language Development." *Indian Journal of Pediatrics* 77 (4): 391–95. doi:10.1007/s12098-010-0044-y.

Tebbenkamp, A. T. N., A. J. Willsey, M. W. State, and N. Sestan. 2014. "The Developmental Transcriptome of the Human Brain: Implications for Neurodevelopmental Disorders." *Current Opinion in Neurology* 27 (2): 149–56.

Thiebaut de Schotten, M., L. Cohen, E. Amemiya, L. W. Braga, and S. Dehaene. 2012. "Learning to Read Improves the Structure of the Arcuate Fasciculus." *Cerebral Cortex* 24 (4): 989–95.

Thormodsen, R., L. M. Rimol, C. K. Tamnes, M. Juuhl-Langseth, A. Holmén, and others. 2013. "Age-Related Cortical Thickness Differences in Adolescents with Early-Onset Schizophrenia Compared with Healthy Adolescents." *Psychiatry Research: Neuroimaging* 214 (3): 190–96. doi:10.1016/j.pscychresns.2013.07.003.

Tomlinson, M., P. Cooper, and L. Murray. 2005. "The Mother–Infant Relationship and Infant Attachment in a South African Periurban Settlement." *Child Development* 76 (5): 1044–54.

Van den Bergh, B. R. 2011. "Developmental Programming of Early Brain and Behaviour Development and Mental Health: A Conceptual Framework." *Developmental Medicine and Child Neurology* 53 (Suppl 4): 19–23.

van den Heuvel, M. P., C. J. Stam, R. S. Kahn, and H. E. Hulshoff Pol. 2009. "Efficiency of Functional Brain Networks and Intellectual Performance." *Journal of Neuroscience* 29 (23): 7619–24.

Yajnik, C. S., S. S. Deshpande, A. A. Jackson, H. Refsum, S. Rao, and others. 2008. "Vitamin B_{12} and Folate Concentrations during Pregnancy and Insulin Resistance in the Offspring: The Pune Maternal Nutrition Study." *Diabetologia* 51 (1): 29–38. doi:10.1007/s00125-007-0793-y.

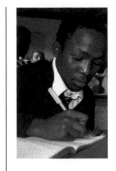

Chapter **11**

Nutrition in Middle Childhood and Adolescence

Zohra Lassi, Anoosh Moin, and Zulfiqar Bhutta

INTRODUCTION

Adolescence is the period between childhood and adulthood. Patton and others (2016) further delineate this period as early adolescence (ages 10–14 years), late adolescence (ages 15–19 years), youth (ages 15–24 years), and young adulthood (ages 20–24 years). Definitions of age groupings and age-specific terminology used in this volume can be found in chapter 1 (Bundy and others 2017). Worldwide, there are nearly 1.8 billion people ages 10–24 years, constituting one-quarter of the total population; 89 percent of young people (ages 10–24 years) live in low- and middle-income countries (LMICs).

Figure 11.1 shows some of the interactions of nutrition and development during the life course. Adolescent development is complex, with puberty, neurocognitive maturity, and social role transitions interacting in complex ways, all with important consequences for nutrition.

Physical Growth and Mental Development

Growth failure and micronutrient inadequacy during childhood and adolescence can delay growth and create high risk of chronic diseases in adulthood. Puberty is accompanied by a growth spurt that increases the requirements for both macronutrients and micronutrients. These higher requirements are balanced by a more efficient use of protein for development rather than energy. For females, pubertal timing is affected by

childhood body mass index (BMI) and percentage of body fat; data for males are inconclusive.

Pubertal timing depends on nutrition during childhood. It also reflects earlier maternal nutrition because appetite control, energy homeostasis, and the pubertal axis are being developed in natal and early postnatal life (Soliman, De Sanctis, and Elalaily 2014). In childhood, stunting (low height for age) and wasting (low weight for height) delay both overall growth and the onset of puberty. In addition, girls born small for gestational age are at risk for insulin resistance, premature pubarche, early menarche, and an attenuated growth spurt. Although increased adiposity is a normal physiologic process that precedes puberty, early weight gains are linked to taller stature in childhood, with a probable increase in growth hormone, insulin-like growth factor, and future obesity, as well as a possible increase in hyperinsulinemia (Viner, Allen, and Patton 2017, chapter 9 in this volume).

Importance of Nutrition in Adolescence

Adolescence is a time of transition when habits are formed that persist into adult life. Good habits, such as exercise and a healthy diet, are likely to bring many benefits, including improved performance in school (Doku and others 2013). Nutritional habits are important, with high intake of processed, energy-dense foods, high BMI, and iron deficiency among the top 20 risk factors of disability-adjusted life years (DALYs) worldwide (WHO 2009).

Corresponding author: Zulfiqar Bhutta, Aga Khan University, Karachi, Pakistan; zulfiqar.bhutta@aku.edu.

Figure 11.1 Nutrition and Related Risk Factors across the Continuum of Care

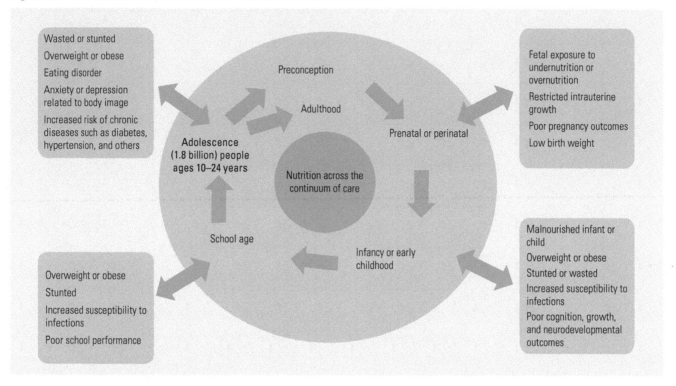

Such factors pose risks for later-life noncommunicable diseases, which are responsible for two of every three deaths globally (Sawyer and others 2012).

Most studies and guidelines on eating behavior are from high-income countries (HICs). The 2010 U.S. dietary guidelines for adolescents (ages 9–18 years), for example, suggest that girls require 1,400–2,400 calories per day and boys require 1,600–3,200 because of their typically larger frames and muscle mass. However, any teenager involved in athletic physical activity can require up to 5,000 calories per day (Caprio and others 1994).

The available studies suggest that adolescents are becoming more independent in their food choices, more likely to be influenced by their peers, and less likely to pick healthy foods (Seymour, Hoerr, and Huang 1997). Other factors that affect their overall nutrition include the kinds of foods available at home, amount of time available to make food (Venter and Winterbach 2010), knowledge of food content (Li and others 2008), and ability to purchase snacks (Ahmed and others 2006). Sociodemographic, behavioral, and environmental factors are also linked to different patterns of adolescent nutrition. Sociodemographic factors include socioeconomic status, age, sex, location, and degree of urbanization. Behavioral factors include patterns of beverage intake, portion sizes, dieting, family dinners, eating in front of and viewing television, and skipping meals (especially breakfast). Environmental factors include eating or buying food prepared outside the home, maternal education and employment, and parental diet (Moreno and others 2014).

Gender norms are often more harmful than beneficial with regard to nutrition and physical activity. Girls are exposed to a culture of overdieting and unhealthy weight loss more often than boys, and many believe that exercise is unfeminine and that athletic women are masculine. Qualities encouraged in sports, such as strength, dominance, and competition, are also considered unfeminine. Spencer, Rehman, and Kirk (2015) found that girls prioritize body image over health. Dror and Allen (2014) reviewed consumption of dairy products in developed countries and found that girls consume less dairy than recommended because they think it causes weight gain, and because their parents either do not consume dairy or do not urge their children to do so, among other reasons. Although the media, parents, and peers can foster negative images, they can also help introduce healthier approaches to weight control and nutrition (Spencer, Rehman, and Kirk 2015).

This chapter discusses the evidence on nutrition for children ages six to nine years and for adolescents, including undernutrition, overweight and obesity, micronutrient deficiencies, nutrition for pregnant adolescents, and eating disorders. Each section discusses the issue and then presents evidence on the effectiveness of interventions to address it. Chapter 3 of this volume (Galloway 2017) discusses global nutrition outcomes at ages 5 to 19.

UNDERNUTRITION

Statistics on undernutrition—including wasting, stunting, anemia, and vitamin A deficiency—in children younger than age five years are well known, but data on undernutrition specifically in adolescents are rare. In the least developed countries, the prevalence of adolescent underweight is 22 percent (UNICEF 2014) and is associated with various health risks. Undernutrition is linked to lower gut immunity, decreased protective secretions, and low innate and acquired immunity (Seidenfeld, Sosin, and Rickert 2004).

Undernourished adolescents have commonly experienced stunted growth in childhood. Undernutrition in early life can result in fewer pancreatic cells that produce insulin. Although this deficit is compensated for in adolescence, with stunted adolescents having more peripheral insulin receptors, this compensation contributes to increased accumulation of fat (Rytter and others 2014). Stunted children, adolescents, and adults have higher rates of later arterial hypertension. Undernutrition in childhood and adolescence also results in constant physiologic and psychologic stress, increasing the production of stress hormones that weaken the body and decreasing the production of thyroid hormones and insulin-like growth factor that regulate growth.

Marshall, Burrows, and Collins (2014) have suggested that dietary intake is generally inadequate for children and adolescents in LMICs (table 11.1), and adolescents do not fulfill their daily nutritional requirements. Furthermore, disparity is high among adolescents from lower socioeconomic profiles as compared with their wealthier counterparts.

Prevalence of Undernutrition

Data on undernutrition in adolescents are underrepresented in global databases, although some smaller studies report regional data. Among adolescents ages 10–14 years, protein energy malnutrition affects 12 girls per 100,000 in Africa and 3 girls per 100,000 in the Eastern Mediterranean (WHO 2014). Matsuzaki and others (2015) studied 722 adolescents and young adults in India from 2003 to 2005 and found mean BMI of 16.8 kilograms/square meter in adolescents and 19.3 kilograms/square meter in young adults. Thomas, Srinivasan, and Sudarshan (2013) studied 409 students in rural India and found that 39 percent were thin (BMI below the 5th percentile for age) and 59 percent were stunted. Lopes and others (2013) studied 523 adolescents (ages 12–18 years) in urban Brazil and found that 9 percent were stunted and 24 percent were overweight, with 36 percent of families having mild and 24 percent having moderate to severe food insecurity. Stunting was associated with low intake of calcium and iron, whereas food insecurity was associated with low intake of protein and calcium. In a study of 23,496 students (ages 11–17 years) conducted in seven African countries (Benin, Djibouti, the Arab Republic of Egypt, Ghana, Malawi,

Table 11.1 Dietary Intake of Children and Adolescents

Study	Findings
Marshall, Burrows, and Collins 2014	Most school-age children in LMICs eat plant-based foods, fewer than 50 percent consume dairy, breakfast is the most often skipped meal, and consumption of processed foods is increasing.
Doku and others 2013; Ochola and Masibo 2014	In Ghana, 31 percent of those ages 12–18 years ate breakfast fewer than four days a week, 56 percent rarely ate fruits, 48 percent rarely ate vegetables, and boys were more physically active than girls.
Barugahara, Kikafunda, and Gakenia 2013	In Uganda, girls ages 11–14 years achieved the World Health Organization daily requirements in the following proportions: 30 percent for folate, 36 percent for energy, 54 percent for iron and riboflavin, 59 percent for protein, 61 percent for vitamin A, 89 percent for vitamin C, and 92 percent for fiber.
Kawade 2012	In India, school-going girls (ages 10–16 years) were deficient in zinc, with 50 percent having cognitive impairments.
Nago and others 2010	In Benin, adolescents (ages 13–19 years) received 40 percent of their daily diet from food prepared outside the home, accounting for 75 percent of their daily energy intake.
Alam and others 2010	In Bangladesh, consumption of nonstaple good-quality food items within the last week were less frequent and correlated positively with the household asset quintile.

Note: LMICs = low- and middle-income countries.

Table 11.2 Summary Estimates of Effectiveness of Interventions for Undernutrition in Adolescence

Study	Intervention	Outcome
Creed-Kanashiro and others 2000	Nine-month intervention consisting of participatory training with community kitchen leaders, educational materials, increased access to heme iron (chicken liver and blood) in first five months	Anemia: RR, 0.32; 95% CI, 0.15 to 0.69 Iron deficiency: RR, 0.78; 95% CI, 0.37 to 1.63
Mann, Kaur, and Bains 2002	Iron (60 milligrams per day) as well as energy supplementation (in the form of pinnies to energy deficient group for three months) Pinnies were prepared from whole wheat flour, semolina, whole soy flour, refined oil, sugar, whole milk powder, and crushed groundnut kernels in the rations. A 60 gram pinni provided 325 kilocalories. The subjects were supplemented with 1.5–3 pinnies according to their energy deficiency.	Hemoglobin: mean difference, –0.10; 95% CI, –0.46 to 0.26

Note: CI = confidence interval; RR = relative risk.

Mauritania, and Morocco), Manyanga and others (2014) found that almost 16 percent of girls and 25 percent of boys were underweight. The highest prevalence of underweight was found in males in Ghana (34 percent), and the lowest was found in females in Egypt (10 percent).

Interventions for Undernutrition

Numerous interventions involving food supplementation have been found to be effective in different age groups, particularly in pregnant women to increase birth weight. However, limited evidence is available for children older than age five years and adolescents. In a study on adolescents (ages 17–19 years) in Peru, Creed-Kanashiro and others (2000) found that a nine-month intervention including participatory training, educational materials, and increased access to heme iron in the first five months reduced anemia. Mann, Kaur, and Bains (2002) supplemented the diet of anemic girls ages 16–20 years in India for three months and found no difference in hemoglobin levels between those consuming adequate and those consuming inadequate calories (table 11.2).

OVERWEIGHT AND OBESITY

Obesity and overweight are consequences of excess food intake, often combined with genetic factors. Childhood obesity and overweight have been linked to severe obesity in adulthood, with a stronger effect on men. Being overweight as an adolescent is strongly associated with obesity as an adult (Ferraro, Thorpe, and Wilkinson 2003). Guo and others (1994) found that white adolescents (age 18 years) with a BMI above the 60th percentile

had a 34 percent (male) and 37 percent (female) chance of being overweight at age 35 years. In Sub-Saharan Africa, being overweight as a child has been linked to significant morbidity and mortality as an adult, with higher BMI associated with type 2 diabetes, hypertension, coronary heart disease (although this effect is not independent of the effect of high adult BMI), asthma, polycystic ovary syndrome, and premature mortality (Park and others 2012; Reilly and Kelly 2011). Furthermore, being above or below a healthy weight has been linked to genetic and environmental factors such as maternal height, age, education, household size, and socioeconomic status (Keino and others 2014).

While undernutrition—especially stunting—continues to be a severe problem, particularly in LMICs, the increasing global trend in child overweight and obesity is alarming because countries have to programmatically deal with the double burden of disease. In rapidly developing and urbanizing societies, diets are becoming more energy dense and processed, yet lacking in fiber and multivitamins, while lifestyles are becoming more sedentary (Popkin 1994). In LMICs, the concern is really the exposure to the nutrient mismatch: starting out with poor fetal nutrition or low birth weight and being overweight in early adulthood, in parallel with the nutrition transition (Adair and Cole 2003; Borja 2013). The role of fetal and early childhood development in establishing risk for noncommunicable disease is discussed in detail in *Disease Control Priorities*, third edition (*DCP3*), volume 5, chapter 6 (Afshin and others 2017), while the policies for addressing unhealthy diet and obesity as risk factors for disease are discussed in Mozaffarian and others (2011), as well as in *DCP3* volume 5, chapter 5 (Bull and others 2017) and chapter 7 (Malik and Hu 2017).

Declining physical activity may also be a factor in increasing childhood overweight and obesity. In 85 countries, no more than 50 percent of boys or girls participated in 60 minutes or more of physical activity per day, with the Middle East and North Africa having the lowest ratios for girls (Patton and others 2012). These changes are accompanied by growth that favors urban over rural areas, with the result that overweight and stunted populations reside in the same country (Popkin 1994; Tzioumis and Adair 2014; Usfar and others 2010). This duality can also be found within the same household or even the same person: when energy-dense food is being consumed in a household, an adult could gain weight but be deficient in micronutrients, while a child could lack adequate calories and nutrients and fail to grow appropriately (Tzioumis and Adair 2014).

Prevalence of Overweight and Obesity

Worldwide, from 1980 to 2013, the prevalence of overweight and obesity combined has risen by 27 percent for adults and 47 percent for children (ages 2–19 years) to 37 percent and 13 percent, respectively (Ng and others 2014). Overweight and obesity increased in both LMICs and HICs during this period, increasing to 23 percent from 16 percent for girls and to 24 percent from 17 percent for boys in HICs, and to 13 percent from 8 percent for girls and boys in LMICs. In LMICs, the highest obesity rates are in the Middle East and North Africa, certain Pacific Islands, Caribbean nations, Chile, Costa Rica, Mexico, and Uruguay (Ng and others 2014).

In Latin America and the Caribbean, between 16.5 million and 21.1 million adolescents (ages 12–19 years) were overweight or obese from 2008 to 2013 (Rivera and others 2014). In China, from 2004 to 2009, the prevalence of overweight in boys ages 12–18 years rose from 7.5 percent to almost 13 percent, sedentary activity increased from 2.2 hours to 3.1 hours per day, and energy intake decreased 19 percent (Seo and Niu 2014). Manyanga and others (2014) studied overweight and obesity in students ages 11–18 years in seven African countries and found that 23 percent of girls were overweight and 4.5 percent were obese, compared with 18 percent and 3 percent, respectively, of boys. The highest rates of overweight in females were in Mauritania (36 percent) and Djibouti (9 percent); the lowest rates of overweight in males were in Ghana (7 percent) and Benin (0.3 percent). In Indonesia, 6 percent of children ages 6–14 years and 19 percent of those ages 15 years and older were overweight or obese (Usfar and others 2010). Ogden and others (2006) found equally high rates in HICs.

Interventions for Overweight and Obesity

Interventions to prevent obesity (lifestyle modification) have been found to yield positive results such as lower blood pressure (Cai and others 2014). However, most of the studies are from HICs. Waters and others (2011) found that interventions focusing on nutritional awareness, increased physical activity, and better-quality diets significantly lowered BMI in children ages 6–12 years. The strongest impact was found for interventions focusing on diet and physical activity that were conducted in community and school settings (Bleich and others 2013). Lobelo and others (2013) reviewed technology-based interventions, such as web-based programs, e-learning, and active video games, for healthy weight management and obesity prevention and found positive effects on diet, physical activity, and psychosocial functioning (table 11.3).

Interventions to manage obesity include methods that seek to impart awareness about healthy nutrition and physical activity, behavioral therapy, and use of

Table 11.3 Summary Estimates of Effectiveness of Interventions for Obesity in High-Income Countries

Study	Intervention	Outcome
Obesity prevention: Bhutta and Lassi 2016	Health promotion and education or counseling on diet, physical activity, lifestyle support, and dietary advice	BMI: SMD, –0.05 (–0.11, –0.01); 16 studies, $N = 14,912$
Obesity management: Bhutta and Lassi 2016	Counseling on diet, physical activity, lifestyle support, and dietary advice	BMI at 6 months follow-up: SMD, –3.02 (–5.08, –0.22); 4 studies, $N = 362$
Obesity management: Bazzano and others 2014	Randomized, parallel-group trial with a low-fat or low-carbohydrate diet, with dietary counseling	Participants with a low-carbohydrate diet had a –3.5 kg (95% CI, –5.6 to –1.4 kg) decrease in weight compared with a –1.5% (95% CI, –2.6% to –0.4%) decrease among participants with a low-fat diet at 12 months

Note: BMI = body mass index; CI = confidence interval; kg = kilogram; SMD = standardized mean difference.

medicine (orlistat, sibutramine, and metformin) or surgery. Such interventions have been found to decrease overweight in children and adolescents. Behavioral interventions lasting 12 months had the most effect on decreasing BMI, followed by behavioral interventions combined with medicine (Whitlock and others 2010). When combined with healthy lifestyle counseling, nutritional interventions were found to improve school performance, with increased physical activity linked to improved function, memory, and mathematics achievement (but not to reading, vocabulary, and language achievement); attention; inhibitory control; or simultaneous processing (Martin and others 2014). For severe obesity, behavioral and surgical interventions were found to lower BMI and improve functioning in adolescents, but surgery outperformed behavioral therapy for at least two years of follow-up (Ells and others 2015).

MICRONUTRIENT DEFICIENCIES

Adolescents need more nutrients than adults because they gain at least 40 percent of their adult weight and 15 percent of their adult height during this period. Inadequate intake can lead to delayed sexual development and slower linear growth (Jacob and Nair 2012).

Cognitive growth also depends on micronutrients; B complex vitamins are important in neural communication, and their absence leads to depression (Black 2008). Vitamin B12, folate, and thiamine are important for neural pathways, and deficiency has been linked to impaired episodic memory and language issues (Black 2008). Iron is required for oligodendrocyte growth and neurotransmitter production, and deficiency affects cognition, memory, and social and motor development (Fretham, Carlson, and Georgeiff 2011). Iodine is involved in structural development, and its absence causes mental retardation (Kapil 2007). Zinc is found in the forebrain and hippocampus, and its deficiency is linked to impaired attention, learning, and memory, as well as to possible development of neuropsychological diseases (Nyaradi and others 2013).

Studies have found inconsistent impact of micronutrient supplementation on children ages 5–15 years in LMICs (Khor and Misra 2012). Iron has been shown to affect weight and mid-arm circumference in children older than age six years (Vucic and others 2013). Vitamin D has been linked to a healthy lipid profile, with higher levels associated with low triglycerides and low total cholesterol, including good ratios of low- to high-density cholesterol (Kelishadi, Farajzadegan, and Bahreynian 2014).

Prevalence of Micronutrient Deficiencies

Iron deficiency anemia is one of the top five causes of years lost to disability (YLDs) and accounts for nearly 50 percent of total YLDs for adolescents (ages 10–19 years). It is the top cause of YLDs in boys and girls ages 10–14 years in South-East Asia and in boys in the Americas (WHO 2009). For 13,113 young people in the Islamic Republic of Iran, older adolescents (ages 14–17 years) had lower than recommended intake of vitamin A, calcium, and phosphorus; younger adolescents (ages 11–16 years) had lower than recommended intake of zinc, calcium, phosphorus, magnesium, and folate; and young adults (ages 18–28 years) had lower than recommended intake of folate, iron, and calcium (Akbari and Azadbakht 2014). In China, children younger than age 18 years were found to be deficient in vitamins A, B12, and K, as well as in iodine, iron, selenium, zinc, and calcium (Akbari and Azadbakht 2014). Children and women, including adolescent girls in resource-poor conditions, are especially vulnerable. Wong and others (2014) found lower than recommended intake of vitamins C and A and riboflavin in Asia, vitamin B6 in Africa, and folic acid in all regions studied. However, in Latin America and the Caribbean, the intake of vitamins A, C, B6, and riboflavin was higher than recommended.

Interventions for Micronutrient Deficiencies

Many children and adolescents have a micronutrient-deficient diet, and appropriate nutrient supplements are needed. Nutrients can be provided via tablets, powders sprinkled on food or mixed in water, and fortified spreads or snacks. Such foods need to have adequate amounts of energy and micronutrients, taste good, be clean and hygienic, and have a long shelf life (Nestel and others 2003). There is some indication that supplementation is helpful for healthy children. Multiple-micronutrient supplementation has been associated with a marginal increase in fluid intelligence and improved academic performance; however, more research is needed (Eilander and others 2010).

Given the persistence of iron-deficiency anemia, vitamin A deficiency, and iodine deficiency, food fortification (iron and iodine in salt), diet modification, and public health and disease control measures (deworming and malaria nets) may be needed (Ahluwalia 2002). In older populations, studies have not supported the use of antioxidant vitamins or mineral supplements (Dangour, Sibson, and Fletcher 2004). However, in children, adolescents, and women, iron supplementation has been found to increase attention, concentration, and intelligence (Falkingham and others 2010). In children younger than

Table 11.4 Summary Estimates of the Effectiveness of Micronutrient Interventions

Study	Intervention	Outcome
Bhutta and Lassi 2016 (adolescents)	Daily iron supplementation	Anemia: RR, 0.60 (0.42, 0.86); 1 study, N = 238
	Weekly iron and folic acid supplementation	Anemia: RR, 0.46 (0.23, 0.94); 4 studies, N = 852
	Vitamin A supplementation	Anemia: RR, 0.73 (0.56, 0.93); 1 study, N = 138
	Calcium supplementation	BMD change: MD, 1.09 (–0.15, 2.33); 1 study, N = 53
		BMD change of hip after one-year supplementation: MD, 1.09 (–0.15, 2.33); 1 study, N = 53
		BMD change of hip after one-year supplementation: MD, 1.17 (–0.45, 2.79); 1 study, N = 53
		Mean birth weight: SMD, 0.47 [–0.17, 1.10]; 2 studies, N = 307
	Vitamin D	Serum 25 hydroxy vitamin D (OH)D levels at three years: MD, 8.8 (–2.68, 20.28); 2 studies, N = 588
	Zinc supplementation	Hemoglobin: SMD, 4.81 (0.47, 8.66); 2 studies, N = 494
		Serum zinc: SMD, 4.28 (2.49, 6.06); 3 studies, N = 805
	Iodine supplementation	Thyroid-stimulating hormone: MD, 0.30 (–0.06, 0.66); 1 study, N = 47
	Multiple micronutrients	Anemia: RR, 0.95 (0.76, 1.18); 1 study, N = 113

Note: BMD = bone mineral density; MD = mean difference; RR = relative risk; SMD = standardized mean difference.

age 18 years, calcium supplementation had a small positive effect on total body and upper-limb bone mineral density (Winzenberg and others 2006), but it did not lower the risk of fracture (Falkingham and others 2010). In pubertal girls, calcium supplementation was associated with increased bone mass during 18 months of intervention (Teegarden and Weaver 1994). Iodine supplementation via salt was found to decrease the risk of goiter, cretinism, low intelligence, and low urinary iodine excretion (Aburto and others 2014). More evidence is needed on supplementation for adolescents (table 11.4).

NUTRITION FOR PREGNANT ADOLESCENTS

Nutrition for adolescents is important given that risk of preterm birth, low birth weight, asphyxia, stillbirth, and neonatal death are higher in adolescents than in young adults (ages 20–24 years) (WHO 2016a). Fall and others (2015) analyzed five longitudinal studies from Brazil, Guatemala, India, the Philippines, and South Africa and reported links between maternal and child undernutrition. They also reported adverse health outcomes in adults, including shorter height; less schooling; lower income or assets; lower–birth weight offspring; higher BMI; and harmful glucose concentrations, lipid profiles, and blood pressure. Undernutrition and low birth weight are further linked with some cancers and mental illnesses.

Overall, stunting is a strong indicator of lower human capital (WHO 2016b).

Adolescent girls are vulnerable to malnutrition secondary to the potential for pregnancy and socioeconomic adversity. Approximately 16 million girls ages 15–19 years give birth each year, accounting for 11 percent of total births and 23 percent of DALYs attributable to pregnancy and childbirth worldwide (WHO 2016a). Half of all births in this age group occur in seven countries: Bangladesh, Brazil, the Democratic Republic of Congo, Ethiopia, India, Nigeria, and the United States. Early pregnancies have significant health, social, and economic repercussions; 10 percent of all maternal deaths occur in adolescents, and 20 countries with the most adolescent maternal deaths account for 82 percent of all maternal deaths (Verguet and others 2017, chapter 28 in this volume; WHO 2016a). The risk of maternal mortality is higher in adolescents than in young adults ages 20–24 years, and 14 percent of all unsafe abortions occur in adolescents (Nove and others 2014). Pregnant adolescents are more likely to leave school; poorer and less educated adolescents are more likely to become pregnant (Nove and others 2014), which can result in transgenerational socioeconomic disadvantage (WHO 2007). Maternal malnutrition; micronutrient deficiency; obesity; gestational diabetes mellitus; and use of alcohol, tobacco, and psychotropic drugs affect mothers and their babies.

Impaired fetal growth, more common in adolescent pregnancies, has been linked to adult diabetes (Sawyer and others 2012).

Interventions during Pregnancy

Interventions for gestational diabetes mellitus in pregnant women have mixed results. Lassi and Bhutta (2015) found that healthy diet, increased physical activity, and strict glycemic control reduced the risk of gestational diabetes, decreased adiposity, and improved pregnancy outcomes in adolescents and women. However, Yin and others (2014) found no significant impact of physical activity on the risk of gestational diabetes. Mohd Yusof and others (2014) found no significant change in the risk of gestational diabetes with similar interventions, but they did find an association between earlier initiation of intervention and underweight babies. Behavioral therapy added to standard antenatal care can lead to lower gestational weight gain—a risk factor for gestational diabetes—in obese women without comorbid conditions (Mohd Yusof and others 2014). These studies do not provide evidence specifically for adolescent mothers.

Many studies have found that micronutrient supplementation during pregnancy is beneficial. Daily iron supplementation increases mean birth weight and decreases the risk of low-birth weight babies, and preventive iron supplementation decreases the risk of maternal anemia and iron deficiency at term (Pena-Rosas and others 2012). An intermittent regimen of iron and folic acid supplementation has been found to be as efficacious as a daily regimen, but with fewer side effects (Fernandez-Gaxiola and De-Regil 2011). No studies have specifically studied supplementation in pregnant adolescents.

Folic acid supplementation during pregnancy helps prevent neural tube defects (De-Regil and others 2010). It has also been found to decrease the incidence of megaloblastic anemia and increase mean birth weight (Lassi and others 2013). The evidence for vitamin A is mixed. Vitamin A decreases the risk of anemia, improves hemoglobin levels during pregnancy, and improves birth weight for women with human immunodeficiency virus, but it has no effect on other outcomes in pregnant women or infants (Thorne-Lyman and Fawzi 2012). Zinc fortification increases zinc serum levels and may improve growth (Das and others 2013). Vitamin D supplementation increases serum levels (Ota and others 2015). Calcium supplementation in both high- and low-dose regimens reduces hypertensive disorders during pregnancy and preterm births and increases birth weight (Hofmeyr,

Belizan, and von Dadelszen 2014). The WHO recommends iodine intake of 250 micrograms per day for pregnant women in iodine-deficient-endemic areas (Zimmermann 2009).

Protein energy supplementation has been found to affect pregnant women in general, especially if they are undernourished. This intervention increases mean birth weight and decreases the risk of low birth weight, small-for-gestational-age births, and stillbirths (Imdad and Bhutta 2012). Again, no studies have been conducted specifically on adolescent mothers. For the majority of micronutrients, evidence could not be found on adolescent populations; therefore, this is an area of research for countries where adolescent pregnancy is still common.

EATING DISORDERS

The American Psychiatric Association (2013) defines an eating disorder as a continuous disturbance of food consumption that leads to either a different pattern of eating or different absorption of food and can cause significant physical or psychological complications. Disorders such as anorexia nervosa, bulimia nervosa, and binge-eating disorder cause nutritional problems including decreased growth, impaired weight gain, and poor oral health (Gonçalves and others 2013). Eating disorders at younger ages (11–17 years) have been linked to eating disorders, overweight, and depression at later ages (17–23 years) (Gonçalves and others 2013).

Anorexia is defined as low self-esteem and a fear of gaining weight; anorexic individuals are frequently severely underweight and amenorrheic (Seidenfeld, Sosin, and Rickert 2004). Anorexia can severely impair bone health, reduce physical and sexual growth, cause hormonal dysfunction, affect cognitive development, and predict future psychological disease (Donaldson and Gordon 2015; Seidenfeld, Sosin, and Rickert 2004). Mortality from anorexia is 12 times higher than mortality from any other cause for American women ages 15–24 years (Herpertz-Dahlmann, Bühren, and Seitz 2011). Bulimia is defined by episodes of binge eating followed by purging through forced vomiting or abuse of diet pills or laxatives and by compensating through excessive exercise (Seidenfeld, Sosin, and Rickert 2004). Adolescents with bulimia have higher suicidal ideation (53 percent of sample) than those with no psychopathology (4 percent) (Sullivan 1995).

Although the majority of the evidence is from HICs, similar patterns have been reported in upper-middle-income countries. Girls are exposed to risk factors beginning in early adolescence. Peer pressure to be thin, thinness as the ideal body image, and dissatisfaction with current body type can increase the chances that adolescents will develop eating disorders (Crow and others 2014). Adolescent girls who binge eat have high functional impairment and comorbid mental health problems. This behavior, along with weight concerns and other behaviors to control weight, were found to be associated with higher BMI two years later in teen girls in the United States (Rohde, Stice, and Marti 2015). Perhaps partly as a result of peer pressure in early adolescence, eating disorders develop most commonly in middle and late adolescence (Portela and others 2012).

Prevalence of Eating Disorders

In 2010, 193.9 million DALYs were attributable to substance abuse and mental disorders (7.4 percent of all DALYs). Eating disorders accounted for 1.2 percent of DALYs attributable to mental and substance abuse. The highest amount of DALYs were reported in persons ages 10–28 years. In the United States, up to 30 million people suffer from eating disorders, with 86 percent of sufferers reporting onset before age 20 years and 43 percent at ages 16–20 years (Whiteford and others 2013). Multiple studies from the United States found that eating disorders were prevalent in 3.6 percent of adolescents and that 63 percent of these individuals had comorbid psychiatric disorders as well (Stice, Marti, and Rohde 2013); lifetime prevalence was 13 percent (Smink and others 2014). For a Dutch cohort of adolescents ages 11–19 years, Smink, van Hoeken, and Hoek (2012) found that lifetime prevalence was 1.7 percent for anorexia, 0.8 percent for bulimia, and 2.3 percent for binge-eating disorder in women; these disorders were rare for men. In the Islamic Republic of Iran, the prevalence of diagnosed eating disorders was 0.25 percent. Boys and girls scored much lower on the eating disorder examination questionnaire when compared with previous studies from Western countries (Nakai and others 2015). Although the occurrence of bulimia nervosa has decreased in recent decades, the overall incidence rate of anorexia nervosa has remained stable (Smink, van Hoeken, and Hoek 2012).

Interventions for Eating Disorders

Interventions that focus on prevention include media literacy and advocacy, psychological education, and self-esteem building (Nakai and others 2015). Interventions that focus on treatment include family therapy, individual therapy, cognitive behavioral therapy, interpersonal psychotherapy, cognitive training, dialectical behavior therapy, and enhanced cognitive behavioral therapy. Only family treatment behavioral therapy has been well established for anorexia. Newer or not well-established therapies include family treatment behavior and supportive individual therapy for bulimia and Internet-delivered cognitive behavioral therapy for binge-eating disorder (Dobbins and others 2013). It is impossible to compare effectiveness because studies use different methods to measure outcomes.

CONCLUSIONS

Malnutrition in adolescence has been a neglected area of research and programming globally. The evidence for effective interventions to address nutritional problems in LMICs is particularly weak. In particular, proven effective responses for stunting, overweight and obesity, and micronutrient deficiencies are not yet available. From HICs, there is some evidence on interventions for eating disorders and obesity, although much further work is needed in these settings as well.

Yet there is an emerging double nutritional threat to child and adolescent health in LMICs. To reduce deficiency-related malnutrition while preventing overweight and obesity, integrated adolescent health programs are needed that prevent infection, improve diet quality, and encourage physical activity. Although the double burden of nutrient deficiency, coupled with overweight and obesity, is increasing in LMICs, policies in most countries focus almost exclusively on undernutrition in multiple forms; only a few countries have implemented national policies to prevent obesity. In view of the rapidly growing number of adolescents who are overweight or obese, the detrimental effects of obesity on health, and the costs to health care systems, programs to monitor and prevent unhealthy weight gain in children and adolescents are urgently needed (Lassi and others 2015).

NOTE

World Bank Income Classifications as of July 2014 are as follows, based on estimates of gross national income (GNI) per capita for 2013:

- Low-income countries (LICs) = US$1,045 or less
- Middle-income countries (MICs) are subdivided:
  a) lower-middle-income = US$1,046 to US$4,125
  b) upper-middle-income (UMICs) = US$4,126 to US$12,745
- High-income countries (HICs) = US$12,746 or more.

REFERENCES

Aburto, N. J., M. Abudou, V. Candeias, and T. Wu. 2014. *Effect and Safety of Salt Iodization to Prevent Iodine Deficiency Disorders: A Systematic Review with Meta-Analyses.* WHO eLibrary of Evidence for Nutrition Actions (eLENA). Geneva: WHO.

Adair, L. S., and T. J. Cole. 2003. "Rapid Child Growth Raises Blood Pressure in Adolescent Boys Who Were Thin at Birth." *Hypertension* 41: 451–56.

Afshin, A., R. Micha, M. Webb, S. Capewell, L. Whitsel, and others. 2017. "Effectiveness of Dietary Policies to Reduce Noncommunicable Diseases." In *Disease Control Priorities* (third edition): Volume 5, *Cardiovascular, Respiratory, and Related Diseases*, edited by D. Prabhakaran, S. Anand, T. Gaziano, J.-C. Mbanya, Y. Wu, and R. Nugent. Washington, DC: World Bank.

Ahluwalia, N. 2002. "Intervention Strategies for Improving Iron Status of Young Children and Adolescents in India." *Nutrition Reviews* 60 (5 Pt 2): S115–17.

Ahmed, F., A. Rahman, A. N. Noor, M. Akhtaruzzaman, and R. Hughes. 2006. "Anaemia and Vitamin A Status among Adolescent Schoolboys in Dhaka City, Bangladesh." *Public Health Nutrition* 9: 345–50.

Akbari, F., and L. Azadbakht. 2014. "A Systematic Review on Diet Quality among Iranian Youth: Focusing on Reports from Tehran and Isfahan." *Archive of Iranian Medicine* 17: 574–84.

Alam, N., S. K, Roy, T. Ahmed, and A. M. Ahmed. 2010. "Nutritional Status, Dietary Intake, and Relevant Knowledge of Adolescent Girls in Rural Bangladesh." *Journal of Health, Population and Nutrition* 28 (1): 86–94.

American Psychiatric Association. 2013. "Feeding and Eating Disorders." In *Diagnostic and Statistical Manual of Mental Disorders*. Washington, DC: American Psychiatric Association. http://www.dsm5.org/documents/eating%20disorders%20fact%20sheet.pdf.

Barugahara, E. I., J. Kikafunda, and W. M. Gakenia. 2013. "Prevalence and Risk Factors of Nutritional Anaemia among Female School Children in Masindi District, Western Uganda." *African Journal of Food, Agriculture, Nutrition, and Development* 13: 7679–92.

Bazzano, L. A., T. Hu, K. Reynolds, L. Yao, C. Bunol, and others. 2014. "Effects of Low-Carbohydrate and Low-Fat Diets: A Randomized Control Trial." *Annals of Internal Medicine* 161 (5): 309–18. doi:10.7326/M14-0180.

Bhutta, Z. A., and Z. S. Lassi. 2016. "Nutrition for Adolescents and Young Women: Recommendations." *Annals of the New York Academy of Sciences*. [Submitted].

Black, M. M. 2008. "Effects of Vitamin B12 and Folate Deficiency on Brain Development in Children." *Food and Nutrition Bulletin* 29 (Suppl 2): S126–31.

Bleich, S. N., J. Segal, Y. Wu, R. Wilson, and Y. Wang. 2013. "Systematic Review of Community-Based Childhood Obesity Prevention Studies." *Pediatrics* 132: e201.

Borja, J. D. 2013. "The Impact of Early Nutrition on Health: Key Findings from the Cebu Longitudinal Health and Nutrition Survey." *Malaysian Journal of Nutrition* 19 (1): 1–8.

Bull, F., S. Goenka, V. Lambert, and M. Pratt. 2017. "Physical Activity for the Prevention of Cardiometabolic Disease." In *Disease Control Priorities* (third edition): Volume 5, *Cardiovascular, Respiratory, and Related Diseases*, edited by D. Prabhakaran, S. Anand, T. Gaziano, J.-C. Mbanya, Y. Wu, and R. Nugent. Washington, DC: World Bank.

Bundy, D. A. P., N. de Silva, S. Horton, G. C. Patton, L. Schultz, and D. T. Jamison. 2017. "Child and Adolescent Health and Development: Realizing Neglected Potential." In *Disease Control Priorities* (third edition): Volume 8, *Child and Adolescent Health and Development,* edited by D. A. P. Bundy, N. de Silva, S. Horton, D. T. Jamison, and G. C. Patton. Washington, DC: World Bank.

Cai, L., Y. Wu, R. F. Wilson, J. B. Segal, M. T. Kim, and others. 2014. "Effect of Childhood Obesity Prevention Programs on Blood Pressure: A Systematic Review and Meta-Analysis." *Circulation* 129 (18): 1832–39.

Caprio, S., G. Cline, S. Boulware, C. Permanente, G. I. Shulman, and others. 1994. "Effects of Puberty and Diabetes on Metabolism of Insulin-Sensitive Fuels." *American Journal of Physiology* 266 (6 Pt 1): E885–91.

Creed-Kanashiro, H. M., T. G. Uribe, R. M. Bartolini, M. N. Fukumoto, T. T. Lopez, and others. 2000. "Improving Dietary Intake to Prevent Anemia in Adolescent Girls through Community Kitchens in a Periurban Population of Lima, Peru." *Journal of Nutrition* 130 (Suppl 2): S459–61.

Crow, S. J., S. A. Swanson, D. Le Grange, E. H. Feig, and K. R. Merikangas. 2014. "Suicidal Behavior in Adolescents and Adults with Bulimia Nervosa." *Comprehensive Psychiatry* 55 (7): 1534–39.

Dangour, A. D., V. L. Sibson, and A. E. Fletcher. 2004. "Micronutrient Supplementation in Later Life: Limited Evidence for Benefit." *Journal of Gerontology Series A: Biological Sciences and Medical Sciences* 59: 659–73.

Das, J. K., R. Kumar, R. A. Salam, and Z. A. Bhutta. 2013. "Systematic Review of Zinc Fortification Trials." *Annals of Nutrition and Metabolism* 62 (Suppl 1): 44–56.

Dobbins, M., H. Husson, K. DeCorby, and R. L. LaRocca. 2013. "School-Based Physical Activity Programs for Promoting Physical Activity and Fitness in Children and Adolescents Aged 6 to 18." *Cochrane Database of Systematic Reviews* 2: CD007651.

Doku, D., L. Koivusilta, S. Raisamo, and A. Rimpelä. 2013. "Socio-Economic Differences in Adolescents' Breakfast Eating, Fruit and Vegetable Consumption and Physical Activity in Ghana." *Public Health Nutrition* 16: 864–72.

Donaldson, A. A., and C. M. Gordon. 2015. "Skeletal Complications of Eating Disorders." *Metabolism* 64: 943–51.

Dror, D. K., and L. H. Allen. 2014. "Dairy Product Intake in Children and Adolescents in Developed Countries: Trends, Nutritional Contribution, and a Review of Association with Health Outcomes." *Nutrition Reviews* 72 (2): 68–81.

Eilander, A., T. Gera, H. S. Sachdev, C. Transler, H. C. van der Knaap, and others. 2010. "Multiple Micronutrient Supplementation for Improving Cognitive Performance in Children: Systematic Review of Randomized Controlled Trials." *American Journal of Clinical Nutrition* 91: 115–30.

Ells, L. J., E. Mead, G. Atkinson, E. Corpeleijn, K. Roberts, and others. 2015. "Surgery for the Treatment of Obesity in

Children and Adolescents." *Cochrane Database of Systematic Reviews* 6: CD011740.

Falkingham, M., A. Abdelhamid, P. Curtis, S. Fairweather-Tait, L. Dye, and others. 2010. "The Effects of Oral Iron Supplementation on Cognition in Older Children and Adults: A Systematic Review and Meta-Analysis." *Journal of Nutrition* 25: 4.

Fall, C. H. D., H. S. Sachdev, C. Osmond, M. C. Restrepo-Mendez, C. Victora, and others. 2015. "Association between Maternal Age at Childbirth and Child and Adult Outcomes in the Offspring: A Prospective Study in Five Low-Middle-Income Countries (COHORTS COLLABORATIONS)." *The Lancet Global Health* 3 (7): e366–77.

Fernandez-Gaxiola, A. C., and L. M. De-Regil. 2011. "Intermittent Iron Supplementation for Reducing Anaemia and Its Associated Impairments in Menstruating Women." *Cochrane Database of Systematic Reviews* 12: CD009218.

Ferraro, K. F., R. J. Thorpe, and J. A. Wilkinson. 2003. "The Life Course of Severe Obesity: Does Childhood Overweight Matter?" *Journal of Gerontology Series B: Psychological Sciences and Social Sciences* 58: S110–19.

Fretham, S. J. B., E. S. Carlson, and M. K. Georgeiff. 2011. "The Role of Iron in Learning and Memory." *Advances in Nutrition* 2: 112–21.

Galloway, R. 2017. "Global Nutrition Outcomes at Ages 5 to 19." In *Disease Control Priorities* (third edition): Volume 8, *Child and Adolescent Health and Development*, edited by Bundy, D. A. P., N. de Silva, S. Horton, D. T. Jamison, and G. C. Patton. Washington, DC: World Bank.

Gonçalves, J. A., E. A. Moreira, E. B. Trindade, and G. M. Fiates. 2013. "Eating Disorders in Childhood and Adolescence." *Revista Paulista de Pediatria* 31: 96–103.

Guo, S. S., A. F. Roche, W. C. Chumlea, J. D. Gardner, and R. M. Siervogel. 1994. "The Predictive Value of Childhood Body Mass Index Values for Overweight at Age 35." *American Journal of Clinical Nutrition* 59: 810–19.

Herpertz-Dahlmann, B., K. Bühren, and J. Seitz. 2011. "Anorexia Nervosa in Childhood and Adolescence: Course and Significance for Adulthood." *Nervenarzt* 82: 1093–99.

Hofmeyr, G. J., J. M. Belizan, and P. von Dadelszen. 2014. "Low-Dose Calcium Supplementation for Preventing Pre-Eclampsia: A Systematic Review and Commentary." *BJOG* 121: 951–57.

Imdad, A., and Z. A. Bhutta. 2012. "Maternal Nutrition and Birth Outcomes: Effect of Balanced Protein-Energy Supplementation." *Paediatric and Perinatal Epidemiology* 26 (Suppl 1): 178–90.

Jacob, J. A., and M. K. Nair. 2012. "Protein and Micronutrient Supplementation in Complementing Pubertal Growth." *Indian Journal of Pediatrics* 79 (Suppl 1): S84–91.

Kapil, U. 2007. "Health Consequences of Iodine Deficiency." *Sultan Qaboos University Medical Journal* 7 (3): 267–72.

Kawade, R. 2012. "Zinc Status and Its Association with the Health of Adolescents: A Review of Studies in India." *Global Health Action* 5: 7353.

Keino, S., G. Plasqui, G. Ettyang, and B. van den Borne. 2014. "Determinants of Stunting and Overweight among Young Children and Adolescents in Sub-Saharan Africa." *Food and Nutrition Bulletin* 35: 167–78.

Kelishadi, R., Z. Farajzadegan, and M. Bahreynian. 2014. "Association between Vitamin D Status and Lipid Profile in Children and Adolescents: A Systematic Review and Meta-Analysis." *International Journal of Food Sciences and Nutrition* 65: 404–10.

Khor, G. L., and S. Misra. 2012. "Micronutrient Interventions on Cognitive Performance of Children Aged 5–15 Years in Developing Countries." *Asia Pacific Journal of Clinical Nutrition* 21 (4): 476–86.

Lassi, Z. S., and Z. A. Bhutta. 2015. "Obesity, Pre-Diabetes, and Diabetes in Adolescents and Women: Evidence-Based Interventions." Nestlé Nutrition Institute Workshops Series.

Lassi, Z. S., R. A. Salam, J. K. Das, J. Wazny, and Z. A. Bhutta. 2015. "An Unfinished Agenda on Adolescent Health: Opportunities for Interventions." *Seminars in Perinatology* 39: 353–60.

Lassi, Z. S., R. A. Salam, B. A. Haider, and Z. A. Bhutta. 2013. "Folic Acid Supplementation during Pregnancy for Maternal Health and Pregnancy Outcomes." *Cochrane Database of Systematic Reviews* 3: CD006896.

Li, M., M. J. Dibley, D. Sibbritt, and H. Yan. 2008. "Factors Associated with Adolescents' Overweight and Obesity at Community, School, and Household Levels in Xi'an City, China: Results of Hierarchical Analysis." *European Journal of Clinical Nutrition* 62: 635–43.

Lobelo, F., I. Garcia de Quevedo, C. K. Holub, B. J. Nagle, E. M. Arredondo, and others. 2013. "School-Based Programs Aimed at the Prevention and Treatment of Obesity: Evidence-Based Interventions for Youth in Latin America." *Journal of School Health* 83: 668–77.

Lopes, T. S., R. Sichieri, R. Salles-Costa, G. V. Veiga, and R. A. Pereira. 2013. "Family Food Insecurity and Nutritional Risk in Adolescents from a Low-Income Area of Rio de Janeiro, Brazil." *Journal of Biosocial Science* 45: 661–74.

Malik, V., and F. Hu. 2017. "Weight Management." In *Disease Control Priorities* (third edition): Volume 5, *Cardiovascular, Respiratory, and Related Diseases*, edited by D. Prabhakaran, S. Anand, T. Gaziano, J.-C. Mbanya, Y. Wu, and R. Nugent. Washington, DC: World Bank.

Mann, S. K., S. Kaur, and K. Bains. 2002. "Iron and Energy Supplementation Improves the Physical Work Capacity of Female College Students." *Food and Nutrition Bulletin* 23: 57–64.

Manyanga, T., H. El-Sayed, D. T. Doku, and J. R. Randall. 2014. "The Prevalence of Underweight, Overweight, Obesity, and Associated Risk Factors among School-Going Adolescents in Seven African Countries." *BMC Public Health* 14: 887.

Marshall, S., T. Burrows, and C. E. Collins. 2014. "Systematic Review of Diet Quality Indices and Their Associations with Health-Related Outcomes in Children and Adolescents." *Journal of Human Nutrition and Dietetics* 27: 577–98.

Martin, A., D. H. Saunders, S. D. Shenkin, and J. Sproule. 2014. "Lifestyle Intervention for Improving School Achievement in Overweight or Obese Children and Adolescents." *Cochrane Database of Systematic Reviews* 3: CD009728.

Matsuzaki, M., H. Kuper, B. Kulkarni, G. B. Ploubidis, J. C. Wells, and others. 2015. "Adolescent Undernutrition and Early Adulthood Bone Mass in an Urbanizing Rural Community in India." *Archives of Osteoporosis* 10: 29.

Mohd Yusof, B. N., S. Firouzi, Z. Mohd Shariff, N. Mustafa, N. A. Mohamed Ismail, and others. 2014. "Weighing the Evidence of Low Glycemic Index Dietary Intervention for the Management of Gestational Diabetes Mellitus: An Asian Perspective." *International Journal of Food Science and Nutrition* 65: 144–50.

Moreno, L. A., F. Gottrand, I. Huybrechts, J. R. Ruiz, M. González-Gross, and others. 2014. "The HELENA (Healthy Lifestyle in Europe by Nutrition in Adolescence) Study 1–3." *Advances in Nutrition* 5: S615–23.

Mozaffarian, D., T. Hao, E. B. Rimm, W. C. Willett, and F. B. Hu. 2011. "Changes in Diet and Lifestyle and Long-Term Gain in Women and Men." *New England Journal of Medicine* 364 (25): 2392–404.

Nago, E. S., C. K. Lachat, L. Huybregts, D. Roberfroid, R. A. Dossa, and others. 2010. "Food, Energy, and Macronutrient Contribution of Out-of-Home Foods in School-Going Adolescents in Cotonou, Benin." *British Journal of Nutrition* 103: 281–88.

Nakai, Y., S. Noma, K. Nin, S. Teramukai, and S. A. Wonderlich. 2015. "Eating Disorder Behaviors and Attitudes in Japanese Adolescent Girls and Boys in High Schools." *Psychiatry Research* 230: 722–24.

Nestel, P., A. Briend, B. de Benoist, E. Decker, E. Ferguson, and others. 2003. "Complementary Food Supplements to Achieve Micronutrient Adequacy for Infants and Young Children." *Journal of Pediatric Gastroenterology and Nutrition* 36: 316–28.

Ng, M., T. Fleming, M. Robinson, B. Thomson, N. Graetz, and others. 2014. "Global, Regional, and National Prevalence of Overweight and Obesity in Children and Adults during 1980–2013: A Systematic Analysis for the Global Burden of Disease Study 2013." *The Lancet* 384 (9945): 766–81.

Nove, A., Z. Matthews, S. Neal, and A. V. Camacho. 2014. "Maternal Mortality in Adolescents Compared with Women of Other Ages: Evidence from 144 Countries." *The Lancet Global Health* 2 (3): e155–64.

Nyaradi, A., J. Li, S. Hickling, J. Foster, W. H. Oddy, and others. 2013. "The Role of Nutrition in Children's Neurocognitive Development, from Pregnancy through Childhood." *Frontiers in Human Neuroscience* 7: 97.

Ochola, S., and P. K. Masibo. 2014. "Dietary Intake of Schoolchildren and Adolescents in Developing Countries." *Annals of Nutrition and Metabolism* 64 (Suppl 2): 24–40.

Ogden, C. L., M. D. Carroll, L. R. Curtin, M. A. McDowell, C. J. Tabak, and others. 2006. "Prevalence of Overweight and Obesity in the United States, 1999–2004." *Journal of the American Medical Association* 295 (13): 1549–55.

Ota, E., R. Mori, P. Middleton, R. Tobe-Gai, K. Mahomed, and others. 2015. "Zinc Supplementation for Improving Pregnancy and Infant Outcome." *Cochrane Database of Systematic Reviews.* 7: CD000230. doi: 10.1002/14651858 .CD000230.pub4.

Park, M. H., C. Falconer, R. M. Viner, and S. Kinra. 2012. "The Impact of Childhood Obesity on Morbidity and Mortality in Adulthood: A Systematic Review." *Obesity Reviews* 13 (11): 985–1000.

Patton, G. C., C. Coffey, C. Cappa, D. Currie, L. Riley, and others. 2012. "Health of the World's Adolescents: A Synthesis of Internationally Comparable Data." *The Lancet* 379 (9826): 1665–75.

Patton, G. C., S. M. Sawyer, J. S. Santelli, D. A. Ross, R. Afifi, and others. 2016. "Our Future: A *Lancet* Commission on Adolescent Health and Well Being." *The Lancet* 387 (10036): 2423–78.

Pena-Rosas, J. P., L. M. De-Regil, T. Dowswell, and F. E. Viteri. 2012. "Daily Oral Iron Supplementation during Pregnancy." *Cochrane Database of Systematic Reviews* 12: CD004736.

Popkin, B. M. 1994. "The Nutrition Transition in Low-Income Countries: An Emerging Crisis." *Nutrition Reviews* 52 (9): 285–98.

Portela, S. M. L., R. J. H. da Costa, G. M. Mora, and R. M. Raich. 2012. "Epidemiology and Risk Factors of Eating Disorder in Adolescence: A Review." *Nutrición Hospitalaria* 27: 391–401.

Reilly, J. J., and J. Kelly. 2011. "Long-Term Impact of Overweight and Obesity in Childhood and Adolescence on Morbidity and Premature Mortality in Adulthood: Systematic Review." *International Journal of Obesity* 35: 891–98.

Rivera, J. Á., T. G. de Cossío, L. S. Pedraza, T. C. Aburto, T. G. Sánchez, and others. 2014. "Childhood and Adolescent Overweight and Obesity in Latin America: A Systematic Review." *The Lancet Diabetes and Endocrinology* 2 (4): 321–32.

Rohde, P., E. Stice, and C. N. Marti. 2015. "Development and Predictive Effects of Eating Disorder Risk Factors during Adolescence: Implications for Prevention Efforts." *International Journal of Eating Disorders* 48: 187–98.

Rytter, M. J., L. Kolte, A. Briend, H. Friis, and V. B. Christensen. 2014. "The Immune System in Children with Malnutrition: A Systematic Review." *PLoS One* 9: e105017.

Sawyer, S. M., R. A. Afifi, L. H. Bearinger, S. Blakemore, B. Dick, and others. 2012. "Adolescence: A Foundation for Future Health." *The Lancet* 379 (9826): 1630–40.

Seidenfeld, M. E., E. Sosin, and V. I. Rickert. 2004. "Nutrition and Eating Disorders in Adolescents." *Mount Sinai Journal of Medicine* 71: 155–61.

Seo, D. C., and J. Niu. 2014. "Trends in Underweight and Overweight/Obesity Prevalence in Chinese Youth, 2004–2009." *International Journal of Behavioral Medicine* 21: 682–90.

Seymour, M., S. L. Hoerr, and Y. L. Huang. 1997. "Inappropriate Dieting Behaviors and Related Lifestyle Factors in Young Adults: Are College Students Different?" *Journal of Nutrition Education* 29: 21–26.

Smink, F. R., D. van Hoeken, and H. W. Hoek. 2012. "Epidemiology of Eating Disorders: Incidence, Prevalence and Mortality Rates." *Current Psychiatric Report* 14 (4): 406–14.

Smink, F. R., D. van Hoeken, A. J. Oldehinkel, and H. W. Hoek. 2014. "Prevalence and Severity of DSM-5 Eating Disorders in a Community Cohort of Adolescents." *International Journal of Eating Disorders* 47: 610–19.

Soliman, A., V. De Sanctis, and R. Elalaily. 2014. "Nutrition and Pubertal Development." *Indian Journal of Endocrinology and Metabolism* 18 (Suppl 1): S39–47.

Spencer, R. A., L. Rehman, and S. F. L. Kirk. 2015. "Understanding Gender Norms, Nutrition, and Physical Activity in Adolescent Girls: A Scoping Review." *International Journal of Behavioral Nutrition and Physical Activity* 12: 6.

Stice, E., C. N. Marti, and P. Rohde. 2013. "Prevalence, Incidence, Impairment, and Course of the Proposed DSM-5 Eating Disorder Diagnoses in an 8-Year Prospective Community Study of Young Women." *Journal of Abnormal Psychology* 122 (2): 445–57.

Sullivan, P. F. 1995. "Mortality in Anorexia Nervosa." *American Journal of Psychiatry* 152 (7): 1073–74.

Teegarden, D., and C. M. Weaver. 1994. "Calcium Supplementation Increases Bone Density in Adolescent Girls." *Nutrition Reviews* 52 (5): 171–73.

Thomas, R., R. Srinivasan, and H. Sudarshan. 2013. "Nutritional Status of Tribal Children and Adolescents in Rural South India: The Effect of an NGO-Delivered Nutritional Programme." *Indian Journal of Pediatrics* 80: 821–25.

Thorne-Lyman, A. L., and W. W. Fawzi. 2012. "Vitamin A and Carotenoids during Pregnancy and Maternal, Neonatal, and Infant Health Outcomes: A Systematic Review and Meta-Analysis." *Paediatric and Perinatal Epidemiology* 26 (Suppl 1): 36–54.

Tzioumis, E., and L. S. Adair. 2014. "Childhood Dual Burden of Under- and Over-Nutrition in Low- and Middle-Income Countries: A Critical Review." *Food and Nutrition Bulletin* 35: 230–43.

UNICEF (United Nations Children's Fund). 2014. *The State of the World's Children 2015.* New York: UNICEF. http://www.unicef.org/publications/files/SOWC_2015_Summary_and_Tables.pdf.

Usfar, A. A., E. Lebenthal, Atmarita, E. Achadi, Soekirman, and others. 2010. "Obesity as a Poverty-Related Emerging Nutrition Problems: The Case of Indonesia." *Obesity Reviews* 11: 924–28.

Venter, I. M., and A. Winterbach. 2010. "Dietary Fat Knowledge and Intake of Mid-Adolescents Attending Public Schools in the Bellville/Durbanville Area of the City of Cape Town." *South African Journal of Clinical Nutrition* 23: 75–83.

Verguet S., A. Nandi, V. Filippi, and D. A. P. Bundy. 2017. "Postponing Adolescent Parity in Developing Countries through Education: An Extended Cost-Effective Analysis." In *Disease Control Priorities* (third edition): Volume 8, *Child and Adolescent Health and Development*, edited by Bundy, D. A. P., N. de Silva, S. Horton, D. T. Jamison, and G. C. Patton. Washington, DC: World Bank.

Viner R., N. Allen, and G. C. Patton. 2017. "Puberty, Developmental Processes, and Health Interventions." In *Disease Control Priorities* (third edition): Volume 8, *Child and Adolescent Health and Development*, edited by D. A. P. Bundy, N. de Silva,

S. Horton, D. T. Jamison, and G. C. Patton. Washington, DC: World Bank.

Vucic, V., C. Berti, C. Vollhardt, K. Fekete, I. Cetin, and others. 2013. "Effect of Iron Intervention on Growth during Gestation, Infancy, Childhood, and Adolescence: A Systematic Review with Meta-Analysis." *Nutrition Reviews* 71 (6): 386–401.

Waters, E., A. de Silva-Sanigorski, B. J. Burford, T. Brown, K. J. Campbell, and others. 2011. "Interventions for Preventing Obesity in Children." *Cochrane Database of Systematic Reviews* 12: CD001871.

Whiteford, H. A., L. Degenhardt, J. Rehm, A. J. Baxter, A. J. Ferrari, and others. 2013. "Global Burden of Disease Attributable to Mental and Substance Use Disorders: Findings from the Global Burden of Disease Study 2010." *The Lancet* 382 (9904): 1575–86.

Whitlock, E. P., E. A. O'Connor, S. B. Williams, T. L. Beil, and K. W. Lutz. 2010. "Effectiveness of Weight Management Interventions in Children: A Targeted Systematic Review for the USPSTF." *Pediatrics* 125: e396–418.

WHO (World Health Organization). 2007. *Adolescent Pregnancy: Unmet Needs and Undone Deeds: A Review of the Literature and Programmes.* Issues in Adolescent Health and Development. Geneva: WHO. http://apps.who.int/iris/bitstream/10665/43702/1/9789241595650_eng.pdf?ua=1&ua=1.

———. 2009. *Global Health Risks: Mortality and Burden of Disease Attributable to Selected Major Risks.* Geneva: WHO. http://www.who.int/healthinfo/global_burden_disease/GlobalHealthRisks_report_full.pdf.

———. 2014. "Data on Death and Disease among Adolescents." WHO, Geneva. http://apps.who.int/adolescent/second-decade/section3/page1/death-&-disease-among-adolescents.html.

———. 2016a. "Adolescent Pregnancy." WHO, Geneva. http://www.who.int/maternal_child_adolescent/topics/maternal/adolescent_pregnancy/en/.

———. 2016b. "Global Nutrition Targets 2025: Stunting Policy Brief." WHO, Geneva. http://thousanddays.org/resource/stunting-policy-brief.

Winzenberg, T. M., K. Shaw, J. Fryer, and G. Jones. 2006. "Calcium Supplementation for Improving Bone Mineral Density in Children." *Cochrane Database of Systematic Reviews* 2: CD005119.

Wong, A. Y., E. W. Chan, C. S. Chui, A. G. Sutcliffe, and I. C. Wong. 2014. "The Phenomenon of Micronutrient Deficiency among Children in China: A Systematic Review of the Literature." *Public Health Nutrition* 17: 2605–18.

Yin, Y. N., X. L. Li, T. J. Tao, B. R. Luo, and S. J. Liao. 2014. "Physical Activity during Pregnancy and the Risk of Gestational Diabetes Mellitus: A Systematic Review and Meta-Analysis of Randomised Controlled Trials." *British Journal of Sports Medicine* 48: 290–95.

Zimmermann, M. B. 2009. "Iodine Deficiency." *Endocrine Reviews* 30 (4): 376–408.

Chapter 12

School Feeding Programs in Middle Childhood and Adolescence

Lesley Drake, Meena Fernandes, Elisabetta Aurino,
Josephine Kiamba, Boitshepo Giyose, Carmen Burbano,
Harold Alderman, Lu Mai, Arlene Mitchell, and Aulo Gelli

INTRODUCTION

Almost every country in the world has a national school feeding program to provide daily snacks or meals to school-attending children and adolescents. The interventions reach an estimated 368 million children and adolescents globally. The total investment in the intervention is projected to be as much as US$75 billion annually (WFP 2013), largely from government budgets.

School feeding may contribute to multiple objectives, including social safety nets, education, nutrition, health, and local agriculture. Its contribution to education objectives is well recognized and documented, while its role as a social safety net was underscored following the food and fuel crises of 2007 and 2008 (Bundy and others 2009). In terms of health and nutrition, school feeding contributes to the continuum of development by building on investments made earlier in the life course, including maternal and infant health interventions and early child development interventions (see chapter 7 in this volume, Alderman and others 2017). School feeding may also help leverage global efforts to enhance the inclusiveness of education for out-of-school children, adolescent girls, and disabled persons, as called for in the Sustainable Development Goals (see chapter 17 in this volume, Graham and others 2017).

Although the *Disease Control Priorities* series focuses on low- and middle-income countries (LMICs), evidence from high-income countries (HICs) is included because of the near universality of school feeding and the insights that inclusion can provide as economies develop. For example, the design of school feeding in countries undergoing the nutrition transition[1] may provide some lessons on how to shift from providing access to sufficient calories to promoting healthful diets and dietary behaviors for children and adolescents (WFP 2013).

Agricultural development has increasingly gained attention. It is clear that to enable the transition to sustainable, scalable government-run programs, the inclusion of the agricultural sector is essential (Bundy and others 2009; Drake and others 2016). Accounting for the full benefits of school feeding through cost-effectiveness and benefit-cost analysis is challenging, similar to other complex interventions, but undertaking this accounting is critical for assessing the tradeoffs with competing investments.

This chapter reviews the evidence about how school feeding meets these objectives and provides some indication of costs in relation to benefits. The costs of the intervention are well established; estimates that encompass all the benefits of school feeding are more challenging. The benefits must be quantified and translated to the same unit to allow for aggregation. Moreover, how school feeding interventions are designed and implemented varies significantly across

Corresponding author: Lesley Drake, Partnership for Child Development, Imperial College London, United Kingdom; lesley.drake@imperial.ac.uk.

countries. Given that delivery of school feeding often involves multiple sectors, common policy frameworks and cross-sectoral coordination are required to achieve maximum benefit (Bundy and others 2009).

Several other chapters in the volume highlight school feeding. These include chapter 11 (Lassi, Moin, and Bhutta 2017), chapter 20 (Bundy and others 2017), chapter 22 (Plaut and others 2017), and chapter 25 (Fernandes and Aurino 2017).

THE GLOBAL PICTURE

Almost all countries practice school feeding (Bundy and others 2009); about one of three primary and lower-secondary schoolchildren benefit, although the number of children varies markedly across countries (figure 12.1). Approximately 18 percent of schoolchildren in low-income countries (LICs) received school meals in 2012, compared with 49 percent in upper-middle-income countries (WFP 2013). On the basis of global estimates of coverage and investment, the authors estimate that an additional investment of US$1.7 billion is needed to support the increase in program coverage in 23 LICs to the levels of upper-middle-income countries—the equivalent of 2 percent to 3 percent of total global investment in school feeding and a 10 percent increase in total beneficiaries.[2] India's Mid-Day Meal Scheme is the largest national school feeding program in the world, serving an estimated 113.8 million children each day (Drake and

others 2016). Brazil's national program, the next largest, provides daily meals to more than 43 million children (Drake and others 2016). China's National Nutrition Improvement Plan provided school meals to 33.5 million children ages 7–15 years across China in 2015 (Liu 2016).

School feeding interventions, most notably implementation modalities of delivery, vary across countries. School feeding may include hot meals, biscuits, or snacks provided in school or as take-home rations, where the households of schoolchildren receive a regular commodity ration on meeting conditions, such as regular attendance. School feeding programs vary in targeting. School meals may be provided free and at reduced, subsidized, or full price. Countries that follow a rights-based approach, such as Brazil and India, provide free school meals to all children in certain age groups. In most LMICs, however, free school meals are targeted geographically to areas with high prevalence of food insecurity and poverty, or individually, based on conditions of vulnerability, such as those in orphanages or disadvantaged households (WFP 2013).

School feeding programs have evolved with levels of development. Many HICs, such as the United States, introduced school feeding programs in the first half of the twentieth century as welfare interventions and to support agricultural markets. More recently, countries such as Brazil have systematically incorporated school feeding procurement with agriculture development interventions. In contrast, national school feeding programs in many LMICs were introduced more recently,

Figure 12.1 School Feeding Participation Worldwide

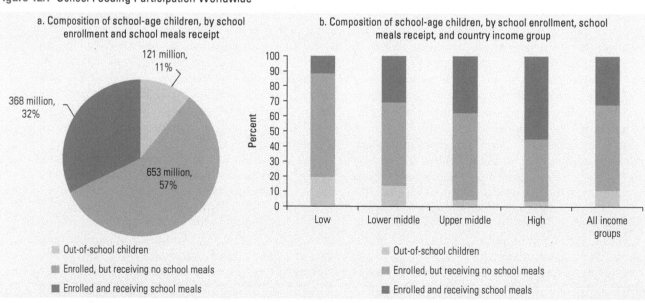

Sources: UNESCO 2014; World Bank 2016.
Note: Primary and lower-secondary schoolchildren only.

with education as the primary objective (Bundy and others 2009) or as a means of social protection in face of crises, given that experience has shown they are relatively easy to scale up during emergencies (Alderman and Bundy 2011). From 2000 to 2012, at least eight LICs launched school feeding programs—six in Sub-Saharan Africa—within the broader framework of the Education for All agenda (WFP 2013). Some of this growth may be due to the inclusion of homegrown school feeding, an approach that sources foods for school meals from local producers or markets, under the food security pillar of the Comprehensive Africa Agriculture Development Programme of 2003 (NEPAD 2003). The number of homegrown school feeding programs has grown steadily in Sub-Saharan Africa since that time (GCNF 2014).

THE EVIDENCE FOR EFFECTIVENESS

This section reviews the large evidence base highlighting the effectiveness of school feeding for multiple outcomes. The evidence suggests that school feeding is a social protection tool that can contribute to education, nutrition, health, and agricultural objectives supporting child and adolescent development (Bundy and others 2009; Jomaa, McDonnell, and Probart 2011). Figure 12.2 presents ways school feeding can affect these outcomes. Homegrown school feeding may also contribute to agricultural development, but not enough evidence exists yet to be incorporated in this review, although box 12.1 presents specific examples.

Design and Implementation Issues

Characteristics such as age, gender, and level of disadvantage may modify the strength of some of these pathways (Kristjansson and others 2009). Moreover, external factors, such as the quality of school inputs, may confound the overall impact of school feeding (Adelman, Gilligan, and Lehrer 2008; Greenhalgh, Kristjansson, and Robinson 2007; Kristjansson and others 2009; chapter 22 in this volume, Plaut and others 2017; Watkins and others 2015). Intervention implementation and study design may also

Figure 12.2 School Feeding Pathways to Shaping Child and Adolescent Development

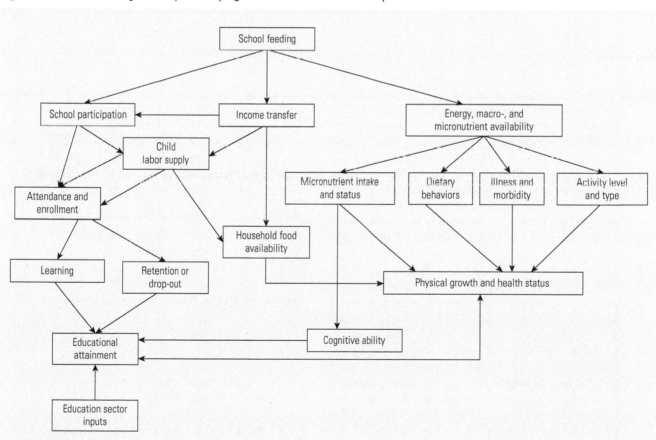

Source: Adapted from Adelman, Gilligan, and Lehrer 2008.

Homegrown School Feeding: Supporting Local Agriculture

The O'Meals program in Nigeria (Osun State Elementary School Feeding and Health Programme) is viewed as a means to combat hunger, increase primary school enrollment, and encourage local and statewide economic growth. The program provides hot, nutritionally balanced school meals daily to more than 252,000 primary schoolchildren. At the same time, it provides employment and income to thousands of local caterers, farmers, and traders, which may indirectly improve their health.

Recently, the menu replaced yam with the more-nutritious cocoyam, and organizers are investigating the introduction of orange-fleshed sweet potato (Drake and others 2016).

In Ghana, preliminary evidence from an impact evaluation of homegrown school feeding suggests sizable gains with regard to income from sales of produce and increases in farming households' agricultural incomes (Aurino and others 2016).

School Meal Planner, Ghana	
Monday	Yam + fish stew + orange
Tuesday	Rice + beans + stew + chicken + orange
Wednesday	Bean porridge + bread + whole egg + banana
Thursday	Rice + egusi garnished with vegetable + chicken + banana
Friday	Cocoyam porridge + vegetable + beef + slice of paw paw

Source: Drake and others 2016.

affect the results. The key issues that can be reflected in the process indicators include consistency of implementation of the intervention over the entire study period, compliance of beneficiaries with the intervention, adequacy of energy transferred, duration of the study, and palatability (Greenhalgh, Kristjansson, and Robinson 2007).

To illustrate this point, table 12.1 presents a selection of parameters for nationally led school feeding programs in 15 countries (Drake and others 2016). Ration design is key, particularly for assessing the quality of the meals and the potential link to local agriculture. The number of school days may enhance the nutritional impact of school feeding, as well as the educational impact, while also influencing the implementation costs.

It is important to understand not only whether school feeding is effective but also the causal chain according to which impact is achieved, which is context specific. This is an important area for further research (Greenhalgh, Kristjansson, and Robinson 2007). More rigorous design evaluations are also needed on government-led school feeding programs, given that the bulk of such evidence is based on school feeding implemented by the World Food Programme (WFP), which may be considerably different. For example, WFP school feeding rations typically include a basic set of foods, such as multifortified corn-soy blend, sugar, and salt, which are internationally procured, in contrast with the rations presented in table 12.1.

Benchmarking School Feeding Programs across Countries

School feeding programs across countries can be benchmarked using the Systems Assessment for Better Education Results (SABER) tool, which is structured around five pillars (Bundy and others 2009; Drake and others 2016):

- Policy frameworks
- Institutional capacity and coordination
- Budget and financing
- Design and implementation
- Community participation.

A national school feeding policy can contribute to sustainability and integration with other policy priorities. Capacity and coordination among relevant institutions

Table 12.1 Government-Led School Feeding Interventions in 15 Countries, Selected Parameters

Country	Income level[a]	Timing	Ration contents	Ration calories	Number of school days	Net enrollment rate, overall (%)	Gender parity index
Botswana	Upper middle	Daily mid-morning hot meal; second meal provided in some districts	Sorghum porridge, stewed canned beef, maize, beans, vegetable oil, bread, milk	572	185	90	0.97
Brazil	Upper middle	Modality varies across states and municipalities	At least 20 percent of daily nutritional needs provided, including three portions of fruits and vegetables	335	200	—	—
Cabo Verde	Lower middle	Hot in-school meal; a glass of milk provided in some schools	Cereals (rice or pasta), beans, oil (vegetable or soya), carrot, fish, Portuguese cabbage	300	—	98	0.92
Chile	Upper middle	Modality varies by age group	Food items vary by vendor but should include meat and fresh fruit and vegetables	850	180	94	0.97
China	Upper middle	Hot meal; mid-morning snacks	Hot dishes include meat and vegetables; snacks include biscuits and bread	810 for meals; 300 for snacks	200	100	0.87
Côte d'Ivoire	Lower middle	Hot meal	Cereals, flours, and legumes	1,141	52	77	0.87
Ecuador	Upper middle	Breakfast meal; milk snack also provided in some schools	Fortified drink composed of wheat flour and soy, granola in flakes, cereal bar, and four types of biscuits	396	—	95	1.00
Ghana	Lower middle	Hot midday meal	Maize, legumes, rice, fish, yams, eggs, groundnuts, vegetables	800	195	76	1.00
India	Lower middle	Hot midday meal	Cereals, pulses, eggs, and fruits	575	200	94	1.03
Kenya[b]	Lower middle	Hot midday meal	Cereals, pulses, vegetable oil, and salt	700	—	82	1.00
Mali	Lower middle	Cooked lunch	Staple foods (millet, sorghum, maize, and rice) with legumes, oil, pulses (such as cowpeas), and meat, fish, or both	735	180	70	0.88
Mexico	Upper middle	Cold or warm breakfast	Skim or partially skim milk, wholemeal cereals, and fresh or dried fruit	395	—	95	1.00
Namibia	Upper middle	Mid-morning meal	Fortified maize meal blend porridge	475	200	86	0.97
Nigeria[c]	Lower middle	Hot midday meal	Includes eggs, fish, and meat	536	—	64	0.92
South Africa	Upper middle	Mid-morning meal	Protein, starch, and a vegetable or fruit	—	182	90	0.95

Sources: Drake and others 2016; World Bank 2016, latest year available for each country.

Note: — = not available. The net enrollment rate is the ratio of children of official school age who are enrolled in school to the population of the corresponding official school age. The gender parity index for gross enrollment ratio in primary education is the ratio of girls to boys enrolled at the primary level in public and private schools.

a. World Bank income level in 2012.

b. School feeding details specific to homegrown school feeding program.

c. Osun State. See box 12.1 for more information about this program.

at the national, regional, and local levels are needed, particularly across different ministries. Channels for financing the program and the implementers, for example, payments to caterers, need to be defined. Communities must be engaged in the program; their contributions, such as firewood, condiments, and meal preparation, may be needed.

Social Protection

School feeding provides a transfer to households in the value of food distributed (Alderman and Bundy 2011). This transfer can reduce a household's food needs; when provided regularly over the school year, it smooths volatility, thereby increasing disposable income to meet other immediate needs or investments. A range of outcomes is possible, including better nutrition. A quasi-experimental design analysis found that India's school feeding program mitigated the effects of drought on physical growth, which had occurred earlier in the lives of the beneficiaries (Singh, Park, and Dercon 2014). In response to the food and fuel price crises of 2007–08, at least 38 LMICs scaled up school feeding programs, in recognition of its potential as a social safety net (WFP 2013). A global review of social safety net programs found that school feeding was one of the largest in estimated number of beneficiaries (World Bank 2014; also see chapter 8 in this volume, Watkins and others 2017).

Several factors determine the effectiveness of school feeding as a social protection tool. One factor is targeting the poorest and most vulnerable households and communities (Alderman and Bundy 2011). The efficiency of geographic targeting is conditioned by the degree to which poverty and food insecurity are concentrated in one or multiple areas, as well as the smallest geographic unit at which targeting can be applied. Poor accessibility to these areas and insufficient infrastructure to deliver school feeding may present barriers. An evaluation from the Lao People's Democratic Republic (Lao PDR) indicated that, because of similar barriers, only one-half to two-thirds of schools eligible for school feeding in select districts actually received school feeding (Buttenheim, Alderman, and Friedman 2011). Rising urban poverty and income inequality may justify individual or school-targeting approaches, although care must be taken to ensure that food provided in targeted schools does not inadvertently draw students from nearby schools receiving no food. Moreover, individual targeting may be challenging if some children in a classroom receive food while other children do not.

A review of eight social protection programs in Latin America and the Caribbean found that school feeding focused on the most disadvantaged households in most countries. However, in some countries such as Guatemala where the poorest children do not attend school, school feeding was less well targeted (Lindert, Skoufias, and Shapiro 2006). We replicated Lindert, Skoufias, and Shapiro (2006) by using data from Malawi, Tanzania, and Uganda. The share of households in the lowest income quintile were more likely to receive school meals, with the largest population share evident in Tanzania (figure 12.3).

In Ghana, the Ministry of Employment and Social Welfare, in a review of targeting in the national school feeding program in 2010, found that higher investment was not consistently made in districts with greater poverty and food insecurity (WFP 2013). The program was retargeted in 2012.

Education

School feeding can promote access to education, as measured by indicators such as enrollment, attendance, and retention (Krishnaratne, White, and Carpenter 2013). Evidence for these links helped identify school feeding as a means for contributing to the Millennium Development Goal 2 of universal enrollment in primary education. Given the links between nutrition status and cognition, school feeding programs, if integrated with interventions to improve education quality, can also contribute to learning and academic achievement (Adelman, Gilligan, and Lehrer 2008; Krishnaratne, White, and Carpenter 2013). Moreover, school feeding may directly or indirectly reduce gender disparities in education outcomes. The following section reviews the evidence, giving greater weight to systematic reviews

Figure 12.3 Targeting Efficiency of School Feeding in Malawi, Tanzania, and Uganda

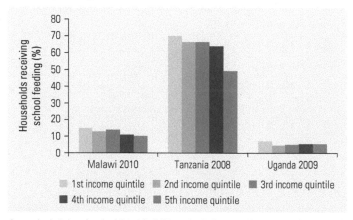

Source: Analysis based on the Atlas of Social Protection: Indicators of Resilience and Equity, World Bank.

and studies with rigorous designs, such as randomized controlled trials.

Access to Education

A review of rigorously designed studies indicated a standardized effect size of 0.156 for enrollment ($p < 0.05$, three studies), 0.449 for drop-out ($p < 0.001$, two studies), and 0.690 for progression ($p < 0.001$, one study) (Krishnaratne, White, and Carpenter 2013). The review did not find statistically significant effects on attendance and learning, although the coefficients were positive (Krishnaratne, White, and Carpenter 2013). In addition to providing an incentive to attend school, evidence indicates that school feeding reduces absenteeism. A review of studies from multiple LMICs found that school feeding was associated with an average of four to six more days attendance at school per year (Kristjansson and others 2009).

The choice of modality may also play an important role. For example, Afridi, Barooah, and Somanathan (2014) showed that monthly attendance increases in response to a switch to a cooked meal from snacks, with modest increases in the state budget in India. Fortified biscuits in Bangladesh improved school enrollment by 14.2 percent, reduced the probability of drop out by 7.5 percent, and raised attendance by about 1.3 days a month (Ahmed 2004). Adelman, Gilligan, and Lehrer (2012) in Northern Uganda, and Kazianga, de Walque, and Alderman (2009) in Burkina Faso found that both school meals and take-home rations effectively increased enrollment. Ahmed and del Ninno (2002) showed that take-home rations for poor households in rural Bangladesh increased school access, with an 8 percent increase in school enrollment and 12 percent increase in attendance.

Moreover, the evidence suggests that school feeding can mitigate gender disparities in school enrollment where girls face greater barriers (Gelli, Meir, and Espejo 2007). In particular, the provision of take-home rations to girls can represent a significant income transfer to households, outweighing the forgone benefits of nonattendance (Bundy and others 2009). The WFP experience suggests that making provision of take-home rations conditional on attendance rates of more than 80 percent was effective, especially in low-resource communities where child labor is common (WFP 2013). In Burkina Faso, the provision of school meals or monthly take-home rations of 10 kilograms of cereal flour conditional on a 90 percent attendance rate increased the enrollment of girls ages 6–12 years by about 6 percent (Kazianga, de Walque, and Alderman 2014).

Learning and Academic Achievement

A smaller but still substantial body of evidence explores the impacts of school feeding on learning and academic achievement. Although some indications of a positive relationship have been documented, other studies have not found statistically significant results. The mixed findings may be due to several factors, including differences in school quality. These differences are consistent with other types of schooling interventions, for which evidence on what works is inconclusive (Glewwe and others 2013).

In Chile, more frequent consumption of dairy products improved education outcomes for primary and secondary students (WHO 1998). Preliminary evidence from Ghana suggests improved learning outcomes for girls in schools where micronutrients were given in the meals. The improvements related to literacy (14 percent), mathematics (13 percent), and reasoning ability (8 percent) (Aurino and others 2016). Other studies, in contrast, have found minimal to no impact of school feeding on academic achievement. Timing of delivery of the feeding and overall learning environments can contribute to explaining the inconsistency of evidence related to school feeding and academic achievement (Powell and others 1998; Vermeersch and Kremer 2004). For instance, Vermeersch and Kremer (2004) attribute their negative finding to the disruptive role of school feeding in the school day, whereas the positive outcome from Powell and others (1998) may be due to the timing of the program (just before the school start). In addition, Chang and others (1996) found that school feeding was associated with improved on-task behaviors in well-organized classrooms but not in disorganized classrooms.

Table 12.2 presents overall average estimates for the impact of school feeding on educational outcomes

Table 12.2 Summary of Educational Impacts of School Feeding

	Overall weighted average effect	Number of studies
Access to schooling		
Enrollment	0.14	7
Attendance	0.09	6
Drop-out	−0.06	3
Completion	0	2
Learning outcomes		
Language arts scores	0.09	8
Math scores	0.10	10
Composite test score	0.14	3

Source: Snilstveit and others 2015.

Note: Weighted average effects are based on the Cohen's index and were estimated based on the standardized mean differences calculated from individual studies. These effects reflect the estimated change in percentile rank for an average student in the control group had he or she received school feeding.

drawing from a systematic review of studies with rigorous design undertaken in LMICs between 1990 and 2015 (Snilstveit and others 2015). These studies primarily included randomized controlled trials, as well as quasi-randomized trials, with adjustments for nonrandom selection to groups such as propensity score matching or regression discontinuity design. Standardized effect sizes were estimated for individual studies, and meta-analysis was used to obtain overall estimates.

Nutrition

The World Health Organization recommends that school feeding programs contribute 30 percent to 45 percent of the recommended daily allowance of energy and nutrients for half-day schools, and 60 percent to 75 percent for full-day schools (WHO 1998). HICs, including Chile, Mexico, the United Kingdom, and the United States, have introduced nutrient-based standards in school feeding programs to enhance the contribution of school meals to recommended dietary intake. Nutrient-based standards are less common in LMICs, however, with the exception of India (Drake and others 2016). A review of national school feeding programs in 12 LMICs indicated that many seek to provide more diversified food baskets that include fresh produce, although this objective is often only aspirational (Aliyar, Gelli, and Hamdani 2015).

School feeding may help children and adolescents receive sufficient nutrients and grow. The inclusion of micronutrient-rich foods or powders may address anemia and support improved cognition (Abizari and others 2012; Abizari and others 2014; Finkelstein and others 2015). School meals may also foster understanding of healthy diets and behaviors that can extend beyond school and throughout life, particularly if nutrition education is incorporated into the program (Kubik and others 2003; Story, Neumark-Sztainer, and French 2002).

However, counteracting factors may weaken these relationships. For example, households may allocate food to siblings not receiving the school meals, possibly offsetting the impact of school feeding on the nutritional status of the target child. Studies analyzing this issue show, nevertheless, that overall energy intake increases almost as much as the transfer provided at school—the flypaper effect (Afridi 2010; Ahmed 2004; IFPRI 2008; Jacoby 2002). In addition, Jacoby (2002) and Ahmed (2004) have shown that children who received snacks shared them with their younger siblings. Few studies have tracked the nutritional status of siblings too young to attend school, however, although Adelman, Gilligan, and Lehrer (2012) and Kazianga, de Walque, and

Alderman (2014) have shown that take-home rations improved weight-for-age by 0.4 standard deviations for the younger siblings of the beneficiaries compared with control groups.

Nutrient Adequacy

Evidence suggests that school feeding can be effective in promoting macronutrient and micronutrient adequacy in the diet (Jomaa, McDonnell, and Probart 2011). For food supplementation programs, evidence from a randomized controlled trial in Kenya showed that the inclusion of meat or milk in the school feeding menus improved plasma vitamin B_{12} concentrations. No other measures of micronutrient status were affected, however, probably because of concurrent incidence of malaria or other infectious diseases (Jomaa, McDonnell, and Probart 2011; Siekmann and others 2003). In a quasi-randomized study, Afridi (2010) found that in the state of Andhra Pradesh in India, the Mid-Day Meal Scheme eliminated daily protein deficiency and decreased calorie deficiency by almost 30 percent and daily iron deficiency by nearly 10 percent (Afridi 2010). Regarding efficacy, Best and others (2011) reported in a review that micronutrient supplementation increased micronutrients and reduced anemia more than supplementation of a single micronutrient or no supplementation.

In 8 out of 10 studies reviewed in Best and others (2011), school feeding raised serum concentrations of iron, iodine, vitamin A, and vitamin B, while improving hemoglobin levels. Two studies identified increased levels of zinc (Nga and others 2009; Winichagoon and others 2006). The impact of school feeding on micronutrient status may depend on the dose, initial micronutrient status, and interactions with other micronutrients supplemented. The iron status of Kenyan schoolchildren was associated with the dosage of iron-fortified flour (Andang'o and others 2007), while a randomized controlled trial in Vietnam showed that only multifortified biscuits reduced anemia more than iron supplementation, which suggests that other micronutrients affect anemia status (Hieu and others 2012).

Food-based strategies in school feeding programs can effectively address micronutrient deficiencies. The introduction of orange-flesh sweet potato in meals, for example, improved vitamin A status in South Africa (van Jaarsveld and others 2005), while consumption of carotene-rich yellow and green leafy vegetables improved vitamin A and hemoglobin concentration and decreased anemia rates in Filipino schoolchildren (Maramag and others 2010). The incorporation of locally available, micronutrient-rich foods may also promote local agriculture. Homegrown school feeding programs follow this approach (box 12.1). A survey of 36 LMICs (mostly Sub-Saharan African) indicated that national sourcing (local purchasing) resulted in the inclusion of more diverse and fresh foods (GCNF 2014).

Last, mixed approaches that combine food supplementation and micronutrient supplementation or food fortification can also promote nutrient adequacy. In Northern Uganda, school meals and take-home rations were found to reduce anemia prevalence in girls ages 10–13 years by 17 to 20 percentage points (Adelman, Gilligan, and Lehrer 2012). In contrast, impacts on anemia were not detected in randomized controlled trials from Burkina Faso and Lao PDR, where the rations did not include multifortified foods (Buttenheim, Alderman, and Friedman 2011; Kazianga, de Walque, and Alderman 2014). The success of these approaches critically depends on the regularity of the supplementation throughout the school year.

Nutrition and Cognition

A large body of literature shows the links between malnutrition, including micronutrient deficiencies, and poor cognition (Glewwe and Miguel 2008; Grantham-McGregor and Ani 2001). In this area, studies have focused on how school feeding can promote cognitive skills such as better attention and short-term memory by reducing deficiencies in iron and other micronutrients. One randomized controlled study found that regular provision of fortified biscuits improved the micronutrient status and cognitive function of children (van Stuijvenberg and others 1999). Two randomized controlled studies from Kenya found that the inclusion of animal source foods improved cognition and child learning, although the magnitude of effects were small (Neumann and others 2003; Whaley and others 2003). Afridi, Barooah, and Somanathan (2013) found that the provision of free meals increased student effort, as measured by their performance in solving puzzles of increasing difficulty, in India.

The timing of the meal may be important. Breakfast programs may support cognitive function during school hours, especially for children who had previously skipped breakfast. Findings from two rigorous studies suggest that eating breakfast improves on-task time (amount of time spent focused on the school activity) and attention (Bro and others 1994; Bro and others 1996). A universal, free breakfast program in Boston public schools in the United States improved school attendance and math achievement, and decreased days tardy for children at nutritional risk as assessed in a pre-post study during a six-month period (Kleinman and

others 2002). Nutritional risk in this study was defined as less than 50 percent of the recommended daily allowance of total energy intake or of two or more micronutrients, or both. A study from Mexico found that children in schools participating in a school breakfast program had higher response speed and memory compared with children from nearby schools that did not participate in the program (Vera Noriega and others 2000). A review did not find that the timing of meal delivery affects cognition, although one study from Israel did find that children performed better shortly after a meal (Vaisman and others 1996).

Anthropometry and Nutrition

A Cochrane review on school feeding (Kristjansson and others 2009) conducted a meta-analysis of three randomized controlled trials in three LMICs: Jamaica (Powell and others 1998), Kenya (Grillenberger and others 2003), and China (Du and others 2004). The meta-analysis found a small yet significant effect on weight (0.39 kilogram, 95 percent confidence interval 0.11, 0.67) and a small nonsignificant effect on height gain (0.38 centimeters, 95 percent confidence interval –0.32, 1.08). The three school feeding programs differed greatly in modality of implementation and target population. In the Jamaica study, 395 children in grades 2–5 were given breakfast for a year (Powell and others 1998). In Kenya, grade 1 schoolchildren were given meat, milk, or an energy supplement for 18 months (Grillenberger and others 2003). In China, the study focused on girls age 10 years who received milk supplementation (Du and others 2004). A more recent review (Watkins and others 2015), which broadened the inclusion criteria by considering studies such as controlled before-and-after studies, found that school feeding had significant effects on weight and height gain.

Micronutrient supplementation and fortified foods delivered through school feeding programs may also affect nutrition outcomes of children. Best and others (2011) reported that 10 studies found that school meals with micronutrient supplementation had statistically significant impacts on micronutrient status even after controlling for baseline status. Findings from several controlled before-and-after studies suggest that micronutrient supplementation may also have statistically significant impacts on height and weight. Table 12.3 summarizes the evidence.

Dietary Behaviors

Schools and school feeding programs, through nutrition education, can serve as a platform for shaping behaviors and food preferences for healthier nutrition

Table 12.3 Summary of Nutrition and Cognitive Impacts of School Feeding

School feeding activity	Anthropometric Status		Micronutrient Status						Cognition
	Height or stunting	Weight or underweight	Iron	Hemoglobin or anemia	Iodine	Vitamin A	Zinc	B vitamins	
In-school meals	+++	+++	+	++	n.a.	+	+	+	+++
Take-home rations	++	++	—	+	n.a.	—	—	—	++
Multiple micronutrient fortification	++	++	+++	+++	+	+++	+++	+	++
Multiple micronutrient powder	++	++	++	++	+	++	++	+	++

Source: Watkins and others 2015.
Note: RCT = randomized controlled trial.
n.a. = not assessed by an RCT; + = evidence from one RCT; ++ = evidence from two RCTs; +++ = evidence from more than two RCTs; — = lack of any evidence.

(Hawkes and others 2015). The development of healthy dietary habits during childhood can also help prevent diet-related diseases later in life, with the evidence showing that dietary habits tend to be persistent from childhood through adulthood (Dunn and others 2000). Dietary diversity may provide an indicator of better diets among children and adolescents. The inclusion of animal-source foods in school snacks increased dietary diversity in Kenya (Murphy and others 2003).

Encouraging lifelong healthy diet choices has so far received more attention in HICs; however, it is increasingly relevant in LMICs, where childhood overweight and obesity are increasing (Lobstein and others 2015). Some studies conducted in HICs found a positive association between school meals and overweight and obesity (Schanzenbach 2009). Others suggest instead that programs targeted to primary-school-age children most effectively reduced obesity, especially when healthy meals were accompanied by communication promoting behavioral change (Corcoran, Elbel, and Schwartz 2014). Initiatives at school that combine healthy eating and active living have been introduced in HICs to support child and adolescent development (De Bourdeaudhuij and others 2011; Herforth and Ahmed 2015; Story, Nanney, and Schwartz 2009). Similar action in LMICs may be needed to respond to the nutrition transition (Faber and others 2014).

Communication materials aimed at changing behavior, alongside school meals, can help inculcate these ideas in schoolchildren and influence household diet. For example, radio jingles and posters were developed in Ghana to complement initiatives undertaken in the Ghana School Feeding Programme to improve nutrition among children, adolescents, and their communities (Gelli and others 2016). Evidence on the impact of nutrition education is scant, particularly in developing countries, and more research is needed.

Agriculture

Initial evidence has shown that home-grown school feeding can change the eating preferences of households, improve community incomes, support smallholder production, and facilitate better market access. Thereby, it has an impact on rural economies. The impact on rural investments and agricultural development has increasingly gained attention through links to the school feeding market. It is also clear that to enable the transition to sustainable, scalable government-run programs, the inclusion of the agricultural sector is critical (Bundy and others 2009; Drake and others 2016).

Initial evidence has shown that homegrown school feeding can not only change eating preferences of households, community incomes, and smalholder production and market access, but can also benefit smallholder farmers and investments in rural economies.

Preliminary findings from an impact evaluation in Ghana show a 33 percent increase in agricultural sales and a strong increase in household income in interventions in which homegrown school feeding is implemented (Aurino and others 2016). However, it is clear that rigorous evidence regarding the impacts that school feeding has on employment and income in the agricultural sector needs to be reinforced (Aurino and others 2016; Drake and others 2016; GCNF 2014; Masset and others 2012).

The following issues need further exploration:

- Transparency in price and payment is key for smallholder trust.
- Timely access to price, quality, and quantity information enhances operational efficiencies of aggregators and market systems.

- Adaptation of quantity and quality requirements and effective communication on them can ease the transition to supplying structured markets.
- The mobile phone platform can allow easier aggregation and management of commodities despite the short period of aggregation.

WEIGHING THE COSTS AGAINST BENEFITS: AN ECONOMIC ASSESSMENT OF SCHOOL FEEDING

This section reviews the literature on quantifiable costs and benefits for an overall assessment of the economics of school feeding. Three issues are particularly salient:

- The heterogeneity in the design and implementation of school feeding interventions across countries underscores the need for standardization when possible. A comparison of costs with benefits is essential for any economic assessment of school feeding or modification to the intervention. For example, retargeting school feeding to the most disadvantaged areas, or shifting from geographic to individual targeting, may reach disadvantaged populations more efficiently.
- Such changes may also entail significant monetary and other costs, including resistance from local government officials whose districts will no longer receive the intervention, or risk of stigma that children and adolescents may experience for receiving free or reduced-price meals if the program is not designed to mitigate that risk.
- Some important drivers of costs may be outside the scope of the intervention, such as global food prices or poor road conditions.

Costs of School Feeding

Costs of school feeding include costs associated with procuring food, transportation and storage, and staff time to monitor program implementation. Some programs hire cooks or caterers to prepare meals; others rely on community volunteers. Communities may provide other, in-kind contributions, such as fresh fruit or vegetables, fuel, condiments, and utensils. The provision of multifortified biscuits and take-home rations entails costs in staffing and delivery. Efficiencies may be gained through integrating school feeding with other school health interventions, such as water, hygiene and sanitation, or deworming (Azomahou, Diallo, and Raymond 2014).

Modality is a key determinant of school feeding costs. On average, school meals, biscuits, and take-home rations cost US$27, US$11, and US$43, respectively, per child per year (Gelli and others 2011). The differences are driven largely by differences in meal size or modality of the transfer; take-home rations cost more because they provide an additional transfer to the household beyond the food delivered in school.

Significant variation in cost is also evident across countries. Drawing from a sample of 74 low-, middle-, and high-income countries, school feeding costs an average of US$173 per child per year, ranging from US$54 in LICs to US$82 in middle-income countries and US$693 in HICs (Gelli and Daryanani 2013). These estimates are standardized for several parameters to support cross-country comparability, including the number of kilocalories in the ration and the number of days school feeding was provided. Food costs were typically the largest component, accounting for more than half of total program costs (Galloway and others 2009; Gelli and others 2011).[3] Although the contributions of communities are not usually reflected in these estimates,[4] they are estimated to be about 5 percent of total cost in LICs, or about US$2 per year (Galloway and others 2009).

The benchmarking of school feeding costs as a percentage of primary school education costs can also support comparability across countries. As table 12.4 shows, school feeding costs become a smaller proportion of primary education costs as the income level of the country increases. For LICs, the share is 68 percent, compared with 19 percent for MICs and 11 percent for HICs.

As gross domestic product increases, the per capita cost of primary school education increases more rapidly than the per capita cost of school feeding, which drives this finding (figure 12.4) (Bundy and others

Table 12.4 School Feeding Costs in 74 Countries

Income level of country	Total cost (US$)	Share of per capita cost of primary education (%)
Low (n = 22)	54	68
Middle (n = 40)	82	19
High (n = 12)	693	11
Total (n = 74)	173	33

Source: Gelli and Daryanani 2013.

Note: n = number of observations.

Figure 12.4 School Feeding and Primary Education Costs per Child per Year

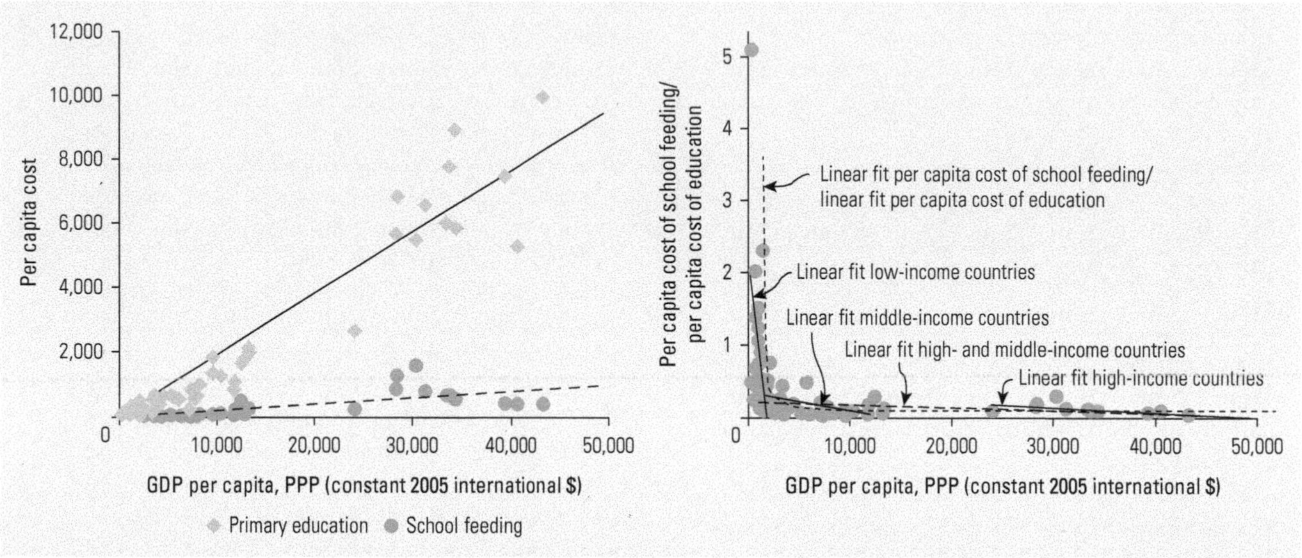

Sources: Bundy and others 2009; Gelli and Daryanani 2013.
Note: GDP = gross domestic product; PPP = purchasing power parity.

2009; Gelli and Daryanani 2013). The high cost of school feeding relative to education is notable, particularly in LICs.

Assessing Costs against Benefits

This section reviews the cost of school feeding by output and outcome. For output, figure B12.2.1 presents the cost of delivering 30 percent of the recommended daily allowances of key micronutrients in 12 countries based on school feeding menus (Drake and others 2016). The composition of school meals varies widely, and diversification may lead to higher costs. Some studies have found positive effects on anthropometric indicators from meat or milk in the meals (Du and others 2004; Grillenberger and others 2003). However, LICs are unlikely to be able to sustain the higher costs of meat, and possibly milk, in meal programs. As economies develop, these food items can be gradually introduced and governments might be able to use schools to encourage the development of dairy sectors. Bangladesh, Rwanda, and Vietnam are encouraging these links through their school feeding programs.

For decentralized programs, setting the appropriate reimbursement rate to meet recommended nutrient levels is critical (Parish and Gelli 2015). Tools such as the School Meals Planner can support the design of costed menus that incorporate nutrient-rich foods (box 12.2). The addition of supplements such as

micronutrient powders to school meals may also increase cost efficiency relative to nutrient content. In Ghana, the provision of micronutrient powders in school meals costs only an estimated additional US$2.92 per child for the entire school year (Stopford and others, forthcoming).

Estimation of the overall cost-effectiveness of school feeding is complicated by the multiple benefits of the intervention and the need to transform the units of different outcomes into the same unit. To simplify the problem, school feeding can be viewed as increasing the quantity and quality of education obtained, with improved nutrition outcomes contributing to quality (Gelli and others 2014). Capturing both education and nutrition outcomes in such calculations is critical for comparisons with other interventions, such as conditional cash transfers,[5] as well as direct schooling investment. Compared with conditional cash transfers, school feeding has high nontransfer costs of approximately 20 percent to 40 percent (Bundy and others 2009).

Previous studies (Jamison and Leslie 1990; Schuh 1981) have hypothesized that the benefit-cost of school feeding programs are attractive. A recent systematic review and meta-analysis (Snilstveit and others 2015) found that school feeding had significant effects on school attendance equivalent to an additional 8 days attended. There were also effects in the expected direction on improving enrollment, decreasing dropout, and improving various measures of attainment

School Meals Planner

The School Meals Planner software and accompanying materials were developed in response to demand from governments to support the design of nutritious, well-balanced meals for homegrown school feeding programs.

The tool is a user-friendly dashboard that helps planning officials who may not be nutritionists (figure B12.2.1). It was adapted to Ghana and tested during the 2014/15 school year. Food composition tables and nutrition recommendations specific to Ghana were developed through high-level political engagement. Officials from 42 districts located across the 10 regions of Ghana designed menus using the School Meals Planner. These menus reached more than 320,000 children.

A set of handy calibrated measures was provided to each school caterer to ensure provision of food quantities listed on the menus. A communication campaign sensitized schools and communities to the health and broader developmental benefits of locally grown, healthy diets.

Figure B12.2.1 The School Meals Planner

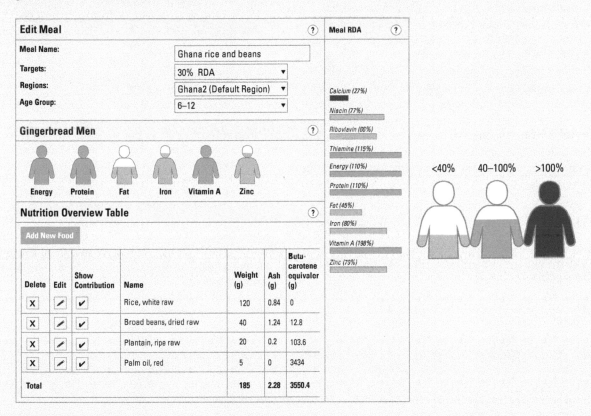

Source: Fernandes and others 2016.
Note: RDA = recommended daily allowance.

(cognitive scores, maths scores, and language arts scores), although none of these was significant. Higher school attendance, in turn, has returns in higher wages upon graduation, and the returns to education in Sub-Saharan Africa are high. Fernandes and Aurino (2017, chapter 25 in this volume) estimate the benefit-cost of the effect of attendance as around 3 for low-income countries, and around 7 for lower-middle-income countries. If there are additional effects of improved cognition, the returns could be even higher.

CONCLUSIONS

School feeding is commonly implemented across low-, middle-, and high-income countries; however, there is significant variation driven by context to a large degree. The research most strongly indicates that school feeding has social protection and educational benefits; more recent studies have explored its nutritional benefits.

School feeding can serve to protect earlier investments in child welfare, buffering the effects of early shocks and contributing to the continuum of interventions from childhood through adolescence and into adulthood. Furthermore, school feeding also has the potential to address emerging issues such as the nutrition transition and could be integrated with other school health interventions, such as deworming, for greater impact.

Homegrown school feeding can not only change eating preferences of households, improve community incomes, and smallholder production and market access, but can also benefit investments in rural economies and contribute to national food security.

Much still needs to be learned about the barriers to these potential benefits. The costs of school feeding vary significantly across countries. An economic modeling exercise indicates that the returns to greater quantity and quality of education are a primary contributor to benefits. Future research is needed on the quantification of benefits to ensure more valid comparisons with other interventions.

NOTES

World Bank Income Classifications as of July 2014 are as follows, based on estimates of gross national income (GNI) per capita for 2013:

- Low-income countries (LICs) = US$1,045 or less
- Middle-income countries (MICs) are subdivided:
  a) lower-middle-income = US$1,046 to US$4,125
  b) upper-middle-income (UMICs) = US$4,126 to US$12,745
- High-income countries (HICs) = US$12,746 or more.

1. The nutrition transition is the rapid transition in LMICs from traditional diets rich in cereals and fiber to westernized diets high in fat, sugars, and animal-source food.
2. Calculation by authors using data from WFP (2013).
3. One study estimated that commodities contributed 57 percent to overall costs (Galloway and others 2009). Gelli and others (2011) found that commodity costs were, on average, 58 percent of total costs, and were highest for take-home rations and biscuit programs (68 percent and 71 percent, respectively).

4. Gelli and Daryanani's (2013) study is an exception because the authors were able to calculate projections for community contributions, where relevant.
5. The value of increased equity in both school feeding and conditional cash transfers is a benefit that is often part of the design but not one that is easily quantified (Alderman, Behrman, and Tasneem 2015).

REFERENCES

Abizari, A., C. Buxton, L. Kwara, J. Mensah-Homiah, M. Armar-Klemesu, and others. 2014. "School Feeding Contributes to Micronutrient Adequacy of Ghanaian School Children." *British Journal of Nutrition* 112 (6): 1019–33.

Abizari, A., D. Moretti, M. B. Zimmermann, M. Armar-Klemesu, and I. D. Brouwer. 2012. "Whole Cowpea Meal Fortified with NaFeEDTA Reduces Iron Deficiency among Ghanaian School Children in a Malaria Endemic Area." *Journal of Nutrition* 142 (10): 1836–42.

Adelman, S., D. Gilligan, and K. Lehrer. 2008. "How Effective Are Food-for-Education Programs? A Critical Reassessment." Food Policy Review No. 9, International Food Policy Research Institute, Washington, DC.

———. 2012. "The Impact of Food for Education Programs on School Participation in Northern Uganda." *Economic Development and Cultural Change* 61 (1): 187–218.

Afridi, F. 2010. "Child Welfare Programs and Child Nutrition: Evidence from a Mandated School Meal Program in India." *Journal of Development Economics* 92 (2): 152–65.

Afridi, F., B. Barooah, and R. Somanathan. 2013. "School Meals and Classroom Effort: Evidence from India." Working Paper, International Growth Centre, London.

———. 2014. "The Mixture as Before? Student Responses to the Changing Content of School Meals in India." IZA Discussion Paper 9924, Institute for the Study of Labor, Bonn.

Ahmed, A. 2004. "Comparing Food and Cash Incentives for Schooling in Bangladesh." International Food Policy Research Institute, Washington, DC.

Ahmed, A., and C. del Ninno. 2002. "The Food for Education Program in Bangladesh: An Evaluation of Its Impact on Educational Attainment and Food Security." Discussion Paper 138, International Food Policy Research Institute, Washington, DC.

Alderman, H., J. Behrman, and A. Tasneem. 2015. "The Contribution of Increased Equity to the Estimated Social Benefits from a Transfer Program." Discussion Paper 1475, International Food Policy Research Institute, Washington, DC.

Alderman, H., J. R. Behrman, P. Glewwe, L. Fernald, and S. Walker. 2017. "Evidence of Impact on Growth and Development of Interventions during Early and Middle Childhood." In *Disease Control Priorities* (third edition): Volume 8, *Child and Adolescent Health and Development*, edited by D. A. P. Bundy, N. de Silva, S. Horton, D. T. Jamison, and G. C. Patton. Washington, DC: World Bank.

Alderman, H., and D. A. P. Bundy. 2011. "School Feeding Programs and Development: Are We Framing the Question Correctly?" *World Bank Research Observer* 27 (2): 204–21.

Aliyar, R., A. Gelli, and S. Hamdani. 2015. "A Review of Nutritional Guidelines and Menu Compositions for School Feeding Programs in 12 Countries." *Frontiers in Public Health* 3: 148. doi: 10.3389/fpubh.2015.00148.

Andang'o, P., S. Osendarp, R. Ayah, C. West, D. Mwaniki, and others. 2007. "Efficacy of Iron-Fortified Whole Maize Flour on Iron Status of Schoolchildren in Kenya: A Randomized Controlled Trial." *The Lancet* 369 (9575): 1799–806.

Aurino, E., C. Adamba, F. Asante, K. M. Bosompem, G. Folson, and others. 2016. "Ghana Home Grown School Feeding Programme. Impact Evaluation Report." Partnership for Child Development, London.

Azomahou, T., F. Diallo, and W. Raymond. 2014. "The Harmony of Programs Package: Quasi-Experimental Evidence on Deworming and Canteen Interventions in Rural Senegal." UNU-MERIT Working Paper, United Nations University, Tokyo.

Best, C., N. Neufingerl, J. del Rosso, C. Transler, T. van den Briel, and others. 2011. "Can Multi-Micronutrient Food Fortification Improve the Micronutrient Status, Growth, Health, and Cognition of Schoolchildren? A Systematic Review." *Nutrition Reviews* 69 (4): 186–204.

Bro, R. T., L. L. Shank, T. F. McLaughlin, and R. L. Williams. 1996. "Effects of a Breakfast Program on On-Task Behavior of Vocational High School Students." *Journal of Education Research* 90 (2): 111–15.

Bro, R. T., L. L. Shank, R. L. Williams, and T. F. McLaughlin. 1994. "The Effects of an In-Class Breakfast Program on Attendance and On-Task Behavior of High School Students." *Child Family Behavior Therapy* 16 (3): 1–8.

Bundy, D. A. P., L. Schultz, B. Sarr, L. Banham, P. Colenso, and others. 2017. "The School as a Platform for Addressing Health." In *Disease Control Priorities* (third edition): Volume 8, *Child and Adolescent Health and Development,* edited by D. A. P. Bundy, N. de Silva, S. Horton, D. T. Jamison, and G. C. Patton. Washington, DC: World Bank.

Bundy, D. A. P., C. Burbano, M. Grosh, A. Gelli, M. Jukes, and L. Drake. 2009. *Rethinking School Feeding. Social Safety Nets, Child Development and the Educational Sector.* Washington, DC: World Bank.

Buttenheim, A., H. Alderman, and J. Friedman. 2011. "Impact Evaluation of School Feeding Programs in Lao PDR." *Journal of Development Effectiveness* 3 (4): 520–42.

Chang, S. M., S. P. Walker, S. Grantham-McGregor, and J. Himes. 1996. "Effect of Breakfast on Classroom Behaviour in Rural Jamaican Schoolchildren." *Food and Nutrition Bulletin* 17 (3): 1–104.

Corcoran, S., B. Elbel, and A. Schwartz. 2014. "The Effect of Breakfast in the Classroom on Obesity and Academic Performance: Evidence from New York City." Working Paper 04-14, Institute for Education and Social Policy, New York.

De Bourdeaudhuij, I., E. Van Cauwenberghe, H. Spittaels, J. M. Oppert, C. Rostami, and others. 2011. "School-Based Interventions Promoting Both Physical Activity and Healthy Eating in Europe: A Systematic Review within the HOPE Project." *Obesity Reviews* 12 (3): 205–16.

Drake, L., A. Woolnough, C. Burbano, and D. A. P. Bundy, eds. 2016. *Global School Feeding Sourcebook. Lessons from 14 Countries.* London: Imperial College Press.

Du, X., K. Zhu, A. Trube, Q. Zhang, G. Ma, and others. 2004. "School-Milk Intervention Trial Enhances Growth and Bone Mineral Accretion in Chinese Girls Aged 10–12 Years in Beijing." *British Journal of Nutrition* 92 (4): 159–68.

Dunn, J., K. Liu, P. Greenland, J. Hilner, and D. Jacobs Jr. 2000. "Seven-Year Tracking of Dietary Factors in Young Adults: The CARDIA Study." *American Journal of Preventive Medicine* 18 (1): 38–45.

Faber, M., S. Laurie, M. Maduna, T. Magudulela, and E. Muehlhoff. 2014. "Is the School Food Environment Conducive to Healthy Eating in Poorly Resourced South African Schools?" *Public Health Nutrition* 17 (6): 1214–23.

Fernandes, M., and E. Aurino. 2017. "Economic Factors in Defining the School-Age Package." In *Disease Control Priorities* (third edition): Volume 8, *Child and Adolescent Health and Development,* edited by D. A. P. Bundy, N. de Silva, S. Horton, D. T. Jamison, and G. C. Patton. Washington, DC: World Bank.

Fernandes, M., R. Galloway, A. Gelli, D. Mumuni, S. Hamdani, and others. 2016. "Enhancing Linkages between Healthy Diets, Local Agriculture and Sustainable Food Systems: The School Meals Planner Package in Ghana." *Food and Nutrition Bulletin* July 19. pii: 0379572116659156.

Finkelstein, J., S. Mehta, S. Udipi, P. S. Ghugre, S. V. Luna, and others. 2015. "A Randomized Trial of Iron-Biofortified Pearl Millet in School Children in India." *Journal of Nutrition* 145 (7): 1576–81.

Galloway, R., E. A. Kristjansson, A. Gelli, U. Meir, F. Espej, and others. 2009. "School Feeding: Outcomes and Costs." *Food and Nutrition Bulletin* 30 (2): 171–82.

GCNF (Global Child Nutrition Foundation). 2014. "XVI Global Child Nutrition Forum. Nutrition in School Feeding Programmes." Executive Summary, GCNF.

Gelli, A., A. Cavallero, L. Minervini, M. Mirabile, L. Molinas, and others. 2011. "New Benchmarks for Costs and Cost-Efficiency for Food Provisions in Schools in Food Insecure Areas." *Food and Nutrition Bulletin* 32 (4): 324–32.

Gelli, A., and R. Daryanani. 2013. "Are School Feeding Programs in Low-Income Settings Sustainable? Insights on the Costs of School Feeding Compared with Investments in Primary Education." *Food and Nutrition Bulletin* 34 (3): 310–17.

Gelli, A., F. Espejo, J. Shen, and E. A. Kristjansson. 2014. "Putting It All Together: Aggregating Impacts of School-Feeding Programs on Education, Health and Nutrition: Two Proposed Methodologies." Working Paper 2014/036, UNU-WIDER, Helsinki, Finland.

Gelli, A., E. Masset, G. Folson, A. Kusi, D. K. Arhinful, and others. 2016. "Evaluation of Alternative School Feeding

Models on Nutrition, Education, Agriculture and Other Social Outcomes in Ghana: Rationale, Randomised Design and Baseline Data." *Trials* 17 (1): 37.

Gelli, A., U. Meir, and F. Espejo. 2007. "Does Provision of Food in School Increase Girls' Enrollment? Evidence from Schools in Sub-Saharan Africa." *Food and Nutrition Bulletin* 28 (2): 149–55.

Glewwe, P., E. Hanushek, S. Humpage, and R. Ravina. 2013. "School Resources and Educational Outcomes in Developing Countries: A Review of the Literature from 1990 to 2010." In *Education Policy in Developing Countries*, edited by P. Glewwe, 13–64. Chicago, IL: University of Chicago Press.

Glewwe, P., and E. Miguel. 2008. "The Impact of Child Health and Nutrition on Education in Less Developed Countries." *Handbook of Development Economics* 4: 3561–606.

Graham, N., L. Schultz, S. Mitra, and D. Mont. 2017. "Disability and Child and Adolescent Development." In *Disease Control Priorities* (third edition): Volume 8, *Child and Adolescent Health and Development*, edited by D. A. P. Bundy, N. de Silva, S. Horton, D. T. Jamison, and G. C. Patton. Washington, DC: World Bank.

Grantham-McGregor, S., and C. Ani. 2001. "A Review of Studies on the Effect of Iron Deficiency on Cognitive Development in Children." *Journal of Nutrition* 131 (2): 649S–68S.

Greenhalgh, T., E. A. Kristjansson, and V. Robinson. 2007. "Realist Review to Understand the Efficacy of School Feeding Programmes." *BMJ* 335 (7665): 858–61.

Grillenberger, M., C. Neumann, S. Murphy, N. Bwibo, P. van't Veer, and others. 2003. "Food Supplements Have a Positive Impact on Weight Gain and the Addition of Animal Source Foods Increases Lean Body Mass of Kenyan Schoolchildren." *Journal of Nutrition* 133 (11): 3957S–64S.

Hawkes, C., T. G. Smith, J. Jewell, J. Wardle, R. A. Hammond, and others. 2015. "Smart Food Policies for Obesity Prevention." *The Lancet* 385 (9985): 2410–21.

Herforth, A., and S. Ahmed. 2015. "The Food Environment, Its Effects on Dietary Consumption, and Potential for Measurement within Agriculture-Nutrition Interventions." *Food Security* 7 (3): 1–16.

Hieu, N. T., F. Sandalinas, A. de Sesmaisons, A. Laillou, N. Tam, and others. 2012. "Multi-Micronutrient-Fortified Biscuits Decreased the Prevalence of Anaemia and Improved Iron Status, Whereas Weekly Iron Supplementation Only Improved Iron Status in Vietnamese Schoolchildren." *British Journal of Nutrition* 108 (8): 1419–27.

IFPRI (International Food Policy Research Institute). 2008. "How Effective Are Food for Education Programs?" IFPRI, Washington, DC.

Jacoby, H. 2002. "Is There an Intrahousehold 'Flypaper Effect'? Evidence from a School Feeding Program." *Economic Journal* 112 (476): 196–221.

Jamison, D. T., and J. Leslie. 1990. "Health and Nutrition Considerations in Education Planning: The Cost and Effectiveness of School-Based Interventions." *Food and Nutrition Bulletin* 12 (3): 204–14.

Jomaa, L. H., E. McDonnell, and C. Probart. 2011. "School Feeding Programs in Developing Countries: Impacts on Children's Health and Educational Outcomes." *Nutrition Reviews* 69 (2): 83–98.

Kazianga, H., D. de Walque, and H. Alderman. 2009. "Educational and Health Impacts of Two School Feeding Schemes. Evidence from a Randomized Trial in Burkina Faso." Policy Research Working Paper 4976, World Bank, Washington, DC.

———. 2014. "School Feeding Programs, Intrahousehold Allocation and the Nutrition of Siblings: Evidence from a Randomized Trial in Rural Burkina Faso." *Journal of Development Economics* 106 (January): 15–34.

Kleinman, R., S. Hall, H. Green, D. Korzec-Ramirez, K. Patton, and others. 2002. "Diet, Breakfast and Academic Performance in Children." *Annals of Nutrition and Metabolism* 46 (1): 24–30.

Krishnaratne, S., H. White, and E. Carpenter. 2013. "Quality Education for All Children? What Works in Education in Developing Countries?" 3ie Working Paper 20, International Initiative for Impact Evaluation, New Delhi.

Kristjansson, B., M. Petticrew, B. MacDonald, J. Krasevec, L. Janzen, and others. 2009. "School Feeding for Improving the Physical and Psychosocial Health of Disadvantaged Students." *Cochrane Database of Systemic Reviews* 7 (1): CD004676.

Kristjansson, E. A., A. Gelli, V. Welch, T. Greenhalgh, S. Liberato, and others. 2015. "Costs, and Cost-Outcome of School Feeding Programmes and Feeding Programmes for Young Children. Evidence and Recommendations." *International Journal of Educational Development* 48 (May): 79–83.

Kubik, M. Y., L. A. Lytle, P. J. Hannan, C. L. Perry, and M. Story. 2003. "The Association of the School Food Environment with Dietary Behaviors of Young Adolescents." *American Journal of Public Health* 93 (7): 1168–73.

Lassi, Z., A. Moin, and Z. Bhutta. 2017. "Nutrition in Middle Childhood and Adoelscence." In *Disease Control Priorities* (third edition): Volume 8, *Child and Adolescent Health and Development*, edited by D. A. P. Bundy, N. de Silva, S. Horton, D. T. Jamison, and G. C. Patton. Washington, DC: World Bank.

Lindert, K., E. Skoufias, and J. Shapiro. 2006. "How Effectively Do Public Transfers Redistribute Income in Latin American Countries?" In *Redistributing Income to the Poor and to the Rich: Public Transfers in Latin America and the Caribbean*, SP Discussion Paper 0605. Washington, DC: World Bank.

Liu, L. M. 2016. "Ministry of Education: Report on the Progress of the Implementation of National Nutrition Improvement Plan for Rural Students in Compulsory Education." Distributed to meeting attendees at the National Seminar on Student Nutrition Improvement, Beijing, China, April 26.

Lobstein, T., R. Jackson-Leach, M. Moodie, K. D. Hall, S. L. Gortmaker, and others. 2015. "Child and Adolescent Obesity: Part of a Bigger Picture." *The Lancet* 385 (9986): 2510–20.

Maramag, C., J. Ribaya-Mercado, P. Rayco-Solon, J. Solon, L. Tengco, and others. 2010. "Influence of Carotene-Rich Vegetable Meals on the Prevalence of Anaemia and Iron Deficiency in Filipino Schoolchildren." *European Journal of Clinical Nutrition* 64 (5): 468–74.

Masset, E., L. Haddad, A. Cornelius, and J. Isaza-Castro. 2012. "A Systematic Review of Agricultural Interventions That Aim to Improve Nutritional Status of Children." *BMJ* 344.

Montenegro, C., and H. Patrinos. 2014. "Comparable Estimates of Returns to Schooling around the World." Policy Research Working Paper 7020, World Bank, Washington, DC.

Murphy, S., C. Gewa, L. Liang, M. Grillenberger, N. Bwibo, and others. 2003. "School Snacks Containing Animal Source Foods Improve Dietary Quality for Children in Rural Kenya." *Journal of Nutrition* 133 (11): 3950S–56S.

NEPAD (New Partnership for Africa's Development). 2003. "The NEPAD Home-Grown School Feeding Programme: A Concept Note." NEPAD, Addis Ababa.

Neumann, C., N. Bwibo, S. Murphy, M. Sigman, S. Whaley, and others. 2003. "Animal Source Foods Improve Dietary Quality, Micronutrient Status, Growth and Cognitive Function in Kenyan School Children: Background, Study Design and Baseline Findings." *Journal of Nutrition* 133 (11): 3941S–49S.

Nga, T. T., P. Winichagoon, M. A. Dijkhuizen, N. C. Khan, E. Wasantwisut, and others. 2009. "Multimicronutrient-Fortified Biscuits Decreased Prevalence of Anemia and Improved Micronutrient Status and Effectiveness of Deworming in Rural Vietnamese School Children." *Journal of Nutrition* 139 (5): 1013–21.

Parish, A., and A. Gelli. 2015. "Managing Trade-Offs in Costs, Diet Quality and Regional Diversity: An Analysis of the Nutritional Value of School Meals in Ghana." *African Journal of Food, Agriculture, Nutrition and Development* 15 (4): 10217–40.

Plaut, D., T. Hill, M. Thomas, J. Worthington, M. Fernandes, and N. Burnett. 2017. "Getting to Education Outcomes: Reviewing Evidence from Health and Education Interventions." In *Disease Control Priorities* (third edition): Volume 8, *Child and Adolescent Health and Development*, edited by D. A. P. Bundy, N. de Silva, S. Horton, D. T. Jamison, and G. C. Patton. Washington, DC: World Bank.

Powell, C., S. Walker, S. Chang, and S. Grantham-McGregor. 1998. "Nutrition and Education: A Randomized Trial of the Effects of Breakfast in Rural Primary Schoolchildren." *American Journal of Clinical Nutrition* 68 (4): 873–79.

Schanzenbach, D. W. 2009. "Does the Federal School Lunch Program Contribute to Childhood Obesity?" *Journal of Human Resources* 44 (3): 683–709.

Schuh, G. E. 1981. "Food Aid and Human Capital Formation." In *Food Aid and Development*, edited by G. O. Nelson and others, 49-60, New York: Agricultural Development Council.

Siekmann, J., L. Allen, N. Bwibo, M. Demment, S. Murphy, and others. 2003. "Kenyan School Children Have Multiple Micronutrient Deficiencies, but Increased Plasma Vitamin B-12 Is the Only Detectable Micronutrient Response to Meat or Milk Supplementation." *Journal of Nutrition* 133 (11): 3972S–80S.

Singh, A., A. Park, and S. Dercon. 2014. "School Meals as a Safety Net: An Evaluation of the Midday Meal Scheme in India." *Economic Development and Cultural Change* 62 (2): 275–306.

Snilstveit, B., J. Stevenson, D. Phillips, M. Vojtkova, E. Gallagher, and others. 2015. "Interventions for Improving Learning Outcomes and Access to Education in Low- and Middle-Income Countries: A Systematic Review." 3ie Systematic Review 24. London: International Initiative for Impact Evaluation (3ie).

Stopford, I., E. Aurino, S. Hamdani, and M. Fernandes. Forthcoming. *A Cost Analysis of Including Micronutrient Powders in the Ghana School Feeding Programme.* Report by the Partnership for Child Development, London.

Story, M., M. S. Nanney, and M. B. Schwartz. 2009. "Schools and Obesity Prevention: Creating School Environments and Policies to Promote Healthy Eating and Physical Activity." *Milbank Quarterly* 87 (1): 71–100.

Story, M., D. Neumark-Sztainer, and S. French. 2002. "Individual and Environmental Influences on Adolescent Eating Behaviors." *Journal of the American Dietetic Association* 102 (3): S40–51.

UNESCO (United Nations Educational, Scientific and Cultural Organization). 2014. "Progress in Getting All Children to School Stalls but Some Countries Show the Way Forward." Policy Paper 14/Fact Sheet 28, UNESCO, New York.

Vaisman N., H. Voet, A. Akivis, and E. Vakil. 1996. "Effect of Breakfast Timing on the Cognitive Functions of Elementary School Students." *Archives of Paediatric and Adolescent Medicine* 150 (10): 1089–92.

van Jaarsveld, P., M. Faber, S. Tanumihardjo, P. Nestel, C. J. Lombard, and others. 2005. "β-Carotene–Rich Orange-Fleshed Sweet Potato Improves the Vitamin A Status of Primary Schoolchildren Assessed with the Modified-Relative-Dose-Response Test." *American Journal of Clinical Nutrition* 81 (5): 1080–87.

van Stuijvenberg, M., J. D. Kvalsvig, M. Faber, M. Kruger, D. J. Kenoyer, and others. 1999. "Effect of Iron-, Iodine-, and Beta-Carotene-Fortified Biscuits on the Micronutrient Status of Primary Schoolchildren: A Randomized Controlled Trial." *American Journal of Clinical Nutrition* 69 (3): 497–503.

Vera Noriega, J. A., S. E. Dominguez Ibáñez, M. O. Peña Ramos, and M. Montiel Carbaja. 2000. "Evaluación de los efectos de un programa de desayunos escolares en atención y memoria." *Archivos Latinoamericano de Nutricion* 5 (1).

Vermeersch, C., and M. Kremer. 2004. "School Meals, Educational Achievement and School Competition: Evidence from a Randomised Evaluation." Policy Research Working Paper 3523, World Bank, Washington, DC.

Viner, R. M., N. B. Allen, and G. C. Patton. 2017. "Puberty, Developmental Processes, and Health Interventions." In *Disease Control Priorities* (third edition): Volume 8, *Child and Adolescent Health and Development*, edited by

D. A. P. Bundy, N. de Silva, S. Horton, D. T. Jamison, and G. C. Patton. Washington, DC: World Bank.

Watkins, K., D. A. P. Bundy, D. T. Jamison, F. Guenther, and A. Georgiadis. 2017. "Evidence of Impact of Interventions on Health and Development during Middle Childhood and School Age." In *Disease Control Priorities* (third edition): Volume 8, *Child and Adolescent Health and Development*, edited by D. A. P. Bundy, N. de Silva, S. Horton, D. T. Jamison, and G. C. Patton. Washington, DC: World Bank.

Watkins, K., A. Gelli, S. Hamdani, E. Masset, C. Mersch, and others. 2015. "Sensitive to Nutrition? A Literature Review of School Feeding Effects in the Child Development Lifecycle." Working Paper Series #16, Home Grown School Feeding. http://www.hgsf-global.org.

WFP (World Food Programme). 2013. *The State of School Feeding*. Rome: WFP.

Whaley, S., M. Sigman, C. Neumann, N. Bwibo, D. Guthrie, and others. 2003. "The Impact of Dietary Intervention on the Cognitive Development of Kenyan School Children." *Journal of Nutrition* 133 (11): 3950S–56S.

WHO (World Health Organization). 1998. "Healthy Nutrition: An Essential Element of a Health-Promoting School." Information Series on School Health—Document Four, WHO, Geneva.

Winichagoon, P., J. E. McKenzie, V. Chavasit, T. Pongcharoen, S. Gowachirapant, and others. 2006. "A Multimicronutrient-Fortified Seasoning Powder Enhances the Hemoglobin, Zinc, and Iodine Status of Primary School Children in North East Thailand: A Randomized Controlled Trial of Efficacy." *Journal of Nutrition* 136 (6): 1617–23.

World Bank. n.d. "Atlas of Social Protection Indicators of Resilience and Equity (ASPIRE)." http://datatopics.worldbank.org/aspire/.

———. 2014. *The State of Social Safety Nets*. Washington, DC: World Bank.

———. 2016. *World Development Indicators*. Washington, DC: World Bank. Retrieved October 2015. http://data.worldbank.org/.

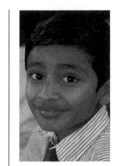

Chapter 13

Mass Deworming Programs in Middle Childhood and Adolescence

Donald A. P. Bundy, Laura J. Appleby, Mark Bradley,
Kevin Croke, T. Deirdre Hollingsworth, Rachel Pullan,
Hugo C. Turner, and Nilanthi de Silva

INTRODUCTION

The current debate on deworming presents an interesting public health paradox. Self-treatment for intestinal worm infection is among the most common self-administered public health interventions, and the delivery of donated drugs through mass drug administration (MDA) programs for soil-transmitted helminths (STHs) exceeds 1 billion doses annually. The clinical literature, especially the older historical work, shows significant impacts of intense STH infection on health; a burgeoning economics literature shows the long-run consequences for development (see, for example, chapter 29 in this volume, Ahuja and others 2017; Fitzpatrick and others 2017). Yet, the literature on clinical trials shows conflicting results, and the resulting controversy has been characterized as the *worm wars*.

The two previous editions of *Disease Control Priorities* contain chapters on STH and deworming programs (Hotez and others 2006; Warren and others 1993). Much of the biological and clinical understanding reflected in those chapters remains largely unchanged. This chapter presents current estimates of the numbers infected and the disease burden attributable to STH infections to illuminate current program efforts, advances in the understanding of epidemiology and program design, and the controversy regarding the measurement of impact.

Definitions of age groupings and age-specific terminology used in this volume can be found in chapter 1 (Bundy, de Silva, and others 2017).

ESTIMATED NUMBER OF INFECTIONS AND DISEASE BURDEN

Three types of STH commonly infect humans: roundworm (*Ascaris lumbricoides*), hookworm (comprising two species, *Ancylostoma duodenale* and *Necator americanus*), and whipworm (*Trichuris trichiura*). Recent use of geographic information systems and interpolated climatic data have identified the distributional limits of STHs on the basis of temperature and rainfall patterns as well as socioeconomic factors (Pullan and Brooker 2012). Globally, in 2010 an estimated 5.3 billion people, including 1 billion school-age children, lived in areas stable for transmission of at least one STH species; 69 percent of these individuals lived in Asia.

Map 13.1 is based on clear limiting relationships observed between infection and climatic factors for each species. For example, experimental and observational findings suggest that transmission is implausible in extremely hot, arid, or cold environments, particularly in Africa and the Middle East (Brooker, Clements, and

Corresponding author: Donald A. P. Bundy, Bill & Melinda Gates Foundation; Seattle, Washington, United States; Donald.bundy@gatesfoundation.org.

Map 13.1 Distribution of Soil-Transmitted Helminth Infection Risk, Applying Climatic Exclusion Limits

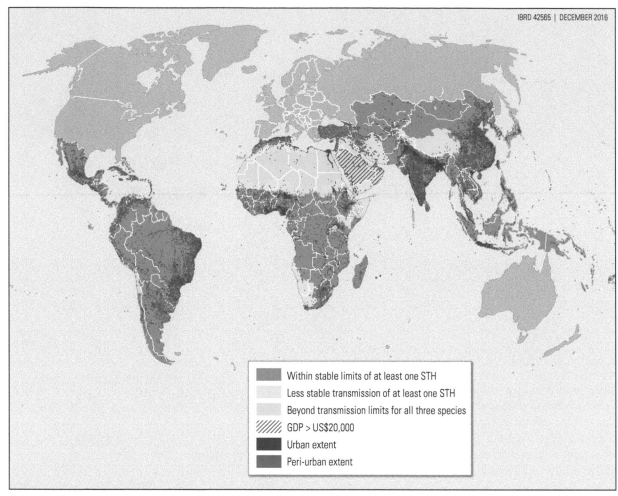

IBRD 42565 | DECEMBER 2016

Within stable limits of at least one STH
Less stable transmission of at least one STH
Beyond transmission limits for all three species
GDP > US$20,000
Urban extent
Peri-urban extent

Source: Adapted from Pullan and Brooker 2012.
Note: Analysis includes only regions considered endemic for STHs. GDP = gross domestic product; STH = soil-transmitted helminth.

Bundy 2006; Brooker and Michael 2000; Pullan and Brooker 2012). Relationships are less clear in Asia, especially for roundworm, for which positive survey data exist even in extremely hot and arid regions of India and Pakistan, perhaps because resistant transmission stages allow for seasonal transmission in environments otherwise hostile for much of the year.

Several attempts have been made to estimate worldwide prevalence of STHs since the first estimates assembled by Norman Stoll in the seminal paper titled "This Wormy World" (Stoll 1947); this section provides revised estimates of the burden of disease for STHs in 2013. The number of persons infected with STHs is generated by applying the revised estimates from 2010 (Pullan and others 2014) to age-stratified population estimates for 2013. These estimates build on a modeling framework that exploits relationships between infection prevalence, intensity, and potential morbidity originally proposed by Chan and Bundy (1999) for use in the first Global Burden of Disease study (Chan 1997). In brief, the age-stratified mean prevalence was estimated for all endemic regions at subnational scales. The approach used to map the mean prevalence of infection within the boundaries of transmission differed by region, determined by the progress in control, environmental associations, and data availability considerations. For Asia, Latin America and the Caribbean, the Middle East and North Africa, and Oceania, empirical estimates were generated directly from the data. For countries within Sub-Saharan Africa—where detailed data were lacking for several countries but where relationships between infection patterns and environmental factors were clearer—a geostatistical space-time modeling framework was used to predict the prevalence of each infection across the continent, following the approach of Hay and others (2009).

For STHs, prevalence alone does not provide a useful measure of potential morbidity because only a small number of infections will be associated with ill health. Instead, morbidity is related to the intensity of infection, with the most intense infections occurring in only a minority of infected individuals (Bundy and Medley 1992). As prevalence increases, the prevalence of high-intensity infections increases at a higher rate, such that high-prevalence communities experience disproportionate amounts of morbidity (Chan and others 1994). Heterogeneity between communities within subnational areas was therefore approximated using modeled distributions, and the number of persons with infection intensities greater than age-dependent thresholds was estimated indirectly for each species. The frequency distributions of worms, and thus the numbers exceeding these thresholds, were estimated using negative binomial distributions that assumed general species-specific aggregation parameters based on data from Brazil, Kenya, and Uganda (Pullan and others 2014). The Institute for Health Metrics and Evaluation then used these estimates to estimate disability-adjusted life years (DALYs) for 2013 (Murray and others 2015).

In 2013, an estimated 0.4 billion children under age 15 years worldwide were infected with at least one species of intestinal nematode, resulting in 1.46 million DALYs. Although the greatest number of DALYs occur in Sub-Saharan Africa and Latin America (map 13.2), a large at-risk population means that the vast majority of total infections occur in Asia, where at least one-fourth of preschool and school-age children are host to at least one STH species (table 13.1). The most important STH infection globally for children is roundworm, reflecting the age distribution of infection. Roundworm is of particular concern for preschool-age children in Sub-Saharan Africa, resulting in 143 DALYs per 100,000 population (table 13.2)—mostly attributable to wasting resulting from high-intensity infections. These figures are substantially lower than previous estimates (de Silva and others 2003), attributable in part to several methodological improvements:

- Limitation of populations at risk to areas suitable for transmission
- Increased availability of contributing survey data
- Generation of estimates at higher spatial resolutions.

Map 13.2 Distribution of DALYs for Soil-Transmitted Helminth Infections, per 100,000 Population

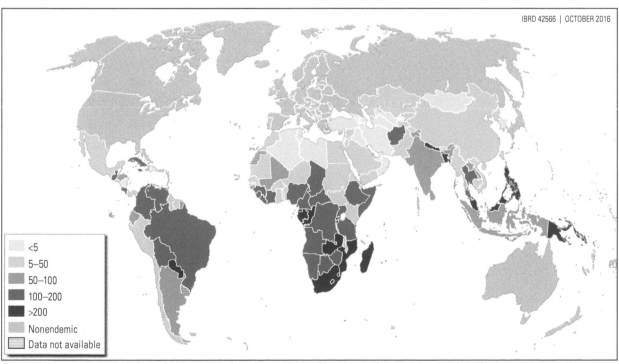

Sources: IHME (Institute for Health Metrics and Evaluation). 2014. "Global Burden of Disease Study 2013: Age-Specific All-Cause and Cause-Specific Mortality 1990–2013." IHME, Seattle, Washington.
Note: DALY = disability-adjusted life year. Soil-transmitted helminths include hookworm, roundworm, and whipworm.

Table 13.1 Total Population, Number of Infected Persons, and Overall Prevalence, 2015

Indicator	Total population (millions)	Number of Persons Infected (millions) (95% CI)				Overall Prevalence (95% CI)			
		Hookworm (millions)	Roundworm (millions)	Whipworm (millions)	Any STH (millions)	Hookworm	Roundworm	Whipworm	Any STH
Preschool age (younger than age five years)									
Middle East and North Africa	55.6	0.3 (0.2–0.3)	1.9 (1.2–2.8)	0.6 (0.4–1.0)	2.5 (1.7–3.7)	0.5 (0.3–0.6)	3.4 (2.2–4.9)	1.2 (0.8–1.7)	4.6 (3.1–6.6)
Latin America and the Caribbean	54.5	1.7 (1.1–2.6)	5.3 (3.1–8.4)	4.6 (2.9–7.1)	10.1 (6.3–14.8)	3.2 (2.0–4.8)	9.7 (5.7–15.4)	8.5 (5.3–13.0)	18.4 (11.6–27.2)
Sub-Saharan Africa	210.7	12.5 (7.7–19.1)	17.8 (10.6–27.8)	13.4 (7.7–21.5)	37.4 (23.1–55.3)	5.9 (3.7–9.1)	8.4 (5.0–13.2)	6.4 (3.7–10.2)	17.7 (11.0–26.3)
East Asia and Pacific	151.0	14.6 (8.9–22.6)	13.4 (7.0–22.5)	12.5 (6.8–20.2)	34.1 (20.2–51.6)	9.6 (5.9–14.9)	8.8 (4.7–14.9)	8.1 (4.5–13.4)	22.6 (13.4–34.2)
South Asia	172.4	7.5 (4.8–11.1)	20.0 (11.8–30.6)	6.8 (4.0–11.0)	30.0 (18.4–43.6)	4.4 (2.8–6.4)	11.6 (6.8–17.8)	4.0 (2.3–6.4)	17.3 (10.7–25.3)
Total	644.2	36.6 (22.7–55.7)	58.4 (33.9–93.0)	37.9 (21.7–60.8)	114.1 (70.0–170.0)	5.7 (3.5–8.7)	9.1 (5.3–14.4)	5.9 (3.4–9.4)	17.8 (10.9–26.4)
School age (ages 5–14 years)									
Middle East and North Africa	94.4	0.7 (0.4–0.9)	5.0 (3.4–7.2)	1.8 (1.2–2.6)	6.8 (4.6–9.6)	0.7 (0.5–1.0)	5.3 (3.6–7.6)	1.9 (1.2–2.8)	7.2 (4.9–10.2)
Latin America and the Caribbean	107.0	4.5 (2.9–6.8)	15.0 (9.4–22.6)	13.0 (8.5–19.2)	27.3 (18.1–38.4)	4.2 (2.7–6.3)	14.0 (8.8–21.1)	12.2 (7.9–17.9)	25.5 (16.9–35.9)
Sub-Saharan Africa	354.3	34.0 (21.6–50.4)	47.2 (30.0–70.1)	36.4 (22.2–55.5)	94.8 (62.7–131.0)	9.6 (6.1–14.2)	13.3 (8.4–19.8)	10.3 (6.3–15.7)	26.7 (17.7–37.0)
East Asia and Pacific	294.0	44.3 (27.8–63.2)	34.2 (18.5–55.8)	32.0 (18.7–50.8)	88.0 (55.1–127.1)	15.1 (9.4–21.5)	11.6 (6.3–19.0)	10.9 (6.4–17.3)	30.0 (18.7–43.2)
South Asia	343.0	24.7 (16.3–35.4)	63.0 (39.1–91.5)	21.7 (12.8–33.7)	90.5 (59.5–124.3)	7.2 (4.7–10.3)	18.3 (11.4–26.7)	6.3 (3.7–9.8)	26.4 (17.3–36.2)
Total	1,192.8	108.2 (68.0–156.6)	164.4 (100.6–249.2)	105.0 (63.3–161.9)	307.4 (200.7–432.4)	8.9 (5.7–13.1)	13.9 (8.4–20.9)	8.8 (5.3–13.6)	25.9 (16.8–36.2)

Source: Adapted from Pullan and others 2014.
Note: CI = confidence interval; STH = soil-transmitted helminth. Numbers in parentheses indicate range at 95 percent confidence interval.

Table 13.2 DALYs per 100,000 Population, by Region and Type of Soil-Transmitted Helminth

	DALYs per 100,000		
	Hookworm	Roundworm	Whipworm
Preschool age (younger than age 5 years)			
Middle East and North Africa	4.2 (2.4–6.4)	14.3 (9.9–19.7)	0.0 (0.0–0.1)
Latin America and the Caribbean	21.8 (13.1–34.1)	34.1 (24.6–46.1)	8.2 (4.3–15.2)
Sub-Saharan Africa	39.7 (25.3–59.7)	143.2 (117.6–173.7)	6.5 (3.7–10.6)
East Asia and Pacific	21.7 (13.4–34.2)	19.7 (13.3–28.9)	7.3 (3.3–14.0)
South Asia	19.3 (11.4–29.8)	43.1 (32.2–58.0)	2.0 (0.9–3.8)
School age (ages 5–14 years)			
Middle East and North Africa	7.3 (4.4–11.0)	4.8 (2.7–8.2)	0.1 (0.0–0.3)
Latin America and the Caribbean	73.7 (47.0–107.7)	19.2 (10.7–31.8)	16.9 (8.7–30.2)
Sub-Saharan Africa	80.7 (51.8–120.2)	33.7 (22.5–49.6)	18.1 (10.0–30.2)
East Asia and Pacific	52.7 (34.0–78.5)	11.6 (6.0–20.9)	14.4 (6.3–28.5)
South Asia	38.1 (22.8–58.4)	36.6 (21.4–60.6)	· 5.2 (2.5–9.5)

Source: Institute for Health Metrics and Evaluation, Global Health Data Exchange, http://ghdx.healthdata.org/.
Note: CI = confidence interval. Numbers in parentheses indicate range at 95 percent CI.

Results are still limited by the paucity of recent data, especially for much of Asia. These prevalence estimates were informed by a comprehensive review of population-based surveys conducted between 1980 and 2010. However, a number of coordinated efforts have been underway recently to scale up and complete the mapping for neglected tropical diseases (NTDs), including STHs. It will be important to ensure that future revisions of the Global Burden of Diseases, Injuries, and Risk Factors Study incorporate these new prevalence estimates when producing revised DALYs for STHs.

Map 13.3 shows the current distribution of STH infections. These infections were historically prevalent in many parts of the world where they are now uncommon. These areas include parts of Europe; Japan; the Republic of Korea; Taiwan, China; and the Caribbean and North America (Mexico and the United States), where sustained control efforts and economic development have led to their elimination, at least as a public health problem (Hong and others 2006; Kobayashi, Hara, and Kajima 2006; Tikasingh, Chadee, and Rawlins 2011). The distribution of worm species also reflects social and environmental factors, with greater transmission of hookworm infection in rural areas, and greater prevalence of roundworm and whipworm in periurban environments (Pullan and Brooker 2012).

The distribution of STH infection is declining, partially as a result of global economic development, declining poverty, and greater access to health services and sanitation programs, especially in poor communities. It seems probable that the targeting of more than 1 billion deworming treatments a year in poor communities has also contributed. More contemporary surveys and joined-up databases are needed for reliable estimates, but crude estimates suggest that the number of school-age children living with worm infection was cut in half from 2010 to 2015.

SCALE OF DEWORMING PROGRAMS

Deworming programs have long been popular with public health teams and the people exposed to infection. Norman Stoll's "This Wormy World" provided a clear vision of the ubiquity of infection and the scale of deworming programs in the then-endemic areas, including the U.S. South (Stoll 1947). Since the beginning of the twentieth century, schools have been viewed as the natural base for programs because they provide an existing infrastructure to reach the age group for whom infection is often most intense and who might benefit the most from deworming at a stage when they are still learning and growing (Bundy, Schultz, and others 2017, chapter 20 in this volume). In Dakar in 2000, at the World Education Forum that relaunched the Education for All program, the role of schools in delivering health programs, including deworming, was reinvigorated by the launch of the global partnership Focusing Resources on Effective School Health (FRESH).

Map 13.3 Distribution of Soil-Transmitted Helminth Infection Prevalence for Children Younger than Age 15 Years, by Species, 2015

a. Hookworm

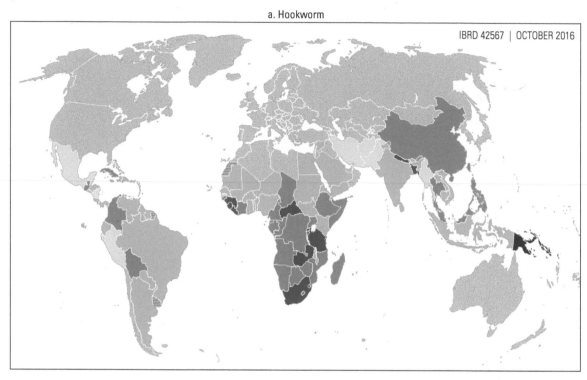

IBRD 42567 | OCTOBER 2016

b. Roundworm

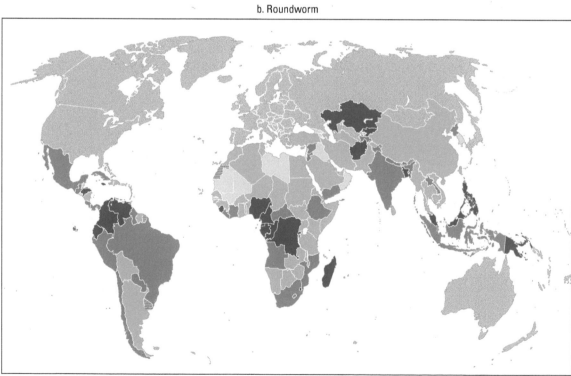

map continues next page

Map 13.3 Distribution of Soil-Transmitted Helminth Infection Prevalence for Children Younger than Age 15 Years, by Species, 2015 *(continued)*

c. Whipworm

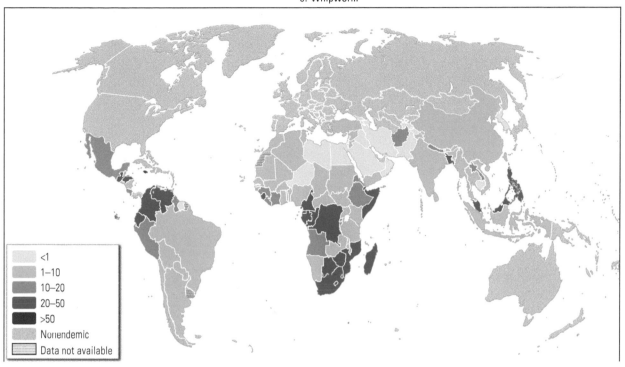

Source: Adapted from Pullan and others 2014 and updated to 2015.
Note: Based on geostatistical models for Sub-Saharan Africa and empirical data for all other regions.

FRESH was given greater vitality a year later when the World Health Assembly endorsed a target of deworming 75 percent of schoolchildren in member states with endemic STH infections. The FRESH principles continue to guide school health programs and are still being used and cited, for example, in the strategic plan for national deworming announced in Ethiopia in 2012.

From these beginnings, deworming, especially school-based deworming, has become a major public health program. In the London Declaration on Neglected Tropical Diseases announced in 2012, 14 pharmaceutical companies committed to donating medicines for 10 of the most prevalent NTDs, including STHs. The specific donations for STHs are targeted at school-age children and comprise 400 million treatments of albendazole (GlaxoSmithKline) and 200 million treatments of mebendazole (Johnson & Johnson). Medicines donated for other purposes, such as ivermectin for onchocerciasis and lymphatic filariasis, are also effective against STHs, and additional albendazole is donated specifically for lymphatic filariasis.

This progress adds up to a substantial volume of treatments efficacious against STHs. In 2015, the latest date for which treatment data are available for all three commonly used anthelmintics, the World Health Organization (WHO) reports that approximately 564 million children (150 million preschool-age children and 416 million school-age children) were treated with albendazole or mebendazole for STHs (WHO 2015a) (table 13.3). While 556.2 million persons (including approximately 36 million preschool-age children and 139 million school-age children) were treated with albendazole under MDA programs targeting elimination of lymphatic filariasis (WHO 2015b), approximately 113.2 million persons were treated with ivermectin under the onchocerciasis elimination program in Africa (WHO 2015a). These figures suggest that in 2015, more than 1 billion persons were treated with drugs that are efficacious against STHs during the course of just one year.

The official estimates of treatment coverage in school-age children continue to show relatively low, albeit rising, levels of coverage, estimated to be about 45 percent in 2014 (figure 13.1 and table 13.3). These estimates are based on the donated drugs provided through WHO mechanisms, expressed as a proportion of the world's school-age children. Both the supply (that is, the numerator) and the demand (that is, the denominator) continue to rise

Table 13.3 Total Number of Preschool-Age and School-Age Children Estimated to Require Preventive Chemotherapy for Soil-Transmitted Helminths, by WHO Region, 2009 and 2015

WHO region	2009			2015		
	Requiring PC for STHs (millions)	Receiving PC for STHs (millions)	Regional coverage (%)	Requiring PC for STHs (millions)	Receiving PC for STHs (millions)	Regional coverage (%)
African	283.8	91.0	32	298.0	153.0	51
Americas	45.5	21.1	46	46.9	24.3	52
Eastern Mediterranean	78.0	2.5	3	74.4	17.9	24
European	4.3	0.4	9	2.3	0.5	23
South-East Asia	372.0	144.8	39	354.4	172.1	49
Western Pacific	99.1	14.1	14	75.2	32.4	43
Total	882.7	273.9	31	851.2	400.2	47

Source: WHO 2011, 2016.
Note: PC = preventive chemotherapy; STHs = soil-transmitted helminths; WHO = World Health Organization.

Figure 13.1 Reported Global Coverage of Preschool- and School-Age Children, 2003–14, with a Projection to the 2020 Target of 75 Percent Coverage

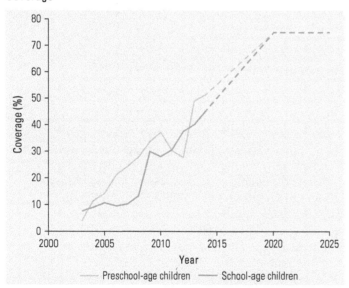

Source: Adapted from figure 1 of Trusscott, Turner, and Anderson 2015. The data on reported coverage are from the World Health Organization, "Neglected Tropical Diseases: PCT Databank," http://www.who.int/neglected_diseases/preventive_chemotherapy/lf/en/.
Note: Figure shows the treatment coverage of preschool-age and school-age children up to 2014. The dashed lines are indicative of the change necessary to reach the goal of 75 percent treatment by 2020.

leading to little change in coverage year over year reported by the WHO. These estimates report the number of doses that are donated specifically for school-based deworming (about 379 million tablets in 2015); they do not report the number of other donated drugs that are efficacious against STHs (an additional 900 million doses in 2014) or the large number of nongovernmental organization and

self-administered treatments in the unprogrammed category that go unreported. The scale of actual treatment of schoolchildren in any year could easily be twice that reported in the official statistics.

HEALTH IMPACT OF WORMS AND DEWORMING

Although the WHO recommends MDA for vulnerable groups, such as children and pregnant women, who live in areas with endemic intestinal worm infection, a series of reviews from both the Cochrane Collaboration (most recently, Taylor-Robinson and others [2015]) and the Campbell Collaboration (Welch and others 2016) argues that there is substantial evidence that mass deworming does not produce health benefits and does not support the use of MDA. How can these two views be reconciled?

Substantial Historical Literature on the Clinical Consequences of STH Infection

The clinical literature, gathered over the early part of the last century, shows significant impacts of intense STH infection on health. Through collation of data from several different studies that described the occurrence of *Ascaris*-induced intestinal obstruction in specific regions of endemic countries, and studies on the community prevalence of ascariasis in the same regions, the incidence of *Ascaris*-induced intestinal obstruction was shown to clearly increase, in a nonlinear fashion, as community prevalence of infection increased (de Silva, Guyatt, and Bundy 1997a). Similar data collations showed patients with acute intestinal obstruction due to ascariasis harbored more than 60 worms in most instances, with a 10-fold higher worm burden in fatal cases. Children younger than age five years were shown to develop obstruction with much smaller worm burdens (de Silva, Guyatt, and Bundy 1997b). A model of the global numbers at risk of morbidity and death due to ascariasis estimated that in 1990, some 11.5 million children were at risk of clinically overt acute illness and that some 200,000 children developed serious complications such as intestinal obstruction, biliary or pancreatic disease, appendicitis, and peritonitis, resulting in about 10,000 deaths each year (de Silva, Chan, and Bundy 1997).

Evidence also points to the effects of *Trichuris* infection on growth and development of infected children, in particular in those children who have a heavy burden of infection. Reports from Jung and Beaver (1951) described dysentery, diarrhea, and colitis in children with *Trichuris* infection; heavily infected children more frequently presented with the more severe symptom of rectal prolapse. This heavy infection can lead to a well-described *Trichuris* dysentery syndrome, characterized by dysentery, anemia, growth retardation, finger clubbing, rectal prolapse, and a specific trichuriasis colitis (Cooper and Bundy 1988). Furthermore, curative treatment for parasite infection leads to rapid alleviation of these symptoms (Cooper and Bundy 1988; Jung and Beaver 1951). Studies have recorded significant catch-up growth in middle childhood—especially ages four to eight years—following curative treatment, with significant increases in height and weight as well as improvements in cognition (Callender and others 1998; Cooper and others 1990; Cooper and others 1995; Nokes and others 1992).

Anemia is associated with trichuriasis colitis and is the defining characteristic of hookworm infection. On maturation and migration to the gut, hookworms attach to the intestinal mucosa and submucosa, rupturing capillaries mechanically as well as through release of anti-clotting agents to maintain blood flow (Hotez and others 2004). The development of anemia is related to infection intensity as well as to the duration of infection and nutritional status of individuals (Crompton and Whitehead 1993; Hall and others 2008). A seminal trial by Stoltzfus and others (1997) showed a significant association between hookworm infection and severe anemia, as well as iron deficiency over and above dietary intake of iron. The authors predicted that eliminating hookworm infections from their study population could lead to a reduction in anemia of 25 percent and severe anemia by as much as 73 percent.

Thus, the pathology for each of these helminth infections can be severe in both immediate effects and medium-term consequences for growth and development. Furthermore, for each of these infections, curative treatment leads to alleviation of the immediate symptoms as well as to accelerated gains in growth and development, indicating that the pathology of worm infection can largely be reversed if treated in a timely manner.

This literature, now largely historical, on clinical trials of patients with known and intense infection compared with untreated controls, offers convincing evidence on both the effect of infection on patients and the benefits of treatment. Such trials should no longer be conducted because it would be unethical to withhold treatment from patients known to be infected.

Impact of Current MDA-Based Trial Design

The majority of deworming trials today are designed quite differently from traditional clinical trials. They are based on the operational design of deworming programs, in which MDA covers all of the target population, usually an age class, living in an area where infection is endemic, with no measure of individual infection status or intensity. Because infection intensity is overdispersed, such that most people have lower-than-average infection and a minority have intense infection (figure 13.2), there will be considerable and unknown variance in the intensity of individual infection. Because the intensity is unknown in any individual, so too is the likelihood of morbidity and the potential scale of benefit from treatment. With the current trial design, the population outcome can only be measured as some average of individual benefits. Even were there to be considerable benefit for the minority of intensely infected individuals, if there is little or no benefit for the majority with light infections then the average effect will be small. The underlying situation across the population is unknowable with current MDA-based trial designs.

To illustrate what the analyses show in practice, we compare two comprehensive analyses drawing on the same small pool of trials available in this area of research. In the first analysis, Taylor-Robinson and others (2015) examined both randomized trials of universal deworming programs, which include children both with and without worms, and studies among groups of infected children already screened and diagnosed. They then conducted formal meta-analysis for eight outcomes: weight, height, middle-upper-arm circumference, triceps skinfold thickness, subscapular skinfold thickness, body mass index, hemoglobin, and school attendance. They concluded that, while *targeted* deworming of infected children may increase weight gain, for mass deworming programs that cover children with and without worms,

Figure 13.2 Distribution of Worm Burden

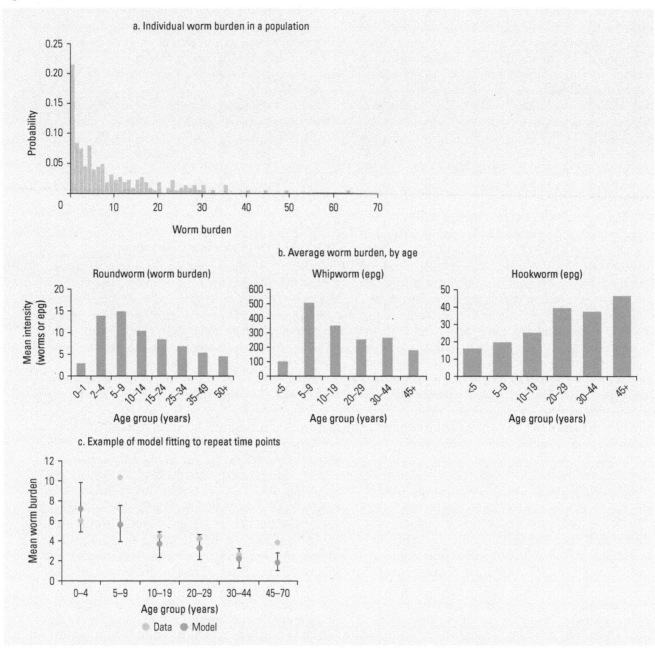

Sources: Panel a, adapted from Hollingsworth, Truscott, and Anderson 2013; panel b, adapted from Truscott and others 2014; panel c, adapted from Truscott, Turner, and Anderson 2015.
Note: epg = eggs per gram of stool. Worm burden indicates the expected number of worms harbored by an individual.

"There is now substantial evidence that [mass treatment of all children in endemic areas] does not improve *average* [emphasis added] nutritional status, hemoglobin, cognition, school performance, or survival" Taylor-Robinson and others (2015, 2). They included a maximum of 11 estimates from 10 trials for weight gain, with many fewer trials for most of the other outcome measures.

In the other analysis, Croke and others (2016) augmented Taylor-Robinson and others' (2015) sample with information from published studies as well as several excluded studies and then conducted meta-analysis on this augmented sample. Focusing on weight gain, for which the number of available studies is greatest, they noted that the appropriate test for the hypothesis of no treatment effect in all cases is a fixed-effect meta-analysis. Using this model, the hypothesis of zero weight gain from deworming was rejected at the 10 percent level using the original data from the Taylor-Robinson and others (2015) study. Using the augmented sample, they found a 0.111 kilogram weight gain ($p < 0.001$) from deworming in a fixed-effects model and a 0.134 kilogram weight gain ($p = 0.01$) in a random-effects model.

Noting that including trials from settings with minimal STH prevalence and mass deworming is not recommended because such a policy may minimize the estimated impact of deworming, they then estimated positive and statistically significant impacts in settings in which the WHO recommends multiple doses of mass treatment annually (greater than 50 percent prevalence), and in settings where the WHO recommends mass deworming at least once per year (greater than 20 percent prevalence). For high- and medium-prevalence areas (greater than 50 percent prevalence of any single STH species), the fixed-effects estimate was 0.157 kilogram, while the random-effects estimate was 0.182 kilogram. For trials in settings with greater than 20 percent prevalence, the fixed-effects estimate was 0.142 kilogram, while the random-effects estimate was 0.148 kilogram.

Accordingly, while Taylor-Robinson and others (2015) highlighted an apparent contradiction between the evidence on treatment of infected individuals (evidence of benefit) and mass treatment (no evidence of benefit), Croke and others (2016) demonstrated that mass deworming also has evidence of benefit, albeit of smaller magnitude than the effects identified in targeted studies. Evidence for this benefit is particularly strong in high- and medium-prevalence settings. The estimated weight gain in these universal treatment studies is notably smaller than in studies of individuals known to be infected—on the order of 0.13 and 0.75 kilogram, respectively—which would be the logical consequence of averaging across a population with an overdispersed distribution of intensity of infection and probability of morbidity.

The similar results but very different conclusions of these two analyses of the same trial datasets may be helpful for understanding the paradoxical literature in the deworming area. Both analyses found effects with targeted treatment trials, as is well documented in the clinical literature. Both analyses found small effects on weight gain (the measure for which most trials are available for meta-analysis) when exploring the effects across whole populations with unknown distribution of infection intensity—finding these effects significant in one analysis and not significant in the other. Resolving this debate requires exploring the distribution of individual morbidity and infection intensity. One important point is that the targeted treatment trials are also the earlier trials: detecting average effects in populations will only become more difficult as infection levels continue to decline.

OPTIMIZING PROGRAM DESIGN BY MODELING POPULATION DYNAMICS

Both chapters on deworming in the earlier editions of *Disease Control Priorities* emphasized the importance of understanding population dynamics as a determinant of good program design (Hotez and others 2006; Warren and others 1993). This section explores how the population dynamics modeling is being used to optimize program design and, in particular, what the modeling says about the value of MDA versus screen and treat and of school-based deworming versus universal coverage.

A common epidemiological feature of STH infections is the overdispersed distribution of worms (figure 13.2, panel a): while many people have a medium to low burden of infection, a minority of people have a high burden of infection. Because of the linear relationship between infection intensity and morbidity, individuals with high burdens are most likely to suffer health impacts of STHs, to contribute the largest number of infectious eggs, and to be reinfected following mass treatment, raising the possibility that targeting these individuals would be the most effective way to control both the health impact and the transmission of STHs. However, this approach has some practical challenges.

- First, commonly used diagnostics—wet smear in saline or Kato-Katz examination of stool samples to count eggs—are poor diagnostics of the underlying worm burden because of both variations in egg output and the nonlinear relationship to worm burden (Anderson and Schad 1985).
- Second, selective diagnosis and treatment involves expensive fieldwork, including collecting and analyzing stool samples and finding, reidentifying, and treating highly infected individuals (see next section on costs).
- Third, the nature of the overdispersed distribution means that a large proportion of the population has to be sampled to detect the few who have to be treated.

The few field studies that have been performed have found that selective treatment of persons with high parasite burden is less effective than mass treatment at reducing population-level prevalence (Asaolu, Holland, and Crompton 1991); that mass treatment is more cost-effective than selective treatment (Holland and others 1996); and that school-based deworming is a highly cost-effective way to reduce anemia (Brooker and others 2008; Guyatt and others 2001) in particular settings, reflecting the results of modeling studies (Guyatt, Bundy, and Evans 1993) and a recent review of costs and cost-effectiveness (Turner and others 2015). Current evidence suggests that the most cost-effective way to reduce high-burden infections in children is through school-based deworming rather than selective treatment.

Epidemiological studies have also found indirect benefits to mass treatment of children, such as reductions in prevalence of infection in untreated adults (Asaolu, Holland, and Crompton 1991; Bundy and others 1990). These indirect effects have been found for roundworm and whipworm, but different effects were found in different settings, reflecting local differences in prevalence and distribution of infection. The population-level impact of a school-based deworming program and the impact on transmission to other members of the community and reinfection after treatment depend on the epidemiology of the parasite, efficacy of the treatments, age distribution of the population, and coverage of the treatment program. For roundworm and whipworm, the highest burden of infection is usually in children (figure 13.2, panel b); therefore, a school-based program covering preschool- and school-age children could have a large impact on transmission, particularly in settings with a high proportion of school-age population, provided the treatment used is effective for whipworm (Chan and others 1994; Turner and others 2016) and prevalence is at moderate to low levels. For hookworm, the burden of infection tends to be higher in adults; therefore, a school-based deworming program is likely to be less effective at reducing both morbidity (Coffeng and others 2015; Truscott, Turner, and Anderson 2015) and transmission at the population level (Anderson, Truscott, and Hollingsworth 2014; Anderson and others 2013; Anderson and others 2015; Chan and others 1994). However, systematically excluding a portion of the community from treatment can undermine elimination programs (Coffeng and others 2015), although it also helps slow the emergence of drug resistance.

Many of these results are from mathematical modeling studies, which have become more complex in recent years. An important development has been the validation of models against repeat time-point data (figure 13.2, panel c); these models are being expanded to include the most recent data (Coffeng and others 2015; Truscott, Turner, and Anderson 2015). Given that coverage of

adults is likely to be required to break transmission, analyses have shown that in many settings the higher cost of coverage is offset by the lower number of rounds required, given that treatment can be stopped when transmission has been permanently interrupted (Lo and others 2015; Turner and others 2015; Turner and others 2016).

This section considers two issues: how treatment can bring down intensity and morbidity, and how treatment might break transmission. Empirical evidence is available for the former, but caution should remain about the latter. Although MDA has proven to be effective with onchocerciasis and lymphatic filariasis, these diseases have much slower epidemic growth rates than do STHs, and both require vectors for transmission rather than fecal contamination of the environment with infective stages.

ESTIMATED COST OF MDA

One of the main arguments for deworming, and the basis of the WHO recommendation for the use of MDA, especially school-based deworming, is the cost-effectiveness arising from an exceptionally low-cost intervention delivered infrequently without the need for costly screening. The value for money of this approach for low-income countries has recently been greatly enhanced by the availability of donated treatments. This section explores the costs in more detail.

MDA offers notable economies of scale (Brooker and others 2008; Evans and others 2011) because the cost per treatment decreases as the number treated rises (figure 13.3, panel a). This effect occurs because some of the most significant costs associated with MDA delivery are fixed and do not depend on the number treated: increasing the number treated therefore reduces the average fixed cost per treatment (Turner and others 2016). These economies of scale may account for much of the observed variation in the costs of delivering NTD treatment (Turner and others 2015).

Table 13.4 lists the costs of STHs delivered through a variety of MDA program designs. Integrating STH programs with other NTD programs or indeed other control programs, such as child health days, can produce economies of scope, by which the average cost per treatment declines as a result of delivering two or more interventions at once (figure 13.3, panel b); for example, integrating NTD programs reduces the overall cost between 16 percent and 40 percent (Evans and others 2011; Leslie and others 2013). Furthermore, the incremental cost of adding deworming into established immunization campaigns or child health days

Figure 13.3 Observed Economies of Scale and Scope Associated with Preventive Chemotherapy

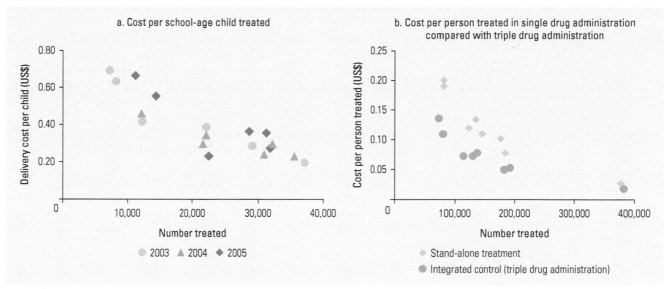

Sources: Panel a, data from Brooker and others 2008; panel b, data from Evans and others 2011.
Note: Triple drug administration refers to the co-administration of albendazole, ivermectin, and praziquantel on a single delivery platform in communities where multiple neglected tropical diseases are prevalent.

Table 13.4 Key Preventive Chemotherapy Costing Studies Using Albendazole and Mebendazole

Study	Country	Target of intervention	Primary distribution method	Results
Brooker and others 2008	Uganda	STHs and SCH	School based (annually)	The overall economic cost per child treated in the six districts was US$0.54, which ranged from US$0.41 to US$0.91 (delivery costs: US$0.19–US$0.69). The overall financial cost per child treated was US$0.39. Costs are in 2005 US$.
Goldman and others 2007	Multicountry study	LF (and STHs indirectly)	Community based (annually)	The financial cost per treatment ranged from US$0.06 to US$2.23. Costs are in 2000–03 US$ (base year 2002).
Evans and others 2011	Nigeria	STHs, SCH, LF, and onchocerciasis	Community based (annually)	In 2008, school-age children in eight local government areas received a single round of ivermectin and albendazole followed at least one week later by praziquantel. The following year, a single round of triple drug administration was given, reducing the programmatic costs for MDA, not including drug and overhead costs, 41 percent (from US$0.078 to US$0.046 per treatment). Costs are in 2008–09 US$.
Goldman and others 2011	Haiti	STHs and LF	School based and community based (annually)	The cost per treatment was US$0.64, including the value of donated drugs. The program cost, excluding the value of the donated drugs, was US$0.42 per person treated. Costs are in 2008–09 US$.
Leslie and others 2011	Niger	STHs and SCH	School based and community based (annually)	The full economic cost of delivering the school-based and community-based treatment was US$0.76 and US$0.46, respectively. Including program costs alone, the values were US$0.47 and US$0.41, respectively. Costs are in 2005 US$.
Leslie and others 2013	Niger	STHs, SCH, LF, and trachoma	School based and community based (annually)	The average economic cost of integrated preventive chemotherapy was US$0.19 per treatment, excluding drug costs. The average financial cost per treatment of the vertical SCH and STH control program (before the NTD programs were integrated) was US$0.10. Costs in are 2009 US$.

table continues next page

Table 13.4 Key Preventive Chemotherapy Costing Studies Using Albendazole and Mebendazole **(continued)**

Study	Country	Target of intervention	Primary distribution method	Results
Boselli and others 2011	Lao PDR	STHs within a child health day campaign	Child health days (annually)	The incremental cost of adding deworming into the national immunization campaign was US$0.03 per treatment (delivery costs: US$0.007). The cost per treatment for the vertical school-based national deworming campaign (targeting school-age children) was US$0.23. Costs are in 2009 US$.
Fiedler and Semakula 2014	Uganda	STHs within a vitamin A supplementation campaign	Child health days (one round)	The average economic cost per child reached by the child health day program was US$0.22 (per round). Costs are in 2010 US$.

Note: LF = lymphatic filariasis; MDA = mass drug administration; NTD = neglected tropical disease; SCH = schistosomiasis; STHs = soil-transmitted helminths. For a more detailed summary of cost data for preventive chemotherapy, see Keating and others (2014) and Turner and others (2015).

with an already developed delivery infrastructure is very small—approximately US$0.03 per treatment (Boselli and others 2011)—and much lower than delivering treatment through vertical national deworming programs (Turner and others 2015); however, it may target younger children only and not access the age group with intense infection. This possibility highlights the critical need to consider the local context of NTD control programs when comparing the reported costs of MDA.

CONCLUSIONS

STH deworming programs are among the largest public health programs in low- and lower-middle-income countries as measured by coverage. The actual scale of these programs is unknown but is substantial; more than 1 billion donated doses of medicines effective against STHs are delivered by formal programs and supplemented by widespread self-treatment and unprogrammed activities. Deworming is one of the most common self-administered treatments in low-income countries; there is no question that there is strong community demand for this intervention. The large majority of formal MDA programs for STHs is school based.

STH infection is declining worldwide, likely reflecting the influence of improved hygiene and sanitation associated with global declines in poverty. The decline also reflects control efforts during the twentieth century that have largely eliminated STHs as a public health problem in previously endemic areas of North America (Mexico and the United States), Japan, Korea, and upper-middle-income countries throughout southern and eastern Asia.

This trend accelerated during the past decade, especially in the poorest countries where infection was previously most intense. Estimates are crude, but suggest that infection prevalence in school-age children was halved between 2010 and 2015. Efforts are underway to provide more extensive and more accurate surveys of infection status, supported by the creation of integrated databases that provide contemporary estimates of infection and treatment coverage. Efforts to monitor the potential emergence of drug resistance in treated populations are also increasing.

Much of the treatment is delivered through schools and targets school-age children. In 2015, India had the largest public health intervention ever conducted in a single day, deworming 89 million schoolchildren during the Annual School Deworming Day. The target for 2016 is 270 million schoolchildren. Modeling suggests that expanding programs to include other age groups might break transmission, and studies are exploring the utility of this approach in practice. Increasingly, countries are combining MDA for lymphatic filariasis and STHs since both use the same anthelmintics.

STH infection has been shown to be associated with clinical and developmental outcomes that are largely reversible by treatment (box 13.1). Both historical and contemporary trials of targeted treatment of individuals known to be infected have also demonstrated benefit from treatment.

WHO Recommendations for the Control of Morbidity Attributable to Soil-Transmitted Helminths

Present recommendations

Since 2001, the World Health Organization (WHO) has recommended, for the prevention and control of the morbidity due soil-transmitted helminth (STH) infection, the implementation of preventive chemotherapy (PC) in the form of periodical, large-scale administration of anthelmintics to population groups at risk of morbidity due to infection.

Children and women of childbearing age are considered the population groups with the highest risk of morbidity from STH infection, because they are in a period of life in which they are particularly vulnerable to nutrient deficiencies associated with infection.

The current recommendation is for treatment once a year when the prevalence of STH infection is more than 20 percent and twice a year when prevalence exceeds 50 percent. The PC strategy is being implemented worldwide; in 2015, more than 50 percent of preschool children and more than 63 percent of school-age children in areas endemic for STHs were treated with anthelmintics.

Updating the recommendations

A WHO Guideline Review Committee (GRC) comprising independent experts met in Geneva in April 2016 to reassess the WHO recommendations on STHs control in light of scientific and programmatic evidence cumulated during the last 15 years of PC interventions. The conclusions of the GRC are presently being finalized and are expected to be published in early 2017.

Source: WHO 2001.

The findings of a small group of more recent clinical trials based on MDA have been controversial. These trials measure average change in health metrics for the whole population treated, irrespective of the infection status of individuals. Since morbidity is related to intensity, and intensity has an overdispersed distribution in populations, the average change in health metrics likely reflects the outcomes for a majority of people who are lightly infected and may derive limited benefit from treatment and for a minority who are more intensely infected and may derive greater benefit. The actual distribution of intensity and infection in these trial populations is unknown because individual screening is not necessary for MDA. The controversy arises because the change when averaged across the whole population is typically small, and there are insufficient data to determine with confidence whether the small size of the change reflects the underlying population distribution or the scale of benefit. An additional factor is that these more recent trials are conducted against the background of successful control efforts and the correspondingly low intensity of infection in most of the study populations. Studies are now being designed that aim to separate these factors.

The controversy in this area has extended from the results themselves to their policy implications. There is general agreement that STH infection can affect health, but disagreement regarding the circumstances that would justify an MDA program. While this debate continues, demand for MDA is continuing in the endemic countries and self-treatment is continuing on a massive scale. The debate would benefit from quantitative policy analysis setting out the population parameters that would and would not justify an MDA approach (see chapter 29 in this volume, Ahuja and others 2017, for an example of how this analysis has been approached from an economic perspective). The trend toward integrated MDA programs that target both lymphatic filariasis and STHs would also change the policy question being asked.

Looking to the future, we can expect infection levels to continue to decline as a result of the combination of high levels of treatment and continuing economic development trends in poor communities. We can also hope for a resolution of the worm wars as methods for assessing impact improve to reflect epidemiological realities, but this goal may be compromised if levels of impact continue to fall with sustained control.

NOTE

World Bank Income Classifications as of July 2014 are as follows, based on estimates of gross national income (GNI) per capita for 2013:

- Low-income countries (LICs) = US$1,045 or less
- Middle-income countries (MICs) are subdivided:
  a) lower-middle-income = US$1,046 to US$4,125
  b) upper-middle-income (UMICs) = US$4,126 to US$12,745
- High-income countries (HICs) = US$12,746 or more.

REFERENCES

Ahuja, A., S. Baird, J. Hamory Hicks, M. Kremer, and E. Miguel. 2017. "The Economics of Mass Deworming Programs." In *Disease Control Priorities* (third edition): Volume 8, *Child and Adolescent Health and Development*, edited by D. A. P. Bundy, N. de Silva, S. Horton, D. T. Jamison, and G. C. Patton. Washington, DC: World Bank.

Anderson, R. M., and G. A. Schad. 1985. "Hookworm Burdens and Faecal Egg Counts: An Analysis of the Biological Basis of Variation." *Transactions of the Royal Society of Tropical Medicine and Hygiene* 79 (6): 812–25.

Anderson, R. M., J. Truscott, and T. D. Hollingsworth. 2014. "The Coverage and Frequency of Mass Drug Administration Required to Eliminate Persistent Transmission of Soil-Transmitted Helminths." *Philosophical Transactions of the Royal Society B Biological Sciences* 369 (1645): 20130435.

Anderson, R. M., J. E. Truscott, R. L. Pullan, S. J. Brooker, and T. D. Hollingsworth. 2013. "How Effective Is School-Based Deworming for the Community-Wide Control of Soil-Transmitted Helminths?" *PLoS Neglected Tropical Diseases* 7 (2): e2027.

Anderson, R. M., H. C. Turner, J. E. Truscott, T. D. Hollingsworth, and S. J. Brooker. 2015. "Should the Goal for the Treatment of Soil Transmitted Helminth (STH) Infections Be Changed from Morbidity Control in Children to Community-Wide Transmission Elimination?" *PLoS Neglected Tropical Diseases* 9 (8): e0003897.

Asaolu, S. O., C. V. Holland, and D. W. T. Crompton. 1991. "Community Control of *Ascaris lumbricoides* in Rural Oyo State, Nigeria: Mass, Targeted, and Selective Treatment with Levamisole." *Parasitology* 103 (2): 291–98.

Boselli, G., A. Yajima, P. E. Aratchige, K. E. Feldon, A. Xeuatvongsa, and others. 2011. "Integration of Deworming into an Existing Immunisation and Vitamin A Supplementation Campaign Is a Highly Effective Approach to Maximise Health Benefits with Minimal Cost in Lao PDR." *International Health* 3 (4): 240–45.

Brooker, S., A. C. A. Clements, and D. A. P. Bundy. 2006. "Global Epidemiology, Ecology, and Control of Soil-Transmitted Helminth Infections." *Advances in Parasitology* 62: 221–61.

Brooker, S., N. B. Kabatereine, F. Fleming, and N. Devlin. 2008. "Cost and Cost-Effectiveness of Nationwide School-Based Helminth Control in Uganda: Intra-Country Variation and Effects of Scaling-Up." *Health Policy and Planning* 23 (1): 24–35.

Brooker, S., and E. Michael. 2000. "The Potential of Geographical Information Systems and Remote Sensing in the Epidemiology and Control of Human Helminth Infections." *Advances in Parasitology* 47: 245–88.

Bundy, D. A. P., M. S. Wong, L. Lewis, and J. Horton. 1990. "Control of Geohelminths by Delivery of Targeted Chemotherapy through Schools." *Transactions of the Royal Society of Tropical Medicine and Hygiene* 84 (1): 115–20.

Bundy, D. A. P., and G. F. Medley. 1992. "Immuno-Epidemiology of Human Geohelminthiasis: Ecological and Immunological Determinants of Worm Burden." *Parasitology* 104 (Suppl): S105–19.

Bundy, D. A. P., L. Schultz, B. Sarr, L. Banham, P. Colenso, and L. Drake. 2017. "The School as a Platform for Addressing Health in Middle Childhood and Adolescence." In *Disease Control Priorities* (third edition): Volume 8, *Child and Adolescent Health and Development*, edited by D. A. P. Bundy, N. de Silva, S. Horton, D. T. Jamison, and G. C. Patton. Washington, DC: World Bank.

Bundy, D. A. P., N. de Silva, S. Horton, G. C. Patton, L. Schultz, and D. T. Jamison. 2017. "Child and Adolescent Health and Development: Realizing Neglected Potential." In *Disease Control Priorities* (third edition): Volume 8, *Child and Adolescent Health and Development*, edited by D. A. P. Bundy, N. de Silva, S. Horton, D. T. Jamison, and G. C. Patton. Washington, DC: World Bank.

Callender, J. E., S. P. Walker, S. M. Grantham-McGregor, and E. S. Cooper. 1998. "Growth and Development Four Years after Treatment for the *Trichuris* Dysentery Syndrome." *Acta Paediatrica* 87 (12): 1247–49.

Chan, M. S. 1997. "The Global Burden of Intestinal Nematode Infections: Fifty Years On." *Parasitology Today* 13 (11): 438–42.

Chan, M. S., and D. A. P. Bundy. 1999. "A Dynamic Model of Intestinal Helminth Control." Schools and Health. http://www.schoolsandhealth.org/SharedDocuments /Misscellaneous/Epiworm.zip.

Chan, M. S., H. L. Guyatt, D. A. P. Bundy, and G. F. Medley. 1994. "The Development and Validation of an Age-Structured Model for the Evaluation of Disease Control Strategies for Intestinal Helminths." *Parasitology* 109 (Pt 3): 389–96.

Coffeng, L. E., R. Bakker, A. Montresor, and S. J. de Vlas. 2015. "Feasibility of Controlling Hookworm Infection through Preventive Chemotherapy: A Simulation Study Using the Individual-Based Wormsim Modelling Framework." *Parasites and Vectors* 8: 541.

Cooper, E. S., and D. A. P. Bundy. 1988. "*Trichuris* Is Not Trivial." *Parasitology Today* 4 (11): 301–6.

Cooper, E. S., D. A. P. Bundy, T. T. MacDonald, and M. H. Golden. 1990. "Growth Suppression in the *Trichuris* Dysentery Syndrome." *European Journal of Clinical Nutrition* 44 (4): 285–91.

Cooper, E. S., E. M. Duff, S. Howell, and D. A. P. Bundy. 1995. "'Catch-up' Growth Velocities after Treatment for *Trichuris* Dysentery Syndrome." *Transactions of the Royal Society of Tropical Medicine and Hygiene* 89 (6): 653.

Croke, K., J. H. Hicks, E. Hsu, M. Kremer, and E. Miguel. 2016. "Does Mass Deworming Affect Child Nutrition? Meta-Analysis, Cost-Effectiveness, and Statistical Power." Working Paper, National Bureau of Economic Research, Cambridge, MA.

Crompton, D. W., and R. R. Whitehead. 1993. "Hookworm Infections and Human Iron Metabolism." *Parasitology* 107 (Suppl): S137–45.

de Silva, N., S. Brooker, P. J. Hotez, A. Montresor, D. Engels, and others. 2003. "Soil-Transmitted Helminth Infections: Updating the Global Picture." *Trends in Parasitology* 19 (12): 547–51.

de Silva, N., M. S. Chan, and D. A. P. Bundy. 1997. "Morbidity and Mortality Due to Ascariasis: Re-Estimation and Sensitivity Analysis of Global Numbers at Risk." *Tropical Medicine and International Health* 2 (6): 519–28.

de Silva, N., H. L. Guyatt, and D. A. P. Bundy. 1997a. "Morbidity and Mortality Due to *Ascaris*-Induced Intestinal Obstruction." *Transactions of the Royal Society of Tropical Medicine and Hygiene* 91 (1): 31–36.

———. 1997b. "Worm Burden in Intestinal Obstruction Caused by *Ascaris lumbricoides*." *Tropical Medicine and International Health* 2 (2): 189–190.

Evans, D., D. McFarland, W. Adamani, A. Eigege, E. Miri, and others. 2011. "Cost-Effectiveness of Triple Drug Administration (TDA) with Praziquantel, Ivermectin, and Albendazole for the Prevention of Neglected Tropical Diseases in Nigeria." *Annals of Tropical Medicine and Parasitology* 105 (8): 537–47.

Fiedler, J. L., and R. Semakula. 2014. "An Analysis of the Costs of Uganda's Child Days Plus: Do Low Costs Reveal an Efficient Program or an Underfinanced One?" *Food and Nutrition Bulletin* 35 (1): 92–104.

Fitzpatrick C., U. Nwankwo, E. Lenk, S. J. de Vlas, and D. A. P. Bundy. 2017. "An Investment Case for Ending Neglected Tropical Diseases." In *Disease Control Priorities* (third edition): Volume 6, *Major Infectious Diseases*. Edited by K. K. Homes, S. Bertozzi, B. R. Bloom, and P. Jha. Washington, DC: World Bank.

Goldman, A. S., M. A. Brady, A. Direny, L. Desir, R. Oscard, and others. 2011. "Costs of Integrated Mass Drug Administration for Neglected Tropical Diseases in Haiti." *American Journal of Tropical Medicine and Hygiene* 85 (5): 826–33.

Goldman, A. S., V. H. Guisinger, M. Aikins, M. L. Amarillo, V. Y. Belizario, and others. 2007. "National Mass Drug Administration Costs for Lymphatic Filariasis Elimination." *PLoS Neglected Tropical Diseases* 1 (1): e67.

Guyatt, H. L., S. Brooker, C. M. Kihamia, A. Hall, and D. A. P. Bundy. 2001. "Evaluation of Efficacy of School-Based Anthelmintic Treatments against Anaemia in Children in the United Republic of Tanzania." *Bulletin of the World Health Organization* 79 (8): 695–703.

Guyatt, H. L., D. A. P. Bundy, and D. Evans. 1993. "A Population Dynamic Approach to the Cost-Effectiveness Analysis of Mass Anthelmintic Treatment: Effects of Treatment Frequency on *Ascaris* Infection." *Transactions of the Royal Society of Tropical Medicine and Hygiene* 87 (5): 570–75.

Hall, A., G. Hewitt, V. Tuffrey, and N. de Silva. 2008. "A Review and Meta-Analysis of the Impact of Intestinal Worms on Child Growth and Nutrition." *Maternal and Child Nutrition* 4 (Suppl 1): 118–236.

Hay, S. I., C. A. Guerra, P. W. Gething, A. P. Patil, A. J. Tatem, and others. 2009. "A World Malaria Map: *Plasmodium falciparum* Endemicity in 2007." *PLoS Medicine* 24: e1000048.

Holland, C. V., E. O'Shea, S. O. Asaolu, O. Turley, and D. W. Crompton. 1996. "A Cost-Effectiveness Analysis of Anthelminthic Intervention for Community Control of Soil-Transmitted Helminth Infection: Levamisole and *Ascaris lumbricoides*." *Journal of Parasitology* 82 (4): 527–30.

Hollingsworth, T. D., J. E. Truscott, and R. M. Anderson. 2013. "Transmission Dynamics of *Ascaris lumbricoides*: Theory and Observation." In *Ascaris: The Neglected Parasite*, edited by C. Holland, 231–62. London: Academic Press.

Hong, S. T., J. Y. Chai, M. H. Choi, S. Huh, H. J. Rim, and others. 2006. "A Successful Experience of Soil-Transmitted Helminth Control in the Republic of Korea." *Korean Journal of Parasitology* 44 (3): 177–85.

Hotez, P. J., S. Brooker, J. M. Bethony, M. E. Bottazzi, A. Loukas, and others. 2004. "Hookworm Infection." *New England Journal of Medicine* 351 (8): 799–807.

Hotez, P. J., D. A. P. Bundy, K. Beegle, S. Brooker, L. Drake, and others. 2006. "Helminth Infections: Soil-Transmitted Helminth Infections and Schistosomiasis." In *Disease Control Priorities in Developing Countries*, second edition, edited by D. T. Jamison, J. G. Breman, A. R. Measham, G. Alleyne, M. Claeson, D. B. Evans, P. Jha, A. Mills, and P. Musgrove, 467–82. Washington, DC: World Bank and Oxford University Press.

IHME (Institute for Health Metrics and Evaluation). 2014. "Global Burden of Disease Study 2013: Age-Specific All-Cause and Cause-Specific Mortality 1990–2013." IHME, Seattle, Washington.

———. 2016. Global Health Data Exchange. http://ghdx.healthdata.org/.

Jung, R. C., and P. C. Beaver. 1951. "Clinical Observations on *Trichocephalus trichurus* (Whipworm) Infestation in Children." *Paediatrics* 8 (4): 548–57.

Keating, J., J. O. Yukich, S. Mollenkopf, and F. Tediosi. 2014. "Lymphatic Filariasis and Onchocerciasis Prevention, Treatment, and Control Costs across Diverse Settings: A Systematic Review." *Acta Tropica* 135: 86–95.

Kobayashi, A., T. Hara, and J. Kajima. 2006. "Historical Aspects for the Control of Soil-Transmitted Helminthiasis." *Parasitology International* 55 (Suppl): S289–91.

Leslie, J., A. Garba, K. Boubacar, Y. Yaye, H. Sebongou, and others. 2013. "Neglected Tropical Diseases: Comparison of the Costs of Integrated and Vertical Preventive Chemotherapy Treatment in Niger." *International Health* 5 (1): 78–84.

Leslie, J., A. Garba, E. B. Oliva, A. Barkire, A. A. Tinni, and others. 2011. "Schistosomiasis and Soil-Transmitted Helminth Control in Niger: Cost-Effectiveness of School-Based and Community-Distributed Mass Drug Administration [Corrected]." *PLoS Neglected Tropical Diseases* 5 (10): e1326.

Lo, N. C., I. I. Bogoch, B. G. Blackburn, G. Raso, E. K. N'Goran, and others. 2015. "Comparison of Community-Wide, Integrated Mass Drug Administration Strategies for Schistosomiasis and Soil-Transmitted Helminthiasis: A Cost-Effectiveness Modelling Study." *The Lancet Global Health* 3 (10): e629–38.

Murray, C. J., R. M. Barber, K. J. Foreman, A. Abbasoglu Ozgoren, F. Abd-Allah, and others. 2015. "Global, Regional and National Disability-Adjusted Life Years (DALYs) for 306 Diseases and Injuries and Health Life Expectancy (HALE) for 188 Countries, 1990–2013: Quantifying the Epidemiological Transition." *The Lancet* 386 (10009): 2145–91.

Nokes, C., S. M. Grantham-McGregor, A. W. Sawyer, E. S. Cooper, B. A. Robinson, and others. 1992. "Moderate to Heavy Infections of *Trichuris trichuria* Affect Cognitive Function in Jamaican School Children." *Parasitology* 104 (3): 539–47.

Pullan, R. L., and S. J. Brooker. 2012. "The Global Limits and Population at Risk of Soil-Transmitted Helminth Infections in 2010." *Parasites and Vectors* 5: 81.

Pullan, R. L., J. L. Smith, R. Jasrasaria, and S. J. Brooker. 2014. "Global Numbers of Infection and Disease Burden of Soil Transmitted Helminth Infections in 2010." *Parasites and Vectors* 7: 37.

Stoll, N. R. 1947. "This Wormy World." *Journal of Parasitology* 33 (1): 1–18.

Stoltzfus, R. J., H. M. Chwaya, J. M. Tielsch, K. J. Schulze, M. Albonico, and others. 1997. "Epidemiology of Iron Deficiency Anemia in Zanzibari Schoolchildren: The Importance of Hookworms." *American Journal of Clinical Nutrition* 65 (1): 153–59.

Taylor-Robinson, D. C., N. Maayan, K. Soares-Weiser, S. Donegan, and P. Garner. 2015. "Deworming Drugs for Soil-Transmitted Intestinal Worms in Children: Effects on Nutritional Indicators, Haemoglobin, and School Performance." *Cochrane Database of Systematic Reviews* 7: CD000371. doi:10.1002/14651858.CD000371.pub6.

Tikasingh, E. S., D. D. Chadee, and S. C. Rawlins. 2011. "The Control of Hookworm in the Commonwealth Caribbean Countries." *Acta Tropica* 120: 24–30.

Truscott, J. E., T. D. Hollingsworth, S. J. Brooker, and R. M. Anderson. 2014. "Can Chemotherapy Alone Eliminate the Transmission of Soil Transmitted Helminths?" *Parasites and Vectors* 7: 266.

Truscott, J. E., H. C. Turner, and R. M. Anderson. 2015. "What Impact Will the Achievement of the Current World Health Organisation Targets for Anthelmintic Treatment Coverage in Children Have on the Intensity of Soil Transmitted Helminth Infections?" *Parasites and Vectors* 8: 551.

Turner, H. C., J. E. Truscott, F. M. Fleming, T. D. Hollingsworth, S. J. Brooker, and others. 2016. "Cost-Effectiveness of Scaling Up Mass Drug Administration for the Control of Soil-Transmitted Helminths: A Comparison of Cost Function and Constant Costs Analyses." *The Lancet Infectious Diseases* 16 (7): 838–46.

Turner, H. C., J. E. Truscott, T. D. Hollingsworth, A. A. Bettis, S. J. Brooker, and others. 2015. "Cost and Cost-Effectiveness of Soil-Transmitted Helminth Treatment Programmes: Systematic Review and Research Needs." *Parasites and Vectors* 8: 355.

Warren, K. S., D. A. P. Bundy, R. M. Anderson, A. R. Davis, D. A. Henderson, and others. 1993. "Helminth Infections." In *Disease Control Priorities in Developing Countries*, first edition, edited by W. H. Mosley, D. T. Jamison, A. R. Measham, and J. L. Bobadilla, 131–60. New York: Oxford University Press.

Welch V. A., E. Ghogomu, A. Hossain, S. Awasthi, Z. Bhutta, and others. 2016. "Deworming and Adjuvant Interventions for Improving the Developmental Health and Well-Being of Children in Low- and Middle-Income Countries: A Systematic Review and Network Meta-Analysis." *Campbell Systematic Reviews* 7.

WHO (World Health Organization). 2001. "World Health Assembly (WHA54.19): Schistosomiasis and Soil-Transmitted Helminth Infections." WHO, Geneva. http://www.who.int/neglected_diseases/mediacentre/WHA_54.19_Eng.pdf?ua=1.

———. 2011. "Soil-Transmitted Helminthiases: Estimates of the Number of Children Needing Preventive Chemotherapy and Number Treated, 2009." *Weekly Epidemiological Record* 25: 257–66.

———. 2015a. "African Programme for Onchocerciasis Control: Progress Report, 2014–2015." *Weekly Epidemiological Record* 90 (49): 661–74.

———. 2015b. "Global Programme to Eliminate Lymphatic Filariasis: Progress Report, 2014." *Weekly Epidemiological Record* 90 (38): 489–504.

———. 2016. "Summary of Global Update on Preventative Chemotherapy Implementation in 2015." *Weekly Epidemiological Record* 91 (39): 456–60.

Malaria in Middle Childhood and Adolescence

Simon J. Brooker, Sian Clarke, Deepika Fernando,
Caroline W. Gitonga, Joaniter Nankabirwa,
David Schellenberg, and Brian Greenwood

INTRODUCTION

The age distribution of cases of malaria is influenced by the intensity of transmission. In areas where the population has low exposure to infection, malaria occurs in all age groups. In high transmission areas, in contrast, the main burden of malaria, including nearly all malaria-related deaths, is borne by young children (figure 14.1). These different age patterns are seen because exposure to repeated malaria infections induces some protection against subsequent attacks; but protection is rarely complete.

The age pattern of clinical malaria is determined by the level of transmission and the consequent level of acquired immunity, so it is sensitive to changes in the level of transmission (Carneiro and others 2010; Snow and others 1997). In many malaria-endemic areas, successful control programs have reduced the level of transmission substantially (Noor and others 2014; O'Meara and others 2010; WHO 2015). Consequently, in such communities, the peak age of clinical attacks of malaria is shifting from very young to older children. In The Gambia, the peak age of hospital admission for severe malaria increased from 3.9 years in 1999–2003 to 5.6 years in 2005–07 (Ceesay and others 2008); similar changes have been seen in Kenya (O'Meara and others 2008).

If the financial support for malaria control continues, further decreases in the intensity of transmission can be anticipated in many highly endemic areas; these decreases will increase the incidence of clinical attacks of malaria, including severe attacks, in school-age children (ages 5–14 years). However, the epidemiology and management of malaria in school-age children has, until recently, received little attention. This chapter reviews the current burden of malaria in school-age children, its clinical consequences, and approaches to controlling the disease in this increasingly vulnerable group. The review focuses largely on Sub-Saharan Africa, in part because this region has the greatest burden of malaria in school-age children, but also because of the lack of information on the impact of malaria in school-age children in other parts of the world, including those where *Plasmodium vivax* is the dominant malaria parasite. An earlier version of the review has been published (Nankabirwa, Brooker, and others 2014). Definitions of age groupings and age-specific terminology used in this volume can be found in chapter 1 (Bundy, de Silva, and others 2017).

PREVALENCE OF MALARIA PARASITEMIA IN SCHOOL-AGE CHILDREN

The burden of malaria in school-age children is poorly defined because this age group is not routinely included in household-based cluster surveys. Information on the prevalence of malaria in this group is derived mainly from school-based surveys and from World Health Organization (WHO) estimates (WHO 2015).

Corresponding author: Brian Greenwood, Faculty of Infectious and Tropical Diseases, London School of Hygiene & Tropical Medicine, London, United Kingdom; brian.greenwood@lshtm.ac.uk.

Figure 14.1 Age Distribution of Cases of Severe Malaria by Intensity of Malaria

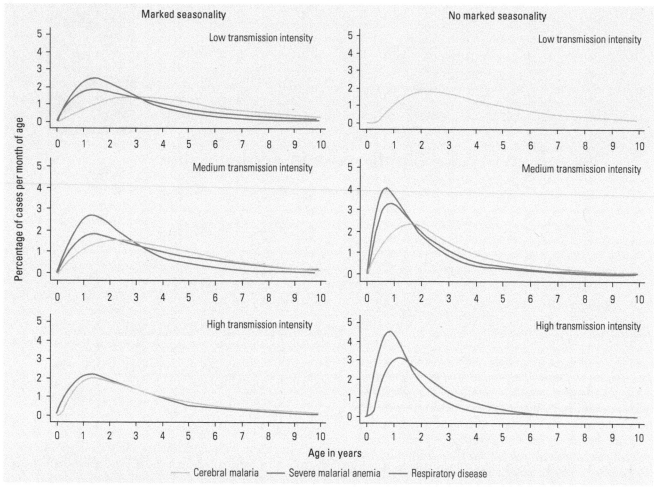

Source: Roca-Feltrer and others 2010.

Note: The figure shows the percentage distribution of each severe malaria syndrome by age for children under age 10 years according to seasonality and transmission intensity, such that the integral of the curve is equal to 100 percent of expected cases.

Understanding the burden of malaria among school-age children is essential to justify investment in school-based malaria control interventions (Bundy and others 2000) and to identify delivery mechanisms to help control malaria in this underserved population.

More than 500 million school-age children worldwide are at risk of malaria infection; 200 million of those at risk live in Sub-Saharan Africa (table 14.1) (Gething and others 2011). Annex 14A, table 14.1 summarizes the results of studies on the prevalence of asymptomatic malaria parasitemia in this population. Map 14.1 shows the frequency with which malaria surveys have been undertaken in school-age children, with an increase in recent years in East Africa. Map 14.2 shows the prevalence observed in school-age children by geographical area.

The majority of malariometric surveys are conducted in children ages 2–10 years. Relatively few studies have been undertaken in older school-age children in Sub-Saharan Africa, and many of those are out of date following improvements in malaria control. In general, higher prevalence rates have been observed in West and Central Africa than in East Africa, but a great deal of heterogeneity has been observed with rates ranging from less than 5 percent to greater than 50 percent in different surveys. Recent studies in Malawi have emphasized the burden of malaria in school-age children and the role that those children play in acting as a reservoir of infection (Mathanga and others 2015; Walldorf and others 2015).

Few reports on the prevalence of asymptomatic malaria in school-age children outside of Sub-Saharan Africa are available (annex 14A, table 14.1). In the Republic of Yemen, Bin Mohanna, Bin Ghouth, and

Table 14.1 Estimated School-Age (5–14 Years) Population at Risk of *Plasmodium falciparum* Malaria in Millions by Region,[a] 2010

Region	Unstable risk	Stable risk	Total
Andean Latin America	1.0	0.6	1.7
Caribbean	2.4	1.8	4.2
Central Asia	0.2	–	0.2
Central Latin America	3.9	2.3	6.2
Central Sub-Saharan Africa	<0.1	26.1	26.1
East Asia	1.6	0.6	2.2
Eastern Sub-Saharan Africa	3.3	80.7	84.0
Middle East and North Africa	4.0	2.5	6.5
Oceania	<0.1	1.4	1.4
South Asia	165.6	98.6	264.3
South-East Asia	37.8	31.6	69.4
Southern Sub-Saharan Africa	2.3	4.8	7.1
Tropical Latin America	4.6	1.7	6.3
Western Sub-Saharan Africa	1.6	86.8	88.4
World	**228.5**	**339.5**	**568.0**

Source: Adapted from Gething and others 2011; data provided by the Malaria Atlas Project (www.map.ox.ac.uk), with thanks to Pete Gething and Zhi Huang, University of Oxford.
Note: – = not applicable. Rows may not add precisely due to rounding.
a. Based on the Global Burden of Disease study, http://www.healthdata.org/sites/default/files/files/GBD_GBD2010_Regions_countries.pdf.

Rajaa (2007) find a prevalence of 13 percent in children ages 6–11 years in the Hajr valley. In Latin America, malaria transmission is restricted to Amazonian areas and is uniformly low. In Brazil, Vitor-Silva and others (2009) find that *P. vivax* was more common than *P. falciparum* among schoolchildren. On the Thai-Burma border, Luxemburger and others (1994) find that 10 percent of school-age children were infected, mainly with *P. falciparum*.

IMPACT OF MALARIA ON THE HEALTH AND DEVELOPMENT OF SCHOOL-AGE CHILDREN

Most school-age children with malaria parasitemia do not have any symptoms because they have acquired some immunity. However, asymptomatic infections can contribute to anemia and impairment of cognitive development. School-age children may be infected with a malaria parasite that expresses antigens to which they have not been exposed and to which they have little or no immunity; the result is the development of symptoms such as fever and, more rarely, severe diseases such as cerebral malaria, life-threatening anemia, and death.

Mortality

The WHO estimates that there were approximately 438,000 (range 236,000–635,000) deaths from malaria in 2015; 90 percent of those deaths occurred in Sub-Saharan Africa (WHO 2015). A comprehensive review of malaria-related deaths between 1980 and 2010 (Murray and others 2012) reports many more deaths than the WHO; the review estimates that 6 percent to 9 percent of malaria deaths occur in children ages 5–14 years, corresponding to an annual figure in the range of 70,000–110,000 deaths. A lower malaria mortality rate was found in school-age children compared with younger children in Bangladesh and Sub-Saharan Africa (Adjuik and others 2006). A similar age pattern was found in India, with an estimated malaria-related death rate of 29 per 1,000 in children ages 5–14 years, compared with 55 per 1,000 in children under age 5 years in 2005 (Dhingra and others 2010).

Incidence of Clinical Malaria in School-Age Children

An estimated 214 million (range 149 million to 303 million) cases of malaria occurred worldwide in 2015; more than 80 percent were in Sub-Saharan Africa (WHO 2015). However, data on the incidence of clinical malaria in school-age children are scarce. Review of the limited

IBRD 42568 | DECEMBER 2016

Legend:
- 1985–1989
- 1990–1994
- 1995–1999
- 2000–2004
- 2005–2009
- 2010–2013

Source: Malaria Atlas Project (MAP), http://www.map.ox.ac.uk.

information published indicates that annual incidence can vary from 0.03 to 2.7 cases per child per year, depending on the transmission setting (annex 14A, table 14.2). The limited data available suggest that it is not unusual for school-age children to experience one clinical attack of malaria severe enough to warrant treatment once every one to two years (Barger and others 2009; Clarke and others 2004; Nankabirwa and others 2010; Rohner and others 2010).

Malaria as a Cause of Anemia in School-Age Children

Anemia is a common problem among school-age children in the tropics. Its etiology is usually multifactorial, and the relative importance of different causes varies from area to area. It is difficult to separate malaria as a causative agent from other factors, such as nutritional deficiencies, helminth infections, and HIV/AIDS, which often coexist in the same communities (Stephenson and others 1985). Many other cross-sectional surveys carried out in highly endemic areas have found a significant

association between the prevalence of anemia and parasitemia, but these studies were conducted mainly among preschool-age children.

The strongest evidence for the role of malaria as a cause of anemia in school-age children comes from the results of intervention studies with trials of intermittent preventive treatment (IPT) in school-age children showing improvement in hemoglobin concentration in both East Africa (Clarke and others 2008; Nankabirwa and others 2010) and West Africa (Barger and others 2009; Clarke and others 2013; Tine and others 2011).

Overall, differentiating the effect of malaria on anemia in school-age children from other confounding factors is difficult; the limited evidence available suggests that it has a significant role. Although administration of supplementary iron can increase the incidence of clinical attacks of malaria in some circumstances, most studies have shown only a modest effect (Ojukwu and others 2009). The WHO and other health authorities (Raiten, Namasté, and Brabin 2011) recommend that iron supplementation is indicated in areas in which iron

Map 14.2 Prevalence of Malaria Parasitemia in School-Age Children in Sub-Saharan Africa
Percent

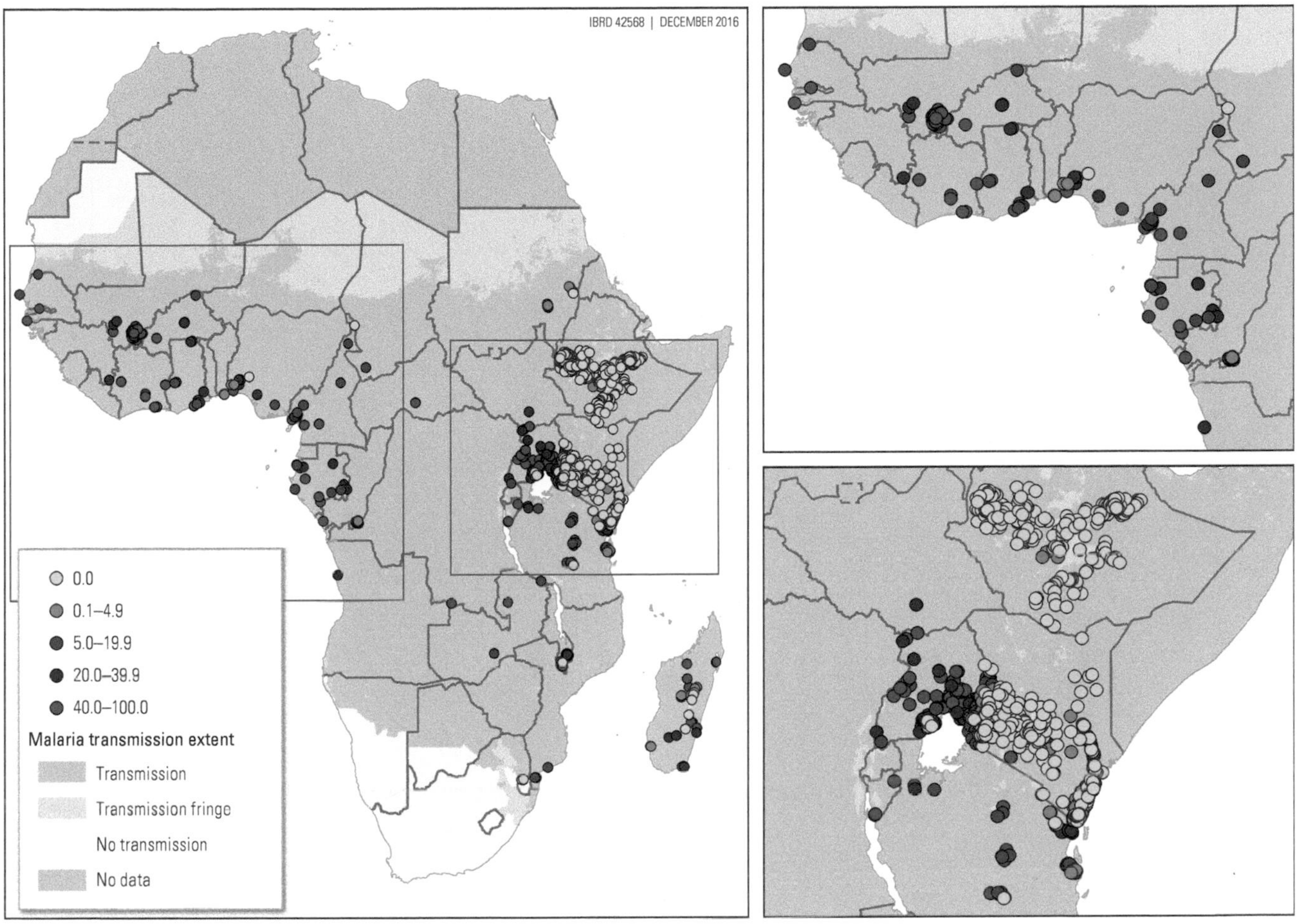

IBRD 42568 | DECEMBER 2016

○ 0.0
◔ 0.1–4.9
◑ 5.0–19.9
◕ 20.0–39.9
● 40.0–100.0

Malaria transmission extent

Transmission
Transmission fringe
No transmission
No data

Source: Malaria Atlas Project (MAP), http://www.map.ox.ac.uk.

deficiency is a major problem, even if these areas are endemic for malaria, provided that malaria control measures, such as distribution of insecticide-treated bednets (ITNs), are put in place at the same time.

Malaria as a Cause of School Absenteeism

The estimated annual loss of school time in Kenya attributable to malaria in 2000 was 4 million to 10 million school days (Brooker and others 2000). Because malaria is an important cause of school absenteeism, preventive efforts should significantly improve school attendance. In a randomized clinical trial in Sri Lanka, Fernando and others (2006) report a 55 percent reduction in malaria incidence and a 62.5 percent reduction in school absenteeism among children who received chloroquine prophylaxis.

Despite the limited number of studies, the available evidence suggests that the cumulative effect of school absenteeism attributable to malaria for children in endemic areas is considerable, preventing children from

achieving their full academic potential and causing a loss to the state with respect to its investment in education.

Impact of Malaria on Cognitive Function

Studies in Africa and Asia provide strong evidence that malaria can impair the cognitive function of school-age children (Fernando, Rodrigo, and Rajapakse 2010; Kihara, Carter, and Newton 2006). Descriptive studies have evaluated the impact of severe malaria, uncomplicated malaria, and asymptomatic parasitemia on various aspects of cognition.

In Kenya, a retrospective assessment of children ages six to nine years who had had an episode of cerebral malaria found significant differences in speech and language and cognition, compared with the healthy control group (Carter, Mung'ala-Odera, and others 2005; Carter, Ross, and others 2005; Carter and others 2006); in Uganda, cerebral malaria was associated with persistent impairment of one or more cognitive domains

Table 14.2 Summary of the Results of Recent Trials of Chemoprevention in School-Age Children

Study setting	Population	Type	Treatment regimen	Study drug	Clinical malaria Percent (95% CI)	Malaria parasitemia Percent (95% CI)	Anemia Percent (95% CI)	Source
Year-round transmission								
Western Kenya	6,735 children ages 5–18 years; 30 schools	IPCs	Treatment once every school term (3 treatments per year)	SP + AQ	Not examined	89 (73–95)	48 (8–71)	Clarke and others 2008
Sierra Leone	591 children ages 6–14 years; 1 school	IPCs	Treatment at month 0 and month 3 (2 treatments per year)	SP	Not examined	No impact	No impact	Rohner and others 2010
Uganda	780 children; 3 schools	IPCs	Single course of treatment; protective efficacy measured after 42 days	SP	Not examined	No impact	No impact	Nankabirwa and others 2010
				SP + AQ	Not examined	48.0 (38.4–51.2)	Mean change Hb +0.37 (0.18–0.56)	
				DP	Not examined	86.1 (79.5–90.6)	Mean change Hb +0.34 (0.15–0.53)	
Uganda	740 children; 1 school	IPCs	Treatment once a school term (4 treatments per year)	DP	No impact	54 (47–60)	No impact	Nankabirwa, Wandera, and others 2014
		IPCs	Treatment once every month (12 treatments per year)	DP	96 (88–99)	94 (92–98)	40 (19–56)	
Highly seasonal transmission								
Mali	262 children ages 5–10 years; 1 village	SMC	Two treatments 8 weeks apart during the malaria season (2 treatments per year)	SP	36 (12–53)	Not examined	Not examined	Dicko and others 2008
Mali	296 children ages 6–13 years; 1 village	SMC	Two treatments 8 weeks apart during the malaria season (2 treatments per year)	SP + AS	66.6	80.7	59.8	Barger and others 2009
				AQ + AS	46.5	75.5	54.1	
Mali	1,815 children ages 6–14 years; 38 schools	IPCs	Single treatment at end of the malaria season (1 treatment per year)	SP + AS	Not examined	99 (98–100)	38 (9–58)	Clarke and others 2013
Senegal	1,000 children under age 10 years; 8 villages	SMC	Two treatments given monthly toward end of malaria season (2 treatments per year)	SP + AQ	79 (10–96)	57 (5–81)	41 (18–58)	Tine and others 2011

Note: AQ = amodiaquine; AS = artesunate; CI = confidence interval; DP = dihydroartemisinin-piperaquine; Hb = hemoglobin; IPCs = intermittent parasite clearance in schools; IST = intermittent screening and treatment; SMC = seasonal malaria chemoprevention; SP = sulphadoxine-pyrimethamine.

(John and others 2008). Similar findings were recorded in Malawian children with retinopathy-positive cerebral malaria (Boivin and others 2011).

Cerebral malaria is not a prerequisite for cognitive impairment as a consequence of malaria infection; studies have suggested that uncomplicated episodes of malaria can adversely affect cognition. Studies in Sri Lanka show that school-age children scored significantly lower on tests of mathematics and language during an episode of clinical malaria than children in the control group (Fernando, de Silva, and Wickremasinghe 2003). In a study in Sri Lanka, Fernando and others (2003) find a negative correlation between mathematical and language skills and a past history of repeated attacks of malaria during the preceding six years among children ages 6–14 years, even after correcting for socioeconomic factors. A history of one or more malaria attacks was associated with poor performance in mathematics and language in a cohort of 198 schoolchildren studied in Brazil (Vitor-Silva and others 2009). A study of school-age children in Mali, where *P. falciparum* malaria predominates, reaches similar conclusions (Thuilliez and others 2010).

Many of the studies considered were primarily descriptive, and their results are open to potential confounding by social or economic factors not included in the analysis. Accordingly, the strongest evidence to support the view that malaria impairs cognitive function comes from intervention trials. In Sri Lanka, a randomized, placebo-controlled, double-blind trial of chloroquine prophylaxis in children ages 6–12 years showed that educational attainment improved and that school absenteeism was reduced significantly ($p < 0.0001$) in children who took chloroquine prophylaxis (Fernando and others 2006). Children in The Gambia ages 3–59 months who were randomized to receive malaria prophylaxis with dapsone-pyrimethamine or placebo during the malaria transmission season for three successive years (Greenwood and others 1988) were reassessed when their mean age was 17 years (Jukes and others 2006). Educational attainment was better in children who had received prophylactic treatment than in the placebo group, but the scores for the cognitive tests were not significantly different between groups. Prophylaxis substantially increased the school enrollment of girls. The intervention also reduced school drop out for students in government schools (Zuilkowski and Jukes 2014).

In a large, stratified, cluster-randomized, double-blind, placebo-controlled trial conducted in schools in Kenya, IPT with sulphadoxine-pyrimethamine plus amodiaquine (SP + AQ) significantly improved sustained attention of schoolchildren ages 10–12 years (Clarke and others 2008). Significant effects on sustained attention are also reported from a trial in schools in southern Mali (Clarke and others 2013).

Overall, these studies strongly suggest that both clinical malaria and asymptomatic parasitemia can adversely affect the cognitive skills of school-age children, but the mechanism by which this occurs remains uncertain.

APPROACHES TO THE CONTROL OF MALARIA IN SCHOOL-AGE CHILDREN

A range of strategies is available for the control of malaria in this age group, delivered through schools or communities. The optimal approach to delivering interventions, including frequency and timing, and their ultimate effectiveness will vary according to the local intensity of malaria transmission. Malaria interventions are best delivered as part of an integrated package, for example, as part of a school health program that also delivers deworming (see chapter 13, Bundy, Appleby, and others [2017]) or school feeding (chapter 12, Drake and others [2017]).

Treatment of Clinical Attacks

Ease of access of school-age children to effective treatment for clinical attacks of malaria is an essential component of any effective national malaria control program. However, in many parts of Sub-Saharan Africa, geographic and financial barriers prevent children from obtaining rapid access to diagnosis and treatment (see volume 6, chapter 14, Babigumira and others 2017).

Schools can play a vital role in ensuring that their pupils obtain rapid access to diagnosis and treatment by providing appropriate health education activities in school, but information about the treatment of malaria is rarely part of the curriculum. A content analysis of school textbooks in nine endemic countries found that most included information on modes of transmission, mosquitoes, and signs and symptoms of malaria, but little about ITNs or the need for prompt and appropriate treatment (Nonaka and others 2012). These findings suggest that improving textbook content in accordance with the national malaria control strategy should become a priority.

Access to prompt treatment can be improved by providing antimalarials to schools and by training teachers to administer antimalarial treatments correctly. In the past, when first-line treatment was either chloroquine or SP given presumptively, training teachers to provide treatment was shown to be feasible and to reduce school absenteeism and malaria deaths (Afenyadu and others 2005; Pasha and others 2003). However, the WHO now recommends diagnosis before any antimalarial treatment is given (WHO 2015). Building on recent efforts to expand diagnosis and treatment of malaria outside of the formal health sector (Ansah and others 2015), an ongoing study in Malawi is evaluating the impact on school attendance and health outcomes of training teachers to use rapid diagnostic tests (RDTs) (Witek-McManus and others 2015). If this approach is effective, operational issues, including supply chains, blood safety, and teacher attrition, will require careful consideration before the strategy is scaled up.

Vector Control

The main methods of vector control of malaria are ITNs, indoor residual spraying (IRS), and reduction of mosquito breeding sites.

Insecticide-Treated Nets

Strong evidence indicates that regular use of ITNs substantially lowers the risks of clinical malaria and all-cause mortality in children under age five years and reduces the burden of malaria among pregnant women (Lengeler 2004; Lim and others 2011). For these reasons, large-scale ITN distribution programs initially focused on these two vulnerable groups. However, following appreciation of the indirect herd effect of a high level of ITN coverage in a community, the development of long-lasting ITNs, and an increase in the financial and political support for ITN programs, there has been a shift from prioritizing vulnerable populations to protecting everyone with an ITN, including school-age children. However, an analysis of household surveys undertaken between 2005 and 2009 in 18 African countries found that school-age children were the group least likely to sleep under an ITN the previous night; between 38 percent and 42 percent of school-age children were unprotected (Noor and others 2009). Similar low ITN usage has been observed among school-age children in Cameroon (Tchinda and others 2012), Kenya (Atieli and others 2011), and Uganda (Pullan and others 2010) (figure 14.2). Substantial progress in population coverage with ITNs has been made since 2000, with more than 50 percent of the population of Sub-Saharan Africa sleeping under ITNs in 2015; nevertheless, ITN use among those ages 5–19 years remains lower than among the population as a whole (WHO 2015). Thus, even in countries with existing national policies of universal access to ITNs, school-based distribution of nets could have a complementary short-term role in addressing this gap.

Few studies have investigated the efficacy of ITNs in school-age children. An early trial among children in a rural boarding school in central Kenya showed that sleeping under an untreated mosquito net following a

Figure 14.2 Age Patterns in the Prevalence of Malaria Parasitemia and of Reported Use of a Bednet on the Previous Night in Uganda.

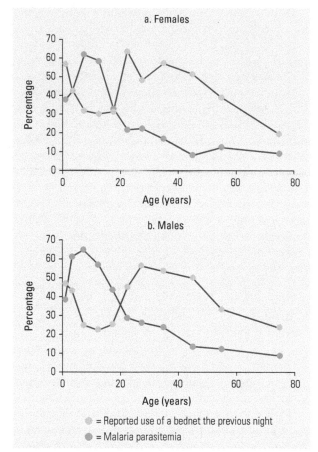

Source: Pullan and others 2010.

round of effective antimalarial treatment reduced the incidence of clinical malaria by 97 percent, but it did not reduce anemia (Nevill and others 1988). A reduction in the incidence of malaria was shown in a randomized trial of children ages 4–15 years in an area of low and unstable transmission on the Thai-Burmese border (Luxemburger and others 1994). In a rural area of western Kenya, where malaria transmission is perennial and high, a community-based trial showed that ITNs halved the prevalence of anemia in girls ages 12–13 years; ITNs were less effective in preventing anemia among girls ages 6–10 years (Leenstra and others 2003). Additional evidence provided by cross-sectional survey data suggests that net use among school-age children is associated with a 71 percent and 43 percent lower risk of *P. falciparum* infection in Somalia (Noor and others 2008) and Uganda (Pullan and others 2010), respectively. An analysis of country-wide data from school surveys in Kenya (Gitonga and others 2012) shows that ITN use was associated with a reduction in the odds of malaria infection and anemia in coastal areas, where malaria transmission is low to moderate, and among boys in western lakeshore Kenya, where transmission is high. In addition, ITN use reduced the risk of parasitemia in the western highland epidemic zones and the risk of anemia in coastal areas where transmission is low.

As children become more independent with increasing age, parents have less control over their bedtimes, where they sleep, and whether they use nets. Education targeted directly to older children, for example, through malaria education in schools, could increase regular use of ITNs among teenage children.

Indoor Residual Spraying

IRS, the application of long-acting insecticides to the walls and roofs of houses and, in some cases, public buildings and domestic animal shelters, is an effective method of malaria control. IRS implemented as a community-wide campaign can achieve substantial reductions in the incidence and prevalence of malaria infection in all age groups (Pluess and others 2010). Repeated IRS campaigns conducted between 1955 and 1959 in the Pare-Taveta area of Tanzania were associated with a reduction in malaria parasitemia from 73 percent to 7 percent in children ages 5–9 years, and from 62 percent to 4 percent in children ages 10–14 years (Draper 1960). Targeted IRS conducted over 12 months in the epidemic-prone Kenyan highlands halved the monthly prevalence of asymptomatic infection in school-age children and reduced the incidence of clinical disease (Zhou and others 2010). Studies that have investigated the impact of combining vector control with ITNs and IRS have produced mixed results, with some showing a benefit and others no added effect.

Reduction of Breeding Sites

Breeding sites of malaria anopheline vector mosquitoes can be controlled in some epidemiological situations through application of larvicides, introduction of predator species, and habitat destruction and drainage (Tusting and others 2013). However, achieving a significant reduction in malaria transmission in many parts of Sub-Saharan Africa is difficult because of the multiplicity and changing nature of breeding sites of the main vector species, such as *Anopheles gambiae* (Fillinger and Lindsay 2011). It is unlikely that encouraging schoolchildren to destroy potential breeding sites of *An. gambiae* in school grounds will have any impact on the prevalence of malaria, although it could help reduce the numbers of other mosquito species, including those that transmit dengue.

Malaria Chemoprevention

The two main approaches to the use of antimalarial drugs to prevent malaria infection are chemoprophylaxis and IPT.

Chemoprophylaxis

Chemoprophylaxis involves the regular administration of antimalarial drugs to those at risk over a sustained period to provide persistent, protective blood levels. Compelling evidence indicates the benefits of chemoprophylaxis in school-age children. A review of trials of malaria chemoprophylaxis in the population of malaria-endemic areas reports significant health impacts in nearly all studies (Prinsens Geerligs, Brabin, and Eggelete 2003). Most of these studies focus on young children, but in 30 of the 36 trials that examined infection rates in children over age five years, reductions in malaria parasitemia ranged from 21 percent to 100 percent (Prinsens Geerligs, Brabin, and Eggelete 2003). A 2008 review confirms these findings (Meremikwu, Donegan, and Esu 2008). Chemoprophylaxis with chloroquine not only reduced the incidence of clinical malaria and absenteeism in Sri Lankan schoolchildren, it also significantly improved educational attainment (Fernando and others 2006).

Intermittent Preventive Treatment

An alternative to chemoprophylaxis is IPT, the periodic administration of a full therapeutic dose of an antimalarial or antimalarial combination to groups at increased risk of malaria. IPT clears existing asymptomatic infections and prevents new infections during the period immediately after treatment when protective blood levels are present. IPT is being evaluated in schoolchildren in two ways: intermittent parasite clearance in schools (IPCs) and seasonal malaria chemoprevention (SMC).

IPCs involves the administration of IPT on a periodic basis to schoolchildren, with the aim of clearing asymptomatic malaria infections and aiding hematologic recovery during the ensuing malaria-free period. Studies that have evaluated IPCs in school-age children are summarized in table 14.2. The first study of IPCs (called IPT in that study), conducted in schools in western Kenya, shows that IPCs with SP + AQ given once a term significantly reduced malaria parasitemia and anemia and significantly improved sustained attention (Clarke and others 2008). However, the spread of parasites resistant to SP, and the consequent withdrawal of SP and AQ in many East African countries, precluded further investigation of IPCs using these drugs in this area. Studies using alternative drugs, including dihydroartemisinin-piperaquine, conducted in a range of settings, show effects on parasitemia, anemia, and clinical malaria similar to those obtained with SP + AQ, with a protective efficacy ranging between 54 percent and 99 percent reduction in malaria infection, and 38 percent to 60 percent reduction in anemia (Barger and others 2009; Clarke and others 2013; Nankabirwa and others 2010).

Several conclusions can be drawn from these studies.

- First, IPCs is highly effective in reducing the burden of malaria among school-age children.
- Second, the medication used for IPCs, and the timing of treatments, needs to be adapted to the local epidemiology.
- Third, IPCs is likely to be most effective in settings where a high proportion of children harbor asymptomatic infections, where malaria is a major cause of anemia, or both.

Seasonal Malaria Chemoprevention

SMC involves administration of treatment on a monthly basis to coincide with the annual peak in malaria transmission. This intervention is highly effective in reducing the incidence of clinical malaria and anemia in young children (Wilson 2011). In 2012, the WHO recommended implementation of SMC for children under age five years in areas of the Sahel subregion of Africa with highly seasonal transmission. This recommendation is being implemented increasingly widely in countries of the Sahel. Although less extensively researched, and not yet recommended by the WHO, evidence suggests that SMC is as effective in school-age children as in children under age five years (Barger and others 2009; Dicko and others 2008; Tine and others 2011, 2014), and Senegal provides SMC to children up to age 10 years.

Intermittent Screening and Treatment

An alternative to IPCs or SMC is intermittent screening and treatment (IST), an intervention in which individuals are screened periodically for malaria infection using an RDT, and those infected (whether symptomatic or not) are treated with a full course of an effective antimalarial agent or combination of agents. A population-based study of IST in Burkina Faso shows no impact on the incidence of clinical malaria in children under age five years or on malaria transmission (Tiono and others 2013); a cluster randomized trial in schools on the coast of Kenya, where transmission is low to moderate, finds no impact on health or cognition (Halliday and others 2014). Possible reasons for the absence of an impact in these studies are the inability of some of the currently available RDTs to detect low-density parasitemia, and the rapid rate of reinfection following treatment in the areas

in which these studies were done. The potential of this approach to control malaria in school-age children needs further investigation.

Vaccination

Development of an effective malaria vaccine has proved to be a major challenge, despite the exploration of many innovative approaches. One vaccine (RTS,S/AS01) has shown partial efficacy in a large-scale Phase 3 clinical trial and was given a positive opinion by the European Medicines Agency in July 2015 (RTS,S Clinical Trials Partnership 2015). However, the duration of protection provided by RTS,S/AS01 is relatively short, and vaccination in early life is unlikely to provide protection that lasts into school age. Only very limited data are available on the safety and immunogenicity of RTS,S/AS01 in school-age children (Bojang and others 2005). RTS,S/AS01 is the most advanced malaria vaccine, but several other vaccines are making steady progress (Schwartz and others 2012); in the longer term, vaccination may have an important role in the prevention of malaria in school-age children.

ECONOMICS OF MALARIA CONTROL IN SCHOOLS

Few economic analyses have evaluated malaria control among school-age children. A 2011 systematic review identified 48 studies that evaluated the cost-effectiveness of malaria interventions (White and others 2011), of which only two were conducted among school-age populations. The first study evaluated the cost-effectiveness of community-wide IRS programs among children ages 2–15 years in southern Mozambique (Conteh and others 2004). The financial costs per person covered in the rural area and peri-urban areas were US$3.86 and US$2.41, respectively. Using health facility records to estimate the number of infections averted, the economic cost per case of malaria parasitemia averted among those ages 2–15 years was US$21.23.

The second study evaluated the cost-effectiveness of IPCs (Temperley and others 2008). The study estimated that the cost of IPCs delivered by teachers was US$1.88 per child per year, with drug and teacher training constituting the largest cost components. The estimated cost per anemia case averted through IPCs was US$29.84, and the estimated cost per case of malaria parasitemia averted was US$5.36 (Temperley and others 2008). Another study investigates the cost of IST delivered through schools and estimates the cost of IST per child screened to be US$6.61 (Drake and others 2011). These estimates of cost and cost-effectiveness fall within the range of per capita costs of other malaria control strategies (White and others 2011), but they are more expensive than school-based deworming programs. However, the simultaneous delivery by teachers of both IPCs and deworming as part of an integrated school health package may yield economies of scope and increase cost-effectiveness. More studies are required on the cost-effectiveness of malaria control in schoolchildren.

It is also important to consider the effect of other ongoing malaria control measures because they will reduce malaria transmission in the wider community. In this situation, mathematical models of malaria can provide insight because they can simultaneously model multiple interventions and take into account the dynamics of malaria transmission, especially the mass effects of community interventions. For example, modeling of the cost-effectiveness of community-wide IST highlighted its value in medium-high transmission settings among school-age children, but only if it was continued indefinitely (Crowell and others 2013). The combined use of mathematical modeling and economic evaluation can help identify which interventions should be targeted specifically toward school-age children and which interventions should be delivered as part of community-wide malaria control.

CONCLUSIONS

On the basis of the available data, some recommendations can be made about the management of malaria in school-age children (box 14.1), but much more needs to be learned about the effectiveness of different approaches (box 14.2).

Better data are needed on the burden of malaria in school-age children. A standardized approach to data collection would improve the ability to monitor progress in this at-risk group. Systems to capture episodes of clinical and fatal malaria in school-age children do not need to be school based, but they should summarize data for this specific risk group.

The potential of serological tests to help in evaluating the burden of malaria in school-age children needs to be studied further. Improved information on the extent of the burden of malaria and on the socioeconomic consequences of malaria in this age group would enhance awareness at multiple levels.

- **Global level**: Policy makers and multilateral funding organizations would pay more attention to this issue.
- **National level**: Interactions among education, health, and potentially other sectors would be catalyzed.

> **Box 14.1**
>
> **Policy Recommendations for the Control of Malaria in School-Age Children**
>
> National malaria control programs need to pay increasing attention to the problem of malaria in school-age children, as the proportion of cases of malaria in older children increases. Education about causes of malaria; its clinical features; and ways of diagnosing, treating, and preventing the infection should be an integral part of the curriculum of all schools in areas where the school-age population is at risk of malaria infection. All school-age children in high-transmission areas need to sleep under insecticide-treated bednets. School-age children who develop clinical malaria need to be able to recognize the nature of their illness and have easy and rapid access to reliable diagnosis and effective treatment, either in their schools or at nearby health facilities.

- **Local and individual levels**: Families that include schoolchildren would be better able to take the necessary steps to prevent and treat malaria.

Operational research is needed to determine how best to raise awareness of the importance of malaria, how to manage it, and how to improve the use of established control measures in this group. Improving the malaria-relevant content of school curricula will help children help themselves and equip them with the understanding needed to accept new approaches to the control of malaria, such as the value of blood testing for parasitological diagnosis to guide appropriate treatment. School-age children can become an important route for disseminating information on malaria control to the rest of the family.

Further studies are needed to understand the potential role of medications in preventing malaria in school-age children. Chemoprophylaxis, SMC, IPCs, and IST may all be beneficial, but it is not clear yet in which settings each might be most effective or cost-effective. Some chemoprevention is likely to be useful in high transmission settings. The cost-effectiveness of chemoprevention is likely to be lower in low transmission settings, where most recipients are unlikely to have malaria. However, the transmission threshold at which to introduce, or withdraw, chemoprevention will only become clear through the modeling of empirical data. The optimal characteristics of drugs for SMC, IPCs, and IST are likely to include low cost, a very good safety profile, exceptional tolerability, long

---

Box 14.2

Key Research Priorities for Malaria in School-Age Children

Epidemiology

- Acquisition of better knowledge of the magnitude and features of malaria in school-age children, especially in areas in which the overall incidence of malaria is declining

Pathogenesis

- Investigation both of the importance of malaria as a cause of anemia in school-age children and of how anemia is caused by the malaria parasite
- Investigation of the mechanisms by which severe, uncomplicated, and asymptomatic malaria impair cognition

Treatment

- Investigation of how malaria can be diagnosed using a rapid diagnostic test and treated effectively by school staff in different settings

Prevention

- Exploration of ways to improve coverage with insecticide-treated bednets among school-age children
- Investigation of the comparative advantages and cost-effectiveness of screening and treatment programs and of intermittent preventive treatment in the prevention of malaria in school-age children in high-risk areas, and investigation of the circumstances that favor either approach
- Exploration of the potential for vaccination to prevent malaria in school-age children

Economic and social consequences

- Acquisition of better knowledge of the socioeconomic consequences of malaria in school-age children, and the costs and benefits of individual malaria control measures in this age group

---

half-life, and single-dose treatment. The development of a rigorous target product profile would help guide the development of drugs suitable for use in the prevention of malaria in school-age children. The potential of IST programs to identify and help not only individuals but also communities at elevated risk of malaria warrants further exploration.

More effective control of malaria is only one part of the drive to improve the health and potential of school-age children. More work is needed to determine how and when to integrate malaria control strategies with other school-based programs at the local and national levels.

ANNEX

The annex to this chapter is as follows. It is available at http://www.dcp-3.org/CAHD.

- Annex 14A. Estimates of Parasitemia and Clinical Disease among School-Aged Children in Africa

NOTES

Portions of this chapter were previously published:

- Nankabirwa J., S. J. Brooker, S. E. Clarke, D. Fernando, C. W. Gitonga, D. Schellenberg, and B. Greenwood. 2014.

"Malaria in school-age children in Africa: an increasing important challenge." Trop med Int Health, 19:1294-1309. © COPYRIGHT OWNER The Authors. Licensed under Creative Commons Attribution (CC BY 4.0) available at: https://creativecommons.org/licenses/by/4.0/.

World Bank Income Classifications as of July 2014 are as follows, based on estimates of gross national income (GNI) per capita for 2013:

- Low-income countries (LICs) = US$1,045 or less
- Middle-income countries (MICs) are subdivided:
  a) lower-middle-income = US$1,046–US$4,125
  b) upper-middle-income (UMICs) = US$4,126–US$12,745
- High-income countries (HICs) = US$12,746 or more

REFERENCES

Adjuik, M., T. Smith, S. Clark, J. Todd, A. Garrib, and others. 2006. "Cause-Specific Mortality Rates in Sub-Saharan Africa and Bangladesh." *Bulletin of the World Health Organization* 84 (3): 181–88.

Afenyadu, G. Y., I. A. Agyepong, G. Barnish, and S. Adjei. 2005. "Improving Access to Early Treatment of Malaria: A Trial with Primary School Teachers as Care Providers." *Tropical Medicine and International Health* 10 (10): 1065–72.

Ansah, E. K., S. Narh-Bana, H. Affran-Bonful, C. Bart-Plange, B. Cundill, and others. 2015. "The Impact of Providing

Rapid Diagnostic Malaria Tests on Fever Management in the Private Retail Sector in Ghana: A Cluster Randomized Trial." *BMJ* 350: h1019.

Atieli, H. E., G. Zhou, Y. Afrane, M. C. Lee, I. Mwanzo, and others. 2011. "Insecticide-Treated Net (ITN) Ownership, Usage, and Malaria Transmission in the Highlands of Western Kenya." *Parasites and Vectors* 4: 113.

Barger, B., H. Maiga, O. B. Traore, M. Tekete, I. Tembine, and others. 2009. "Intermittent Preventive Treatment Using Artemisinin-Based Combination Therapy Reduces Malaria Morbidity among School-Aged Children in Mali." *Tropical Medicine and International Health* 14 (7): 784–91.

Bin Mohanna, M. A., A. S. Bin Ghouth, and Y. A. Rajaa. 2007. "Malaria Signs and Infection Rate among Asymptomatic Schoolchildren in Hajr Valley, Yemen." *Eastern Mediterranean Health Journal* 13 (1): 35–40.

Boivin, M. J., M. J. Gladstone, M. Vokhiwa, G. L. Birbeck, J. G. Magen, and others. 2011. "Development Outcomes in Malawian Children with Retinopathy-Positive Cerebral Malaria." *Tropical Medicine and International Health* 16 (3): 263–71.

Bojang, K. A., F. Olodude, M. Pinder, O. Ofori-Anyinam, L. Vigneron, and others. 2005. "Safety and Immunogenicity of RTS,S/AS02A Candidate Malaria Vaccine in Gambian Children." *Vaccine* 23 (32): 4148–57.

Brooker, S., H. Guyatt, J. Omumbo, R. Shretta, L. Drake, and J. Ouma. 2000. "Situation Analysis of Malaria in School-Aged Children in Kenya—What Can Be Done?" *Parasitology Today* 16 (5): 183–86.

Bundy, D. A. P., S. Lwin, J. S. Osika, J. McLaughlin, and C. O. Pannenborg. 2000. "What Should Schools Do about Malaria?" *Parasitology Today* 16 (5): 181–82.

Bundy, D. A. P., L. Appleby, M. Bradley, K. Croke, T. D. Hollingsworth, and others. 2017. "Mass Deworming Programs in Middle Childhood and Adolescence." In *Disease Control Priorities* (third edition): Volume 8, *Child and Adolescent Health and Development*, edited by D. A. P. Bundy, N. de Silva, S. E. Horton, D. T. Jamison, and G. C. Patton. Washington, DC: World Bank.

Bundy, D. A. P., N. de Silva, S. Horton, G.C. Patton, L. Schultz, and D. T. Jamison. 2017. "Child and Adolescent Health and Development: Realizing Neglected Potential." In *Disease Control Priorities* (third edition): Volume 8, *Child and Adolescent Health and Development*, edited by D. A. P. Bundy, N. de Silva, S. Horton, D. T. Jamison, and G. C. Patton. Washington, DC: World Bank.

Carneiro, I., A. Roca-Feltrer, J. T. Griffin, L. Smith, M. Tanner, and others. 2010. "Age-Patterns of Malaria Vary with Severity, Transmission Intensity and Seasonality in Sub-Saharan Africa: A Systematic Review and Pooled Analysis." *PLoS One* 5 (2): e8988.

Carter, J. A., J. A. Lees, J. K. Gona, G. Murira, K. Rimba, and others. 2006. "Severe *falciparum* Malaria and Acquired Childhood Language Disorder." *Developmental Medicine and Child Neurology* 48 (1): 51–57.

Carter, J. A., V. Mung'ala-Odera, B. G. Neville, G. Murira, N. Mturi, and others. 2005. "Persistent Neurocognitive Impairments Associated with Severe *falciparum* Malaria in Kenyan Children." *Journal of Neurology, Neurosurgery and Psychiatry* 76 (4): 476–81.

Carter, J. A., A. J. Ross, B. G. Neville, E. Obiero, K. Katana, and others. 2005. "Developmental Impairments Following Severe *falciparum* Malaria in Children." *Tropical Medicine and International Health* 10 (1): 3–10.

Ceesay, S. J., C. Casals-Pascual, J. Erskine, S. E. Anya, N. O. Duah, and others. 2008. "Changes in Malaria Indices between 1999 and 2007 in The Gambia: A Retrospective Analysis." *The Lancet* 372 (9649): 1545–54.

Clarke, S. E., S. Brooker, J. K. Njagi, B. Estembale, E. Muchini, and others. 2004. "Malaria Morbidity among School Children Living in Two Areas of Contrasting Transmission in Western Kenya." *American Journal of Tropical Medicine and Hygiene* 71 (6): 732–38.

Clarke, S. E., M. C. Jukes, J. K. Njagi, L. Khasakhala, B. Cundill, and others. 2008. "Effect of Intermittent Preventive Treatment of Malaria on Health and Education in Schoolchildren: A Cluster-Randomised, Double-Blind, Placebo-Controlled Trial." *The Lancet* 372 (9644): 127–38.

Clarke, S., S. Rouhani, S. Diarra, M. Bamadio, R. Jones, and others. 2013. "The Impact of Intermittent Parasite Clearance on Malaria, Anaemia, and Cognition in Schoolchildren: New Evidence from an Area of Highly Seasonal Transmission." *Tropical Medicine and International Health* 18 (Suppl 1): 64.

Conteh, L., B. L. Sharp, E. Street, A. Barreto, and S. Konar. 2004. "The Cost and Cost-Effectiveness of Malaria Vector Control by Residual Insecticide House-Spraying in Southern Mozambique: A Rural and Urban Analysis." *Tropical Medicine and International Health* 9 (1): 125–32.

Crowell, V., O. J. Briët, D. Hardy, N. Chitnis, N. Maire, and others. 2013. "Modelling the Cost-Effectiveness of Mass Screening and Treatment for Reducing *Plasmodium falciparum* Malaria Burden." *Malaria Journal* 12: 4.

Dhingra, N., P. Jha, V. P. Sharma, A. A. Cohen, R. M. Jotkar, and others. 2010. "Adult and Child Malaria Mortality in India: A Nationally Representative Mortality Survey." *The Lancet* 376 (9754): 1768–74.

Dicko, A., S. Sagara, M. S. Sissoko, O. Guindo, A. L. Diallo, and others. 2008. "Impact of Intermittent Preventive Treatment with Sulphadoxine-Pyrimethamine Targeting the Transmission Season on the Incidence of Clinical Malaria in Children in Mali." *Malaria Journal* 7: 123.

Drake, L., M. Fernandes, E. Aurino, J. Kiamba, B. Giyose, and others. 2017. "School Feeding Programs in Middle Childhood and Adolescence." In *Disease Control Priorities* (third edition): Volume 8, *Child and Adolescent Health and Development*, edited by D. A. P. Bundy, N. de Silva, S. Horton, D. T. Jamison, and G. C. Patton. Washington, DC: World Bank.

Drake, T., G. Okello, K. Njagi, K. E. Halliday, M. C. Jukes, and others. 2011. "Cost Analysis of School-Based Intermittent Screening and Treatment of Malaria in Kenya." *Malaria Journal* 10: 273.

Draper, C. C. 1960. "Effect of Malaria Control on Haemoglobin Levels." *BMJ* 1 (5184): 1480–83.

Fernando, D., D. de Silva, R. Carter, K. N. Mendis, and R. Wickremasinghe. 2006. "A Randomized, Double-Blind, Placebo-Controlled, Clinical Trial of the Impact of Malaria Prevention on the Educational Attainment of School Children." *American Journal of Tropical Medicine and Hygiene* 74 (3): 386–93.

Fernando, D., D. de Silva, and R. Wickremasinghe. 2003. "Short-Term Impact of an Acute Attack of Malaria on Cognitive Performance of Schoolchildren Living in a Malaria-Endemic Area of Sri Lanka." *Transactions of the Royal Society of Tropical Medicine and Hygiene* 97 (6): 633–39.

Fernando, S. D., D. M. Gunawardena, M. R. S. S. Bandara, D. de Silva, R. Carter, and others. 2003. "The Impact of Repeated Malaria Attacks on the School Performance of Children." *American Journal of Tropical Medicine and Hygiene* 69 (6): 582–88.

Fernando, S. D., C. Rodrigo, and S. Rajapakse. 2010. "The 'Hidden' Burden of Malaria: Cognitive Impairment Following Infection." *Malaria Journal* 9: 366.

Fillinger, U., and S. W. Lindsay. 2011. "Larval Source Management for Malaria Control in Africa: Myths and Reality." *Malaria Journal* 10: 353.

Gething, P. W., A. P. Patil, D. L. Smith, C. A. Guerra, I. R. Elyazar, and others. 2011. "A New World Malaria Map: *Plasmodium falciparum* Endemicity in 2010." *Malaria Journal* 10: 378.

Gitonga, C. W., T. Edwards, P. N. Karanja, A. M. Noor, R. W. Snow, and S. J. Brooker. 2012. "*Plasmodium* Infection, Anaemia and Mosquito Net Use among School Children across Different Settings in Kenya." *Tropical Medicine and International Health* 17 (7): 858–70.

Greenwood, B. M., A. M. Greenwood, A. K. Bradley, R. W. Snow, P. Byass, and others. 1988. "A Comparison of Two Strategies for Control of Malaria within a Primary Health Care Programme in The Gambia." *The Lancet* 1 (8595): 1121–27.

Halliday, K. E., G. Okello, E. L. Turner, K. Njaqi, C. Mcharo, and others. 2014. "Impact of Intermittent Screening and Treatment for Malaria among Schoolchildren in Kenya: A Cluster Randomised Trial." *PLoS Medicine* 11: e1001594.

John, C. C., P. Bangirana, J. Byarugaba, R. O. Opoka, R. Idro, and others. 2008. "Cerebral Malaria in Children Is Associated with Long-Term Cognitive Impairment." *Pediatrics* 122 (1): 92–99.

Jukes, M. C., M. Pinder, E. L. Grigorenko, H. B. Smith, G. Walraven, and others. 2006. "Long-Term Impact of Malaria Chemoprophylaxis on Cognitive Abilities and Educational Attainment: Follow-up of a Controlled Trial." *PLoS Clinical Trials* 1: e19.

Kihara, M., J. A. Carter, and C. R. J. C. Newton. 2006. "The Effect of *Plasmodium falciparum* on Cognition: A Systematic Review." *Tropical Medicine and International Health* 11 (4): 386–97.

Leenstra, T., P. A. Phillips-Howard, S. K. Kariuki, W. A. Hawley, J. A. Alaii, and others. 2003. "Permethrin-Treated Bed Nets in the Prevention of Malaria and Anemia in Adolescent Schoolgirls in Western Kenya." *American Journal of Tropical Medicine and Hygiene* 68 (Suppl 4): 86–93.

Lengeler, C. 2004. "Insecticide-Treated Bed Nets and Curtains for Preventing Malaria." *Cochrane Database of Systematic Reviews* 3: CD000363.

Lim, S. S., N. Fullman, A. Stokes, N. Ravishankar, F. Masiye, and others. 2011. "Net Benefits: A Multicountry Analysis of Observational Data Examining Associations between Insecticide-Treated Mosquito Nets and Health Outcomes." *PLoS Medicine* 8: e1001091.

Luxemburger, C., W. A. Perea, G. Delmas, C. Pruja, B. Pecoul, and A. Moren. 1994. "Permethrin-Impregnated Bed Nets for Prevention of Malaria in Schoolchildren on the Thai-Burmese Border." *Transactions of the Royal Society of Tropical Medicine and Hygiene* 88 (2): 155–59.

Mathanga, D. P., K. E. Halliday, M. Verney, A. Bauleni, J. Sande, and others. 2015. "The High Burden of Malaria among Primary Schoolchildren in Southern Malawi." *American Journal of Tropical Medicine and Hygiene* 93 (4): 779–89.

Meremikwu, M. M., S. Donegan, and E. Esu. 2008. "Chemoprophylaxis and Intermittent Treatment for Preventing Malaria in Children." *Cochrane Database of Systematic Reviews* 2: CD003756.

Murray, C. J., L. C. Rosenfeld, S. S. Lim, K. G. Andrews, K. J. Foreman, and others. 2012. "Global Malaria Mortality between 1980 and 2010: A Systematic Analysis." *The Lancet* 379 (9814): 413–31.

Nankabirwa, J., S. J. Brooker, S. E. Clarke, D. Fernando, C. W. Gitonga, and others. 2014. "Malaria in School-Age Children in Africa: An Increasingly Important Challenge." *Tropical Medicine and International Health* 19 (11): 1294–309.

Nankabirwa, J., B. Cundill, S. Clarke, N. Kabatereine, P. J. Rosenthal, and others. 2010. "Efficacy, Safety, and Tolerability of Three Regimes for Prevention of Malaria: A Randomized, Placebo-Controlled Trial in Ugandan Schoolchildren." *PLoS One* 5: e13438.

Nankabirwa, J. I, B. Wandera, P. Amuge, N. Kiwanuka, G. Dorsey, and others. 2014. "Impact of Intermittent Preventive Treatment with Dihydroartemisinin-Piperaquine on Malaria in Ugandan Schoolchildren: A Randomized, Placebo-Controlled Trial." *Clinical Infectious Diseases* 58 (10): 1404–12.

Nevill, C. G., W. M. Watkins, J. Y. Carter, and C. G. Munafu. 1988. "Comparison of Mosquito Nets, Proguanil Hydrochloride, and Placebo to Prevent Malaria." *BMJ* 297 (6645): 401–3.

Nonaka, D., M. Jimba, T. Mizoue, J. Kobayashi, J. Yasuoka, and others. 2012. "Content Analysis of Primary and Secondary School Textbooks Regarding Malaria Control: A Multi-Country Study." *PLoS One* 7: e36629.

Noor, A. M., D. K. Kinyoki, C. W. Mundia, C. W. Kabaria, J. W. Mutua, and others. 2014. "The Changing Risk of *Plasmodium falciparum* Malaria Infection in Africa: 2000–10: A Spatial and Temporal Analysis of Transmission Intensity." *The Lancet* 383 (9930): 1739–47.

Noor, A. M., V. C. Kirui, S. J. Brooker, and R. W. Snow. 2009. "The Use of Insecticide Treated Nets by Age:

Implications for Universal Coverage in Africa." *BMC Public Health* 9: 369.

Noor, A. M., G. Moloney, M. Borle, G. W. Fegan, T. Shewchuk, and others. 2008. "The Use of Mosquito Nets and the Prevalence of *Plasmodium falciparum* Infection in Rural South Central Somalia." *PLoS One* 3: e2081.

Ojukwu, J. U., J. U. Okebe, D. Yahav, and M. Paul. 2009. "Oral Iron Supplementation for Preventing or Treating Anaemia among Children in Malaria-Endemic Areas." *Cochrane Database of Systematic Reviews* 3: CD006589.

O'Meara, W. P., P. Bejon, T. W. Mwangi, E. A. Okiro, N. Peshu, and others. 2008. "Effect of a Fall in Malaria Transmission on Morbidity and Mortality in Kilifi, Kenya." *The Lancet* 372 (9649): 1555–62.

O'Meara, W. P., J. N. Mangeni, R. Steketee, and B. Greenwood. 2010. "Changes in the Burden of Malaria in Sub-Saharan Africa." *Lancet Infectious Diseases* 10 (8): 545–55.

Pasha, O., J. Del Rosso, M. Mukaka, and D. Marsh. 2003. "The Effect of Providing Fansidar (Sulfadoxine-Pyrimethamine) in Schools on Mortality in School-Age Children in Malawi." *The Lancet* 361 (9357): 577–78.

Pluess, B., F. C. Tanser, C. Lengeler, and B. L. Sharp. 2010. "Indoor Residual Spraying for Preventing Malaria." *Cochrane Database of Systematic Reviews* 4: CD006657.

Prinsens Geerligs, P. D., B. J. Brabin, and T. A. Eggelete. 2003. "Analysis of the Effects of Malaria Chemoprophylaxis in Children on Haematological Responses, Morbidity and Mortality." *Bulletin of the World Health Organization* 81: 205–16.

Pullan, R. L., H. Bukirwa, S. G. Staedke, R. W. Snow, and S. Brooker. 2010. "*Plasmodium* Infection and Its Risk Factors in Eastern Uganda." *Malaria Journal* 9: 2.

Raiten, D. J., S. Namasté, and B. Brabin. 2011. "Considerations for the Safe and Effective Use of Iron Interventions in Areas of Malaria Burden—Executive Summary." *International Journal of Vitamin and Nutritional Research* 81 (1): 57–71.

Roca-Feltrer, A., I. Carneiro, L. Smith, J. R. Schellenberg, B. Greenwood, and others. 2010. "The Age Patterns of Severe Malaria Syndromes in Sub-Saharan Africa across a Range of Transmission Intensities and Seasonality Settings." *Malaria Journal* 9: 282.

Rohner, F., M. B. Zimmermann, R. J. Amon, P. Vounatsou, A. B. Tschannen, and others. 2010. "In a Randomized Controlled Trial of Iron Fortification, Anthelmintic Treatment, and Intermittent Preventive Treatment of Malaria for Anemia Control in Ivorian Children, Only Anthelmintic Treatment Shows Modest Benefit." *Journal of Nutrition* 140 (3): 635–41.

RTS,S Clinical Trials Partnership. 2015. "Efficacy and Safety of RTS,S/AS01 Malaria Vaccine with or without a Booster Dose in Infants and Children in Africa: Final Results of a Phase 3, Individually Randomised, Controlled Trial." *The Lancet* 386 (9988): 31–45.

Schwartz, L., G. V. Brown, B. Genton, and V. S. Moorthy. 2012. "A Review of Malaria Vaccine Clinical Projects Based on the WHO Rainbow Table." *Malaria Journal* 11: 11.

Snow, R. W., J. A. Omumbo, B. Lowe, C. S. Molyneux, J.-O. Obiero, and others. 1997. "Relation between Severe Malaria Morbidity in Children and Level of *Plasmodium falciparum* Transmission in Africa." *The Lancet* 349 (9066): 1650–54.

Stephenson, L. S., M. C. Latham, K. M. Kurz, S. N. Kinoti, M. L. Oduori, and others. 1985. "Relationships of *Schistosoma hematobium*, Hookworm and Malarial Infections and Metrifonate Treatment to Hemoglobin Level in Kenyan School Children." *American Journal of Tropical Medicine and Hygiene* 34 (3): 519–28.

Tchinda, V. H., A. Socpa, A. A. Keundo, F. Zeukeng, C. T. Seumen, and others. 2012. "Factors Associated to Bed Net Use in Cameroon: A Retrospective Study in Mfou Health District in the Centre Region." *Pan African Medical Journal* 12: 112.

Temperley, M., D. H. Mueller, J. K. Njagi, W. Akhwale, S. E. Clarke, and others. 2008. "Costs and Cost-Effectiveness of Delivering Intermittent Preventive Treatment through Schools in Western Kenya." *Malaria Journal* 7: 196.

Thuilliez, J., M. S. Sissoko, O. B. Toure, P. Kamate, J. C. Berthélemy, and O. K. Doumbo. 2010. "Malaria and Primary Education in Mali: A Longitudinal Study in the Viallage of Donéguébougou." *Social Science and Medicine* 71 (2): 324–34.

Tine, R. C. K., B. Faye, C. T. Ndour, J. L. Ndiaye, M. Ndiaye, and others. 2011. "Impact of Combining Intermittent Preventive Treatment with Home Management of Malaria in Children Less than 10 Years in a Rural Area of Senegal: A Cluster Randomized Trial." *Malaria Journal* 10: 358.

Tine, R. C. K., C. T. Ndour, B. Faye, M. Cairns, K. Sylla, and others. 2014. "Feasibility, Safety and Effectiveness of Combining Home Based Malaria Management and Seasonal Malaria Chemoprevention in Children Less than 10 Years in Senegal: A Cluster-Randomised Trial." *Transactions of the Royal Society of Tropical Medicine and Hygiene* 108 (1): 13–21.

Tiono, A. B., A. Ouédraogo, B. Ogutu, A. Diarra, S. Coulibaly, and A. Gansané. 2013. "A Controlled, Parallel, Cluster-Randomised Trial of Community-Wide Screening and Treatment of Asymptomatic Carriers of *Plasmodium falciparum* in Burkina Faso." *Malaria Journal* 12: 79.

Tusting, L. S., J. Thwing, D. Sinclair, U. Fillinger, J. Gimnig, and others. 2013. "Mosquito Larval Source Management for Controlling Malaria." *Cochrane Database of Systematic Reviews* 8: CD008923. doi:10.1002/14651858.

Vitor-Silva, S., R. C. Reyes-Lecca, T. R. A. Pinheiro, and M. V. G. Lacerda. 2009. "Malaria Is Associated with Poor School Performance in an Endemic Area of the Brazilian Amazon." *Malaria Journal* 8: 230.

Walldorf, J. A., L. M. Cohee, J. E. Coalson, A. Bauleni, K. Nkanaunena, and others. 2015. "School-Age Children Are a Reservoir of Malaria Infection in Malawi." *PLoS One* 10: e0134061.

White, M. T., L. Conteh, R. Cibulskis, and A. C. Ghani. 2011. "Costs and Cost-Effectiveness of Malaria Control Intervention: A Systematic Review." *Malaria Journal* 10: 337.

Wilson, A. L. on behalf of the IPTc Taskforce. 2011. "A Systematic Review and Meta-Analysis of the Efficacy and Safety of Intermittent Preventive Treatment of Malaria in Children (IPTc)." *PLoS One* 6: e16976.

Witek-McManus, S., D. P. Mathanga, M. Verney, A. Mtali, D. Ali, and others. 2015. "Design and Implementation of a Training Programme for School Teachers in the Use of Malaria Rapid Diagnostic Tests as Part of a Basic First Aid Kit in Southern Malawi." *BMC Public Health* 15: 904.

WHO (World Health Organization) 2015. *Guidelines for the Treatment of Malaria*. 3rd ed. Geneva: WHO.

Zhou, G., A. K. Githeko, N. Minakawa, and G. Yan. 2010. "Community-Wide Benefits of Targeted Indoor Residual Spray for Malaria Control in the Western Kenya Highland." *Malaria Journal* 9: 67.

Zuilkowski, S. S., and M. C. H. Jukes. 2014. "Early Childhood Malaria Prevention and Children's Patterns of School Leaving in The Gambia." *British Journal of Educational Psychology* 84: 483–501.

School-Based Delivery of Vaccines to 5- to 19-Year Olds

D. Scott LaMontagne, Tania Cernuschi, Ahmadu Yakubu,
Paul Bloem, Deborah Watson-Jones, and Jane J. Kim

INTRODUCTION

Significant progress has been achieved in the social, economic, educational, and health status of many populations. Compared with previous generations, the educational status of those born after 1990 has improved, as reflected in higher rates of school enrollment, especially in low- and middle-income countries (LMICs) (UNESCO 2014). Countries have started to expand their immunization programs beyond infants to young children, adolescents, and adults, with the goal of preventing, controlling, and where possible, eliminating vaccine-preventable diseases (WHO 2013a).

The combination of increased school attendance and expanded target populations for vaccines has created a rich opportunity for exploring vaccine delivery in schools (annex 15A, figure 15A.1). Meningitis, measles, hepatitis B, tetanus toxoid (TT), and human papillomavirus (HPV) are examples of vaccines offered in schools, either as routine primary or booster vaccinations or through campaigns for catch-up strategies or disease control (Grabowsky and others 2005; Mackroth and others 2010; WHO 2012a). These vaccines have demonstrated efficacy in preventing significant morbidity and mortality among school-age children, adolescents, and adults (Mehlhorn, Balcer, and Sucher 2006; WHO 2009). Understanding country experiences with the operational and logistical factors that have enabled successful delivery of vaccines through school-based programs—and the challenges encountered—can provide salient lessons for other countries, irrespective of income status. This chapter highlights the promise of school-based delivery of vaccines in LMICs, using the experience of TT and HPV vaccine delivery as examples. Definitions of age groupings and age-specific terminology used in this volume can be found in chapter 1 (Bundy and others 2017).

TETANUS AND HPV EPIDEMIOLOGY AND PREVENTION

Tetanus

Tetanus is caused by the bacterium *Clostridium tetani*, the spores of which are widespread in the environment (Black, Huber, and Curlin 1980). The bacterium is introduced into umbilical stump tissue during unclean delivery or unclean cord care practices, or occasionally at the site of traditional surgery and deep penetrating wounds. The disease is caused by the action of a neurotoxin produced by the bacteria when they grow in the absence of oxygen. Tetanus is characterized by muscle spasms, initially in the jaw. As the disease progresses, mild stimuli may trigger generalized tetanic seizure-like activity, which contributes to serious complications and eventually to death unless supportive treatment is given (Black, Huber, and Curlin 1980).

Vaccines containing TT are the primary prevention strategy against infection and have been in use

Corresponding author: D. Scott LaMontagne, PATH, Seattle, WA, United States; slamontagne@path.org.

for decades. Both the efficacy and the effectiveness of the TT vaccine are well documented (Newell and others 1971). TT vaccines, particularly the widespread expansion of maternal tetanus immunization services, have been largely responsible for the marked reduction in neonatal tetanus deaths, from 787,000 deaths in 1988 to 49,000 by 2013 (Liu and others 2015; Vandelaer and others 2003).

According to the World Health Organization (WHO), effective and full immunization against the tetanus infection requires five doses between infancy and adolescence (WHO 2006). An additional dose during the first pregnancy will protect a woman and her fetus throughout this and future pregnancies, provided that she has received all previous recommended doses (Rahman and others 1982). Countries have been using TT vaccines, including school-based vaccination, as a main strategy to eliminate maternal and neonatal tetanus and to maintain elimination status. The success of such strategies has been demonstrated in Tanzania (WHO 2013c).

Cervical Cancer

Cervical cancer is caused by several types of HPV (zur Hausen 1977). Two types, 16 and 18, account for approximately 70 percent of all cases (Denny and others 2015; Ferlay and others 2010). This virus is sexually transmitted, and most people are exposed within the first few years of engaging in sexual relations (Moscicki 2007). If the infection persists long term, women can develop precancerous lesions; if left untreated, these lesions can develop into cervical cancer (zur Hausen 1977). The progression from infection to disease takes, on average, 20 years. Globally, there are more than 528,000 new cases of cervical cancer and more than 266,000 deaths each year among women; more than 85 percent of the disease burden occurs in LMICs (Ferlay and others 2010).

Cervical cancer can be prevented through either primary prevention (vaccination) or secondary prevention (screening and treatment) (Denny and others 2015). Vaccines against HPV are effective when administered to individuals not yet exposed to HPV vaccine types, which for most people is before sexual debut (Denny and others 2015). Screening through cervical smears (Papanicolaou or Pap smears), visual inspection with acetic acid, or HPV DNA (deoxyribonucleic acid)-based testing is effective in detecting precancerous lesions that can be treated. Accordingly, HPV vaccination is recommended for girls ages 9–13 years (WHO 2014b), and screening is recommended for adult women generally beginning at age 25 or 30 years to age 49 years (Denny and others 2015).

Prevention

Both TT and HPV vaccinations have been demonstrated to be cost-effective in schools (Goldie and others 2008; Griffiths and others 2004). Targeting children at the beginning and end of primary school for booster doses of TT vaccines and targeting young adolescents before completing primary school for HPV vaccines have been two successful delivery strategies (LaMontagne and others 2011; Steinglass 1998). Young adolescents ages 9–11 years produce higher levels of antibodies to HPV vaccines, which are maintained at higher levels over time, compared with older adolescents (Block and others 2006). Additionally, delivering HPV vaccines at this young age generally ensures that girls receive the vaccine before sexual exposure to HPV (Moscicki 2007; WHO 2014b).

Since adolescents do not regularly attend health facilities, schools may offer advantages for reaching this population (Mackroth and others 2010). Increasingly high levels of primary school enrollment and attendance throughout LMICs have created an opportunity to identify and efficiently reach a large proportion of the population eligible for school-based vaccination (Grabowsky and others 2005; UNESCO 2014). Schools can also be used to leverage additional services or interventions (Broutet and others 2013) that might be needed by the age groups receiving TT or HPV vaccine, such as antihelmintics for deworming, vision screening, and bednet distribution (Broutet and others 2013).

PROGRAM DESIGN FOR SCHOOL-BASED VACCINE DELIVERY OF TT AND HPV VACCINES

TT Vaccine Delivery Strategies

The childhood tetanus immunization schedule recommended by the WHO includes five doses:

- Primary series of three doses of DTP (diphtheria/tetanus/pertussis) or other tetanus-containing vaccine, such as DTwP (diphtheria/tetanus/whole pertussis) or DTaP/TDaP (diphtheria/tetanus/acellular pertussis) given before age one year
- Booster dose of a TT vaccine at ages four to seven years
- Second booster dose between ages 12 and 15 years (WHO 2006).

Resources available through existing school health services are used to give the TT booster doses in adolescence while ensuring that out-of-school children are also served through routine activities of national immunization programs (WHO 2008b).

Many low- and lower-middle-income countries implement some school-based vaccination (annex 15A, table 15A.1), targeting the school grades where the largest proportion of children are found. Several countries have conducted household and school-based surveys to tabulate age-by-grade distributions to determine which grade is most appropriate for capturing the largest proportion of children—ages 4–7 years or ages 12–15 years. Indonesia found that most children ages 6–9 years are enrolled in grades one to three (Kim-Farley and others 1987). Nepal and Tunisia determined that entry in primary school was the optimal time to provide TT vaccination (Vandelaer, Partridge, and Suvedi 2009; WHO 2008c).

An email survey was sent to all 192 WHO member countries in 2008 (WHO-UNICEF 2009). Of the 143 countries responding, 61 countries (43 percent) reported conducting some school-based immunization. Among these 61 countries, the TT-containing vaccine was one of the interventions given; 41 countries (67 percent) start from primary school grade 1, and 54 percent target ages 9–13 years. Data from the 2012 WHO-UNICEF Expanded Programme on Immunization Joint Reporting Form indicate that, among 86 low- and lower-middle-income countries, 21 countries (24 percent) administer TT-containing vaccines; 10 of these countries deliver the vaccine in grade 1, and 16 deliver TT vaccines through grade 6 (on average, capturing children ages 12–15 years) (WHO-UNICEF 2013). The relatively low levels of school vaccination in these countries, combined with increasing school enrollment, particularly among girls, suggests an untapped opportunity to increase vaccination coverage through school-based programs.

Information, education, and communication components are essential in ensuring the success of school-based TT vaccination in LMICs. Parents and community leaders need to know why the children are being vaccinated; have resources for further information, as well as know when the vaccination activities will take place; and understand what to do if their children miss the vaccine. To prevent rumors that TT vaccination is connected to fertility control and to address the immunity gap that results in lack of a second opportunity for TT vaccination in adolescent boys and adult men, both boys and girls are often vaccinated. Information on the protection conferred by the vaccine against tetanus caused by injuries during sports, planting, and other activities helps achieve community acceptance (Steinglass 1998). The active engagement, collaboration, and training of the ministries of health and education on the requirements of the school-based TT vaccination are crucial (WHO 2008c).

HPV Vaccine Delivery Strategies

The WHO recommends that the HPV vaccine be given to girls between ages 9 and 13 years, including immuno-compromised individuals (WHO 2014b). As of early 2016, three HPV vaccines are available—a quadrivalent vaccine (Gardasil, Merck & Co.), a bivalent vaccine (Cervarix, GlaxoSmithKline), and a nonavalent vaccine (Gardasil9, Merck & Co.). Licensure recommendations vary by country; in general, Gardasil and Gardasil9 are registered for use in females ages 9–26 years in 130 and 39 countries, respectively. In some countries, these two HPV vaccines are also registered for use in males of the same age for the prevention of genital warts. Cervarix is generally registered for use in females ages 9–44 years in more than 120 countries; it is not registered for males because no clinical trial of the efficacy of this vaccine in males has been conducted.

Although all HPV vaccines were licensed for a three-dose schedule, the European Medicines Agency (EMA) (EMA 2013, 2014) and the WHO Strategic Advisory Group of Experts on Immunization recently concluded there was sufficient evidence for the bivalent and quadrivalent HPV vaccines to recommend a two-dose schedule for young immunocompetent adolescent girls up to age 14 years, with a minimum interval of six months between doses (WHO 2014c). As of early 2016, 46 countries had adopted the revised two-dose schedule, or schedules with two initial doses and a delayed third-dose booster after five years, for young immunocompetent adolescent girls in their national immunization programs (Brotherton and Bloem 2015; Institute of Social and Preventive Medicine 2014).

As of early 2016, HPV vaccination is part of the recommended national schedule in nearly 80 countries or territories, of which approximately 25 percent are low- or middle-income (comprising both lower-middle and upper-middle income) countries. As of June 2016, 89 countries and territories have HPV vaccination on a national schedule (map 15.1; annex 15A, table 15A.2). However, an additional 37 LMICs have piloted the introduction of the vaccine in one or more urban and rural districts, 20 of which are in Sub-Saharan Africa (annex 15A, table 15A.3).

Based on experiences with pilot demonstration programs, school-based vaccination is most often used as the primary delivery strategy, usually accompanied by a secondary strategy based in health centers to reach out-of-school and underserved girls (Ladner and others 2012; LaMontagne and others 2011; Paul and Fabio 2014; Watson-Jones and others 2012). Countries introducing HPV vaccines through schools seem to use grade- and age-based eligibility equally (Gallagher and others 2016; LaMontagne and others 2011; Paul and Fabio 2014).

Map 15.1 HPV National Vaccine Introduction Globally, June 2016

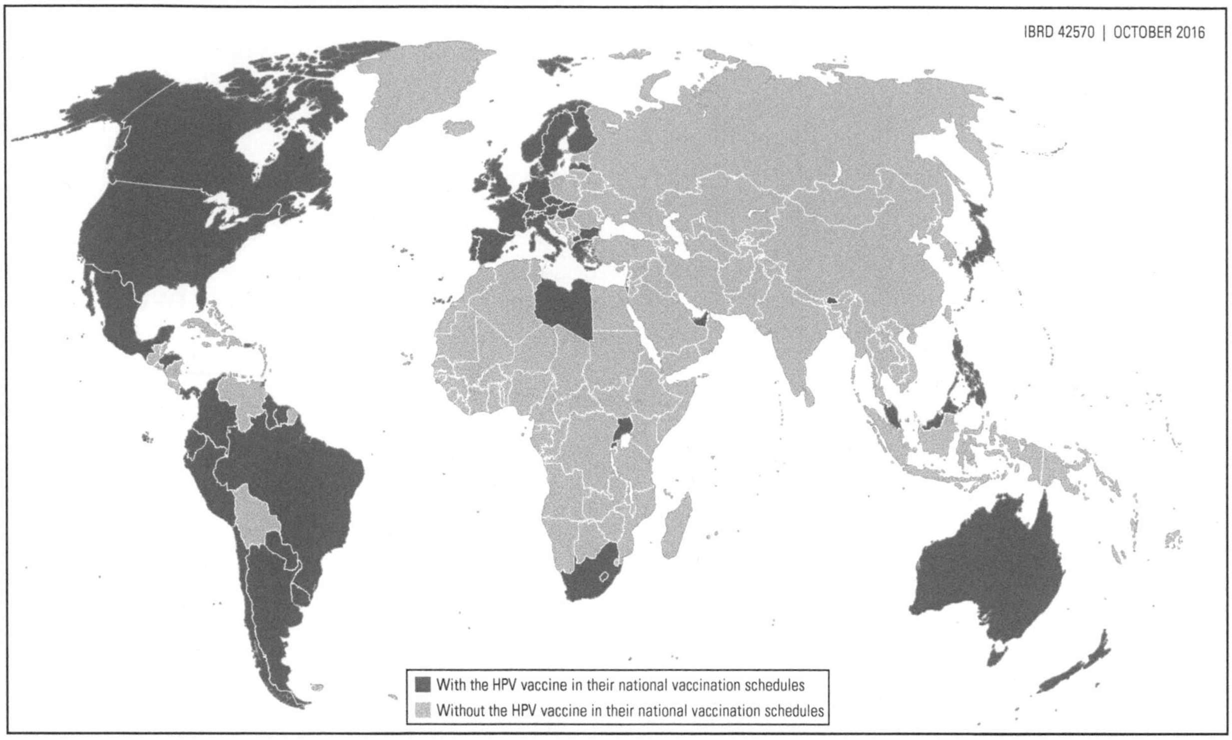

IBRD 42570 | OCTOBER 2016

■ With the HPV vaccine in their national vaccination schedules
▨ Without the HPV vaccine in their national vaccination schedules

Note: HPV = human papillomavirus.

Several elements make HPV vaccine delivery unique. These considerations may create operational challenges for implementation (WHO 2014a).

- There is often lack of awareness of cervical cancer and of HPV infection as a causal agent (Rama and others 2010).
- Unlike other immunization programs that target infants of both genders, HPV vaccination is targeted to girls ages 9–13 years (before sexual debut) (WHO 2014b).
- Because the recommended age group for HPV vaccination may not routinely attend health facilities, and visits by health workers to schools for vaccination may be one-time events, such as vaccination campaigns, delivery platforms and strategies used for HPV vaccine delivery may be new for LMICs (WHO 2012b).
- Consent procedures for HPV vaccines are not standardized; both opt-in and opt-out are used (Cover and others 2012; Moodley and others 2013; WHO 2014a).

HPV vaccination can be integrated with other health services for this underserved age group, which may enhance the efficiency and sustainability of vaccination programs (Broutet and others 2013; Mugisha and others 2015; Watson-Jones and others 2016). Some countries also use the opportunity to sensitize girls and women to the importance of adhering to the screening guidelines, the delivery of cervical cancer screening of adult women, or other child health programs (Wamai and others 2012).

HPV vaccination requires special attention to social mobilization and communication efforts to ensure acceptability and high coverage (Bingham, Drake, and LaMontagne 2009). In most low- and lower-middle-income countries, messages were disseminated through meetings in schools and communities, during home visits, and through written materials and radio announcements (Kabakama and others 2016; LaMontagne and others 2011). In Rwanda, Uganda, and Vietnam, teachers play an important role in communication efforts (Binagwaho and others 2012; Galagan and others 2013). The WHO encourages all countries to develop communication strategies with multisectoral stakeholders and engage communities at the start of planning the program (WHO 2013b). Among LMICs that have completed pilot delivery of HPV vaccine, all have chosen to focus messages on cervical cancer prevention and the importance of vaccination rather than to stress the sexual transmission of HPV because these messages have been proven to be the most important for parental acceptability (Bingham, Drake, and LaMontagne 2009; Kabakama and others 2016; LaMontagne and others 2011).

Some pilot programs followed extensive informed consent processes (Moodley and others 2013). In others, the government used the same consenting procedures applied to other vaccines, including those delivered to children up to age 17 years, principally through an opt-out or implied consent approach (LaMontagne and others 2011). Pending developments that could facilitate easier delivery of HPV vaccines to young adolescent populations include expanded in-country licensure for delivery to boys (Markowitz and others 2012), alternative dosing schedules for three-dose regimens (Esposito and others 2011; LaMontagne and others 2013), and the recent approval of two-dose schedules for immunocompetent adolescent girls younger than age 15 years (WHO 2014c). Moreover, opportunities for reduced procurement prices through Gavi, the Vaccine Alliance and the Pan American Health Organization Revolving Fund, as well as potential cost reductions through the pooled purchase for middle-income countries by the United Nations Children's Fund, are likely to increase the number of countries that will introduce HPV vaccines by 2020 (Gavi, the Vaccine Alliance 2016).

EVIDENCE OF EFFECTIVE SCHOOL-BASED DELIVERY OF HPV AND TT VACCINES

TT Vaccine

Although some country programs have added delivery of TT vaccines to those as young as age 10 years, documentation of the implementation method, successes, and challenges has been largely absent in the literature. Among the 27 low- and lower-middle-income countries administering TT-containing vaccines in schools, 19 have reported coverage data (WHO-UNICEF 2013). In Indonesia, consistently high coverage of more than 95 percent of children enrolled in schools has been reported (Kim-Farley and others 1987; WHO-UNICEF 2013). Sri Lanka monitors the proportion of schools reached for immunization in each province, and 92 percent of all schools were covered by 2005 (WHO 2008b). Data from the 2014 WHO-UNICEF Joint Reporting Form show nine additional countries (Afghanistan, the Arab Republic of Egypt, Honduras, Mongolia, Mozambique, Nepal, Sierra Leone, Tonga, and Vanuatu) reported coverage levels for TT-containing vaccines of more than 80 percent for the population targeted in schools between 2011 and 2013 (WHO-UNICEF 2014). However, the lack of adequate documentation of TT-containing vaccines in schools continues to be a major obstacle to meaningful conclusions about school-based delivery for this intervention. A summary of facilitators and barriers to TT-containing vaccine delivery in schools is provided in annex 15A, table 15A.4.

HPV Vaccine

Schools have been a primary delivery strategy for HPV vaccine in a number of LMICs (Gallagher and others 2016; Ladner and others 2012; LaMontagne and others 2011; Raesima and others 2015). The rising levels of primary school attendance in many LMICs has enhanced this delivery approach (UNESCO 2014). The vaccine is usually offered at specific times during the school year, and school-based delivery may be combined with outreach or health facility vaccine delivery. High three-dose coverage (75 percent to 100 percent) has been achieved in pilot studies and demonstration programs using school-based delivery strategies, which is similar to the coverage levels achieved in national programs that also used school-based delivery (Brotherton and Bloem 2015; Markowitz and others 2012; Sinka and others 2013). A systematic review of HPV vaccine delivery experiences in 47 LMICs reported coverage levels of 70 percent or greater in the vast majority of programs that used a school-based delivery component (Gallagher and others 2016). Differences in coverage between the previously recommended three-dose schedule and the revised two-dose schedule were not observed; however, only 10 countries had reported coverage data from two-dose delivery. Further information about the possible impact of fewer doses on feasibility of school-based HPV vaccine delivery will be available in future years as this schedule becomes established.

Countries implementing school-based programs need to decide whether to establish age- or grade-based eligibility. A demonstration project in Tanzania found significantly higher coverage with grade-based vaccination, compared with age-based vaccination, at slightly lower cost (Watson-Jones and others 2012). Bhutan has reported national coverage of more than 90 percent through school-based delivery (Dorji and others 2015). A summary of facilitators and barriers to HPV vaccine delivery in schools can be found in annex 15A, table 15A.5.

COSTS AND COST-EFFECTIVENESS OF SCHOOL-BASED TT AND HPV VACCINE DELIVERY

Consideration of the costs and cost-effectiveness of school-based vaccination programs are instrumental in decisions for national introduction and scale-up (WHO 2006, 2014b). Given the shortage of routine health services for adolescents (UNICEF 2007), the opportunities to leverage existing programs are limited (Broutet and others 2013; WHO 2008a). Accordingly, the incremental costs associated with implementation and delivery of TT and HPV vaccinations, both targeted to adolescents, are expected to be high relative to new childhood interventions. School-based delivery of vaccines provides an opportunity to access young adolescent populations who may not attend regular health services. To date, the empirical data on the added costs of school-based vaccination programs have been limited, with little to no coverage of TT vaccination (Griffiths and others 2004). However, several demonstration studies have emerged on the financial and economic costs of school-based HPV vaccination (Levin and others 2013; Levin and others 2014; Levin and others 2015).

Costs of HPV Vaccine Delivery

Several published studies have estimated the incremental costs of school-based HPV vaccine delivery in Bhutan, India, Peru, Tanzania, Uganda, and Vietnam, which are all LMICs (Levin and others 2015). Each of the analyses distinguished financial costs, reflecting actual expenditures, from economic costs, including the value of donated and shared resources, to more fully assess the opportunity costs of the HPV vaccination program. Results from three studies largely resulted in consistent estimates for economic and financial costs per HPV vaccine dose and per fully immunized girl (table 15.1; Levin and others 2013). In these studies, the incremental

financial cost ranged from US$1.65 to US$2.25 per dose and US$4.96 to US$7.49 per fully immunized girl for a three-dose vaccination schedule. The economic costs were higher, ranging from US$2.11 to US$4.62 per dose and US$6.37 to US$16.10 per fully immunized girl. A two-dose vaccine schedule would reduce both financial and economic costs per fully immunized girl, but start-up costs are expected to be similar. As hypothesized, these costs are higher than the delivery costs of other routine immunizations reported in LMICs, which have ranged between US$0.75 and US$1.40 per dose, depending upon vaccine, country, and year of implementation (Brenzel and others 2006).

Specific findings from the studies also suggested interesting trends in the cost of HPV vaccine delivery mechanisms. For example, Quentin and others (2012) found that HPV vaccine delivery in urban schools was cheaper than delivery in rural schools, mainly due to higher costs of procurement and transport to rural areas. Irrespective of location, grade-based delivery was less costly by roughly 30 percent than age-based delivery in schools because of higher coverage and number of eligible girls. Hutubessy and others (2012) found that the recurrent costs for delivering HPV vaccines in schools were higher than delivery in health facilities by US$1.65 for three doses per eligible girl (US$0.55 per dose). Similarly, Levin and others (2013) found that school-based delivery had higher economic costs than an integrated (school and health center) approach or delivery solely in a health center, mainly due to the additional personnel and transportation costs required to reach the schools.

Table 15.1 Financial and Economic Costs for School-Based HPV Vaccine Delivery Using a Three-Dose Schedule (Excluding Vaccine Cost), 2013

U.S. dollars

	Tanzania (Hutubessy and others 2012)	Tanzania (Quentin and others 2012)	Peru (Levin and others 2013)	Uganda (Levin and others 2013)	Vietnam (Levin and others 2013)
Program scale	Scaled-up national program	Scaled-up regional program	Demonstration project	Demonstration project	Demonstration project
Method of estimation	Projected (using WHO C4P tool)	Projected	Microcosting approach	Microcosting approach	Microcosting approach
Financial cost, per dose	2.2	2.3	2.2	2.2	1.7
Financial cost, per FIG	7.5	7.1	6.5	6.9	5.0
Economic cost, per dose	4.6	4.0	4.1	3.2	2.1
Economic cost, per FIG	16.1	12.7	12.4	10.4	6.4

Note: FIG = fully immunized girl for recommended three-dose schedules at the time of study; HPV = human papillomavirus; WHO C4P tool = World Health Organization Cervical Cancer Prevention and Control Costing tool. Methods for estimating costs differed across studies, except in Peru, Uganda, and Vietnam.

Main Contributors to Costs

Head-to-head comparison of the main cost contributors across all settings was precluded by differences in categorizations of costs across studies. The cost of procurement, including receiving and transporting vaccines to the appropriate locations, was the largest cost component of scaled-up delivery of HPV vaccination in schools (46 percent to 70 percent of financial costs) (Hutubessy and others 2012; Quentin and others 2012). Of the remaining costs, service delivery, comprising health worker salary and allowances; social mobilization, comprising information, education, and communication (IEC); and supervision of vaccinations were important contributors to the total delivery costs (LSHTM and PATH, forthcoming).

In one study, costs were broadly categorized as start-up costs (for example, social mobilization and IEC, training, and microplanning) and recurrent (for example, personnel) costs (Levin and others 2013). Start-up costs of school-based vaccination programs were a large share of the total financial cost per dose (69 percent in Peru, 41 percent in Uganda, and 72 percent in Vietnam). When shared and donated resources were taken into account, start-up costs were far lower at 36 percent, 27 percent, and 56 percent of the total economic cost per dose, respectively.

The cost estimates may not be widely generalizable to other countries because the unit costs were setting specific. Accordingly, the experience of school-based delivery of HPV vaccines may not be generalizable to other adolescent vaccines such as TT, although the same principles may well apply. Furthermore, simultaneous delivery of TT and HPV vaccines in schools—to the same or different age cohorts or grades—may allow for the sharing of cost drivers, such as transport, which can reduce delivery costs.

Cost-Effectiveness of HPV Vaccination

According to several cost-effectiveness analyses in LMICs, HPV vaccination of preadolescent girls is likely to be good value for money, even at the higher cost of school-based delivery (Levin and others 2015). Several studies have estimated that the economic cost per fully vaccinated girl for a three-dose vaccination schedule was I\$25 (25 international dollars) when the vaccine cost was US\$5 per dose (Goldie and others 2008). At this vaccine cost, under assumptions of lifelong high vaccine efficacy against HPV-16/18 cervical cancers, the analyses found that HPV vaccination was very cost-effective in most LMICs, according to a cost-effectiveness threshold of per capita gross domestic product (GDP) (Fesenfeld, Hutubessy, and Jit 2013). At lower vaccine costs that

are more reflective of the subsidized price of HPV vaccines for countries eligible through Gavi, the Vaccine Alliance (for example, US\$0.55–US\$2.00 per dose), HPV vaccination was found to be cost-saving or had attractive cost-effectiveness ratios well below per capita GDP (Goldie and others 2008; Kim and others 2013; Levin and others 2015). In these analyses, the most influential drivers of cost-effectiveness were the cost per vaccinated girl (including vaccine price and delivery costs), vaccine coverage and efficacy, overall cancer and genital warts disease burden, and assumptions about the discount rate. With the recent change in the recommended schedule for HPV vaccine among young immunocompetent adolescent girls from three doses to two and increased flexibility in the interval between doses, adjustments to the cost and cost-effectiveness assumptions and analyses are likely to result in an increasingly favorable cost scenario for school-based delivery in a wider range of LMICs.

The question of male HPV vaccination has been evaluated in several high-income countries, but only a few cost-effectiveness analyses have addressed this question in LMICs, and the conclusions have been mixed. In Brazil (Kim, Andres-Beck, and Goldie 2007) and Vietnam (Sharma, Sy, and Kim 2015), including males in the HPV vaccination program yielded marginal health gains relative to vaccinating girls only. While the analysis in Vietnam found that at a low vaccine cost, vaccinating boys had a cost-effectiveness ratio below per capita GDP, both studies concluded that increasing coverage in girls was more cost-effective than extending coverage to boys. In contrast, in Mexico (Insinga and others 2007), the quadrivalent HPV vaccine in both girls and boys was found to be very cost-effective when including genital warts and cervical cancer benefits. As in analyses from high-income countries, the cost-effectiveness of male HPV vaccination depends heavily on the achievable HPV vaccine uptake in females, vaccine price, and health conditions (such as male and female cancers) included in the analysis.

Overall, these findings imply that at the estimated total cost of delivering HPV vaccination in schools, HPV vaccination of preadolescent girls is good value for money, but that vaccination of boys is less certain.

Summary of Cost-Effectiveness Analyses

Although the evidence on the cost of HPV vaccine delivery in LMICs is emerging, findings from a number of studies in selected settings affirm that the cost of school-based delivery of HPV vaccination is slightly higher relative to other traditional and new infant immunizations. Reaching a target group not routinely served by national immunization programs may require new or modified delivery strategies (LaMontagne and others 2011; WHO 2014b); more intensive IEC activities (Galagan and others 2013; WHO 2013b); and additional logistics and staff time, resulting in higher start-up and recurrent costs. An analysis from Tanzania concluded that the financial cost of introducing HPV vaccination for a three-dose schedule to 26 regions over a five-year period (2011–15) was an estimated US$11.9 million, excluding vaccine cost; or US$40.9 million with vaccine at an unsubsidized price of US$5 per dose (Hutubessy and others 2012). To the extent that scaling up a program to the national level would result in economies of scale; or that the vaccination program could be integrated as part of an existing, efficient program; or that the vaccination schedule would be reduced from three doses to two, both financial and economic costs of HPV vaccine delivery may be lower than what has been estimated in these smaller-scale studies. Countries will need to commit substantial resources to initiate, scale up, and sustain HPV vaccination programs.

Based on the start-up and recurrent cost estimates of school-based delivery from published studies, the majority of cost-effectiveness analyses have found HPV vaccination to be good value for money, even in the poorest countries. Securing a low vaccine cost and achieving high vaccine uptake and adherence in adolescent girls will maximize the return on investment of school-based HPV vaccination in any setting.

CONCLUSIONS

School-based delivery of vaccines is a viable approach for the control of infections and diseases that cause significant morbidity and mortality. Increasing school enrollment and attendance by children and adolescents, particularly girls, has changed the landscape for health service delivery, providing an excellent opportunity to capture large proportions of populations eligible for TT-containing, HPV, and other vaccines. To ensure equitable access for the most vulnerable populations, school-based delivery of vaccines must be complemented by strategies to reach those not attending school, such as mobile teams, outreach, and provision of vaccines at health facilities.

The wide variety of experiences using schools to deliver TT-containing vaccines in 27 LMICs or HPV vaccines in 47 LMICs has provided valuable lessons about the factors that have resulted in success. Pilot programs have been useful in providing countries with the opportunity to test new delivery strategies and learn what works well in their contexts. Community acceptance can be achieved through effective sensitization and mobilization efforts. Feasible delivery strategies for

LMICs, especially using two-dose schedules, can be implemented and reach high coverage. And a strong case for the cost-effectiveness of using schools as a location for adolescent vaccinations has been documented.

Government ownership, endorsement, and financial support; active and sustained involvement and leadership from ministries of health and education; and broad-based community support from health workers, teachers, community leaders, civil society, parents, and adolescents are critical elements in the success and sustainability of any vaccine delivery program, but especially those using schools.

Delivery of TT-containing and HPV vaccines is an opportunity to regalvanize school health programs and build a stronger foundation for the delivery of other important health interventions. A holistic approach combining vaccine delivery with other interventions may help sustain both and has the potential to lead to improvements in the overall health of children and adolescents.

ANNEX

The annex to this chapter is as follows. It is available at http://www.dcp-3.org/CAHD.

- Annex 15A. Supplemental Figures and Tables for School-Based Vaccinations

NOTES

Tania Cernuschi, MSc, MPH, represented Gavi, the Vaccine Alliance Secretariat, Geneva, Switzerland, at the time this work was performed.

World Bank Income Classifications as of July 2014 are as follows, based on estimates of gross national income (GNI) per capita for 2013:

- Low-income countries (LICs) = US$1,045 or less
- Middle-income countries (MICs) are subdivided:
  a) lower-middle-income = US$1,046 to US$4,125
  b) upper-middle-income (UMICs) = US$4,126 to US$12,745
- High-income countries (HICs) = US$12,746 or more.

REFERENCES

Binagwaho, A., C. M. Wagner, M. Gatera, C. Karema, C. T. Nutt, and others. 2012. "Achieving High Coverage in Rwanda's National Human Papillomavirus Vaccination Programme." *Bulletin of the World Health Organization* 90: 623–28.

Bingham, A., J. K. Drake, and D. S. LaMontagne. 2009. "Sociocultural Issues in the Introduction of Human Papillomavirus Vaccines in Low-Resource Settings." *Archives of Pediatric and Adolescent Medicine* 163 (5): 455–61.

Black, R. E., D. H. Huber, and G. T. Curlin. 1980. "Reduction of Neonatal Tetanus by Mass Immunization of Non-Pregnant Women: Duration of Protection Provided by One or Two Doses of Aluminium-Adsorbed Tetanus Toxoid." *Bulletin of the World Health Organization* 58 (6): 927–30.

Block, S. L., T. Nolan, C. Sattler, E. Barr, K. E. Giacoletti, and others. 2006. "Comparison of the Immunogenicity and Reactogenicity of a Prophylactic Quadrivalent Human Papillomavirus (Types 6, 11, 16, and 18) L1 Virus-Like Particle Vaccine in Male and Female Adolescents and Young Adult Women." *Pediatrics* 118 (5): 2135–45.

Brenzel, L., L. J. Wolfson, J. Fox-Rusby, M. Miller, and N. A. Halsey. 2006. "Vaccine-Preventable Diseases." In *Disease Control Priorities in Developing Countries* (second edition): edited by D. T. Jamison, J. G. Breman, A. R. Measham, G. Alleyne, M. Claeson, D. B. Evans, P. Jha, A. Mills, and P. Musgrove, 389–412. Washington, DC: Oxford University Press and World Bank.

Brotherton, J. M. L., and P. J. N. Bloem. 2015. "HPV Vaccination: Current Global Status." *Current Obstetrics and Gynecology Reports* 26. doi:10.1007/s13669-015-0136-9.

Broutet, N., N. Lehnertz, G. Mehl, A. V. Camacho, P. Bloem, and others. 2013. "Effective Health Interventions for Adolescents that Could Be Integrated with Human Papillomavirus Vaccination Programs." *Journal of Adolescent Health* 53 (1): 6–13.

Bundy D. A. P., N. de Silva, H. Horton, G. C. Patton, L. Schultz, and D. T. Jamison. 2017. "Child and Adolescent Health and Development: Realizing Neglected Potential." In *Disease Control Priorities* (third edition): Volume 8, *Child and Adolescent Health and Development,* edited by D. A. P. Bundy, N. de Silva, S. Horton, D. T. Jamison, and G. C. Patton. Washington, DC: World Bank.

Cover, J. K., N. Q. Nghi, D. S. LaMontagne, D. T. Huyen, N. T. Hien, and others. 2012. "Acceptance Patterns and Decision-Making for Human Papillomavirus Vaccination among Parents in Vietnam: An In-Depth Qualitative Study Post-Vaccination." *BMC Public Health* 12: 629.

Denny, L., R. Herrero, C. Levin, and J. J. Kim. 2015. "Cervical Cancer." In *Disease Control Priorities* (third edition): Volume 3, *Cancer,* edited by H. Gelband, P. Jha, R. Sankaranarayanan, and S. Horton, 69–84. Washington, DC: World Bank.

Dorji, T., U. Tshomo, S. Phuntsho, T. D. Tamang, T. Tshokey, and others. 2015. "Introduction of a National HPV Vaccination Program into Bhutan." *Vaccine* 33 (31): 3726–30.

EMA (European Medicines Agency). 2013. "Assessment Report [for Bivalent HPV Vaccine]." Report EMA/789820/2013. http://www.ema.europa.eu/docs/en_GB/document_library/EPAR_-_Assessment_Report_-_Variation/human/000721/WC500160885.pdf.

———. 2014. "Assessment Report [for Quadrivalent HPV Vaccine]." Report EMA/CHMP/66618/2014. http://www.ema.europa.eu/docs/en_GB/document_library/EPAR_-_Assessment_Report_-_Variation/human/000732/WC500167944.pdf.

Esposito, S., V. Birlutiu, P. Jarcuska, A. Perino, S. C. Man, and others. 2011. "Immunogenicity and Safety of Human Papillomavirus-16/18 AS04-Adjuvanted Vaccine Administered According to an Alternative Dosing Schedule Compared with the Standard Dosing Schedule in Healthy Women Aged 15 to 25 Years." *Pediatric Infectious Disease Journal* 30 (3): e49–55.

Ferlay, J., H. R. Shin, F. Bray, D. Forman, C. Mathers, and others. 2010. "Estimates of Worldwide Burden of Cancer in 2008: GLOBOCAN 2008." *International Journal of Cancer* 15: 127 (12): 2893–917.

Fesenfeld, M., R. Hutubessy, and M. Jit. 2013. "Cost-Effectiveness of Human Papillomavirus Vaccination in Low and Middle Income Countries: A Systematic Review." *Vaccine* 31 (37): 3786–804.

Galagan, S. R., P. Paul, L. Menezes, and D. S. LaMontagne. 2013. "Influences on Parental Acceptance of HPV Vaccination in Demonstration Projects in Uganda and Vietnam." *Vaccine* 31 (30): 3072–78.

Gallagher, K. E., S. Kabakama, N. Howard, S. Mounier-Jack, U. K. Griffiths, and others. 2016. "Lessons Learnt from Human Papillomavirus (HPV) Vaccine Demonstration Projects and National Programmes." London School of Hygiene & Tropical Medicine. https://researchonline.lshtm.ac.uk.

Gavi, the Vaccine Alliance. 2016. "Human Papillomavirus Vaccine Support." http://www.gavi.org/support/nvs/human-papillomavirus/.

Goldie, S. J., M. O'Shea, N. G. Campos, M. Diaz, S. Sweet, and others. 2008. "Health and Economic Outcomes of HPV 16, 18 Vaccination in 72 GAVI-Eligible Countries." *Vaccine* 26 (32): 4080–93.

Grabowsky, M., T. Nobiya, M. Ahun, R. Donna, M. Lengor, and others. 2005. "Distributing Insecticide-Treated Bednets during Measles Vaccination: A Low-Cost Means of Achieving High and Equitable Coverage." *Bulletin of the World Health Organization* 83 (3): 195–201.

Griffiths, U. K., L. J. Wolfson, A. Quddus, M. Younus, and R. A. Hafiz. 2004. "Incremental Cost-Effectiveness of Supplementary Immunization Activities to Prevent Neonatal Tetanus in Pakistan." *Bulletin of the World Health Organization* 82: 643–51.

Hutubessy, R., A. Levin, S. Wang, W. Morgan, M. Ally, and others. 2012. "A Case Study Using the United Republic of Tanzania: Costing Nationwide HPV Vaccine Delivery in Low and Middle Income Countries Using the WHO Cervical Cancer Prevention and Control Costing Tool." *BMC Medicine* 10: 136.

Insinga, R. P., E. J. Dasbach, E. H. Elbasha, A. Puig, and L. M. Reynales-Shigematsu. 2007. "Cost-Effectiveness of Quadrivalent Human Papillomavirus (HPV) Vaccination in Mexico: A Transmission Dynamic Model-Based Evaluation." *Vaccine* 26 (1): 128–39.

Institute of Social and Preventive Medicine. 2014. "Evidence Based Recommendations on Human Papilloma Virus (HPV) Vaccines Schedules." Background paper for World Health Organization Strategic Advisory Group of Experts (SAGE) discussions, University of Bern. http://www.who.int/immunization/sage/meetings/2014/april/1_HPV_Evidence_based_recommendationsWHO_with_Appendices2_3.pdf?ua=1.

Kabakama, S., K. E. Gallagher, N. Howard, S. Mounier-Jack, H. E. D. Burchett, and others. 2016. "Social Mobilisation, Consent and Acceptability: A Review of Human Papillomavirus Vaccination Procedures in Low- and Middle-Income Countries." *BMC Public Health* 16: 834.

Kim, J. J., B. Andres-Beck, and S. J. Goldie. 2007. "The Value of Including Boys in an HPV Vaccination Programme: A Cost-Effectiveness Analysis in a Low-Resource Setting." *British Journal of Cancer* 97 (9): 1322–28.

Kim, J. J., N. G. Campos, M. O'Shea, M. Diaz, and I. Mutyaba. 2013. "Model-Based Impact and Cost-Effectiveness of Cervical Cancer Prevention in Sub-Saharan Africa." *Vaccine* 31 (Suppl 5): F60–72.

Kim-Farley, R., T. I. Soewarso, A. Karyadi, and M. Adhyatma. 1987. "Assessing the Impact of the Expanded Programme on Immunization: The Example of Indonesia." *Bulletin of the World Health Organization* 65 (2): 203–6.

Ladner, J., M. H. Besson, R. Hampshire, L. Tapert, M. Chirenje, and others. 2012. "Assessment of Eight HPV Vaccination Programs Implemented in Lowest Income Countries." *BMC Public Health* 12: 370.

LaMontagne, D. S., S. Barge, N. T. Le, E. Mugisha, M. E. Penny, and others. 2011. "Human Papillomavirus Vaccine Delivery Strategies that Achieved High Coverage in Low- and Middle-Income Countries." *Bulletin of the World Health Organization* 89: 821B–30B.

LaMontagne, D. S., V. D. Thiem, V. M. Huong, Y. Tang, and K. M. Neuzil. 2013. "Immunogenicity of Quadrivalent HPV Vaccine among Girls 11 to 13 Years of Age Vaccinated Using Alternative Dosing Schedules: Results 29–32 Months after Third Dose." *Journal of Infectious Diseases* 208 (8): 1325–34.

Levin, A., S. A. Wang, C. Levin, V. Tsu, and R. Hutubessy. 2014. "Costs of Introducing and Delivering HPV Vaccines in Low and Lower Middle Income Countries: Inputs for GAVI Policy on Introduction Grant Support to Countries." *PLoS One* 9 (6): e101114.

Levin, C. E., M. Sharma, Z. Olson, S. Verguet, J. F. Shi, S.-M. Wang, Y.-L. Qiao, D. T. Jamison, and J. J. Kim. 2015. "An Extended Cost-Effectiveness Analysis of Publicly Financed HPV Vaccination to Prevent Cervical Cancer in China." In *Disease Control Priorities* (third edition): Volume 3, *Cancer*, edited by H. Gelband, P. Jha, R. Sankaranarayanan, and S. Horton, 295–305. Washington, DC: World Bank.

Levin, C. E., H. Van Minh, J. Odaga, S. S. Rout, D. N. Ngoc, and others. 2013. "Delivery Cost of Human Papillomavirus Vaccination of Young Adolescent Girls in Peru, Uganda and Viet Nam." *Bulletin of the World Health Organization* 91 (8): 585–92.

Liu, L., S. Oza, D. Hogan, J. Perin, I. Rudan, and others. 2015. "Global, Regional, and National Causes of Child Mortality in 2000–13, with Projections to Inform Post-2015 Priorities: An Updated Systematic Analysis." *The Lancet* 385 (9966): 430–40.

LSHTM (London School of Hygiene and Tropical Medicine) and PATH. Forthcoming. "Lessons Learnt from Human Papillomavirus (HPV) Vaccine Demonstration Projects and National Programmes in Low- and Middle-Income Countries." Technical Research Report. Summary results available at http://www.rho.org/HPVlessons. Full report to be available on the LSHTM website.

Mackroth, M. S., K. Irwin, J. Vandelaer, J. Hombach, and L. O. Eckert. 2010. "Immunizing School-Age Children and Adolescents: Experience from Low- and Middle-Income Countries." *Vaccine* 28 (5): 1138–47.

Markowitz, L. E., V. Tsu, S. L. Deeks, H. Cubie, S. A. Wang, and others. 2012. "Human Papillomavirus Vaccine Introduction: The First Five Years." *Vaccine* 30S: F139–48.

Mehlhorn, A. J., H. E. Balcer, and B. J. Sucher. 2006. "Update on Prevention of Meningococcal Disease: Focus on Tetravalent Meningococcal Conjugate Vaccine." *Annals of Pharmacotherapy* 40 (4): 666–73.

Moodley, I., N. Tathiah, V. Mubaiwa, and L. Denny. 2013. "High Uptake of Gardasil Vaccine among 9–12-Year-Old Schoolgirls Participating in an HPV Vaccination Demonstration Project in KwaZulu-Natal, South Africa." *South African Medical Journal* 103 (5): 313–17.

Moscicki, A. B. 2007. "HPV Infections in Adolescents." *Disease Markers* 23 (4): 229–34.

Mugisha, E., D. S. LaMontagne, A. R. Katahoire, D. Murokora, E. Kumakech, and others. 2015. "Feasibility of Delivering HPV Vaccine to Girls Aged 10 to 15 Years in Uganda." *African Health Sciences* 15 (1): 33–41.

Newell, K. W., D. R. Leblanc, G. Edsall, L. Levine, H. Christensen, and others. 1971. "The Serological Assessment of a Tetanus Toxoid Field Trial." *Bulletin of the World Health Organization* 45 (6): 773–85. http://europepmc.org/articles/PMC2427996/pdf/bullwho00199-0079.pdf.

Paul, P., and A. Fabio. 2014. "Literature Review of HPV Vaccine Delivery Strategies: Considerations for School- and Non-School Based Immunization Program." *Vaccine* 32 (3): 320–26.

Quentin, W., F. Terris-Prestholt, J. Changalucha, S. Soteli, J. W. Edmunds, and others. 2012. "Costs of Delivering Human Papillomavirus Vaccination to School Girls in Mwanza Region, Tanzania." *BMC Medicine* 10: 137.

Raesima, M. M., S. E. Forhan, A. C. Voetsch, S. Hewitt, S. Hariri, and others. 2015. "Human Papillomavirus Vaccination Coverage among School Girls in a Demonstration Project: Botswana, 2013." *Morbidity and Mortality Weekly Report* 64 (40): 1147–49.

Rahman, M., L. C. Chen, J. Chakraborty, M. Yunus, A. I. Chowdhury, and others. 1982. "Use of Tetanus Toxoid for the Prevention of Neonatal Tetanus. Reduction of Neonatal Mortality by Immunization of Non-Pregnant and Pregnant Women in Rural Bangladesh." *Bulletin of the World Health Organization* 60 (2): 261–67.

Rama, C. H., L. L. Villa, S. Pagliusi, M. A. Andreoli, M. C. Costa, and others. 2010. "Awareness and Knowledge of HPV, Cervical Cancer and Vaccines in Young Women after First Delivery in São Paulo, Brazil: A Cross-Sectional Study." *BMC Women's Health* 10: 35. http://www.biomedcentral.com/1472-6874/10/35.

Sharma, M., S. Sy, and J. J. Kim. 2016. "The Value of Male HPV Vaccination in Preventing Cervical Cancer and Genital Warts in a Low-Resource Setting." *British Journal of Obstetrics and Gynaecology* 123 (6): 917–26.

Sinka, K., K. Kavanagh, R. Gordon, J. Love, A. Potts, and others. 2013. "Achieving High and Equitable Coverage of Adolescent HPV Vaccine in Scotland." *Journal of Epidemiology and Community Health* 68 (1): 57–63.

Steinglass, R. 1998. "Using Childhood Booster Doses to Maintain the Elimination of Neonatal Tetanus." Based on a paper delivered at the World Health Organization Neonatal Tetanus Elimination Technical Consultation, Geneva, 1997. Published for the U.S. Agency for International Development (USAID) by the Basic Support for Institutionalizing Child Survival (BASICS) Project, Arlington, VA.

UNESCO (United Nations Educational, Scientific and Cultural Organization). 2014. *Education for All Global Monitoring Report 2013/14. Teaching and Learning: Achieving Quality for All*. ED.2013/WS/29. Paris: UNESCO.

UNICEF (United Nations Children's Fund). 2007. *State of the World's Children 2008: Child Survival*. New York: UNICEF. http://www.unicef.org/sowc08/docs/sowc08.pdf.

Vandelaer, J., M. Birmingham, F. Gasse, M. Kurian, C. Shaw, and others. 2003. "Tetanus in Developing Countries: An Update on the Maternal and Neonatal Tetanus Elimination Initiative." *Vaccine* 21 (24): 3442–45.

Vandelaer, J., J. Partridge, and B. K. Suvedi. 2009. "Process of Neonatal Tetanus Elimination in Nepal." *Journal of Public Health* 31 (4): 561–65. http://jpubhealth.oxfordjournals.org/content/31/4/561.full.

Wamai, R. G., C. A. Ayissi, G. O. Oduwo, S. Perlman, E. Welty, and others. 2012. "Assessing the Effectiveness of a Community-Based Sensitization Strategy in Creating Awareness about HPV, Cervical Cancer and HPV Vaccine among Parents in North West Cameroon." *Journal of Community Health* 37 (5): 917–26.

Watson-Jones, D., K. Baisley, R. Ponsiano, F. Lemme, P. Remes, and others. 2012. "Human Papillomavirus Vaccination in Tanzanian Schoolgirls: Cluster-Randomized Trial Comparing 2 Vaccine-Delivery Strategies." *Journal of Infectious Diseases* 206 (5): 678–86.

Watson-Jones, D., S. Lees, J. Mwanga, N. Neke, J. Changalucha, and others. 2016. "Feasibility and Acceptability of Delivering Adolescent Health Interventions alongside HPV Vaccination in Tanzania." *Health Policy and Planning* 31 (6): 691–99.

WHO (World Health Organization). 2006. "Tetanus Vaccine." Position Paper. *Weekly Epidemiological Record* 81 (2): 198–208. http://www.who.int/wer/2006/wer8120.pdf?ua=1.

———. 2008a. *Promoting Adolescent Sexual and Reproductive Health through Schools in Low Income Countries*. Information Brief, Geneva: WHO. http://www.who.int/maternal_child_adolescent/documents/who_fch_cah_adh_09_03/en/index.html.

———. 2008b. *School Immunization Programme in Sri Lanka; 26 May-2 June 2008*. Geneva: WHO.

———. 2008c. *Tunisia School Immunization Report*. Geneva: WHO.

———. 2009. "Hepatitis B Vaccines." Position paper. *Weekly Epidemiological Record* 40 (84): 405–20. http://www.who.int/wer/2009/wer8440.pdf?ua=1.

———. 2012a. *MenA Campaign in Ghana (9–18 October): Highlights from Upper West Region*. Geneva: WHO. http://www.afro.who.int/en/ghana/press-materials/item/5040-mena-campaign-in-ghana-09-18-october-2012-highlights-from-upper-west-region.html.

———. 2012b. *Report of the HPV Vaccine Delivery Meeting: Identifying Needs for Implementation and Research*. Geneva: WHO. http://screening.iarc.fr/doc/WHO_IVB_12.09_eng.pdf.

———. 2013a. *Global Vaccine Action Plan 2011–2020*. Geneva: WHO.

———. 2013b. *HPV Vaccine Communication: Special Considerations for a Unique Vaccine*. WHO/IVB/13.12. Geneva: WHO.

———. 2013c. "Validation of Maternal and Neonatal Tetanus Elimination in United Republic of Tanzania, 2012." *Weekly Epidemiological Record* 88 (3): 313–20.

———. 2014a. "Considerations Regarding Consent in Vaccinating Children and Adolescents between 6 and 17 Years Old." WHO/IVB/14.04. WHO, Geneva.

———. 2014b. "Human Papillomavirus Vaccines." Position paper. *Weekly Epidemiological Record* 43 (89): 465–92. http://www.who.int/wer/2014/wer8943.pdf?ua=1.

———. 2014c. "Summary of the SAGE April 2014 Meeting." http://www.who.int/immunization/sage/meetings/2014/april/report_summary_april_2014/en/.

WHO-UNICEF. 2009. "Potential Role of School-Based Immunization in Protecting More Children: Results of email Survey." Presented at the Fourth Annual Global Immunization Meeting, New York, February.

———. 2013. *Expanded Programme on Immunization Joint Reporting Form (2012 data)*. http://www.who.int/immunization/monitoring_surveillance/routine/reporting/reporting/en/.

———. 2014. *Expanded Programme on Immunization Joint Reporting Form (2013 data)*. http://www.who.int/immunization/monitoring_surveillance/routine/reporting/reporting/en/.

zur Hausen, H. 1977. "Human Papillomaviruses and Their Possible Role in Squamous Cell Carcinomas." *Current Topics in Microbiology and Immunology* 78: 1–30.

Chapter 16

Promoting Oral Health through Programs in Middle Childhood and Adolescence

Habib Benzian, Renu Garg, Bella Monse,
Nicole Stauf, and Benoit Varenne

INTRODUCTION

Oral diseases are among the most common diseases worldwide, particularly for school-age children and adolescents. They pose significant public health problems for all countries and entail substantial health, social, and economic impacts. Simple and effective interventions exist to prevent most oral diseases. The school setting, among others, plays an important role.

This chapter describes oral disease control priorities for school-age children and adolescents ages 5–19 years. Oral diseases and effective population-based interventions are highlighted in two other chapters in the *Disease Control Priorities* (third edition) series: chapter 10 in volume 1 (Niederman, Feres, and Ogunbodede 2015) and chapter 5 in volume 3 (Sankaranarayanan and others 2015). Definitions of age groupings and age-specific terminology used in this volume can be found in chapter 1 (Bundy and others 2017).

ORAL DISEASES AND CONDITIONS AFFECTING CHILDREN AND ADOLESCENTS

School-age children and adolescents are affected by a range of oral diseases and conditions. This chapter focuses on tooth decay (dental caries) as it is the most common disease with the highest global burden. It also includes oral injuries and trauma, as well as noma (a destructive gangrene affecting orofacial soft and hard tissues with high mortality), as significant but neglected oral conditions. Other oral diseases, which are partly discussed in other volumes, include simple gingivitis and periodontitis, congenital malformations, fluorosis of teeth in areas of high fluoride concentrations in drinking water, oral mucosa lesions that are often symptoms of other systemic diseases, and simple malocclusions.

Tooth Decay

Tooth decay affects about 3.1 billion people. The prevalence of tooth decay in permanent teeth ranked 1st and in deciduous teeth ranked 10th among 291 diseases analyzed in the Global Burden of Disease study (Marcenes and others 2013). The highest burden of tooth decay is in upper-middle-income countries, and the lowest is in low-income countries (LICs) (figure 16.1), although these averages mask large variations among countries within each income category. Between 40 percent and 90 percent of 12-year-old children in low- and middle-income countries (LMICs) suffer from tooth decay (FDI World Dental Federation 2015); tooth decay is also a problem in high-income countries (HICs). In the United States, tooth decay in children is four times more common than asthma (CDC 2004). Across all country income groups, the majority of decay remains untreated, ranging from 52 percent in HICs to almost 100 percent in LICs.

Corresponding author: Habib Benzian, Department of Epidemiology and Health Promotion, College of Dentistry, New York University, New York, United States; habib.benzian@mac.com.

Figure 16.1 Average Number of Teeth Affected by Tooth Decay in 12-Year-Olds, by Country Income Group, Latest Data Available, 2000–14

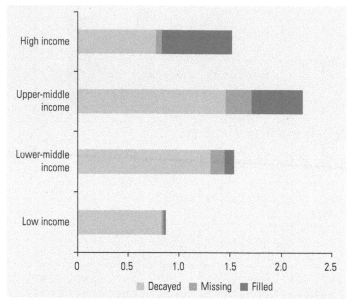

Source: FDI World Dental Federation 2015.
Note: The data are based on the WHO Oral Health Country/Area Profile Project (http://www.mah.se /capp/), which is the only authoritative source of international data on tooth decay. The DMFT index is generally used to report tooth decay in epidemiological studies. The index records the number of decayed (D), missing (M), and filled (F) teeth (T). A DMFT score of 1.0 means that 1 of the 32 permanent teeth is decayed, missing, or filled.

Tooth decay can develop once the first teeth erupt. Toothache as the main symptom is highly prevalent among all age groups, ranging between 15 percent and 45 percent in different studies (Boeira and others 2012; Hayes and others 2013; Kassebaum and others 2015; Miotto, Barcellos, and Lopes 2013; Noro and others 2014). The decay process may progress to total tooth destruction and exposure of the pulp—causing severe pain, infection, and systemic reactions—which may be fatal as a result of septicemia (Kawashita, Kitamura, and Saito 2011).

Severe tooth decay may also affect child growth and nutrition, with significant impacts on psychosocial well-being, contributing to reduced quality of life and educational opportunities (Espinoza and others 2013; Leal and others 2012; Ramos-Jorge and others 2014; Sheiham 2006). Studies from LMICs such as Brazil, the Islamic Republic of Iran, the Philippines, South Africa, and Thailand, show that tooth decay negatively affects social interactions and the self-esteem of children and adolescents (Kakoei and others 2013; Miotto, Barcello, and Lopes 2013; Naidoo, Chikte, and Sheiham 2001). It is also among the most frequent reasons for school and work absenteeism (Department of Education 2008; Krisdapong and others 2013). An estimated 59 million

hours of school were lost because of oral health problems in 1989 in the United States, confirming such impacts in high-income settings (U.S. DHHS 2000).

Growing evidence suggests that severe tooth decay and malnutrition are associated. Children with severe dental caries are at increased risk for undernutrition and failure to thrive because pain, chronic infection, and abscesses from decayed teeth impair their appetite, ability to chew, diet, and sleep (Sheiham 2006). Conversely, prevention and treatment can contribute to reduced malnutrition and undernutrition; underweight children with severe tooth decay show rapid weight gain once destroyed teeth are extracted (Benzian, Monse, and others 2011; Duijster and others 2013; Sheiham 2006).

The association between dental caries and obesity is more complex. Both diseases share common risk factors, such as overconsumption of sugar-laden foods and beverages. Studies confirm an association between obesity and caries for the permanent dentition, but the causal direction of the association requires more examination (Hayden and others 2013). Evolving evidence suggests that food-related preventive interventions addressing dental caries also provide benefits for reducing obesity and vice versa.

Oral Injuries and Trauma

Oral injuries and trauma include fractures of facial bones, as well as fractures, dislocations, and loss of teeth. Orofacial injuries may be a result of traffic accidents, sport injuries, abuse, or violence. They account for 5 percent of injuries among all age groups, even though oral structures represent only 1 percent of body surface. Oral injuries are more frequent in the first 10 years of life, with more boys affected than girls. The likelihood of oral injuries decreases with age, but the incidence of trauma to the head and neck increases (Andersson 2013). Estimates indicate that 30 percent of children show signs of trauma to their deciduous teeth; 20 percent are affected by trauma to their permanent, mostly anterior, teeth. Oral injuries and trauma have significant physical, psychosocial, and economic impacts and are major public health problems. Dental treatment is necessary in about half of all trauma cases involving permanent teeth. The annual direct costs of dental trauma are between US$3.6 million and US$9.0 million in 2012 dollars per 1 million inhabitants per year (Borum and Andreasen 2001).

Noma

Noma is a disease characterized by severe gangrenous destruction of soft and hard tissues of the mouth and face. It predominantly affects children under age six years in Sub-Saharan Africa. Noma progresses rapidly from a small lesion to major destruction. The disease is rare but has significant impacts on the lives of those affected; mortality is between 70 percent and 90 percent. Survivors suffer lifelong impairments to speaking or eating because of significant tissue destruction. Victims and their families are often stigmatized, with increased risk of poverty for affected households (Marck 2013; Ogbureke and Ogbureke 2010).

Noma is most prevalent in Burkina Faso, Ethiopia, Mali, Niger, Nigeria, and Senegal; however, because of unreliable documentation, there are no accurate epidemiologic data. The etiology of noma is associated with malnutrition, insufficient access to improved sanitation, cohabitation with animals, and compromised immune systems. This confluence of etiologic factors can be disrupted; if diagnosed at early stages, simple and effective treatment, consisting of disinfection and hygiene measures combined with antibiotics, is possible. However, by the time patients receive care, noma is often in advanced stages. Surviving children usually require costly and complex surgery, which is either unavailable or unaffordable. Informing at-risk population groups, especially mothers, about simple oral and other hygiene improvements, balanced nutrition, and early detection of potential lesions can help prevent noma.

RISK FACTORS, SOCIAL DETERMINANTS, INEQUALITIES, AND DISEASE TRENDS

The many factors that influence oral health include individual, environmental, family, community, and broader societal factors. For children and adolescents, high sugar intake and insufficient oral hygiene are the leading risk factors for poor oral health, while behavioral and environmental influences affect the likelihood of oral injuries and trauma.

The risk factors for oral diseases and major noncommunicable diseases (NCDs) overlap; these include, for example, unhealthy diet and the consumption of tobacco and alcohol. This overlap provides the basis for integrated prevention strategies through the common risk factor approach (Sheiham and Watt 2000), one of the cornerstones of oral health promotion.

High Sugar Consumption

A diet characterized by frequent and high intake of sugary food or sugar-sweetened beverages (SSBs) increases the risk of developing tooth decay. Free sugars include all sugars added to foods and drinks by manufacturers, cooks, or consumers, as well as sugars naturally present in honey, syrups, and fruit juices. High sugar consumption is often combined with an unhealthy diet characterized by, for example, low fruit and vegetable intake and overconsumption of foods with high fat and salt content (Alzahrani and others 2014); it is thus closely linked to the leading causes of major NCDs, such as diabetes and obesity. To reduce the likelihood of dental caries, obesity, and diabetes, the World Health Organization (WHO) Guideline on Sugars Intake (WHO 2015) recommends that less than 10 percent of the daily energy intake come from sugar. Further benefits may be achieved by reducing consumption to less than 5 percent (five teaspoons per day) of total daily energy intake (Moynihan and Kelly 2014).

Alcohol and Tobacco Use

Children and adolescents are increasingly exposed to other risk factors that may lead to oral diseases later in life, particularly oral cancer. Tobacco use in all its forms is the main risk factor for oral cancer, and harmful alcohol consumption further amplifies the risk. Although exposure in HICs is decreasing as a result of effective regulations, the challenges in LMICs are increasing. The average age of smoking initiation has dropped from 15–17 years to 13–14 years; high rates of tobacco and alcohol use are increasingly common. Up to 20 percent of 15-year-olds in LMICs use tobacco, and more than 50 percent of 13-year-olds in the United States have tried alcohol. In the Philippines, 30 percent of those ages 11–16 years reported alcohol use in the past month. These habits may persist and deepen during adulthood (Ahlström and Österberg 2004; Bach 2015; Lillard and Christopoulou 2015; Peltzer and Pengpid 2015). Electronic nicotine delivery systems have grown in popularity. Although the evaluation of their health effects is still ongoing, indications of their harm include the induction of children and adolescents to smoking and nicotine addiction, with its negative impact on adolescent brain development.

Changing Consumption Patterns

Moreover, global demographic changes, rapid urbanization, the economic transition from low-income status to lower-middle-income status, and migration streams within and between countries are influencing consumption patterns for many populations. In recent decades, the proportion of the population living in middle-income countries has grown from 26.7 percent in 1990 to 72 percent in 2012. During the same period, the proportion of people living in LICs decreased from 57.7 percent to 11.7 percent. Although these shifts have brought major advances in general development (Jamison and others 2013), they have also modified population exposure to risk factors for diseases. In particular, these changes have increased the consumption of sugar, fat, and salt. Accordingly, the disease burden in LMICs has shifted from a focus on infectious diseases to a predominance of NCDs (Popkin, Adair, and Ng 2012).

Oral diseases are part of this global transition (figure 16.1), as exemplified by changes in disability-adjusted life years (DALYs[1]) caused by tooth decay in Sub-Saharan Africa. From 1990 to 2012, the global average increase in disease burden of dental caries, as measured in DALYs, was 34.5 percent; for most countries in this region, however, it was between 42 percent and 78 percent (Dye and others 2013; Kassebaum and others 2015).

CHALLENGES TO EFFECTIVE ORAL HEALTH PROMOTION IN LMICs

Countries that have traditionally emphasized prevention and control of oral diseases, particularly in schools (such as Hong Kong SAR, China; Scandinavian countries; and Switzerland) have been able to achieve substantial improvements in oral health status with high rates of caries-free children. In LMICs, however, despite the growing oral disease burden, designing and implementing effective oral health promotion strategies has proved challenging for several reasons:

- Communicable diseases and diseases with high mortality receive priority over NCDs and oral diseases (Benzian, Hobdell, and others 2011; Piva and Dodd 2009).
- There is reluctance to view oral health in the context of systemic health care and to include it as part of comprehensive health care services and related infrastructure.
- Reliable information on the oral disease burden, which is often not integrated into national health surveillance, is lacking, resulting in the unavailability of up-to-date epidemiological data, even though standardized survey tools exist (FDI World Dental Federation 2015; Petersen and others 2005)
- Evidence-based and population-wide preventive strategies that take into account the broader determinants of health are absent (Watt 2007).
- Priority is given to curative clinical approaches, which are generally costly and associated with access barriers. Oral diseases are considered the fourth most expensive health condition and result in high out-of-pocket payments, particularly in LMICs (Kandelman and others 2012).

PREVENTION AND HEALTH PROMOTION TO IMPROVE ORAL HEALTH

The development of effective prevention and oral health promotion strategies, in conjunction with pain relief and emergency services, may be the most realistic strategy for LMICs based on available resources and ethical considerations (Frencken, Holmgren, and van Palenstein Helderman 2002). This section discusses oral health promotion in school settings, including related supportive policies, as a cost-effective area for government and public health intervention.

Making Schools Healthy Places

Children and adolescents spend significant time in school, which is a key setting for promoting oral and general health. Net primary school enrollment rates worldwide for both genders have increased steadily for decades and averaged 89 percent in 2013 (UNESCO 2015). Reaching a majority of children through primary schools may be possible without requiring complex additional health structures. Oral health interventions can be used as entry points for wider integration with other health activities, including the potential to address broader determinants of health (Macnab and Kasangaki 2012). Building skills and providing services, together with improving the conditions of the school environment, have the potential to influence lifelong knowledge, attitudes, health status, and behaviors of children.[2]

Schools are also influential model institutions in their communities and may facilitate participatory approaches that involve parents and the wider community in health promotion. Creating health-promoting schools requires school-level commitment as well as policy guidance to encourage risk-reduction measures, such as banning smoking or foods with high sugar content on the premises (Bundy 2011), or providing clean and healthy environments that include sustained access to safe water, sanitation, and hygiene (Emory University Center for Global Safe Water and UNICEF 2013).

Research on the effects of oral health promotion in schools comes primarily from HICs, but evidence from LMICs is growing (Haleem and others 2016; Macnab 2015; Monse and others 2013; Petersen and others 2015). Several supportive policy frameworks exist to guide countries in developing school health strategies. The Focusing Resources on Effective School Health approach provides a conceptual framework and guides national policies; its principles also apply to oral health promotion in schools (World Education Forum 2000).

The WHO Health Promoting Schools framework includes technical guidance for oral health programs (Macnab 2015), although a recent Cochrane review revealed limited evidence for sustained impact and called for better implementation and research (Langford and others 2014). Building on both concepts, the Fit for School Action Framework provides practical implementation guidance and integrates daily, skills-based oral health activities with other school-based priority interventions (box 16.1) (Benzian and others 2012).

Reducing Risk Exposure

Reducing Sugar Consumption. Public institutions, especially schools, should not only raise awareness of but also provide healthy food and beverage options. Some 370 million children worldwide receive school meals each day, providing opportunities to offer healthy choices low in free sugars, fat, and salt, thereby reducing the risk for tooth decay, obesity, and related chronic conditions (Vandevijvere and others 2015).

Canteens or vendors on or near school premises typically offer snacks and SSBs. Schools may consider limiting or prohibiting the sale of sugary foods and SSBs on school premises, along with providing healthy alternatives. Advertisements for and sponsorship of unhealthy foods and drinks may also be banned from schools (New Zealand Beverage Guidance Panel 2014; Patel and Hampton 2011; Wilder and others 2015).

On a policy level, the introduction of taxes on unhealthy products such as SSBs, regulations for transparent food labeling, and restrictions on marketing to children and adolescents may contribute to reducing risk exposure (Rayner, Scarborough, and Briggs 2015).

Banning Tobacco and Alcohol Products. A review of school-based tobacco prevention initiatives in 40 LMICs confirmed that only bans reduced smoking rates; educational interventions alone had no significant effect (Agaku and others 2015). Accordingly, an appropriate policy would be to ban the sale, marketing, and sponsorship of tobacco and alcohol products for children and adolescents in general and on school premises in particular (Saraf and others 2012).

Improving Safety and Protection. Although it is impossible to prevent all oral injuries and trauma, certain measures can make schools safer. For example, avoiding injury-prone installations, such as sharp edges or places for high climbing, can help prevent falls, oral injuries, and trauma (Glendor 2009). Wearing mouth protection can reduce the risk of trauma from contact sports, but it requires sufficient resources. Road safety on the way to school and enforced use of proper helmets

---

Box 16.1

Integrated School Health: The Fit for School Programme

The Fit for School Programme is implemented by the Ministries of Education in Cambodia, Indonesia, the Lao People's Democratic Republic, and the Philippines, with support from Deutsche Gesellschaft für Internationale Zusammenarbeit (GIZ) GmbH. As the recipient of an award from the World Health Organization, the World Bank, and the United Nations Development Programme for innovation in global health, the model integrates an oral health intervention into a school health program addressing prevalent diseases in school-age children. Students brush their teeth with fluoride toothpaste as a daily group activity, combined with group handwashing with soap.

This approach helps familiarize children with healthy habits and reduces other hygiene-related diseases (Monse and Benzian 2011). Research in participating schools has shown that daily group toothbrushing with fluoride toothpaste has prevented 17.3 percent of new caries lesions (Monse and others 2013). However, results depend on implementation quality. Under controlled conditions, reviews show a preventive power of up to 25 percent for toothbrushing with fluoride toothpaste (Marinho and others 2009). The Fit for School Programme costs US$0.60 per child per year in supplies and reduces absentee rates due to illness.

Source: Marinho and others 2003.

---

for cycling and use of motorbikes or similar vehicles are measures to reduce the frequency and severity of dental and craniofacial trauma.

Strategies to Promote Oral Health

Skills-Based Oral Health Promotion. Oral health promotion in schools has traditionally focused on educational approaches that transfer knowledge about disease or healthy behavior. However, evidence suggests that these approaches alone have limited long-term effects. Instead, a focus on activities that develop children's skills, hygiene practices, and habits is more successful in improving individual oral health behaviors (Cooper and others 2013; Hopkins and others 2007; Kay and Locker 1998; Peters and others 2009).

Skills-based oral health education includes daily group toothbrushing with fluoride toothpaste at school. Group activities are fun for children and enforce healthy social norms, which are effective drivers of oral hygiene behavior

(Claessen and others 2008). Toothbrushing in a group while using appropriate washing facilities is a practical way to facilitate implementation with little extra workload for supervising teachers. Because these activities do not require the involvement of health professionals, they can be readily integrated into the daily school schedule.

Promoting Access and Use of Appropriate Fluorides. Ample evidence demonstrates that use of fluorides is the most effective method for preventing dental caries in populations. The WHO, the FDI World Dental Federation, and the International Association for Dental Research, and the Chinese Stomatological Association (2007) strongly recommend twice-daily toothbrushing with fluoride toothpaste (box 16.2) for the following reasons:

- Prevention of tooth decay by using fluoride is the most realistic way to reduce the burden of tooth decay in populations.
- Fluoride toothpaste remains the most widespread, significant, and rigorously evaluated form of fluoride used globally.
- Fluoride toothpaste is generally safe to use.

The most efficient and effective way to improve use of fluoride in schools is integrating toothbrushing with fluoride toothpaste as a routine activity into the daily school schedule (Petersen and others 2015). Other sources of fluoride may include brushing with high-fluoride-containing gel once a week or application of fluoride varnish by trained health workers in schools. In HICs, the application of fissure sealants may be considered. These procedures require adequate infrastructure, staff, and resources, which are beyond the means of most LMICs. Moreover, as with many health interventions, robust cost-effectiveness data from large-scale implementation are lacking (Isman 2010; Marinho and others 2013).

The institutionalization of such activities requires supportive structures on several levels (Benzian and others 2012). On a policy level, improving access to and use of appropriate fluorides requires reducing taxation of fluoride toothpaste, increasing taxation of toothpaste without fluoride to discourage its use, and strengthening national regulations for the quality and labeling of fluoride toothpaste.

Oral Health Care Services. Generally, provision of health services at schools is costly and challenging to sustain. Referral systems are often deficient, even in HICs (Pine 2007); primary oral health care in LMICs is generally challenged by low numbers of oral health professionals, lack of infrastructure and supplies, or high access barriers posed by costs and transportation (Petersen 2014).

Depending on available resources, schools may offer oral health care services in the form of an attached dental clinic or regular visits of oral health professionals or trained community health workers. Basic treatment, such as pain relief and emergency care, may be provided on site or through referral to nearby health facilities. Teachers may preselect children with dental problems. Screening without provision of basic care to children in need is considered unethical.

A study using data from 1999 estimated that, for 1 billion children in LMICs (ages 6–18 years), restorative oral care would cost more than US$860 billion (Yee and Sheiham 2002), an amount exceeding the capacities of any health care system. The direct treatment costs of oral disease in 2010 (all age groups and countries combined) were estimated to be US$300 billion, with HICs spending US$244 billion and the United States and Canada alone spending US$120 billion (Listl and others 2015). These findings highlight dramatic inequalities in oral health care expenditure, reflecting low service availability in LMICs. They also show that a focus on costly clinical oral health care is not a realistic option in these settings. Delivery of dental procedures is discussed in chapter 1 of volume 1 in this series (Mock and others 2015).

Strengthening Surveillance and Research

Oral disease surveillance in LMICs should be strengthened and integrated with national surveillance systems to improve epidemiological information on the disease

---

Box 16.2

Principles of Toothbrushing with Fluoride Toothpaste

- Brush teeth at least twice a day for two minutes with fluoridated toothpaste (1,200–1,500 parts per million fluoride concentration). Children up to age six years should use only a pea-sized amount of toothpaste.
- Brush preferably after meals, especially breakfast, and before going to bed.
- Do not swallow toothpaste; spit out the slurry after brushing, without rinsing with water.
- Parents and teachers should supervise toothbrushing so that children do not swallow toothpaste.
- Rinse toothbrush after use, store it in an upright position, allow it to air dry, and ensure that it does not touch other toothbrushes or surfaces to avoid cross-contamination.
- Visit a dental or health professional for routine check-ups and in cases of discomfort, pain, or discoloration of the teeth.

burden for better advocacy and effective action (Varenne 2015). A number of opportunities exist for integrating oral health data into ongoing international collaborative surveys such as the Global School-Based Student Health Survey, the Global Youth Tobacco Survey, and the WHO STEPs surveys for NCDs. Oral health–specific modules exist for each of these surveys, but they are not regularly applied or reported.

More evidence is also needed to better understand what interventions are effective and under what conditions. Applied research and rigorous evaluation of approaches, projects, and programs may help identify effective and appropriate strategies. Furthermore, research results need to be accessible and presented in a format that can inform policy decisions, particularly for effective school health interventions (Benzian and others 2012).

Supportive Policies for Oral Health

Advocacy at the global and national levels to highlight the burden and consequences of oral diseases among children and adolescents may help prioritize interventions for prevention and control. Approaches with good evidence and cost-effectiveness, as well as skills-based oral health education, may strengthen healthy lifelong behaviors. Strategies addressing the social determinants and common risk factors of oral diseases require policies promoting oral health as part of the general health sector, as well as other sectors such as education, agriculture, transportation, commerce and trade, housing, and water and sanitation, to establish health-conducive environments and healthy nutrition. The emerging regional and national action plans addressing NCDs may provide opportunities for integration of simple, sustainable, and scalable oral health interventions.

Strengthening Intersectoral Collaboration

School-based health promotion is an intersectoral challenge, with stakeholders mainly from the education; health; and water, sanitation, and hygiene sectors; but also from other sectors that jointly address key determinants of health. Task-sharing and leveraging the existing workforce may reduce costs and facilitate implementation. Defining clear roles and responsibilities for all involved stakeholders, including parents and the community, is crucial to ensuring successful and sustainable implementation.

CONCLUSIONS

Worldwide, children and adolescents suffer from a significant and largely preventable burden of oral diseases, particularly dental caries. The consequences affect well-being and quality of life, general health, school performance, and social interactions. Preventing oral diseases with simple and cost-effective population-wide interventions is possible, even in resource-constrained LMICs (Geneau and others 2010), and schools are ideal platforms for reaching children. Recommended approaches require action at the school, community, and policy levels, and include the following:

- Prioritization of schools as health-promoting settings where skills-based and high-impact interventions, such as daily toothbrushing with fluoride toothpaste, can be implemented as part of integrated school health
- Increased advocacy to emphasize the burden and consequences of oral diseases to prioritize interventions for prevention and control in LMICs
- Development of concepts, practical implementation models, evaluation tools, and related national capacity for cost-effective best-buy interventions to address caries and other priority oral diseases in LMICs.

The disease and risk factor trends indicate that inaction is likely to increase the challenges. Although most evidence is from HICs, further research may strengthen the links between concept, policy, and action. Such an agenda needs consensus from stakeholders and organizations active in the prevention and control of oral diseases to better prioritize oral diseases in LMICs. Only then can advocacy, science, strengthening of capacities, and technical assistance go hand in hand to have a significant effect on the global burden of oral diseases (Benzian, Hobdell, and others 2011).

DISCLAIMER

Renu Garg and Benoit Varenne are staff members of the World Health Organization (WHO), and Bella Monse is a staff member of the Gesellschaft für Internationale Zusammenarbeit (GIZ) GmbH. The authors alone are responsible for the views expressed in this publication, since they do not necessarily represent the decisions, policies, or views of the WHO or of GIZ.

NOTES

World Bank Income Classifications as of July 2014 are as follows, based on estimates of gross national income (GNI) per capita for 2013:

- Low-income countries (LICs) = US$1,045 or less

- Middle-income countries (MICs) are subdivided:
  a) lower-middle-income = US$1,046 to US$4,125
  b) upper-middle-income (UMICs) = US$4,126 to US$12,745
- High-income countries (HICs) = US$12,746 or more.

1. The DALY is a measure of overall disease burden, expressed as the number of years lost due to ill-health, disability, or early death.
2. The measures described for the school context are equally relevant for the kindergarten and preschool contexts, even if these settings are not explicitly mentioned.

REFERENCES

Agaku, I. T., E. M. Obadan, O. O. Odukoya, and O. Olufajo. 2015. "Tobacco-Free Schools as a Core Component of Youth Tobacco Prevention Programs: A Secondary Analysis of Data from 43 Countries." *European Journal of Public Health* 25 (2): 210–15.

Ahlström, S., and E. Österberg. 2004. *International Perspectives on Adolescent and Young Adult Drinking*. Bethesda, MD: National Institute on Alcohol Abuse and Alcoholism.

Alzahrani, S. G., R. G. Watt, A. Sheiham, M. Aresu, and G. Tsakos. 2014. "Patterns of Clustering of Six Health-Compromising Behaviours in Saudi Adolescents." *BMC Public Health* 14: 1215.

Andersson, L. 2013. "Epidemiology of Traumatic Dental Injuries." *Journal of Endodontics* 39: S2–S5.

Bach, L. 2015. "The Path to Tobacco Addiction Starts at Very Young Ages." Factsheet. Campaign for Tobacco Free Kids, Washington, DC.

Benzian, H., M. Hobdell, C. Holmgren, R. Yee, B. Morse, and others. 2011. "Political Priority of Global Oral Health: An Analysis of Reasons for International Neglect." *International Dental Journal* 61: 124–30.

Benzian, H., B. Monse, V. Belizario, A. Schratz, M. Sahin, and others. 2012. "Public Health in Action: Effective School Health Needs Renewed International Attention." *Global Health Action* 5: 14870.

Benzian, H., B. Monse, R. Heinrich-Weltzien, M. Hobdell, J. Mulder, and others. 2011. "Untreated Severe Dental Decay: A Neglected Determinant of Low Body Mass Index in 12-Year-Old Filipino Children." *BMC Public Health* 11: 558.

Boeira, G. F., M. B. Correa, K. G. Peres, M. A. Peres, I. S. Santos, and others. 2012. "Caries Is the Main Cause for Dental Pain in Childhood: Findings from a Birth Cohort." *Caries Research* 46: 488–95.

Borum, M., and J. Andreasen. 2001. "Therapeutic and Economic Implications of Traumatic Dental Injuries in Denmark: An Estimate Based on 7549 Patients Treated at a Major Trauma Centre." *International Journal of Paediatric Dentistry* 11: 249–58.

Bundy, D. A. P., N. de Silva, S. Horton, G. C. Patton, L. Schultz, and D. T. Jamison. 2017. "Child and Adolescent Health and Development: Realizing Neglected Potential." In *Disease Control Priorities* (third edition): Volume 8, *Child and Adolescent Health and Development*, edited by Bundy, D. A. P., N. de Silva, S. Horton, D. T. Jamison, and G. C. Patton. Washington, DC: World Bank.

Bundy, D. A. P. 2011. *Rethinking School Health: A Key Component of Education for All*. Directions in Development Series. Washington, DC: World Bank.

CDC (Centers for Disease Control and Prevention). 2004. "Children's Oral Health." Factsheet. Division of Oral Health, CDC, Atlanta, GA.

Claessen, J.-P., S. Bates, K. Sherlock, F. Seearsand, and R. Wright. 2008. "Design Interventions to Improve Tooth Brushing." *International Dentistry Journal* 58 (S5): 307–20.

Cooper, A. M., L. A. O'Malley, S. N. Elison, R. Armstrong, G. Burnside, and others. 2013. "Primary School-Based Behavioural Interventions for Preventing Caries." *Cochrane Database of Systematic Reviews* 5: CD009378.

Department of Education. 2008. *National Oral Health Survey among the Public School Population in the Philippines*. Manila: Department of Education.

Duijster, D., A. Sheiham, M. H. Hobdell, G. Itchon, and B. Monse. 2013. "Associations between Oral Health-Related Impacts and Rate of Weight Gain after Extraction of Pulpally Involved Teeth in Underweight Preschool Filipino Children." *BMC Public Health* 13: 533.

Dye, C., T. Mertens, G. Hirnschall, W. Mpanju-Shumbusho, R. D. Newman, and others. 2013. "WHO and the Future of Disease Control Programmes." *The Lancet* 381 (9864): 413–18.

Emory University Center for Global Safe Water and UNICEF (United Nations Children's Fund). 2013. *Equity of Access to WASH in Schools*. New York, NY: UNICEF.

Espinoza, I., W. M. Thomson, J. Gamonal, and O. Arteaga. 2013. "Disparities in Aspects of Oral-Health-Related Quality of Life among Chilean Adults." *Community Dentistry and Oral Epidemiology* 41: 242–50.

FDI World Dental Federation. 2015. "The Challenge of Oral Diseases: A Call for Global Action." In *Oral Health Atlas* (second edition), edited by H. Benzian and D. Williams. Geneva: FDI.

Frencken, J. E., C. Holmgren, and W. van Palenstein Helderman. 2002. *Basic Package of Oral Care (BPOC)*. Nijmengen, Netherlands: WHO Collaborating Centre for Oral Health Care Planning and Future Scenarios, University of Nijmengen.

Geneau, R., D. Stuckler, S. Stachenko, M. McKee, S. Ebrahim, and others. 2010. "Raising the Priority of Preventing Chronic Diseases: A Political Process." *The Lancet* 376 (9753): 1689–98.

Glendor, U. 2009. "Aetiology and Risk Factors Related to Traumatic Dental Injuries: A Review of the Literature." *Dental Traumatology* 25: 19–31.

Haleem, A., M. K. Khan, S. Sufia, S. Chaudhry, M. I. Siddiqui, and others. 2016. "The Role of Repetition and Reinforcement in School-Based Oral Health Education: A Cluster Randomized Controlled Trial." *BMC Public Health* 16: 2.

Hayden, C., J. O. Bowler, S. Chambers, R. Freeman, G. Humphris, and others. 2013. "Obesity and Dental Caries in Children:

A Systematic Review and Meta-Analysis." *Community Dental and Oral Epidemiology* 41: 289–308.

Hayes, A., A. Azarpazhooh, L. Dempster, V. Ravaghi, and C. Quinonez. 2013. "Time Loss Due to Dental Problems and Treatment in the Canadian Population: Analysis of a Nationwide Cross-Sectional Survey." *BMC Oral Health* 13: 17.

Hopkins, G. L., D. McBride, H. H. Marshak, K. Freier, J. V. Stevens, and others. 2007. "Developing Healthy Kids in Healthy Communities: Eight Evidence-Based Strategies for Preventing High-Risk Behaviour." *Medical Journal of Australia* 186: S70–73.

Isman, R. 2010. "Dental Sealants: A Public Health Perspective." *Journal of the California Dental Association* 38: 735–45.

Jamison, D. T., L. H. Summers, G. Alleyne, K. J. Arrow, S. Berkley, and others. 2013. "Global Health 2035: A World Converging within a Generation." *The Lancet* 382 (9908): 1898–955.

Kakoei, S., M. Parirokh, N. Nakhaee, F. Jamshidshirazi, M. Rad, and others. 2013. "Prevalence of Toothache and Associated Factors: A Population-Based Study in Southeast Iran." *Iran Endodontic Journal* 8: 123–28.

Kandelman, D., S. Arpin, R. J. Baez, P. C. Baehni, and P. E. Petersen. 2012. "Oral Health Care Systems in Developing and Developed Countries." *Periodontology* 60 (1): 98–109.

Kassebaum, N. J., E. Bernabe, M. Dahiya, B. Bhandari, C. J. Murray, and others. 2015. "Global Burden of Untreated Caries: A Systematic Review and Metaregression." *Journal of Dental Research* 94 (5): 650–58.

Kawashita, Y., M. Kitamura, and T. Saito. 2011. "Early Childhood Caries." *International Journal of Dentistry* 2011: 725320.

Kay, E., and D. Locker. 1998. "A Systematic Review of the Effectiveness of Health Promotion Aimed at Improving Oral Health." *Community Dental Health* 15: 132–44.

Krisdapong, S., P. Prasertsom, K. Rattanarangsima, and A. Sheiham. 2013. "School Absence Due to Toothache Associated with Sociodemographic Factors, Dental Caries Status, and Oral Health–Related Quality of Life in 12- and 15-Year-Old Thai Children." *Journal of Public Health Dentistry* 73: 321–28.

Langford, R., C. P. Bonell, H. E. Jones, T. Pouliou, S. M. Murphy, and others. 2014. "The WHO Health Promoting School Framework for Improving the Health and Well-Being of Students and Their Academic Achievement." *Cochrane Database of Systematic Reviews* 4: CD008958.

Leal, S. C., E. M. Bronkhorst, M. Fan, and J. E. Frencken. 2012. "Untreated Cavitated Dentine Lesions: Impact on Children's Quality of Life." *Caries Research* 46: 102–6.

Lillard, D., and R. Christopoulou. 2015. *Life-Course Smoking Behaviour: Patterns and National Context in Ten Countries.* Oxford, U.K.: Oxford University Press.

Listl, S., J. Galloway, P. A. Mossey, and W. Marcenes. 2015. "Global Economic Impact of Dental Diseases." *Journal of Dental Research* 94: 1355–61.

Macnab, A. J. 2015. "Children's Oral Health: The Opportunity for Improvement Using the WHO Health Promoting School Model." *Advances in Public Health* 2015: 1–6.

Macnab, A. J., and A. Kasangaki. 2012. "'Many Voices, One Song': A Model for an Oral Health Programme as a First Step in Establishing a Health Promoting School." *Health Promotion International* 27: 63–73.

Marcenes, W., N. J. Kassebaum, E. Bernabe, A. Flaxman, M. Naghavi, and others. 2013. "Global Burden of Oral Conditions in 1990–2010: A Systematic Analysis." *Journal of Dental Research* 92: 592–97.

Marck, K. W. 2013. "Noma: A Neglected Enigma." *The Lancet Global Health* 1: e58–59.

Marinho, V. C. C., J. P. T. Higgins, S. Logan, and A. Sheiham. 2003. "Fluoride Toothpastes for Preventing Dental Caries in Children and Adolescents." *Cochrane Database of Systematic Reviews* 1: CD002278.

Marinho, V. C. C., H. V. Worthington, T. Walsh, and J. E. Clarkson. 2013. "Fluoride Varnishes for Preventing Dental Caries in Children and Adolescents." *Cochrane Database of Systematic Reviews* 7: CD002279.

Miotto, M. H., L. A. Barcellos, and Z. V. Lopes. 2013. [Dental Pain as a Predictor of Absenteeism among Workers in a Juice Factory in Southeastern Brazil]. *Cien Saude Colet* 18: 3183–90.

Mock, C. E., P. Conkar, A. Gawande, D. T. Jamison, M. E. Kruk, and H. T. Debas. 2015. "Essential Surgery: Key Messages of this Volume." In *Disease Control Priorities* (third edition): Volume 1, *Essential Surgery*, edited by H. T. Debas, P. Donkor, A. Gawande, D. T. Jamison, M. E. Kruk, and C. N. Mock. Washington, DC: World Bank.

Monse, B., and H. Benzian. 2011. "The Philippine Fit for School Programme." In *Rethinking School Health*, edited by D. A. P. Bundy, 168–73. Washington, DC: World Bank.

Monse, B., E. Naliponguit, V. J. Belizario, A. Schratz, and others. 2013. "The Fit for School Health Outcome Study: A Longitudinal Survey to Assess Health Impacts of an Integrated School Health Programme in the Philippines." *BMC Public Health* 13: 256.

Moynihan, P. J., and S. A. Kelly. 2014. "Effect on Caries of Restricting Sugars Intake: Systematic Review to Inform WHO Guidelines." *Journal of Dental Research* 93: 8–18.

Naidoo, S., U. M. Chikte, and A. Sheiham. 2001. "Prevalence and Impact of Dental Pain in 8–10-Year-Olds in the Western Cape." *South African Dental Journal* 56: 521–23.

New Zealand Beverage Guidance Panel. 2014. "Policy Brief: Options to Reduce Sugar Sweetened Beverage (SSB) Consumption in New Zealand." *Pacific Health Dialogue* 20: 98–102.

Niederman, R., M. Feres, and E. Ogunbodede. 2015. "Dentistry." In *Disease Control Priorities* (third edition): Volume 1, *Essential Surgery*, edited by H. T. Debas, P. Donkor, A. Gawande, D. T. Jamison, M. Kruk, and C. N. Mock. Washington, DC: World Bank.

Noro, L. R., A. G. Roncalli, F. I. J. Mendes, K. C. Lima, and A. K. Teixeira. 2014. "Toothache and Social and Economic Conditions among Adolescents in Northeastern Brazil." *Cien Saude Colet* 19: 105–14.

Ogbureke, K., and E. Ogbureke. 2010. "Noma: A Preventable 'Scourge' of African Children." *Open Dentistry Journal* 4: 201–6.

Patel, A. I., and K. E. Hampton. 2011. "Encouraging Consumption of Water in School and Child Care Settings: Access, Challenges, and Strategies for Improvement." *American Journal of Public Health* 101 (8): 1370–79.

Peltzer, K., and S. Pengpid. 2015. "Health Risk Behaviour among In-School Adolescents in the Philippines: Trends between 2003, 2007 and 2011: A Cross-Sectional Study." *International Journal of Environmental Research Public Health* 13 (1): 73.

Peters, L. W., G. Kok, G. T. Ten Dam, G. J. Buijs, and T. G. Paulussen. 2009. "Effective Elements of School Health Promotion across Behavioral Domains: A Systematic Review of Reviews." *BMC Public Health* 9: 182.

Petersen, P. E. 2014. "Strengthening of Oral Health Systems: Oral Health through Primary Health Care." *Medical Principles and Practice* 23 (Suppl 1): 3–9.

Petersen, P. E., D. Bourgeois, D. Bratthall, and H. Ogawa. 2005. "Oral Health Information Systems: Towards Measuring Progress in Oral Health Promotion and Disease Prevention." *Bulletin of the World Health Organization* 83: 686–93.

Petersen, P. E., J. Hunsrisakhun, A. Thearmontree, S. Pithpornchaiyakul, J. Hintao, and others. 2015. "School-Based Intervention for Improving the Oral Health of Children in Southern Thailand." *Community Dental Health* 32: 44–50.

Pine, C. 2007. "Designing School Programmes to be Effective Vehicles for Changing Oral Hygiene Behaviour. *International Dental Journal* 57: 377–81.

Piva, P., and R. Dodd. 2009. "Where Did All the Aid Go? An In-Depth Analysis of Increased Health Aid Flows over the Past 10 Years." *Bulletin of the World Health Organization* 87: 930–39.

Popkin, B. M., L. S. Adair, and S. W. Ng. 2012. "Global Nutrition Transition and the Pandemic of Obesity in Developing Countries." *Nutrition Reviews* 70: 3–21.

Ramos-Jorge, J., I. A. Pordeus, M. L. Ramos-Jorge, L. S. Marques, and S. M. Paiva. 2014. "Impact of Untreated Dental Caries on Quality of Life of Preschool Children: Different Stages and Activity." *Community Dental and Oral Epidemiology* 42: 311–22.

Rayner, M., P. Scarborough, and A. Briggs. 2015. "Public Health England's Report on Sugar Reduction." *BMJ* 351: h6095. doi: http://dx.doi.org/10.1136/bmj.h6095.

Sankaranarayanan, R., K. Ramadas, H. Amarasinghe, S. Subramanian, and N. Johnson. 2015. "Oral Cancer: Prevention, Early Detection, and Treatment." In *Disease Control Priorities* (third edition): Volume 3, *Cancer*, edited by H. Gelband, P. Jha, R. Sankaranarayanan, and S. Horton. Washington, DC: World Bank.

Saraf, D. S., B. Nongkynrih, C. S. Pandav, S. K. Gupta, B. Shah, and others. 2012. "A Systematic Review of School-Based Interventions to Prevent Risk Factors Associated with Noncommunicable Diseases." *Asia Pacific Journal of Public Health* 24: 733–52.

Sheiham, A. 2006. "Dental Caries Affects Body Weight, Growth and Quality of Life in Pre-School Children." *British Dental Journal* 201: 625–26.

Sheiham, A., and R. G. Watt. 2000. "The Common Risk Factor Approach: A Rational Basis for Promoting Oral Health." *Community Dentistry and Oral Epidemiology* 28: 399–406.

UNESCO (United Nations Educational, Scientific and Cultural Organization). 2015. *Education Data*. Institute for Statistics.

U.S. DHHS (United States Department of Health and Human Services). 2000. *Oral Health in America: A Report of the Surgeon General*. Rockville, MD: National Institutes of Health, National Institute of Dental and Craniofacial Research.

Vandevijvere, S., C. Dominick, A. Devi, and G. Swinburn. 2015. "The Healthy Food Environment Policy Index: Findings of an Expert Panel in New Zealand." *Bulletin of the World Health Organization* 93: 294–302.

van Palenstein, H. W., C. Holmgren, B. Monse, and H. Benzian. 2015. "Caries Prevention and Control in Low- and Middle-Income Countries." In *Dental Caries: The Disease and Its Clinical Management*, edited by O. Fejerskov, B. Nyvad, and E. Kidd, 405. New York: Wiley-Blackwell.

Varenne, B. 2015. "Integrating Oral Health with Non-Communicable Diseases as an Essential Component of General Health: WHO's Strategic Orientation for the African Region." *Journal of Dental Education* 79 (5 Suppl): S32–37.

Watt, R. G. 2007. "From Victim Blaming to Upstream Action: Tackling the Social Determinants of Oral Health Inequalities." *Community Dental and Oral Epidemiology* 35: 1–11.

Wilder, J. R., L. M. Kaste, A. Handler, T. Chapple-McGruder, and K. M. Rankin. 2015. "The Association between Sugar-Sweetened Beverages and Dental Caries among Third-Grade Students in Georgia." *Journal of Public Health Dentistry* 76 (1): 76–84.

WHO (World Health Organization). 2015. *Guideline: Sugars Intake for Adults and Children*. Geneva: WHO.

WHO, FDI World Dental Federation, International Association for Dental Research, and Chinese Stomatological Association. 2007. "Beijing Declaration: Achieving Dental Health through Fluoride in China and South East Asia." Conference on Dental Health through Fluoride in China and South East Asia, Beijing, China, September 18–19.

World Education Forum. 2000. *Focusing Resources on Effective School Health (FRESH): A FRESH Start to Improving the Quality and Equity of Education*. Dakar, Senegal: World Education Forum.

Yee, R., and A. Sheiham. 2002. "The Burden of Restorative Dental Treatment for Children in Third World Countries." *International Dental Journal* 52 (1): 1–9.

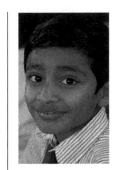

Chapter 17

Disability in Middle Childhood and Adolescence

Natasha Graham, Linda Schultz,
Sophie Mitra, and Daniel Mont

INTRODUCTION

Worldwide, people with disabilities have difficulty accessing education, health services, and employment. Disability is an economic development issue because it is linked to poverty: disability may increase the risk of poverty, and poverty may increase the risk of disability (Sen 2009). A growing body of evidence indicates that children with disabilities and their families are more likely than their peers to experience economic disadvantage, especially in low- and middle-income countries (LMICs).

Approximately 15 percent of the world's adult population lives with some form of disability (WHO and World Bank 2011). Children ages 0–14 years account for slightly less than 6 percent of persons with disabilities globally, but the number of disabled children is grossly underestimated in LMICs (UNICEF 2008). The estimates for prevalence of disability among children fall in a wide range because the methods for identifying them in surveys have varied (Cappa, Petrowski, and Njelesani 2015). This variation results from the complexity of identifying childhood disability (Meltzer 2010, 2016). However, new international standards offer hope for good quality, internationally comparable data moving forward.

This chapter expands on a central theme of this volume: the need for a multisectoral approach to addressing the complex interactions between child and adolescent development and physical and mental health.

In particular, we have focused on the relationship with education—the gateway to participating fully in society, securing a livelihood, and capitalizing on the opportunities that society offers. Children with disabilities are less likely to attend school; when they do attend school, they are less likely to stay in school and be promoted (Filmer 2005; Mizunoya, Mitra, and Yamasaki 2016; WHO and World Bank 2011). They account for a large proportion of children who do not complete a primary education, reducing their employment opportunities and productivity in adulthood (Burchardt 2005; Filmer 2008; Mete 2008).

The literature has focused on advocacy, reflecting the relative neglect of this important area. This focus is beginning to change, at least with regard to the availability of information, and efforts to provide more quantitatively rigorous information are increasing (see, for example, WHO and World Bank 2011). However, information for children and adolescents ages 5–19 years is notably lacking, especially from LMICs. In this age group, the focus has been on schoolchildren and the development consequences of excluding children from education. In the absence of a comprehensive economic analysis or review of disability and development in children and adolescents, this chapter makes extensive use of case studies, which document real-world efforts in LMICs to address disability in this age group in poor communities.

Corresponding author: Daniel Mont, Center for Inclusive Policy, Washington, DC, United States; danielmont01@gmail.com.

Through the use of these case studies, this chapter provides examples of how deprivations can become disability if children are excluded from school in LMICs. The case studies emphasize interventions to ensure that children with disabilities gain access to education, and they examine the design of supportive education systems and the use of school health programs to address the needs of children with impairments. Most assessments have focused on physical disability, especially mobility, and they provide this specific perspective on barriers to education. Little is known about these common forms of disability in LMICs; even less is known about the impact of socio-behavioral constraints, such as those associated with autism, which we know to be prevalent and important constraints in high-income countries (HICs). This chapter explores this issue in a case study of a rare program in a lower-middle-income country in Sub-Saharan Africa. Definitions of age groupings and age-specific terminology used in this volume can be found in chapter 1 (Bundy, de Silva, and others 2017).

DISABILITY DEFINITIONS AND MEASUREMENTS

Disability can be defined and measured in several ways. Traditionally, disability was considered a medical issue to prevent or cure (medical model). Later, disability came to be considered a social construct that required societal changes (social model). More recently, interactional models of disability have been developed that combine both medical and social determinants and courses of action. In this bio-psychosocial model, disability is seen as emerging from the interaction between impairments and the environment; environment is understood as going beyond the physical environment to include the cultural and institutional environments. Several inter-actional models are available (Mitra 2006; Shakespeare 2006); the most influential is the one underlying the International Classification of Functioning, Disability and Health (ICF) (WHO 2002). In the ICF, disability refers to the negative aspects of the interaction between the individual with a health condition and the context of the person (such as physical and attitudinal). Under the ICF, disability is used as an umbrella term for impairments, activity limitations, and participation restrictions. In addition to theoretical definitions for these models, various definitions of disability are used by statistical agencies that collect information on censuses and surveys, as well as by legislative and political bodies to determine eligibility for disability programs or coverage under disability rights laws. The UN Convention on the Rights of Persons with Disabilities uses a concept of disability consistent with the social model.[1]

The differing nuances of the word *disability* and the differing cultural contexts within which people operate have made internationally comparable data on the incidence, distribution, and trends difficult to obtain. Where children are involved, further complexities arise. For example, survey questions developed for adults but used for children may skew the results (WHO and World Bank 2011), and caregivers who complete surveys may not accurately portray children's experiences (Chamie 1994). The setting for data collection can also affect the prevalence estimates for children. For example, HICs often identify disability in medical or educational settings, but many LMICs do not have formal services for identifying children with disabilities (Cappa, Petrowski, and Njelesani 2015).

Progress is being made with respect to measuring disability in an internationally comparable manner, and the United Nations Children's Fund (UNICEF) and the Washington Group on Disability Statistics (WG) have developed a survey for identifying children with disabilities. Data using the child functioning module, or *child questionnaire* have been finalized and ready for use.

The WG has also developed questions for adults that have already been adopted in censuses, general surveys, and disability-specific surveys, creating a growing evidence base for work on disability and development (Altman 2016). Both the WG's adult and the child measures define people with disabilities as those with functional and basic activity limitations that put them at risk of social exclusion due to barriers in the environment (Altman 2016).

Various ethical considerations arise when collecting data on children with disabilities. Data on children come from surveys of mothers or primary caretakers. Caretakers who have responded to questions about children's difficulties functioning might expect that the questions will be followed by services, and a second-stage assessment needs to be linked to service delivery. Another concern is the issue of labeling a child as having a disability. This labeling can cause shame to families in some cultures and can create expectations that limit children. Fortunately, the newer approach to disability identification in surveys, as in the UNICEF/WG instrument, lessens the impact of this issue significantly. The word *disability* is never used, and children are never labeled as having a disability. Children are identified only anonymously in statistical analyses, rather than on a case-by-case basis in person.

This chapter defines disability by a person's functional, activity, and participation limitations based on his or her physical, cultural, and policy environments. The concept of disability is not solely equated with a medical diagnosis; it encompasses an environment that restricts a person's activity and participation. A lack of assistive devices, an inaccessible physical environment, negative attitudes, and stereotypes all prevent people from participating in society on an equal basis. Because this chapter is a literature review, it also uses the definitions underlying the studies under review, which may be different from the above definition.

PREVALENCE BY AGE AND TYPE OF DISABILITY

The estimated prevalence of childhood disability varies substantially across and within countries, depending on questionnaires and study designs under use. The prevalence estimates in this chapter are not definitive but rather a reflection of available data. A literature review by Cappa, Petrowski, and Njelesani (2015) found that the prevalence of childhood disability in LMICs ranged from less than 1 percent to almost 50 percent. Unfortunately, census data are not good sources of data on disability among children because census questions—even the short set of WG questions recommended for use in censuses by the United Nations Statistical Commission—are not effective in identifying children with developmental disabilities. A special child-functioning survey module is needed to accurately assess disability status, and this module would be too long for use in censuses.

Despite the shortcomings of the measures used to date, there are a number of estimates of disability prevalence among children. Based on the latest Global Burden of Disease (GBD) data (IHME 2016), on average, a greater percentage of children ages 0–14 years in LMICs are estimated to have a disability compared with children of the same age group in HICs (table 17.1). The IHME statistics define disability in a particular way because it is used as the basis for the estimation of disability-adjusted life years. Disability in this context includes the acute, often temporary, and typically reversible disability that arises from, for example, an episode of influenza, a bout of malaria, or a broken limb, as well as the chronic, often permanent, and typically irreversible conditions within the more usual definitions of disability. As a result, the IHME definition leads to estimates that suggest a much larger proportion of the population is affected.

UNICEF (2005) estimates that 150 million children and adolescents younger than age 18 years live with disability. Mizunoya, Mitra, and Yamasaki (2016), using the WG questions for adults, found that the median prevalence stands at 0.8 percent and 1 percent for primary- and secondary-school-age children, respectively, in 15 LMICs. Disability prevalence in primary-school-age children did not surpass 1.5 percent in 12 of 15 countries, but it was much higher in 3 countries (2.9 percent in Uganda; 4.5 percent in South Africa, and 5.0 percent in Maldives). Disability prevalence rates in secondary-school-age children do not exceed about 2.0 percent in 13 of 15 countries. None of these disability prevalence estimates for children is satisfactory, and more research and data collection are needed in this area.

The GBD estimates are inferred from data on health conditions and impairments alone, using available data on distributions of limitations that may result from health conditions and impairments. Mizunoya, Mitra, and Yamasaki (2016) used a questionnaire developed for adults, which is known to be unable to identify certain disabilities that prevail among children, such as developmental disabilities.

There are many types of disability, with varying degrees of severity. A disability can be physical, cognitive, psychosocial, communicative, or sensory. The nature of the causes of the impairments associated with these disabilities can vary significantly by country context, as can the types of barriers that children with those disabilities face. Attention to the type of disability can add a good deal of depth to the analyses of disability data and the development and implementation of disability policies. *Disease Control Priorities in Developing Countries*, second edition, discusses discuss loss of vision and hearing (Frick and others 2006) as well as learning and developmental disabilities (Durkin and others 2006).

Unfortunately, good-quality data on the type of disability—especially data that are internationally comparable—are difficult to obtain (Cappa, Petrowski, and Njelesani 2015; Maulik and Darmstadt 2007). That is one reason that UNICEF and the WG have developed a module on childhood disability. Even data using the Ten Question Screening Instrument adopted in UNICEF's Multiple Indicator Cluster Survey are of limited use in this regard for several reasons. First, the instrument was not designed for complete disaggregation by type of disability. Second, it was designed as part of a two-stage process. The first stage was to cast a wide net to capture all children who might possibly be identified as having a disability, to be followed by more detailed assessment. The second stage, however, is rarely done, which presumably creates false positives for studies using only the Ten Question Screening Instrument. There is no reason to believe that the false positives in the dataset have the same distribution by type of disability as the true positives. Where follow-up assessments have been used (for example, the 2013 Two-Stage Child Disability Study in Bhutan undertaken by the Bhutan National Statistics Bureau), however, there have been questions about their quality because they require personnel with specific training. The Bhutan report notes that some level of issues arose with the cognitive follow-up assessments.

Table 17.1 Estimated Point Prevalence of Disability and Severity among Children and Adolescents Ages 0–14 across WHO Regions

percent

Sex and age group (years)	World	High-income countries	Low- and Middle-Income Countries, WHO Region					
			Africa	Americas	Eastern Mediterranean	Europe	South-East Asia	Western Pacific
No disability								
Male 0–14	30	37	22	31	35	36	30	32
Female 0–14	30	37	22	30	33	36	30	31
Very mild disability								
Male 0–14	12	11	13	11	11	13	12	11
Female 0–14	11	12	13	11	11	13	11	11
Mild disability								
Male 0–14	18	15	20	19	18	17	21	19
Female 0–14	20	17	22	21	20	19	23	20
Moderate disability								
Male 0–14	22	23	23	21	19	20	21	21
Female 0–14	22	22	23	21	20	20	20	21
Severe disability								
Male 0–14	15	12	18	15	14	12	15	14
Female 0–14	14	10	17	14	14	11	14	13
Very severe disability								
Male 0–14	2	2	3	2	2	2	2	2
Female 0–14	2	2	3	3	2	2	2	2

Source: IHME 2016.

Note: High-income countries includes Asia Pacific and North America. Western Pacific includes East Asia, South Asia, Central Asia, Oceania, Australasia, and the Western Pacific.

Comparison problems arise in HICs as well. As table 17.2 shows, data on disability among children and adolescents from Australia and the United States are not comparable; the age categories are different as are the categories of types of disabilities assessed. One common result, even with these differences, is that boys have a higher rate of disability. This is a common finding across almost all child disability surveys.

Using its 10-question Multiple Indicator Cluster Survey, UNICEF screened more than 200,000 children ages two to nine years in 20 countries for risk of disability (UNICEF 2008). Between 14 percent and 35 percent of children screened positive for risk of disability in most countries (UN Statistics Division 2010). However, this finding is an overestimate because the questions were designed to be a first-stage screen to be followed by a more detailed assessment that was not conducted.

The surveys revealed important trends in disability risk among children. For example, children in ethnic minority groups, from poorer households, and with limited early childhood education were more likely than their peers to screen positive for disability (UNICEF 2008). Weight and nutrition are risk factors as well (Groce and others 2013). Low birth weight and a lack of essential dietary nutrients, such as iodine or folic acid, are associated with incidence and prevalence of disability (Hack, Klein, and Taylor 1995; UNICEF 2008; Wang and others 1997). The proportion of children at risk for disability increases among children with severe stunting and nutrient deprivation (UNICEF 2008). An estimated 200 million children younger than age five years do not reach their full cognitive, social, and emotional development potential (Grantham-McGregor and others 2007).

Table 17.2 Prevalence of Disability by Type of Disability, Australia and the United States
percent

| | Australia | | | United States | | |
| | Ages 0–14 years | | | Ages 5–17 years | | |
	Boys	Girls	All	Boys	Girls	All
Intellectual or learning	5.2	2.0	3.7	—	—	—
Remembering	—	—	—	5.3	2.8	4.1
Psychiatric	1.5	0.7	1.1	—	—	—
Sensory or speech	4.0	2.1	3.1	—	—	—
Hearing	—	—	—	0.6	0.6	0.6
Vision	—	—	—	0.9	0.8	0.8
Physical	4.2	3.1	3.7	0.7	0.6	0.6
Acquired brain injury	0.5	0.2	0.3	—	—	—
Going outside the home	—	—	—	2.2	1.8	2.0
Dressing	—	—	—	1.2	0.7	0.9
Total	9.6	5.4	7.6	6.5	4.0	5.3

Sources: AIHW 2004; American Community Survey 2014, https://www.census.gov/people/disability.

Note: — = not available. The columns sum to more than the total because some children have multiple disabilities and so are included in more than one row.

DISABILITY AND SOCIOECONOMIC INEQUALITIES: DETERMINANTS, CONSEQUENCES, AND CORRELATION

Disability is both a determinant and a consequence of socioeconomic inequalities. Children in poor families or communities, in LMICs especially, are exposed to poverty-related risk factors that may contribute to the onset of health conditions associated with disability. Low birth weight and cumulative deprivations from malnutrition (Black and others 2008; UNICEF 2008), lack of clean water, and inadequate sanitation can manifest in developmental disabilities (Rauh, Landrigan, and Claudio 2008). In addition, lack of access to health services may convert a health condition into a disability. Finally, a child with a disability might experience further issues that exacerbate the severity of his or her disability (Krahn, Hammond, and Turner 2006). First, certain resources, such as clean water and sanitation or health clinics, may be inaccessible. Second, individuals with disabilities may be subjected to discrimination within their families and receive a disproportionately low share of familial resources (Rosales-Rueda 2014).

Growing evidence suggests a correlation between poverty and disability among children and adults with disability (WHO and World Bank 2011). Overall, in LMICs the evidence points to individuals with disability often being economically worse off in educational attainment; the evidence is more mixed with regard to employment,

household assets, and expenditures (Mitra, Posarac, and Vick 2013; Mizunoya and Mitra 2013). However, several studies have provided growing evidence that disability is associated with a higher likelihood of experiencing multiple deprivations simultaneously (Mitra, Posarac, and Vick 2013; Trani and Canning 2013; Trani and others 2015; Trani and others 2016). Although the nature of deprivations may vary across countries, they may include employment, health, educational attainment, household material well-being, social participation, or psychological well-being.

Even with the same levels of income, people with disabilities and their households are likely to be effectively poorer than people without disabilities and their households. This trend is in part due to the direct costs of disability, for example, higher health and transportation costs (Braithwaite and Mont 2009; Cullinan, Gannon, and Lyons 2011; Zaidi and Burchardt 2005). Researchers have attempted to quantify the extra cost of living with a disability, but the findings vary considerably. The costs of disability accounted for an estimated 9 percent of income in Vietnam, 14 percent in Bosnia and Herzegovina, and 11 percent to 69 percent in the United Kingdom (Braithwaite and Mont 2009; Zaidi and Burchardt 2005).

The direct and indirect costs related to disability can worsen social and economic well-being through many channels, including the costs associated with medical care, assistive devices, personal support, and exclusion from employment (Jenkins and Rigg 2003). People with disabilities can be poorer because of the loss of work productivity resulting from various factors including their exclusion from the workforce, as well as from the more limited labor participation of their family members who might have care-giving responsibilities (Buckup 2009; Palmer and others 2015). The estimated cost of lost productivity due to exclusion from employment among individuals with disabilities is as high as 7 percent of gross domestic product (Buckup 2009). Many of the direct and indirect costs could be reduced if inaccessible environments were more inclusive (WHO and World Bank 2011). This two-way causality between disability and socioeconomic deprivations may also combine with other factors, such as violence and conflict, that may lead to both disability and poverty simultaneously.

Educational opportunities may mitigate some of the associations between disability and poverty. In a cross-country study of 13 LMICs, disability was associated with a higher probability of being poor, but this correlation was no longer statistically significant once educational attainment was controlled for, suggesting that education could mediate this association (Filmer 2008).

DISABILITY AND EDUCATION

Many children with disabilities have been excluded from mainstream educational opportunities in many parts of the world. Education is particularly important for disabled children, who are often stigmatized or excluded. School attendance helps dispel the misconceptions about disability that serve as barriers to inclusion in other spheres (Bundy 2011). Education bolsters human capital, minimizes barriers to entering the workforce, and improves economic earning potential.

Inclusive education is based on the belief that all children can learn and should have access to a curriculum and necessary adaptations to ensure meaningful educational attainment. Support for inclusive education is gaining momentum in LMICs, with a few countries adapting strategies to fit the local context. Durkin and others (2006) examine interventions likely to improve child development and educational outcomes for children in LMICs. At present, no country has a fully inclusive system (WHO and World Bank 2011).

School Attendance

A large body of evidence shows that adults with disabilities in LMICs have lower educational attainment than adults without disabilities: Bulgaria, Georgia, Moldava, Romania (Mete 2008); 15 countries (Mitra, Posarac, and Vick 2013); Vietnam (Mont and Cuong 2011); Afghanistan and Zambia (Trani and Loeb 2012); Morocco and Tunisia (Trani and others 2015); India (World Bank 2007); 51 LMICs and HICs (WHO and World Bank 2011).

This association, consistently found among adults, may result from lower school attendance among children with disabilities, or it may be due to more frequent onsets of disability among adults with limited educational attainment, for example, via malnutrition, lack of access to health care, and risky working conditions.

There is a small but growing literature on school attendance and disability in LMICs. Much of this literature is descriptive and documents the extent of the gap in school attendance across disability status (Filmer 2008; Trani and Canning 2013). Filmer (2008) documents gaps in school attendance across disability status in 13 LMICs from 1992 to 2005, ranging from 10 percent to 60 percent in middle childhood (ages 6–11 years), and 15 percent to 58 percent in adolescence (ages 12–17 years), although the measures of disability vary substantially. Studies in Malawi, Namibia, Zambia, and Zimbabwe found that, while only 9 percent to 18 percent of nondisabled children older than age five years had never attended school, 24 percent to 39 percent of disabled children had never done so (Eide and Loeb 2006; Eide, van Rooy, and Loeb 2003; Eide and others 2003; Loeb and Eide 2004). In India, close to 40 percent of disabled children were not enrolled in school, compared with 8 percent to 10 percent of children in Scheduled Tribes or Castes (World Bank 2007).

Mizunoya, Mitra, and Yamasaki (2016) explored the gap in enrollment in primary and secondary education between children with and without disabilities using the WG measure for adults. Using nationally representative datasets from 15 LMICs, they found consistent and statistically significant disability gaps in both primary and secondary education in all countries. A household fixed effects model shows that disability reduces the probability of school attendance by a median of 30.9 percentage points, and that neither the individual characteristics nor their socioeconomic and unobserved household characteristics explain the disability gap. This finding indicates that general poverty reduction policies through social transfers to the poor will not contribute to closing the disability gap in schooling. Finally, Mizunoya, Mitra, and Yamasaki (2016) found that the disability gaps for primary-school-age children follow an inverted U-shape relationship with gross national income (GNI) per capita. This result suggests that, as GNI per capita rises and more resources become available for improving access to education, children without disabilities increasingly attend school, whereas the situation of children with disabilities may improve only slowly.

Among children with disabilities, enrollment rates differ according to type of impairment. In Burkina Faso, disabled children were more than twice as likely not to attend school as other children, but only 10 percent of deaf children were in school, compared with 40 percent of children with other physical disabilities (UNESCO 2010). In India, more than 50 percent of children with mental disabilities were enrolled, compared with 70 percent of children with poor vision, presumably because both physical access and their ability to communicate with teachers is higher for the latter group (Mont 2014).

Barriers to Education

Beyond enrollment and regular attendance, studies show that children with disabilities are more successful in schools that are accessible for all learners (Dessemontent, Bless, and Morin 2012; Kalambouka and others 2007; Lindsay 2007; Ruijs and Peetsma 2009). Common barriers to education include gaps in policy regarding inclusive education, including limited resources, insufficient number of trained teachers, lack of adaptive learning materials, and inaccessible facilities:

- *Accessible facilities.* Building accessible schools is vital to making the transition to inclusive education. Children who use wheelchairs need ramps to enter the school, elevators to attend classes on upper floors, and accessible toilets. Building an accessible school costs barely 1 percent more than building an inaccessible school (Steinfeld 2005), but retrofitting an inaccessible school is considerably more expensive. Incorporating universal design in the floor plan enables schools to include disabled children and minimizes the need for separate schools.
- *Teacher capacity.* Many LMICs educate children with disabilities in separate classrooms or mainstream them into regular classrooms but provide little support. Teacher training and access to specialists are at the core of full inclusion, but very few receive training in inclusive education through either pre- or in-service training (Ferguson 2008; Odom, Buysse, and Soukakou 2011). Children also have limited access to specialists and teaching assistants. Effective programs often include training in inclusive education for administrators at the school, district, and national levels and have the resources, personnel, and discretion to implement changes suitable to the local context.
- *Curriculum design.* A hallmark of inclusive education is having a child-centered curriculum (McLeskey, Waldron, and Redd 2014; Rose, Meyer, and Hitchcock

2005). Curricula in many countries are not adapted to the learning needs, challenges, and strengths of individual children. Inclusive education policies can benefit all children because such policies are intended to respond to individual differences and abilities.
- *Environmental barriers outside the school system.* Schools exist within an environmental context, and exclusion may result from barriers not within the school's purview. These barriers can include, for example, inaccessible transportation, poor provision of assistive devices, and inaccessible health clinics that make the health of children with disabilities more fragile. Exclusion can also result from parents being less willing to send their children to school because of low expectations of the utility of that education or from feelings of shame.

Addressing these issues requires both policy- and school-level changes, as well as an action plan (McGregor and Vogelsberg 1998; Bundy 2011). Perhaps the most important requirement is school- and policy-level leadership committed to educating all children.

Several avenues are available for financing special needs education. Brazil used the national budget to establish a special national fund; Pakistan allocated funding from its national budget to finance a special education network of schools. Nicaragua and Panama dedicate a fixed amount of the overall education budget, 0.92 percent and 2.3 percent, respectively, to special needs education. Chile and Mexico cover the financial costs of special needs institutions, including materials, training, and teaching aids. Denmark, Finland, Hungary, and New Zealand help individuals offset the additional costs of educating a child with special needs. Switzerland and the United States have implemented combined approaches (Hartman 1992; Parrish 1994).

MEASURING ECONOMIC RETURNS OF INCLUSIVE INTERVENTIONS

Measuring the economic returns to inclusive education is complex because the costs are incurred in the short term, but the benefits accrue in the long term. Rigorous evaluations and economic analyses of how to invest in inclusive education programs or the returns generated by inclusive education are not yet available. As a result, the return on investment, children's income potential, and the increase in caretaker productivity are not well known.

In Nepal, education has a bigger impact on the future earnings of children with disabilities than on those of other children (Lamichhane and Sawada 2013). Gains in functional capacity can be largest when interventions occur early in children's development. Early detection of developmental delays can improve development and school readiness (WHO and UNICEF 2011). Removing barriers early can minimize the compounding effects of multiple barriers. One approach is to use education as an equalizing platform, especially in the formative years.

The returns to inclusive education, rehabilitation services, or any other intervention depend on future barriers that individuals with disabilities will face as adults. If significant barriers to employment are coupled with discrimination, transportation difficulties, and weak labor laws, the return on childhood interventions may be small.

Following this line of reasoning, countries with fewer barriers to adult activities will gain higher returns from child services. One sectoral reform by itself may not have a substantial return, but improving inclusion in multiple sectors creates synergies that will increase those returns in the future.

CASE STUDIES

These six case studies provide a nuanced look at both the progress in and the barriers to improving educational provision and participation for children with disabilities. They illustrate how the first steps to inclusive education have been taken in different settings. Observing the positive effects of inclusive education in schools and in communities can spur the development of equitable policies in other sectors.

Case Study 1. Vision, Learning, and Free Eyeglasses

Elisabetta Aurino, Lesley Drake, Paul Glewwe, Imran Khan, and Kristine West contributed this case study.

Poor vision can affect the development of children and adolescents and the economic prosperity of a country, costing the world more than US$200 billion a year (Fricke and others 2012).[2] However, data on the prevalence of visual impairments in school-age children and adolescents are limited and varied. In one 2004 study, 1 percent of school-age children ages 5–15 years (almost 13 million) were visually impaired (Resnikoff and others 2008). Country-specific estimates range from 1 percent in Malawi (Lee 2016), to 13 percent in China (Glewwe, Park, and Zhao 2016), and 31 percent in high-poverty school districts in the United States (Glewwe, West, and Lee 2015).

Poor vision may lead to poor educational outcomes (Bundy and others 2003). Primary schoolchildren in Northeast Brazil with poor vision had a 10 percentage point higher probability of dropping out and an 18 percentage point higher probability of repeating a grade (Gomes-Neto and others 1997). In rural China, poor vision lowered students' academic performance 0.2–0.3 standard deviation, equivalent to a loss of 0.3 year of schooling (Glewwe, Park, and Zhao 2016). In high-poverty counties in the United States, students with poor vision who received free screening and eyeglasses had a 3.4 and 5.0 percentage point higher probability of passing standardized tests in reading and math, respectively, than similar students in control schools.

Skilled eye care personnel and infrastructure are lacking in LMICs, and schools have become a platform for delivering eye care services in various contexts (Limburg, Kansara, and d'Souza 1999; Sharma and others 2008; Wedner and others 2000; Zhang and others 2011). In Cambodia, teachers were trained to assess whether children and adolescents needed an eye examination (Ormsby and others 2012). Within four weeks, fewer than 100 teachers screened 13,175 students and referred 44 to a team of refractionists, who provided ready-made or customized glasses.

The costs per child were minimal, including operational costs (travel, per diems, training), vision screening kits, and glasses (about US$2–US$3 for ready-made and US$3–US$7 for custom-made glasses). Teachers' time was covered by their salaries, while equipment was borrowed. The cost of eyeglasses can vary by the type of glasses and the region or country. In eight delivery models, eyeglasses cost between US$2.59 and US$7.06 per pair (Wilson 2011). Costs were similar in Zanzibar (Laviers and others 2010). In China, costs ranged between US$2 and US$15 (Glewwe, Park, and Zhao 2016). In the United States, screenings cost about US$2, and examinations and glasses cost about US$100 (Glewwe, West, and Lee 2015).

Baltussen, Naus, and Limburg (2009) modeled the cost-effectiveness of interventions to determine the prevalence of visual impairment by age and enrollment in Africa, America, Asia, and Europe. They also evaluated cost-effectiveness for 10 years and found that annual screening was more cost-effective for adolescents (ages 11–15 years) than for children (ages 5–10 years) because of differences in prevalence and enrollment. Screening at broad age intervals was more cost-effective than screening at single age intervals.

Sustainability and other constraints can be challenging. Eyeglasses need to be replaced regularly, especially in children. Supply constraints relate to lack of trained personnel and poor eye care infrastructure. Demand constraints include lack of awareness of need and societal views that eyewear is unattractive (Kodjebacheva, Maliski, and Coleman 2015). In China, take-up was 65 percent, while in the United States it was 75 percent. The main impediment in all studies was failure to gain parental permission for the exam.

In summary, school-based approaches provide an economically attractive intervention to correct visual impediments that hinder child development.

Case Study 2. Childhood Disability, Education, and Poverty in Vietnam

Daniel Mont contributed this case study.

The WG is the international standard setter for measuring disability at the national level. It identifies the likelihood of disability using the ICF. The questionnaire identifies difficulties that people have in undertaking basic activities (box 17.1). It is also useful for disaggregating socioeconomic indicators by disability status (Loeb 2016).

In 2006, Vietnam based disability questions on the WG questionnaire and included them in the Vietnam Household Living Standards Survey, which was administered to a nationally representative sample of households. The result was a high-quality dataset on both disability and socioeconomic indicators (Mont and Nguyen 2013b).

The poverty rate in Vietnam was 22 percent for people with disabilities and 15 percent for people without disabilities (Mont and Cuong 2011). The poverty gap was even higher for younger people. Poverty was nearly twice as high for children with disabilities, after adjusting for the extra costs of living with a disability, as for other children (table 17.3).

Having a childhood disability was also associated with having less education. Children with disabilities were 41 percent less likely to attend school; excluding children with mild disabilities, that figure rose to 47 percent. Overall, having a disability in childhood was found to significantly reduce the chances of completing

school for older children and adolescents regardless of the definition of disability or type of school. Having a childhood disability also lowered the level of completed education. Moreover, having a parent with a disability reduced the chances that children without disabilities would attend school (Mont and Nguyen 2013a).

Including the WG questions on both the census and household survey allowed for small-area estimation of the relationship between poverty and disability. The poverty gap between households with and without a disabled member varied significantly and was lower in areas with better infrastructure and health care services (Mont and Nguyen 2013b).

This dataset from Vietnam adds weight to the relationship between disability and poverty. As the questionnaires are administered more widely, policy makers can better determine where the link between disability and poverty is strongest and what the most promising and appropriate avenues are for designing interventions to weaken that link.

Case Study 3. Disability-Inclusive School Health and Nutrition Programs

Sergio Meresman and Cai Heath contributed this case study.

School health and nutrition programs have increasingly been recognized for their educational impact on the most vulnerable learners (PCD 2015). Inclusive education encompasses children who have difficulty seeing or hearing, limited mobility, or difficulty learning in classrooms designed for children without disabilities. *Disability-inclusive school health and nutrition* refers to educational approaches designed to meet the needs of all children who are vulnerable to dropping out or being excluded from education,

---

Box 17.1

Washington Group Short Set of Questions on Disability

The next questions ask about difficulties you may have doing certain activities because of a HEALTH PROBLEM.

1. Do you have difficulty seeing, even if wearing glasses?
2. Do you have difficulty hearing, even if using a hearing aid?
3. Do you have difficulty walking or climbing steps?
4. Do you have difficulty remembering or concentrating?

5. Do you have difficulty (with self-care such as) washing all over or dressing?
6. Using your usual (customary) language, do you have difficulty communicating, for example, understanding or being understood?

Possible responses for all questions are no difficulty, some difficulty, a lot of difficulty, and cannot do at all.

Table 17.3 Poverty Rates for People in Vietnam, with and without Disabilities, 2006
percent

Current age (years)	People without disabilities	People with disabilities	People with disabilities after accounting for extra costs of living with a disability
5–18	19.3	31.1	36.2
19–40	15.1	24.7	31.4
41–62	9.2	11.9	15.3
Older than 62	14.5	17.0	22.8

Source: Mont and Cuong 2011.

Table 17.4 Pillars of the FRESH Framework

FRESH pillar	Key concepts for inclusion	Practical implications
Equitable school health policies	Inclusive development; universal design	Gather and disaggregate data on children with disabilities; require adequate and sustainable funding; make policy makers aware and trained
A safe learning environment	Physical access; stigma-free environment	Follow accessibility standards; promote human rights, equity, and diversity to remove attitudinal barriers
Skills-based health education	Curriculum adaptations; information, education, and communication materials in accessible formats (Braille, sign language, easy reading)	Adapt methodologies and content to the learning needs of all children; provide accessible learning materials
School-based health and nutrition services	Inclusive delivery of health and nutrition services; cross-sector collaboration; integrated approaches to programming	Train teachers and health workers in inclusive school health and nutrition; provide health screening and appropriate assistive devices; conduct high-quality context analysis; support inclusive homegrown school feeding programs; provide inclusive water, sanitation, and hygiene programming; engage families and organizations to support outreach and delivery of services

Source: Meresman and others 2015.
Note: FRESH = Focusing Resources on Effective School Health.

including children with disabilities, orphans, migrants, those affected by human immunodeficiency virus/acquired immune deficiency syndrome (HIV/AIDS), those who do not speak the language used in the classroom or who belong to a different religion or caste, and those who are sick, hungry, or not excelling academically.

In 2000, the Education for All goals and Focusing Resources on Effective School Health (FRESH) framework were launched at the World Education Forum in Dakar (FRESH Initiative 2000). The framework outlines approaches that support effective school health programming (table 17.4).

The FRESH framework is helpful for designing and implementing disability-inclusive school programs because it addresses the needs of the learners from multiple angles. For more information on FRESH, see chapter 20 in this volume on school as a platform for addressing health (Bundy, Schultz, and others 2017).

Although a disability-inclusive approach to school health and nutrition programming is a recent concept, the need for these strategies in education sector planning has long been apparent. Kenya's 2005–10 Education Sector Plan identified two key gaps: a lack of clear guidelines on the implementation of an all-inclusive education policy and a lack of reliable data on children with special needs (Republic of Kenya 2005). Zanzibar's 2008–16 Education Sector Plan noted, "Enrollment of children with special needs is low [and] this results in insufficient support to people with special needs." Key strategies included designing all education interventions in a disability-inclusive manner, collecting more accurate data, and improving training for teachers (Government of Zanzibar 2007).

School health and nutrition programs are becoming more disability inclusive. In Kenya the government's homegrown school feeding program (discussed in chapter 12 in this volume, Drake and others 2017) sought to improve targeting and data collection for all vulnerable children, sensitize teachers and parents, and provide vocational training to improve economic outcomes (PCD 2013).

Case Study 4. Early Childhood Monitoring to Screen for Disability in the Lao People's Democratic Republic

Sally Brinkman contributed this case study.

The Lao People's Democratic Republic is a predominantly rural low-income country. More than two-thirds of the country's 6.5 million people live in rural areas, where the poverty rate is almost 30 percent (Lao Population and Housing Census 2015; Lao Statistics Bureau 2014). Most rural children have never seen a doctor, and less than one-fifth of the population lives in villages with health centers; three in four villages have primary schools (Lao Population and Housing Census 2015). Little is known about the situation of children with disabilities (Evans and others 2014).

In April 2014, the Early Childhood Education Program received funding to improve child development and school readiness and establish a monitoring system to measure child development. The program includes a two-phase process. First-phase screening is part of a population-wide system for monitoring childhood development. Second-phase screening is provided to children who were identified in the first phase as having a disability or impairment (World Bank 2014).

The project is collecting baseline data using the WG short set of questions on disability, with data to be collected on an estimated 6,500 children across five provinces. The results will demonstrate the questionnaire's effectiveness in Lao PDR and determine the prevalence of childhood disability—both important steps in filling the current knowledge gap regarding children with disabilities.

The most likely impediment to scale-up of the program will be the expense and service capacity needs associated with second-phase screening, which must be covered by the health care system, nongovernment agencies, or families. Analyzing the results of first-phase screening against the diagnostic tests to assess the costs of scaling up to the national level will be important.

Case Study 5. Autism Spectrum Disorders: Providing Inclusive Education in Kilifi, Kenya

Amina Abubakar, Andy Shih, Joseph Gona, and Amy Daniels contributed this case study.

The prevalence of autism spectrum disorders has grown considerably in recent decades. Today an estimated 1 in 68 children in the United States has autism (CDC 2014), and estimated prevalence is comparable in other regions (Elsabbagh and others 2012). Autism is typically a lifelong condition characterized by impaired social interaction and communication and the presence of restrictive or repetitive behavior. Children with autism are significantly more likely to have intellectual disabilities and other mental and physical conditions than other children. Autism can severely affect the quality of life of autistic persons and their caregivers.

In the United States, autism was estimated to cost US$1.4 million for individuals over a lifetime and US$137 billion for society per year (Buescher and others 2014). Less is known about the costs of autism in LMICs (Wang and others 2012; Xiong and others 2011).

In Kenya, inclusive education has been a major government policy for many years, but most children with disabilities continue to receive their education in special schools and units (Adoyo 2007; Kenya Ministry of Education 2009). To investigate some of the factors that have hindered the success of inclusive education, Autism Speaks conducted a small qualitative survey of stakeholders, including teachers, placement officers, and representatives of a community-based organization, in Kilifi, Kenya. The discussions centered on the challenges facing the mainstreaming agenda and the steps that could be taken to facilitate inclusive education. Questions were asked about children with autism, although the interview also touched on other forms of disability.

The survey revealed that inclusive education in Kilifi faces four principal challenges: teacher-related problems (lack of training; poor attitude toward inclusion), family obstacles (preference for separate education; tendency to delay the start of school for children with disability), inadequate resources (inadequate facilities; large class sizes), and government policies (motivation allowances for teachers in special units but not for teachers with disabled students in regular schools; former practice of basing school resources on test results). Teachers in mainstream schools identified lack of adequate training for handling children with disabilities as the major hindrance to inclusive education.

What needs to be done to facilitate inclusive education in Kenya and other low-resource settings? Participants from the study highlighted four areas that have the potential to be scaled up in Kenya and other countries:

- Train and provide teachers in mainstream schools with the skills required to handle students with special needs

- Ensure that children with limited mobility can move around the school comfortably
- Initiate parent-based interventions aimed at raising awareness and encouraging them to time school matriculation properly, reinforce skill-building techniques at home, and become engaged in inclusive education efforts
- Make special needs education mandatory for all teacher trainees and critically evaluate the current teacher education curriculum in colleges and universities to ensure an all-inclusive curriculum.

Taking steps to implement the policy and provide adequate infrastructural support for learners with special needs will contribute toward a more inclusive educational setting in Kilifi, Kenya, specifically, and in other low-resource settings more generally.

Case Study 6. Targeting HIV Prevention and Sexual Health Education for Young People with Hearing Loss in Brazil and Uruguay

Sergio Meresman contributed this case study.

Persons with disabilities are at high risk of HIV/AIDS exposure and are disproportionately affected by the epidemic in communities worldwide (World Bank 2003). The main drivers of the epidemic are strongly associated with disability, including a high prevalence of poverty (Inclusion International 2006; Watermeyer 2006), lack of education (Helander 1999; Muthukrishna 2006; World Bank 2003), and lack of access to sexual and reproductive health education or services (DenBoer 2008; Katoda 1993; WHO and UNFPA 2009). Once persons with disabilities become infected, many structural and social factors linked with disability significantly decrease the likelihood that they will receive the treatment, care, and support available to other people living with HIV/AIDS (World Bank 2004).

Because of the misconception that individuals with disability are not exposed to sexual violence and abuse and not at risk of contracting sexually transmitted infections (Berman Bieler and Meresman 2010), prevention campaigns and educational programs frequently overlook this population, making it more vulnerable to the risks of transmission (Groce 2003). A long chain of barriers and taboos—combined with the poverty and exclusion that disproportionately affect persons with disabilities and their families—deprives disabled persons of access to sexuality education suited to their age and needs, to HIV/AIDS programs, and to health services in general.

In South America, the deaf and hard-of-hearing population is one of the largest groups omitted from HIV/AIDS education. In Uruguay, a country with more than 30,000 people who have severe hearing impairments or are deaf (MIDES 2011), most children and adolescents with disabilities attend school but are not involved in health and sexuality education programs (Meresman and others 2015). In Brazil, a country with more than 5 million people who have impaired hearing (CONADIS 2010), HIV/AIDS education has involved marginalized communities for many years, but materials in sign language and inclusive programming have yet to be developed.

Since 2010, the Inter-American Institute on Disability and Inclusive Development, the Center for Health Promotion, and the Partnership for Child Development have been working with deaf organizations in Brazil and Uruguay to promote inclusive approaches to HIV/AIDS education and information on reproductive health. This partnership established the Everyone's School (Escola de Todos) Program, which is administered in collaboration with the national education and health authorities and the national HIV/AIDS programs in both countries. Everyone's School provides access to reproductive health and HIV/AIDS education in sign language for deaf youth. Educational resources were prepared by deaf participants and distributed throughout the deaf community in Brazil and Uruguay. The set included posters, postcards, and quick response (QR) code messages—a digital media platform that is increasingly being used in inclusive school health and nutrition projects—aimed at deaf people. Two workshops were conducted. In each, about 20 participants adapted and translated key messages on health, prevention, and effective condom use into Brazilian and Uruguayan sign language.

As a result of the positive outcomes of the Everyone's School Program, task forces were created with the goal of improving accessibility to programs and services. Such interest spawned new initiatives, including an inclusive prevention grant made available by the National Prevention Program of Uruguay to support training and to design accessible campaigns around sexually transmitted diseases and unwanted pregnancies. A group of deaf youth trained in the initial program is preparing to implement the new initiative.

CONCLUSIONS

The definition of disability has changed over the years and is now commonly used to describe the interaction between impairments and the physical, cultural, and institutional environments. Progress on defining disability has not been matched by efforts to provide standardized estimates of the prevalence of disability. The differing nuances used by statistical agencies, legislative, and political bodies has made it difficult to collect comparable data on prevalence and severity of disability in both LMICs and in HICs, alike.

Education is the gateway into society, but that gateway is not fully open to children with disabilities. Developing polices that equalize the opportunity to receive a quality education requires a deeper understanding of the scope and nature of children with disabilities' exclusion and the barriers they face. Recent development in how we conceptualize and measure disability are beginning to make a difference in our ability to do that.

Introducing inclusive education is the start of a process to increase the ability of individuals with disabilities to participate in their communities. The path to implementing and achieving inclusive education is complex and is likely to be country specific. However, meaningful steps can be taken at all stages of development.

Establishing inclusive education may be slow, but cross-sectoral collaborations will be critical to achieving progress and to documenting and disseminating successes. The impacts of disability are cross-sectoral, and an approach that focuses on a single sector will be less successful than an approach that takes into account the full range of challenges facing a disabled child. Policies that promote access to education will be more fruitful if school-to-work transition programs are in place to promote employment and inclusion for people with disabilities.

Several publications and reports have outlined key actions that governments can take to support children with disabilities (Thomas and Burnett 2013; UNICEF 2013, 2015). The following actions, which are in line with the recommendations of these publications and those outlined in the *World Report on Disability* (WHO and World Bank 2011) and in the *State of the World's Children 2013* (UNICEF 2013), should form part of a successful platform designed to meet the needs of all learners:

- Undertake situational analyses to better understand the nature and scope of the barriers children with disabilities face when it comes to attending school. These studies should rely on the bio-psychosocial model of disability that conceptualizes disability as arising from the interaction between a children's impairments and the environmental barriers they face.
- Promote inclusive education for children with disabilities at all levels, including early childhood education, and review national policies in relevant sectors— health, education, and social—to ensure that they are aligned with international conventions and commitments and inclusive of children with disabilities

- Collect high-quality data about disability and the school environment via administrative data systems consistent with international standards to fill gaps and monitor progress on the education of children with disabilities.
- Analyze sector-wide strategies, programs, and budgets to determine whether they include concrete actions to support children with disabilities and their families
- Develop, implement, and monitor a comprehensive multisector national strategy and plan of action for children with disabilities that addresses family support, community awareness and mobilization, human resources capacity, coordination, and service provision
- Establish clear lines of responsibility and mechanisms for coordination, monitoring, and reporting across sectors
- Ensure that an inclusive education strategy and action plan are part of the education sector plan, including building or retrofitting schools that are accessible for children with disabilities; creating accessible curricula and learning materials, processes, and assessments; and training teachers to foster a commitment to inclusion in schools and communities
- Evaluate and identify gaps in service delivery, advocate for and seek sustainable financial and technical support to address the gaps identified, and link the collection of disability data with service provision

NOTES

World Bank Income Classifications as of July 2014 are as follows, based on estimates of gross national income (GNI) per capita for 2013:

- Low-income countries (LICs) = US$1,045 or less
- Middle-income countries (MICs) are subdivided:
  a) lower-middle-income = US$1,046 to US$4,125
  b) upper-middle-income (UMICs) = US$4,126 to US$12,745
- High-income countries (HICs) = US$12,746 or more.

1. In the Convention on the Rights of Persons with Disabilities, "Persons with disabilities include those who have long-term physical, mental, intellectual or sensory impairments which in interaction with various barriers may hinder their full and effective participation in society on an equal basis with others."
2. The authors wish to thank Hasan Minto, Vilay Pillay, and David Wilson of the Brien Holden Vision Institute for information regarding the cost of glasses.

REFERENCES

Adoyo, P. O. 2007. "Educating Deaf Children in an Inclusive Setting in Kenya: Challenges and Considerations." *Electronic Journal for Inclusive Education* 2 (2): 8.

AIHW (Australia Institute of Health and Welfare). 2004. *Children with Disabilities in Australia, AIHW Catalogue Number DIS 38.* Australia: AIHW.

Altman, B. M. 2016. *International Measurement of Disability: Purpose, Method, and Application; the Work of the Washington Group on Disability Statistics.* New York: Springer.

Baltussen, R., J. Naus, and H. Limburg. 2009. "Cost-Effectiveness of Screening and Correcting Refractive Errors in School Children in Africa, Asia, America, and Europe." *Health Policy* 89 (2): 201–15.

Berman Bieler, R., and S. Meresman. 2010. *Cuatro Principios Fundamentales Para la Inclusión de Personas con Discapacidad.* Panamá: SICA-SISCA.

Black, R. E., L. H. Allen, Z. A. Bhuttz, L. E. Caulfield, M. de Onis, and others. 2008. "Maternal and Child Undernutrition: Global and Regional Exposures and Health Consequences." *The Lancet Special Series* 371 (9608): 243–60.

Braithwaite, J., and D. Mont. 2009. "Disability and Poverty: A Survey of World Bank Poverty Assessments and Implications." *ALTER—European Journal of Disability Research* 3 (3): 219–32.

Buckup, S. 2009. "The Price of Exclusion: The Economic Consequences of Excluding People with Disabilities from the World of Work." Employment Working Paper 43, International Labour Organization, Geneva.

Buescher, A. V., Z. Cidav, M. Knapp, and D. S. Mandell. 2014. "Costs of Autism Spectrum Disorders in the United Kingdom and the United States." *JAMA Pediatrics* 168 (8): 721–28.

Bundy, D. A. P., N. de Silva, S. Horton, G. C. Patton, L. Schultz, and D. T. Jamison. 2017. "Child and Adolescent Health and Development: Realizing Neglected Potential." In *Disease Control Priorities* (third edition): Volume 8, *Child and Adolescent Health and Development,* edited by D. A. P. Bundy, N. de Silva, S. Horton, D. T. Jamison, and G. C. Patton. Washington, DC: World Bank.

Bundy, D. A. P., A. Joshi, M. Rowlands, and Y. T. Kung. 2003. *EnVISIONing Education in Low-Income Countries.* Washington, DC: World Bank.

Bundy, D. A. P., L. Schultz, B. Sarr, L. Banham, P. Colenso, and others. 2017. "The School as a Platform for Addressing Health in Middle Childhood and Adolescence." In *Disease Control Priorities* (third edition): Volume 8, *Child and Adolescent Health and Development,* edited by D. A. P. Bundy, N. de Silva, S. Horton, D. T. Jamison, and G. C. Patton. Washington, DC: World Bank.

Bundy, D. A. P. 2011. *Rethinking School Health: A Key Component of Education for All.* Directions in Development. Washington, DC: World Bank. doi:10.1596/978-0-8213-7907-3.

Burchardt, T. 2005. *The Education and Employment of Disabled Young People: Frustrated Ambition.* Bristol: Policy Press.

Cappa, C., N. Petrowski, and J. Njelesani. 2015. "Navigating the Landscape of Child Disability Measurement: A Review of Available Data Collection Instruments." *ALTER—European Journal of Disability Research* 9 (4): 317–30.

CDC (Centers for Disease Control and Prevention). 2014. "Prevalence of Autism Spectrum Disorder among Children Aged 8 Years: Autism and Developmental Disabilities Monitoring Network, 11 Sites, United States, 2010." *Surveillance Summaries* 63 (SS02): 1–21.

Chamie, M. 1994. "Can Childhood Disability Be Ascertained Simply in Surveys?" *Epidemiology* 5 (3): 273–75.

CONADIS (National Council for Disabilities). 2010. *National Council for Disabilities (CONADIS).* Annual Report, Brazil.

Cook J., K. D. Frick, R. Baltussen, S. Resnikoff, A. Smith, J. Mecaskey, and P. Kilima. 2006. "Loss of Vision and Hearing." In *Disease Control Priorities in Developing Countries* (second edition), edited by D. T. Jamison, J. G. Breman, A. R. Measham, G. Alleyne, M. Cleason, D. B. Evans, P. Jha, A. Mills, and P. Musgrove. Washington, DC: Oxford University Press and World Bank.

Cullinan, J., B. Gannon, and S. Lyons. 2011. "Estimating the Extra Cost of Living for People with Disabilities." *Health Economics* 20 (5): 582–99.

DenBoer, J. W. 2008. Book review of "The Facts of Life—and More: Sexuality and Intimacy for People with Intellectual Disabilities." *Sexuality and Disability* 26 (1): 51–53.

Dessemontent, R. S., G. Bless, and D. Morin. 2012. "Effects of Inclusion on the Academic Achievement and Adaptive Behaviour of Children with Intellectual Disabilities." *Journal of Intellectual Disability Research* 56 (6): 579–87.

Drake, L., M. Fernandes, E. Aurino, J. Kiamba, B. Giyose, and others. 2017. "School Feeding Programs in Middle Childhood and Adolescence." In *Disease Control Priorities* (third edition): Volume 8, *Child and Adolescent Health and Development,* edited by D. A. P. Bundy, N. de Silva, S. Horton, D. T. Jamison, and G. C. Patton. Washington, DC: World Bank.

Durkin M. S., H. Schneider, V. S. Pathania, K. B. Nelson, G. C. Solarsh, N. Bellows, R. M. Scheffler, and K. J. Hofman. 2006. "Learning and Developmental Disabilities." In *Disease Control Priorities in Developing Countries* (second edition), edited by D. T. Jamison, J. G. Breman, A. R. Measham, G. Alleyne, M. Cleason, D. B. Evans, P. Jha, A. Mills, and P. Musgrove. Washington, DC: Oxford University Press and World Bank.

Eide, A. H., and M. E. Loeb. 2006. "Living Conditions among People with Activity Limitations in Zambia." A National Representative Study, SINTEF Health Research, Oslo, Norway.

Eide, A. H., S. Nhiwathiwa, J. Muderedzi, and M. E. Loeb. 2003. "Living Conditions among People with Activity Limitations in Zimbabwe." A Regional Representative Survey, SINTEF Health Research, Oslo, Norway.

Eide, A. H., G. van Rooy, and M. E. Loeb. 2003. "Living Conditions among People with Activity Limitations in Namibia." A National Representative Survey, SINTEF Health Research, Oslo, Norway.

Elsabbagh, M., G. Divan, Y. J. Koh, Y. S. Kim, S. Kauchali, and others. 2012. "Global Prevalence of Autism and Other Pervasive Developmental Disorders." *Autism Research* 5 (3): 160–79.

Evans, P., S. Shah, A. Huebner, S. Sivasubramaniam, C. Vuthy, and others. 2014. "A Population-Based Study on the

Prevalence of Impairment and Disability among Young Cambodian Children." *Disability, CBR, and Inclusive Development* 25 (2): 5–20.

Ferguson, L. 2008. "International Trends in Inclusive Education: The Continuing Challenge to Teach One and Everyone." *European Journal of Special Needs Education* 23 (2): 109–20.

Filmer, D. 2005. "Disability, Poverty and Schooling in Developing Countries: Results from 11 Household Surveys." Social Protection Discussion Paper Series 0539, World Bank, Washington, DC.

———. 2008. "Disability, Poverty, and Schooling in Developing Countries: Results from 14 Household Surveys." *World Bank Economic Review* 22 (1): 141–63.

FRESH Initiative. 2000. *Focusing Resources on Effective School Health: A FRESH Approach for Achieving Education for All.* Paris: UNESCO.

Fricke, T. R., B. A. Holden, D. A. Wilson, G. Schlenther, K. S. Naidoo, and others. 2012. "Global Cost of Correcting Vision Impairment from Uncorrected Refractive Error." *Bulletin of the World Health Organization* 90 (10): 728–38.

Glewwe, P., A. Park, and M. Zhao. 2016. "A Better Vision for Development: Eyeglasses and Academic Performance in Rural Primary Schools in China." *Journal of Development Economics* 122 (September): 170–82. doi:10.1016/j.jdeveco.2016.05.007.

Glewwe, P., K. West, and J. Lee. 2015. "The Impact of Providing Vision Screening and Free Eyeglasses on Academic Outcomes: Evidence from a Randomized Trial in Title 1 Elementary Schools in Florida." Working Paper, Department of Applied Economics, University of Minnesota, St. Paul, MN.

Gomes-Neto, J. B., E. A. Hanushek, R. Helio Leite, and R. C. Frota-Bezzera. 1997. "Health and Schooling: Evidence and Policy Implications for Developing Countries." *Economics of Education Review* 16 (3): 271–82.

Government of Zanzibar. 2007. *Zanzibar Education Development Programme (ZEDP) 2008/09–2015/16.* Final Draft. Zanzibar City: Government of Zanzibar.

Grantham-McGregor, S., Y. B. Cheung, S. Cueto, P. Glewwe, L. Richter, and others. 2007. "Developmental Potential in the First Five Years for Children in Developing Countries." *The Lancet* 369 (9555): 60–70.

Groce, N. E. 2003. "HIV/AIDS and People with Disability." *The Lancet* 361 (9367): 1401–02.

Groce, N. E., M. Kerac, A. Farkas, W. Schultink, and R. B. Bieler. 2013. "Inclusive Nutrition for Children and Adults with Disabilities." *The Lancet Global Health* 1 (4): e18–81.

Hack, M., N. K. Klein, and H. G. Taylor. 1995. "Long-Term Developmental Outcomes of Low Birthweight Infants." *Future of Children* 5 (1): 176–96.

Hartman, W. T. 1992. "State Funding Models for Special Education." *Remedial and Special Education* 13 (6): 47–58.

Helander, E. 1999. *Prejudice and Dignity: An Introduction to Community-Based Rehabilitation.* 2nd ed. New York: UNDP.

IHME (Institute for Health Metrics and Evaluation). 2016. GBD Compare. https://vizhub.healthdata.org/gbd-compare.

Inclusion International. 2006. *Hear Our Voices: A Global Report; People with Intellectual Disabilities and Their Families Speak Out on Poverty and Exclusion.* London: Inclusion International.

Jenkins, S. P., and J. A. Rigg. 2003. "Disability and Disadvantage: Selection, Onset, and Duration Effects." Paper 74, Centre for Analysis of Social Exclusion, London School of Economics, London.

Kalambouka, A., P. Farrell, P. Dyson, and I. Kaplan. 2007. "The Impact of Placing Pupils with Special Educational Needs in Mainstream Schools on the Achievement of Their Peers." *Educational Research* 49 (4): 365–82.

Katoda, H. 1993. "Parents' and Teachers' Praxes of and Attitudes to the Health and Sex Education of Young People with Mental Handicaps: A Study in Stockholm and Tokyo." *Journal of Intellectual Disability Research* 37 (2): 115–29.

Kenya Ministry of Education. 2009. *The National Special Needs Education Policy Framework.* Nairobi: Government of Kenya.

Kodjebacheva, G. D., S. Maliski, and A. L. Coleman. 2015. "Use of Eyeglasses among Children in Elementary School: Perceptions, Behaviors, and Interventions Discussed by Parents, School Nurses, and Teachers during Focus Groups." *American Journal of Health Promotion* 29 (5): 324–31.

Krahn, G. L., L. Hammond, and A. Turner. 2006. "A Cascade of Disparities: Health and Health Care Access for People with Intellectual Disabilities." *Mental Retardation and Developmental Disabilities Research Reviews* 12 (1): 70–82.

Lamichhane, K., and Y. Sawada. 2013. "Disability and Returns to Education in a Developing Country." *Economics of Education Review* 37 (December): 85–94.

Lao Population and Housing Census. 2015. "Provisional Report." Ministry of Planning and Investment, Lao Statistics Bureau, Vientiane.

Lao Statistics Bureau. 2014. *Poverty Profile in Lao PDR: Poverty Report for the Lao Consumption and Expenditure Survey, 2012–2013.* Vientiane Capital: Ministry of Planning and Investment, Australian Aid, and the World Bank.

Laviers, H. R., F. Omar, H. Jecha, G. Kassim, and C. Gilbert. 2010. "Presbyopic Spectacle Coverage, Willingness to Pay for Near Correction, and the Impact of Correcting Uncorrected Presbyopia in Adults in Zanzibar, East Africa." *Investigative Ophthalmology and Visual Science* 51 (2): 1234–41.

Lee, J. 2016. *The Effect of Eyeglasses Provision on Childhood Education in Malawi: Implementation Report.* Department of Applied Economics, University of Minnesota.

Limburg, H., H. T. Kansara, and S. d'Souza. 1999. "Results of School Eye Screening of 5.4 Million Children in India: A Five-Year Follow-Up Study." *Acta Ophthalmologica Scandinavica* 77 (3): 310–14.

Lindsay, G. 2007. "Educational Psychology and the Effectiveness of Inclusive Education/Mainstreaming." *British Journal of Educational Psychology* 77 (Pt 1):1–24.

Loeb, M. E. 2016. "An Analysis of International Census/Survey Data Using the Short Set of Disability Questions Developed by the Washington Group on Disability Statistics." In *International Measurement of Disability: Purpose, Method and Application,* edited by M. B. Altman. New York: Springer.

Loeb, M. E., and A. H. Eide. 2004. "Living Conditions among People with Activity Limitations in Malawi." Federation of Disability Organizations in Malawi, Blantyre, Malawi.

Maulik, P. K., and G. L. Darmstadt. 2007. "Childhood Disability in Low- and Middle-Income Countries: Overview of Screening, Prevention, Services, Legislation, and Epidemiology." *Pediatrics* 120 (Suppl 1): S1–55.

McGregor, G., and R. T. Vogelsberg. 1998. *Inclusive Schooling Practices: Pedagogical and Research Foundations, a Synthesis of the Literature that Informs Best Practices about Inclusive Schooling.* Baltimore, MD: Brookes Publishing.

McLeskey, J., N. L. Waldron, and L. Redd. 2014. "A Case Study of a Highly Effective, Inclusive Elementary School." *Journal of Special Education* 48 (1): 59–70.

Meltzer, H. 2010. "Disability among Children: A Statistical Perspective." http://www.cdc.gov/nchs/data/washington _group/meeting4/WG4_Session5_Paper2.pdf.

———. 2016. "The Challenges of Conducting National Surveys of Disability among Children." In *International Measurement of Disability: Purpose, Method and Application: The Work of the Washington Group on Disability Statistics*, edited by M. B. Altman. Social Indicators Series. New York: Springer.

Meresman, S., S. Bagree, L. Drake, C. Heath, J. Kiamba, and N. Graham. 2015. "Inclusive School Health and Nutrition Programmes: A Roadmap for Mainstreaming Disability into the FRESH Agenda." Partnership for Child Development Working Paper Series #1, Imperial College London, Inter-American Institute on Disability and Inclusive Development, and World Bank.

Mete, C., ed. 2008. *Economic Implications of Chronic Illness and Disability in Eastern Europe and the Former Soviet Union.* Washington, DC: World Bank.

MIDES (Ministry of Social Development). 2011. *National Census.* Montevideo, Uruguay: Ministry of Social Development.

Miguez, M. N., S. Meresman, M. Larrandaburu, O. D. Pedemonte, L. F. Pellejero, and others. 2013. "Health and Inclusion: Nothing about us without Us." *Journal of the Multidisciplinary Network on Disability.*

Mitra, S. 2006. "The Capability Approach and Disability." *Journal of Disability Policy Studies* 16 (4): 236–47.

Mitra, S., A. Posarac, and V. Vick. 2013. "Disability and Poverty in Developing Countries: A Multidimensional Study." *World Development* 41 (January): 1–18.

Mizunoya, S., and S. Mitra. 2013. "Is There a Disability Gap in Employment Rates in Developing Countries?" *World Development* 42: 28–43.

Mizunoya, S., S. Mitra, and I. Yamasaki. 2016. "Towards Inclusive Education: The Impact of Disability on School Attendance in Developing Countries." Innocenti Working Paper No. 2016-03, UNICEF Office of Research, Florence.

Mont, D. 2014. "Childhood Disability and Poverty." Working Paper 25, Leonard Cheshire Disability and Inclusive Development Centre, University College, London.

Mont, D., and N. V. Cuong. 2011. "Disability and Poverty in Vietnam." *World Bank Economic Review* 25 (2): 323–59.

Mont, D., and C. V. Nguyen. 2013a. "Does Parental Disability Matter for Child Education? Evidence from Vietnam." *World Development* 48 (August): 88–107.

———. 2013b. "Spatial Variation in the Disability-Poverty Correlation: Evidence from Vietnam." Working Paper 20, Leonard Cheshire Disability and Inclusive Development Centre, University College, London.

Muthukrishna, N. 2006. "Mapping Barriers to Basic Education in the Context of HIV and AIDS: A Report on Research Conducted in the Richmond District, KwaZulu-Natal." University of KwaZulu-Natal, School of Education and Development, Scottsville.

Odom, S. L., V. Buysse, and E. Soukakou. 2011. "Inclusion for Young Children with Disabilities: A Quarter Century of Research Perspectives." *Journal of Early Intervention* 33 (4): 344–56.

Ormsby, G. M., A.-L. Arnold, L. Busija, M. Mörchen, T. S. Bonn, and J. E. Keeffe. 2012. "The Impact of Knowledge and Attitudes on Access to Eye-Care Services in Cambodia." *Asia-Pacific Journal of Ophthalmology* 1 (6): 331–35.

Palmer, M., N. Groce, D. Mont, O. H. Nguyen, and S. Mitra. 2015. "The Economic Lives of People with Disabilities in Vietnam." *PLoS One* 10 (7): e0133623.

Parrish, T. B. 1994. "Fiscal Policies in Special Education: Removing Incentives for Restrictive Placements." Policy Paper 4, Center for Special Education Finance, American Institutes for Research, Palo Alto, CA.

PCD (Partnership for Child Development). 2013. *Annual Report 2012–2013.* PCD, Imperial College, London. http:// schoolsandhealth.org.

———. 2015. "Inclusive School Health and Nutrition Programs: A Roadmap for Mainstreaming Disability into the FRESH Agenda." Working Paper 1, PCD, Imperial College, London.

Rauh, V. A., P. J. Landrigan, and L. Claudio. 2008. "Housing and Health: Intersection of Poverty and Environmental Exposures." *Annals of the New York Academy of Sciences* 1136: 276–88.

Republic of Kenya. 2005. *Kenya Education Sector Support Programme, 2005–2010.* Nairobi: Ministry of Education Science and Technology.

Resnikoff, S., D. Pascolini, S. P. Mariotti, and G. P. Pokharel. 2008. "Global Magnitude of Visual Impairment Caused by Uncorrected Refractive Errors in 2004." *Bulletin of the World Health Organization* 86 (1): 63–70.

Rosales-Rueda, M. F. 2014. "Family Investment Responses to Childhood Health Conditions: Intrafamily Allocation of Resources." *Journal of Health Economics* 37 (September): 41–57.

Rose, D., A. Meyer, and C. Hitchcock, eds. 2005. *The Universally Designed Classroom: Accessible Curriculum and Digital Technologies.* Cambridge, MA: Harvard Education Press.

Ruijs, N., and T. Peetsma. 2009. "Effects of Inclusion on Students with and without Special Educational Needs Reviewed." *Educational Research Review* 4 (2).

Sen, A. 2009. *The Idea of Justice.* Cambridge, MA: Belknap Press of Harvard University Press.

Shakespeare, T. 2006. *Disability Rights and Wrongs.* New York: Routledge.

Sharma, A., L. Li, Y. Song, K. Choi, D. S. Lam, and others. 2008. "Strategies to Improve the Accuracy of Vision Measurement by Teachers in Rural Chinese Secondary Schoolchildren: Xichang Pediatric Refractive Error Study (X-PRES) Report No. 6." *Archives of Ophthalmology* 126 (10): 1434–40.

Steinfeld, E. 2005. *Education for All: The Cost of Accessibility.* Washington, DC: World Bank.

Thomas, M., and N. Burnett. 2013. *Exclusion from Education: The Economic Cost of Out of School Children in 20 Countries.* Washington, DC: Results for Development and Educate a Child.

Trani, J.-F., P. Bakhshi, S. Myer Tlapek, D. Lopez, and F. Gall. 2015. "Disability and Poverty in Morocco and Tunisia: A Multidimensional Approach." *Journal of Human Development and Capabilities* 16 (4): 518–48. doi:10.1080/19452829.2015.1091808.

Trani, J.-F., and T. I. Canning. 2013. "Child Poverty in an Emergency and Conflict Context: A Multidimensional Profile and an Identification of the Poorest Children in Western Darfur." *World Development* 48: 48–70.

Trani, J.-F., J. Kuhlberg, T. Cannings, and D. Chakkal. 2016. "Multidimensional Poverty in Afghanistan: Who Are the Poorest of the Poor?" *Oxford Development Studies* 44 (2): 220–45. doi:10.1080/13600818.2016.1160042.

Trani, J.-F., and M. E. Loeb. 2012. "Poverty and Disability: A Vicious Circle? Evidence from Afghanistan and Zambia." *Journal of International Development* 24 (Suppl 1): S19–52.

UN (United Nations) Statistics Division. 2010. *Workshop on Millennium Development Goals Monitoring.* Geneva: United Nations Statistics Division.

UNESCO (United Nations Educational, Scientific and Cultural Organization). 2010. *Reaching the Marginalized EFA Global Monitoring Report 2010.* Paris: UNESCO.

UNICEF (United Nations Children's Fund). 2005. *The State of the World's Children 2006: Excluded and Invisible.* New York: UNICEF.

———. 2008. "Monitoring Child Disability in Developing Countries: Results from the Multiple Indicator Cluster Surveys." Division of Policy and Practice, UNICEF, New York.

———. 2013. *The State of the World's Children 2013: Children with Disabilities.* New York: UNICEF.

———. 2015. *Fixing the Broken Promise of Education for All: Findings from the Global Initiative on Out-of-School Children.* New York: UNICEF.

Wang, J., M. Harris, B. Amos, M. Li, X. Wang, and others. 1997. "A Ten-Year Review of the Iodine Deficiency Disorders Program of the People's Republic of China." *Journal of Public Health Policy* 18 (2): 219–41.

Wang, J., X. Zhou, W. Xia, C. H. Sun, L. J. Wu, and others. 2012. "Parent-Reported Health Care Expenditures Associated with Autism Spectrum Disorders in Heilongjiang Province, China." *BMC Health Services Research* 12 (7).

Watermeyer, B., ed. 2006. *Disability and Social Change: A South African Agenda.* Cape Town: HSRC Press.

Wedner, S. H., D. A. Ross, R. Balira, L. Kayi, and A. Foster. 2000. "Prevalence of Eye Diseases in Primary School Children in a Rural Area of Tanzania." *British Journal of Ophthalmology* 84 (11): 1291–97.

WHO (World Health Organization). 2002. *Towards a Common Language for Functioning, Disability, and Health: International Classification of Functioning, Disability, and Health.* Geneva: WHO.

WHO and UNFPA (United Nations Population Fund). 2009. "Promoting Sexual and Reproductive Health for Persons with Disabilities." Guidance Note, WHO, Geneva.

WHO and UNICEF (United Nations Children's Fund). 2012. "Early Childhood Development and Disability." Discussion Paper, WHO, Geneva.

WHO and World Bank. 2011. *World Report on Disability.* Washington, DC: WHO and World Bank.

Wilson, D. A. 2011. "Efficacious Correction of Refractive Error in Developing Countries." PhD thesis, University of New South Wales, Kensington.

World Bank. 2003. "Youth with Disability: Issues and Challenges." Social Protection Unit, World Bank, Washington, DC.

———. 2004. *HIV/AIDS and Disability: Capturing Hidden Voices: The Yale/World Bank Global Survey on Disability and HIV/AIDS.* Washington, DC: World Bank.

———. 2007. *People with Disabilities in India: From Commitments to Outcomes.* New Delhi: Human Development Unit, South Asia Region.

———. 2014. *Lao People's Democratic Republic: Early Childhood Education Project.* Washington, DC: World Bank Group.

Xiong, N., L. Yang, Y. Yu, J. Hou, J. Li, and others. 2011. "Investigation of Raising Burden of Children with Autism, Physical Disability, and Mental Disability in China." *Research in Developmental Disabilities* 32 (10): 306–11.

Zaidi, A., and T. Burchardt. 2005. "Comparing Incomes when Needs Differ: Equivalization for the Extra Costs of Disability in the UK." *Review of Income and Wealth* 51 (1): 89–114.

Zhang, M., R. Zhang, M. He, W. Liang, X. Li, and others. 2011. "Self Correction of Refractive Error among Young People in Rural China: Results of Cross-Sectional Investigation." *BMJ* 343: d4767.

Chapter 18

Health and Disease in Adolescence

Nicola Reavley, George C. Patton, Susan M. Sawyer,
Elissa Kennedy, and Peter Azzopardi

INTRODUCTION

Rising adolescent health problems, such as road traffic injuries (RTIs), mental disorders, and substance use disorders, are an increasing cause for concern in countries that have otherwise reduced maternal mortality and boosted child survival (Patton and others 2009). Moreover, with aging populations and a convergence to a disease burden dominated by noncommunicable diseases (NCDs) in later life, adolescent health risks, such as tobacco use, physical inactivity, obesity, substance use, and poor diet, assume greater significance (Jamison and others 2013). Adolescence is defined as ages 10–19 years. Definitions of age groupings and age-specific terminology used in this volume can be found in chapter 1 (Bundy and others 2017).

Better adolescent health requires matching interventions to health profiles, focusing on the important social determinants of health during the adolescent years, considering adolescent development and neurodevelopment, and addressing gender and equity.

The Sustainable Development Goals will put a greater focus on adolescents as recipients of interventions and as decision makers and implementation partners in health-related issues. Although the Millennium Development Goals increased the focus on sexual and reproductive health among adolescents and young adults ages 15–24 years, other areas of health risks and problems received far less attention, and health gains have been weaker among adolescents than among other age groups.

When reading this chapter, it is important to remember that nearly all of the data and evidence come from studies of programs in high-income countries (HICs). We cannot say with any certainty the extent to which the results presented here apply to low- and middle-income countries (LMICs). This lack of research is a particular challenge in planning and selecting interventions for this age group and helps to emphasize the need for much more research into the health of adolescents in LMICs.

MATCHING INTERVENTIONS TO HEALTH PROFILES

Matching interventions to health profiles is critical to achieving a significant improvement in adolescent health. Health profiles vary among and within countries, largely reflecting progress through the epidemiological transition that follows economic development and the demographic transition. In multiburden countries that have yet to pass through this transition, diseases of poverty predominate, including undernutrition, major sexual and reproductive health problems, and infectious diseases (see also chapter 21, figure 21.1, Sawyer and others 2017). In injury-excess countries, high levels of unintentional injury or violence and high adolescent birth rates are recorded, while NCD-predominant countries have high rates of mental and substance use disorders and chronic physical illness. Chapter 5 in this volume

Corresponding author: Nicola Reavley, Melbourne School of Population and Global Health, University of Melbourne, Melbourne, Australia; nreavley@unimelb.edu.au.

(Patton, Azzopardi, and others 2017) provides further details on the categorization of disease burdens and methods used to derive the three categories of countries.

Addressing the Social Determinants of Adolescent Health

As in any age group, economic and social conditions influence adolescent health. Social determinants that improve adolescent health include policies and environments that support access to education and employment, delay marriage and childbearing, provide universal health coverage, and create opportunities to enhance youth autonomy, decision-making capacity, and human rights (Sawyer and others 2012). These determinants lie largely outside of health services, as do the interventions necessary to address them. Accordingly, the settings for health actions extend from health services, schools, and education to families and communities, places of employment, road transportation, the media, and structural, legal, and policy environments. Chapter 21 in this volume describes these platforms in more detail (Sawyer and others 2017).

Considering Adolescent Development and Neurodevelopment

Adolescent development and our understanding of it are changing. The age of onset of puberty is decreasing, yet the age at which mature social roles are achieved is increasing, and adolescence is lasting longer (NRC and IOM 2005). Interventions for adolescent health need to consider this developmental trajectory; strategies suited to younger adolescents may be inappropriate or ineffective with older adolescents or young adults (Viner and others 2012). Moreover, neuroscience has revealed adolescent neurodevelopment to be particularly dynamic and strongly influenced by social and nutritional environments as well as by exposures to behaviors such as substance use (Blakemore and Mills 2014). The decision making of adolescents, including that affecting health, differs from that of adults. Adolescents are more influenced by peers and often seek out and are more influenced by exciting, arousing, and stressful situations (Steinberg 2008). To maximize effectiveness, interventions for adolescent health need to consider such decision-making processes and provide opportunities for adolescents to exercise self-determination.

Focusing on Gender and Equity

Better adolescent health also requires focusing on gender, since strategies that are effective and appropriate for girls may be less effective for boys, and vice versa. In addition, considering the impact of interventions on equity is critical. For example, school-based interventions may increase inequity, as they do not reach adolescents who are not in school. Addressing gender disparities in access and targeting more resources to disadvantaged adolescents (including ethnic minorities; lesbian, gay, bisexual, or transsexual youth; persons with disabilities; and persons who are homeless or in juvenile detention) are critical to closing equity gaps.

METHODS

We conducted a series of systematic reviews to assess current knowledge on the effectiveness of prevention interventions outside formal health care settings across nine areas of health[1] (see figure 21.1 in chapter 21 by Sawyer and others 2017). We included both specific health outcomes and health risks. Some responses (for example, policy measures such as taxation, or legislation such as gun control) are not directly targeted at young people but may have particular benefits for them compared with other age groups. Other actions target adolescents directly.

From March 15 to March 30, 2015, we searched the peer-reviewed literature and websites of key organizations. Annex 18A offers further details on the inclusion and exclusion criteria, classification of levels of evidence, appraisal of quality, and synthesis methods.

SEXUAL AND REPRODUCTIVE HEALTH, INCLUDING HIV/AIDS

More than any other area of health, a country's cultural, religious, legal, political, and economic contexts affect the sexual and reproductive health of adolescents, and actions for sexual and reproductive health need to take these contexts into account. The evidence suggests that implementing multicomponent interventions that act in two or more settings improves sexual and reproductive health and reduces the impact of human immunodeficiency virus/acquired immune deficiency syndrome (HIV/AIDS): structural or policy settings, community settings (including schools), and health services (annex 18B, table 18B.1). For example, high-quality, comprehensive sex education is more likely to prevent pregnancy and reduce the prevalence of sexually transmitted infections (STIs) or HIV/AIDS if it is combined with the provision of contraceptives (Chin and others 2012; Oringanje and others 2009). Legislation to protect adolescents from early marriage and pregnancy is more likely to be effective if accompanied by actions to encourage favorable community and professional attitudes (Gottschalk and Ortayli 2014). Although evidence exists to show the impact on safe-sex behaviors of interventions to promote universal health coverage, relatively little exists to show their impact on STI or HIV/AIDS prevalence (Denno, Hoopes, and Chandra-Mouli 2015). The quality of training for providers is likely to be an important factor in the success of such interventions, and studies targeting marginalized or vulnerable adolescents, including those not in school, are needed (Chandra-Mouli and others 2015).

INFECTIOUS AND VACCINE-PREVENTABLE DISEASES

Vaccination against infectious diseases has received far less attention in adolescents than in children. Yet adolescents are also important for ensuring completion of immunization schedules (such as measles-rubella and hepatitis B vaccine), administering booster doses (such as diphtheria-tetanus), and ensuring primary immunization (such as for human papillomavirus). Rubella vaccination is important for adolescent girls given intergenerational risks, although hepatitis B vaccine is important for both genders, given its adult burden. Other vaccines to consider according to local prevalence of disease and cost are tuberculosis, influenza, and meningitis vaccines.

Lack of basic knowledge has hindered responses to common infectious diseases in adolescents. In contrast to diarrheal disease in children, the etiological agents, proportion of vaccine-preventable morbidity and mortality, and comorbidities are largely unknown in adolescents. Similarly, adolescent tuberculosis has received little attention, even though it is the leading contributor to the burden of infectious disease in young adults in multiburden countries (Snow and others 2015).

Adolescents in Sub-Saharan Africa also carry a substantial burden of malaria. In high-transmission areas, rates are higher in adolescent girls than in boys, with pregnant girls experiencing additional risks (Desai and others 2007). In endemic regions, people are exposed to malaria earlier in life and more frequently. In these settings, partial immunity develops relatively early, and the risk of severe malaria in adolescence declines. However, in areas of lower transmission, clinical disease is more common in adolescents and young adults. As infection in endemic areas is controlled and the development of childhood immunity becomes less likely, the risk of malaria in adolescents and young adults increases (Lalloo, Olukoya, and Olliaro 2006). In low-transmission regions, the incidence of malaria among adolescents reflects their use of individual preventive interventions, such as insecticide treated bednets. A study from Nigeria, where an estimated 50 percent of the community experiences an episode of malaria each year, showed that only 8.5 percent of students ages 13–18 years reported sleeping under insecticide treated bednets (Udonwa, Gyuse, and Etokidem 2010).

UNDERNUTRITION

No adolescent-specific evidence exists of the benefit of interventions for the prevention of undernutrition. Interventions do not typically target adolescents alone or report age-disaggregated outcomes. However, good evidence exists about interventions targeting nutrition-related risks that commonly affect adolescents. These risks include iron-deficiency anemia, protein-energy malnutrition, and other micronutrient deficiencies. Energy and iron requirements increase during puberty and are required for optimal growth (Haider 2006).

Interventions to reduce protein-energy malnutrition, including balanced protein-energy supplementation (Bhutta and others 2013), cash transfers (DFID 2012), and improved household food storage systems (Masset and others 2011), may be particularly beneficial in adolescents (Prentice and others 2013). As adolescence is a period of rapid growth, it is plausible that interventions that support catch-up growth in young children might also promote catch-up growth in stunted adolescents, although further research is required to confirm this (Reinhardt and Fanzo 2014).

The additional iron necessary to meet menstruation-related needs places adolescent girls at increased risk of iron-deficiency anemia. Iron fortification of staple foods, such as flour, can reduce iron deficiency anemia at a population level by up to 63 percent and has been shown to be cost-effective (DFID 2012). Interventions addressing food insecurity may also improve iron levels (Bhutta and others 2013).

Adolescent Pregnancy

Adolescent pregnancy places girls at increased risk of undernutrition; children born to adolescent girls are more likely to have low birth weight, independent of socioeconomic or maternal preconception nutritional status (Gibbs and others 2012). Preconception interventions, such as multiple-micronutrient supplementation or iron and folic acid supplementation continuing into pregnancy, deworming to reduce nutrient loss, and antenatal nutrition counseling and education, can play a role in preventing undernutrition and poor health outcomes in offspring (Bhutta and others 2013). Delaying first pregnancies, spacing subsequent births, and increasing young women's access to education and health care or control over household resources are likely to be central in preventing adversity (Bushamuka and others 2005; Chandra-Mouli, Camacho, and Michaud 2013). Delaying the first pregnancy is essential in stunted adolescent girls (King 2003).

UNINTENTIONAL INJURY

Much of the disease burden of adolescent unintentional injury is related to RTIs. Adolescents and young adults, particularly those in LMICs, are at high risk; they are more likely to be vulnerable road users, such as pedestrians, cyclists, and motorcyclists (Peden and others 2004). Moreover, in young men in particular, developmental immaturity, risky behavior, and poor decision making increase the risks (Toroyan and Peden 2007).

In HICs, improvements in road design, equipment and maintenance, traffic control, vehicle design and protective devices, driver training and regulation, police enforcement and sanctions, public education and information, and postcrash care have significantly reduced the burden of injury, including in adolescents (WHO and ExpandNet 2013). Chapter 3 in volume 7 discusses RTIs in more detail (Bachani and others 2017). More targeted actions include the following:

- *Graduated licensing systems* that extend the learning period, increase low-risk supervised driving, and regulate exposure to high-risk settings, such as driving at night without supervision, driving with other young passengers, or using alcohol during an initial licensing period (Simpson 2003). Robust testing of competence before issuing licenses is generally an essential element.
- *Legislation and enforcement of mandatory helmet wearing for motorcyclists* in countries where a high proportion of adolescents and young adults ride motorcycles (Norton and others 2006).
- *Investment in pedestrian safety* in regions where pedestrian injuries are common, such as Sub-Saharan Africa. Effective actions include the imposition of lower speed limits on lengths of road where pedestrians mix with other traffic and enforcement of these limits (Afukaar 2003), regulation including police enforcement of the behavior of drivers and riders at pedestrian crossings (Elvik and Vaa 2009), improved pedestrian facilities such as footpaths and crossings (Forjuoh 2003), separation of pedestrians

and vehicles (Retting, Ferguson, and McCartt 2003), and increased visibility of pedestrians (Porchia and others 2014).

Although education programs have shown some benefits (Williams 2006), school-age driver education programs that focus on selecting driving instructors and offering theory and practical tests should be avoided, as they may encourage earlier driving and lead to greater risk of accident (Roberts and Kwan 2001).

Intersectoral coordination, underpinned by strong information systems, clear governance, civil society advocacy, and a capacity to implement effectively within different sectors, is central to achieving reductions in RTIs.

VIOLENCE

Violent behavior in adolescents and young adults develops because of complex interactions among individual, relationship, community, and societal factors (Krug and others 2002). Individual risk factors include substance use, impulsivity, low educational attainment, and childhood aggression. Relationship risk factors include peer involvement in problem behavior, family conflict, poor family management, child abuse, and pro-violent parental attitudes and behavior. Communities with poor social cohesion, low socioeconomic status, high residential mobility, drug trafficking, and unemployment also increase the risk of violence. Societal risk factors include inequality, availability of weapons, and laws and cultural norms that support violence.

Adolescent-specific violence prevention strategies are implemented in three principal settings: schools, communities, and families, and policy interventions are most often targeted to the broader community (WHO 2010a) (annex 18B, table 18B.2). Universal school-based interventions have shown some evidence of effectiveness in reducing violent or aggressive behavior (Fagan and Catalano 2013; Hahn and others 2007), with similar impacts in schools in areas characterized by lower socioeconomic status and high crime rates (Hahn and others 2007).

School-based interventions are likely to be more effective in at-risk adolescents, with beneficial effects in mixed groups and boys-only groups (Limbos and others 2007; Mytton and others 2006; Park-Higgerson and others 2008). Family-focused interventions seek to promote parent-child communication and improve parenting skills, such as providing children with information about the positive and negative consequences of their behavior (Fagan and Catalano 2013; Woolfenden, Williams, and Peat 2002). Some interventions use a combined family and school approach (Fagan and Catalano 2013). Although good evidence exists of the impact of parenting interventions targeted to younger children (Furlong and others 2012), less research has been conducted among adolescents. However, family-focused and family- and school-based interventions have shown beneficial effects (Fagan and Catalano 2013). Limited evidence exists on the effectiveness of community-based social development interventions that target risk factors for violence (Fagan and Catalano 2013; Sethi and others 2010).

Most evidence of the effectiveness of policy interventions comes from studies conducted in the broader population. Reducing the availability and harmful use of alcohol and reducing the access to weapons (for example, laws against owning and carrying weapons, fines for carrying weapons, policies on school-based weapons) have been shown to reduce violence in adolescents and young adults (Krug and others 2002; WHO 2010a).

Reducing the violence-related burden of disease in young people is likely to require a multifaceted approach that is integrated with policies directed at social and political risk factors, such as inequality, lack of access to education, unemployment, availability of weapons and laws, and cultural norms that support violence (WHO 2010a). This is likely to be particularly important in countries in which many adolescents are not in school.

Early adolescence is a period in which gender role differences intensify and boys and girls begin to explore intimate relationships. Interventions at this stage offer opportunities to promote attitudes and behaviors that reduce the risk of interpersonal and sexual violence.

Evidence for the prevention of intimate-partner and sexual violence in adolescents and young adults is largely lacking. In many cases, particularly in LMICs, studies are of poor quality, with small sample sizes, varied outcome measures, and short follow-up periods. The most common types of interventions targeted to this age group are educational and skills-based interventions, which can be effective in changing attitudes but which appear to have little impact on violent behavior (Fellmeth and others 2013). Moreover, most of these interventions have been implemented in schools and tertiary institutions in HICs, particularly the United States. Community-based programs to promote gender-equitable norms are the most common interventions in LMICs, but the evidence for their effectiveness is mixed (Lundgren and Amin 2015).

Programs are needed that more fully address the risk factors for intimate-partner and sexual violence, alcohol misuse, family-derived attitudes to violence, and social norms, such as those that condone violence and gender inequality. They need to be tailored to local contexts, include families where appropriate, target persons at high risk, and be subject to rigorous evaluation (Ellsberg and others 2015; Whitaker and others 2006). Legislative and judicial responses are important, but they are unlikely to reduce intimate-partner and sexual violence in isolation (Ellsberg and others 2015).

MENTAL DISORDERS

Most mental disorders begin before age 25 years, most often at ages 11–18 years (Kessler and others 2005). Although not all adolescent mental health problems persist into adulthood, particularly if the episodes are brief, those that do often have lifelong impacts (Copeland and others 2011; Patton and others 2014). This has led to increased emphasis on early intervention, either in primary health care or, in some countries, through adolescent-focused mental health services (McGorry, Bates, and Birchwood 2013). Although access to health services has increased in some places, evidence that these increases have led to detectable improvements in adolescent mental health is largely lacking (Jorm 2015).

Although prevention of mental disorders is increasingly seen as a public health priority, evaluation studies have focused mainly on taking effective clinical treatments, such as cognitive-behavioral therapies, and applying them to the general population of adolescents or to at-risk subgroups to test if they prevent the development of disorders. A systematic meta-review and meta-analysis of randomized controlled trials of prevention interventions for depression or anxiety in children and adolescents showed that these interventions produced a minimal to moderate reduction in symptoms in the short term, but no effect beyond 12 months of follow-up (Stockings and others 2016).

Innovative approaches are needed, including those that focus on developmental mental health risks such as bullying and interpersonal violence. Exploration is also needed into the role of digital and social media as risk factors and as potential avenues for preventive interventions (Nesi and Prinstein 2015).

SUICIDE

The risk factors for suicide in adolescents include suicidal behavior in families, depression, alcohol abuse, use of hard drugs, mental health problems, suicidal behavior of friends, family discord (especially for females), poor peer relationships, living apart from parents, antisocial behavior (especially in females), sexual abuse, physical abuse, and unsupportive parents (Evans, Hawton, and Rodham 2004). Contagion—when a suicidal act increases the likelihood of other suicides in a community—is a further factor in up to 60 percent of suicides in adolescents and young adults (Hazell 1993). Deliberate self-harm is also common in adolescents, particularly in females, and heightens the risks for subsequent suicide (Hawton, Zahl, and Weatherall 2003).

Adolescent suicide prevention strategies typically include one or more of the following goals: increased help-seeking for suicidal thoughts and behaviors; identification and referral of at-risk young people by health professionals, teachers, parents, or peers; reduction of risk factors for suicide; and promotion of mental health (Gould and others 2003). School-based interventions are the most commonly evaluated interventions in the adolescent age group; although some evidence shows that universal interventions improve attitudes toward suicide (Cusimano and Sameem 2011; Katz and others 2013; Klimes-Dougan, Klingbeil, and Meller 2013; Robinson and others 2013), these gains are unlikely to be maintained at follow-up, and iatrogenic effects remain largely untested (Robinson and others 2013). Gatekeeper training, which teaches specific groups of people to identify people at high risk of suicide and refer them for treatment, also improves knowledge and attitudes toward suicide and builds confidence in providing help (Katz and others 2013; Klimes-Dougan, Klingbeil, and Meller 2013; Miller, Eckert, and Mazza 2009; Robinson and others 2013).

Evidence is mixed on the effectiveness of universal school-based interventions, gatekeeper training, public education and mass media interventions, screening or intervention-after-suicide programs (Andriessen 2014), and clinical treatments (Robinson, Hetrick, and Martin 2011) on help-seeking behavior, help-giving behavior, suicidal ideation, or suicide attempts in adolescents.

Evidence from studies among the broader population suggests that training health practitioners to recognize depression and evaluate suicide risks and restricting access to lethal methods show some benefits for preventing suicide (Mann and others 2005).

Many studies of suicide prevention interventions are of poor quality, and evidence for effective interventions to prevent suicide in young people is largely lacking, particularly in LMICs. Reducing the suicide-related burden of disease in young people is likely to require a multifaceted approach that focuses on restricting access to means and training health practitioners, particularly in depression and substance use (Burns and Patton 2000; Gould and others 2003; Robinson, Hetrick, and Martin 2011). Help-seeking behavior is likely to differ between males and females, and future evaluations of preventive actions should address gender differences (Klimes-Dougan, Klingbeil, and Meller 2013). Chapter 9 in volume 4 addresses this issue in more depth (Vijayakumar and others 2015).

PHYSICAL HEALTH AND HEALTH RISKS

Prevention of Overweight and Obesity

The prevalence of overweight and obesity in a population commonly increases in mid-adolescence and continues into early adulthood (Ng and others 2014). Because adolescent obesity strongly predicts adult obesity and associated morbidity, preventing obesity in adolescence is essential (Whitaker and others 1997), particularly when considering the maternal and intergenerational health risks of obesity in young women (Ruager-Martin, Hyde, and Modi 2010).

Modifiable risks for obesity also change rapidly across adolescence. Physical activity commonly decreases, and sedentary behavior increases (Dumith and others 2011); adolescents have greater autonomy in their choice of food and are more likely to eat outside of the home, increasing the likelihood that they will choose less healthy food (Niemeier and others 2006). Exposure to media influences and susceptibility to the marketing of processed foods also intensify (Jordan, Kramer-Golinkoff, and Strasburger 2008).

In summary, although the evidence for interventions to reduce body mass index and increase physical activity in adolescents is mixed, multicomponent interventions incorporating support for increased physical activity and education about the importance of a healthy diet and physical activity are more likely to be effective (Clemmens and Hayman 2004; Crutzen 2010; De Bourdeaudhuij and others 2011; Murillo Pardo and others 2013; Pearson, Braithwaite, and Biddle 2015; Seo and Sa 2010) (annex 18B, table 18B.3). Further research is needed to explore obesity prevention interventions that capitalize on other aspects of adolescence, including peer and social network influences. Further research is also needed to explore the impact of gender on the response to obesity prevention interventions, since it is likely that gender becomes increasingly important during adolescence (Rees and others 2006). Barriers to participation may be greater for girls than for boys and may include sensitivity regarding body image, a focus on competitive sports, and inadequate facilities in schools, such as changing rooms and showers (Camacho-Miñano, LaVoi, and Barr-Anderson 2011; Pearson, Braithwaite, and Biddle 2015; Rees and others 2006).

Further research is also needed into interventions targeting adolescents and young adults who are not in educational settings, are from minority groups, or are disadvantaged (De Meester and others 2009; Rees and others 2006; Stice, Shaw, and Marti 2006; van Sluijs, McMinn, and Griffin 2008). However, policy approaches such as taxing unhealthy foods and beverages, reducing fast-food advertising, and front-of-pack, traffic-light nutrition labeling are more likely to work best and be cost-effective (Gortmaker and others 2011; Laska and others 2012).

Alcohol, Illicit Drugs, and Tobacco

Alcohol

Consumption of alcohol often begins and then increases during adolescence, with some evidence suggesting that adolescents are starting at increasingly early ages (Francis and others 2014). Early initiation of alcohol use is linked to binge drinking, heavy drinking, and alcohol-related problems in adolescence and adulthood (Bonomo and others 2004). Evidence suggests that early consumption may impair neurological development (Ewing, Sakhardande, and Blakemore 2014).

Although evidence suggests that interventions in schools and family settings have achieved small but significant impacts on alcohol consumption and alcohol-related harm (Foxcroft and Tsertsvadze 2011a, 2011b; Smit and others 2008), regulatory or statutory enforcement interventions are likely to show the greatest benefit in preventing harmful use (Martineau and others 2013), as shown in annex 18B, table 18B.4. Regulating access to alcohol through age restrictions on purchases is particularly effective for preventing alcohol-related harm in adolescents and young adults. However, most of this evidence is from HICs; interventions should be tailored to the local context, taking into consideration the level of alcohol consumption, age- and gender-related drinking patterns, and level of harm (WHO 2010b). Chapter 7 in volume 4 provides more detail on this issue (Medina-Mora and others 2015).

Illicit Drugs

As with alcohol, adolescence is a time when most people are first exposed to drugs and start using them. School-based interventions aim to prevent drug use, delay initiation, or prevent regular use (see annex 18B, table 18B.5). However, interventions that provide information alone are not likely to be effective in reducing use, although evidence shows that programs with a social competence approach have significant but minimal benefits (Carney and others 2014; Faggiano and others 2014). Evidence also shows that brief interventions have small but significant effects on substance use, with greater benefits if delivered in an individual format and over multiple sessions (Barnett and others 2012). Evidence is mixed about the effectiveness of

family-based (Kumpfer, Alvarado, and Whiteside 2003), community-level (Gates and others 2006; Strang and others 2012), and online (Champion and others 2013; Wood and others 2014) interventions, and some evidence supports using screening and motivational interventions in health care settings (Barnett and others 2012; Jensen and others 2011). Further studies are needed, particularly in LMICs. However, since the effects of such programs are small, they should form part of more comprehensive strategies for preventing drug use. Mass media interventions are unlikely to be effective (Ferri and others 2013).

Treatment and rehabilitation services and strategies to minimize harm have been the main focus in reducing the consequences of illicit drug use. Harm minimization strategies are essential in preventing the transmission of blood-borne viruses, including HIV/AIDS and hepatitis, and may include needle and syringe exchange programs, drug substitution programs that switch users from black market drugs to legal drugs dispensed by health professionals, HIV/AIDS testing and counseling, prevention and services for the management of STIs, overdose prevention, and education relating to wound and vein care (WHO and ExpandNet 2011). Strategies need to be tailored to the local context, including patterns of use and levels of harm.

Tobacco Use

As most adult smokers began smoking in adolescence, regular tobacco use in adolescence increases the likelihood of associated adult and intergenerational health risks. Whether or not an adolescent initiates tobacco use depends on diverse factors, such as gender; concerns with body weight; attitudes to smoking; parental, peer, and community smoking; socioeconomic status; and level of education (Warren and others 2009). School- (Thomas, McLellan, and Perera 2013), family- (Thomas and others 2015), community- (Carson and others 2011), and media-based (Brinn and others 2010) interventions can be beneficial, but the effects are small (annex 18B, table 18B.6). There is good evidence that policies to control tobacco are associated with lower prevalence of smoking in young people. These policies include age restrictions on purchase, taxation and pricing, smoke-free-air laws, and funding for tobacco control programs (Farrelly and others 2013; Wakefield and Chaloupka 2000). The Framework Convention on Tobacco Control provides clear guidance on the minimum standards governing the production, sale, distribution, advertisement, and taxation of tobacco that are needed to protect adolescents and young adults from the harms of smoking.

CONCLUSIONS

Major gaps in the evidence base for effective actions in many health areas reflect the relative lack of investment in adolescent health programs, especially in LMICs. For example, for health areas such as undernutrition and RTIs, no adolescent-specific evidence has been gathered through systematic reviews. Even in the area of sexual and reproductive health, the evidence from systematic reviews is limited on what might need to be done differently to allow adolescents to access interventions that are effective in adults (Mavedzenge, Luecke, and Ross 2014).

However, because the social and environmental determinants of health among adolescents and young adults vary widely, intersectoral and multicomponent interventions offer the best opportunity to improve adolescent health. For example, school- and health-service-based interventions to prevent early marriage and pregnancy are more likely to succeed if accompanied by interventions that generate community support, such as public hearings, meetings, and fairs (Gottschalk and Ortayli 2014). School-based interventions that go beyond teaching health education in classrooms to encompass changes to the curriculum and the wider social environment, as well as engagement with families and the community, are more likely to improve sexual health, reduce violence, and decrease smoking-related outcomes (Blank and others 2010; Harden and others 2009; Langford and others 2014). In the broader population, intersectoral action has been central to public health gains in HICs, including reducing RTIs and helping to control tobacco use (Elvik and Vaa 2009; Farrelly and others 2013).

With the exception of sexual and reproductive health, available evidence is mostly from HICs, particularly the United States. Implementation in other countries, in particular in LMICs, is uncertain. As effective interventions will only have benefits if widely implemented, consideration must be given to local contexts, including culture, beliefs, knowledge, lifestyles, and health systems. Effective implementation and scale up require a systematic approach to addressing these factors and to achieving a balance between desired outcomes and implementation constraints. It also requires involving all stakeholders and engaging existing system capacities, wherever possible, rather than imposing additional burdens (WHO and ExpandNet 2010). Ongoing monitoring and evaluation of interventions in different contexts are critical to building the evidence base (Milat and others 2013).

Within any country, marked differences exist in health between different regions and adolescent groups, with poverty, gender, and social marginalization important determinants. Although groups such as ethnic minorities; lesbian, gay, bisexual or transsexual youths; persons with disabilities; and youth who are homeless or in juvenile detention have the greatest health needs, scant evidence exists to suggest the effectiveness of interventions across the spectrum of disadvantage. Some interventions may not reach vulnerable groups and may actually worsen inequities. Interventions should therefore be designed and implemented with an equity lens to ensure that benefits extend to the most hard-to-reach adolescents and young adults (O'Neill and others 2014). Scaling up should also give careful consideration to gender, race, ethnicity, sexuality, geography, socioeconomic status, and disability (Chandra-Mouli, Lane, and Wong 2015).

Finally, nearly all of the data and evidence come from studies of programs in HICs. We cannot say with any certainty the extent to which the results presented here apply to LMICs. This lack of research is a particular challenge in planning and selecting interventions for adolescents and emphasizes the need for much more research into the health of adolescents in LMICs.

ANNEXES

The annexes to this chapter are as follows. They are available at http://www.dcp-3.org/CAHD.

- Annex 18A. Methods
- Annex 18B. Evidence of Effectiveness and Cost-Effectiveness of Sexual and Reproductive Health Interventions, including HIV

NOTES

World Bank Income Classifications as of July 2014 are as follows, based on estimates of gross national income (GNI) per capita for 2013:

- Low-income countries (LICs) = US$1,045 or less
- Middle-income countries (MICs) are subdivided:
  a) lower-middle-income = US$1,046 to US$4,125
  b) upper-middle-income (UMICs) = US$4,126 to US$12,745
- High-income countries (HICs) = US$12,746 or more.

1. The nine areas of health included in this chapter are infectious and vaccine-preventable diseases; undernutrition; HIV/AIDS; sexual and reproductive health; unintentional injuries; violence; physical disorders; mental disorders; and substance use disorders.

REFERENCES

Afukaar, F. K. 2003. "Speed Control in Developing Countries: Issues, Challenges, and Opportunities in Reducing Road Traffic Injuries." *Injury Control and Safety Promotion* 10 (1–2): 77–81. doi:10.1076/icsp.10.1.77.14113.

Andriessen, K. 2014. "Suicide Bereavement and Postvention in Major Suicidology Journals: Lessons Learned for the Future of Postvention." *Crisis* 35 (5): 338–48. doi:10.1027/0227-5910/a000269.

Bachani, A. M., M. Peden, G. Gururaj, R. Norton, and A. A. Hyder. 2017. "Road Traffic Injuries." In *Disease Control Priorities* (third edition): Volume 7, *Injury Prevention and Environmental Health*, edited by C. N. Mock, O. Kobusingye, R. Nugent, and K. Smith. Washington, DC: World Bank.

Barnett, E., S. Sussman, C. Smith, L. A. Rohrbach, and D. Spruijt-Metz. 2012. "Motivational Interviewing for Adolescent Substance Use: A Review of the Literature." *Addictive Behaviors* 37 (12): 1325–34.

Bhutta, Z. A., J. K. Das, A. Rivzi, M. F. Gaffey, N. Walker, and others. 2013. "Evidence-Based Interventions for Improvement of Maternal and Child Nutrition: What Can Be Done and at What Cost?" *The Lancet* 382 (9890): 452–77. doi:10.1016/s0140-6736(13)60996-4.

Blakemore, S. J., and K. L. Mills. 2014. "Is Adolescence a Sensitive Period for Sociocultural Processing?" *Annual Review of Psychology* 65 (September 6): 187–207. doi:10.1146/annurev-psych-010213-115202.

Blank, L., S. K. Baxter, N. Payne, L. R. Guillaume, and H. Pilgrim. 2010. "Systematic Review and Narrative Synthesis of the Effectiveness of Contraceptive Service Interventions for Young People, Delivered in Educational Settings." *Journal of Pediatric and Adolescent Gynecology* 23 (6): 341–51. doi:10.1016/j.jpag.2010.03.007.

Bonomo, Y. A., G. Bowes, C. Coffey, J. B. Carlin, and G. C. Patton. 2004. "Teenage Drinking and the Onset of Alcohol Dependence: A Cohort Study Over Seven Years." *Addiction* 99 (12): 1520–28.

Brinn, M. P., K. V. Carosn, A. J. Esterman, A. B. Chung, B. J. Smith, and others. 2010. "Mass Media Interventions for Preventing Smoking in Young People." *Cochrane Database of Systematic Reviews* 11: CD001006. doi:10.1002/14651858.CD001006.pub2.

Bundy, D. A. P., N. de Silva, S. Horton, G. C. Patton, L. Schultz, and D. T. Jamison. 2017. "Child and Adolescent Health and Development: Realizing Neglected Potential." In *Disease Control Priorities* (third edition): Volume 8, *Child and Adolescent Health and Development,* edited by D. A. P. Bundy, N. de Silva, S. Horton, D. T. Jamison, and G. C. Patton. Washington, DC: World Bank.

Burns, J. M., and G. C. Patton. 2000. "Preventive Interventions for Youth Suicide: A Risk Factor-Based Approach." *Australian and New Zealand Journal of Psychiatry* 34 (3): 388–407.

Bushamuka, V. N., S. de Pee, A. Talukder, and M. Bloem. 2005. "Impact of a Homestead Gardening Program on Household Food Security and Empowerment of Women in Bangladesh." *Food and Nutrition Bulletin* 26 (1): 17–25.

Camacho-Miñano, M. J., N. M. LaVoi, and D. J. Barr-Anderson. 2011. "Interventions to Promote Physical Activity among Young and Adolescent Girls: A Systematic Review." *Health Education Research* 26 (6): 1025–19.

Carney, T., B. J. Myers, J. Louw, and C. Okwundu. 2014. "Brief School-Based Interventions and Behavioural Outcomes for Substance-Using Adolescents." *Cochrane Database of Systematic Reviews* 2: CD008969. doi:10.1002/14651858.CD008969.pub2.

Carson, K. V., M. P. Brinn, N. A. Labiszewski, A. J. Esterman, A. B. Chang, and others. 2011. "Community Interventions for Preventing Smoking in Young People." *Cochrane Database of Systematic Reviews* 7: CD001291. doi:10.1002/14651858.CD008969.pub2.

Champion, K. E., N. C. Newton, E. L. Barrett, and M. Teesson. 2013. "A Systematic Review of School-Based Alcohol and Other Drug Prevention Programs Facilitated by Computers or the Internet." *Drug and Alcohol Review* 32 (2): 115–23. doi:10.1111/j.1465-3362.2012.00517.x.

Chandra-Mouli, V., A. V. Camacho, and P. A. Michaud. 2013. "WHO Guidelines on Preventing Early Pregnancy and Poor Reproductive Outcomes among Adolescents in Developing Countries." *Journal of Adolescent Health* 52 (5): 517–22.

Chandra-Mouli, V., C. Lane, and S. Wong. 2015. "What Does Not Work in Adolescent Sexual and Reproductive Health: A Review of Evidence on Interventions Commonly Accepted as Best Practices." *Global Health Science and Practice* 3 (3): 333–40.

Chandra-Mouli, V., J. Svanemyr, A. Amin, H. Fogstad, L. Say, and others. 2015. "Twenty Years after International Conference on Population and Development: Where Are We with Adolescent Sexual and Reproductive Health and Rights?" *Journal of Adolescent Health* 56 (Suppl 1): S1–6. doi:10.1016/j.jadohealth.2014.09.015.

Chin, H. B., T. S. Sipe, R. Elder, S. L. Mercer, S. K. Chattopadhyay, and others. 2012. "The Effectiveness of Group-Based Comprehensive Risk-Reduction and Abstinence Education Interventions to Prevent or Reduce the Risk of Adolescent Pregnancy, Human Immunodeficiency Virus, and Sexually Transmitted Infections: Two Systematic Reviews for the Guide to Community Preventive Services." *American Journal of Preventive Medicine* 42 (3): 272–94. doi:10.1016/j.amepre.2011.11.006.

Clemmens, D., and L. L. Hayman. 2004. "Increasing Activity to Reduce Obesity in Adolescent Girls: A Research Review." *Journal of Obstetric, Gynecologic, and Neonatal Nursing* 33 (6): 801–08.

Copeland, W., L. Shanahan, E. J. Costello, and A. Angold. 2011. "Cumulative Prevalence of Psychiatric Disorders by Young Adulthood: A Prospective Cohort Analysis from the Great Smoky Mountains Study." *Journal of the American Academy of Child and Adolescent Psychiatry* 50 (3): 252–61.

Crutzen, R. 2010. "Adding Effect Sizes to a Systematic Review on Interventions for Promoting Physical Activity among European Teenagers." *International Journal of Behavioral Nutrition and Physical Activity* 7 (April 16): 29–29. doi:10.1186/1479-5868-7-29.

Cusimano, M. D., and M. Sameem. 2011. "The Effectiveness of Middle and High School-Based Suicide Prevention Programmes for Adolescents: A Systematic Review." *Injury Prevention* 17 (1): 43–49. doi:10.1136/ip.2009.025502.

De Bourdeaudhuij, I., E. Van Cauwenberghe, H. Spittaels, J. M. Oppert, C. Rostami, and others. 2011. "School-Based Interventions Promoting Both Physical Activity and Healthy Eating in Europe: A Systematic Review within the HOPE Project." *Obesity Reviews* 12 (3): 205–16. doi:10.1111/j.1467-789X.2009.00711.x.

De Meester, F., F. J. van Lenthe, H. Spittaels, N. Lien, and I. De Bourdeaudhuij. 2009. "Interventions for Promoting Physical Activity among European Teenagers: A Systematic Review." *International Journal of Behavioral Nutrition and Physical Activity* 6 (December 6): 82–82. doi:10.1186/1479-5868-6-82.

Denno, D. M., A. F. Hoopes, and V. Chandra-Mouli. 2015. "Effective Strategies to Provide Adolescent Sexual and Reproductive Health Services and to Increase Demand and Community Support." *Journal of Adolescent Health* 56 (Suppl 1): S22–41. doi:10.1016/j.jadohealth.2014.09.012.

Desai, M., F. O. ter Kuile, F. Nosten, R. McGready, K. Asamoa, and others. 2007. "Epidemiology and Burden of Malaria in Pregnancy." *The Lancet Infectious Diseases* 7 (2): 93–104.

DFID (Department for International Development). 2012. *The Neglected Crisis of Undernutrition: Evidence for Action.* London: DFID.

Dumith, S. C., D. P. Gigante, M. R. Domingues, and H. W. Kohl III. 2011. "Physical Activity Change during Adolescence: A Systematic Review and a Pooled Analysis." *International Journal of Epidemiology* 40 (3): 685–98. doi:10.1093/ije/dyq272.

Ellsberg, M., D. J. Arango, M. Morton, F. Gennari, S. Kiplesund, and others. 2015. "Prevention of Violence against Women and Girls: What Does the Evidence Say?" *The Lancet* 385 (9977): 1555–66. doi:10.1016/S0140-6736(14)61703-7.

Elvik, R., and T. Vaa, eds. 2009. *The Handbook of Road Safety Measures,* second edition. Bingley, U.K.: Emerald Group Publishing.

Evans, E., K. Hawton, and K. Rodham. 2004. "Factors Associated with Suicidal Phenomena in Adolescents: A Systematic Review of Population-Based Studies." *Clinical Psychology Review* 24 (8): 957–79. doi:10.1016/j.cpr.2004.04.005.

Ewing, S. W., A. Sakhardande, and S. J. Blakemore. 2014. "The Effect of Alcohol Consumption on the Adolescent Brain: A Systematic Review of MRI and fMRI Studies of Alcohol-Using Youth." *NeuroImage: Clinical* 5 (July 5): 420–37.

Fagan, A. A., and R. F. Catalano. 2013. "What Works in Youth Violence Prevention: A Review of the Literature." *Research on Social Work Practice* 23 (2): 141–56. doi:10.1177/1049731512465899.

Faggiano, F., S. Minozzi, E. Versino, and D. Buscemi. 2014. "Universal School-Based Prevention for Illicit Drug Use." *Cochrane Database of Systematic Reviews* 12: CD003020. doi:10.1002/14651858.CD003020.pub3.

Farrelly, M. C., B. R. Loomis, B. Han, J. Gfroerer, N. Kuiper, and others. 2013. "A Comprehensive Examination of the Influence of State Tobacco Control Programs and Policies on Youth Smoking." *American Journal of Public Health* 103 (3): 549–55. doi:10.2105/AJPH.2012.300948.

Fellmeth, G. L., C. Heffernan, J. Nurse, S. Habibula, and D. Sethi. 2013. "Educational and Skills-Based Interventions for Preventing Relationship and Dating Violence in Adolescents

and Young Adults." *Cochrane Database of Systematic Reviews* 6: CD004534. doi:10.1002/14651858.CD004534.pub3.

Ferri, M., E. Allara, A. Bo, A. Gasparrini, and F. Faggiano. 2013. "Media Campaigns for the Prevention of Illicit Drug Use in Young People." *Cochrane Database of Systematic Reviews* 6: CD009287. doi:10.1002/14651858.CD009287.pub2.

Forjuoh, S. N. 2003. "Traffic-Related Injury Prevention Interventions for Low-Income Countries." *Injury Control and Safety Promotion* 10 (1–2): 109–18. doi:10.1076/icsp.10.1.109.14115.

Foxcroft, D. R., and A. Tsertsvadze. 2011a. "Universal School-Based Prevention Programs for Alcohol Misuse in Young People." *Cochrane Database of Systematic Reviews* 5: CD009113. doi:10.1002/14651858.CD009113.

———. 2011b. "Universal Family-Based Prevention Programs for Alcohol Misuse in Young People." *Cochrane Database of Systematic Reviews* 9: CD009308. doi:10.1002/14651858.CD009308.

Francis, J. M., H. Grosskurth, J. Changalucha, S. H. Kapiga, and H. A. Weiss. 2014. "Systematic Review and Meta-Analysis: Prevalence of Alcohol Use among Young People in Eastern Africa." *Tropical Medicine and International Health* 19 (4): 476–88. doi:10.1111/tmi.12267.

Furlong, M., S. McGilloway, T. Bywater, J. Hutchings, S. M. Smith, and others. 2012. "Behavioural and Cognitive-Behavioural Group-Based Parenting Programmes for Early-Onset Conduct Problems in Children Aged 3 to 12 Years." *Cochrane Database of Systematic Reviews* 2: CD008225. doi:10.1002/14651858.CD008225.pub2.

Gates, S., J. McCambridge, L. A. Smith, and D. R. Foxcroft. 2006. "Interventions for Prevention of Drug Use by Young People Delivered in Non-School Settings." *Cochrane Database of Systematic Reviews* 1: CD005030.

Gibbs, C. M., A. Wendt, S. Peters, and C. J. Hoque. 2012. "The Impact of Early Age at First Childbirth on Maternal and Infant Health." *Paediatric and Perinatal Epidemiology* 26 (Suppl 1): 259–84.

Gortmaker, S. L., B. A. Swinburn, D. Levy, R. Carter, P. L. Mabry, and others. 2011. "Changing the Future of Obesity: Science, Policy, and Action." *The Lancet* 378 (9793): 838–47. doi:10.1016/S0140-6736(11)60815-5.

Gottschalk, L. B., and N. Ortayli. 2014. "Interventions to Improve Adolescents' Contraceptive Behaviors in Low- and Middle-Income Countries: A Review of the Evidence Base." *Contraception* 90 (3): 211–25. doi:10.1016/j.contraception.2014.04.017.

Gould, M. S., T. Greenberg, D. M. Velting, and D. Shaffer. 2003. "Youth Suicide Risk and Preventive Interventions: A Review of the Past 10 Years." *Journal of the American Academy of Child and Adolescent Psychiatry* 42 (4): 386–405.

Hahn, R., D. Fuqua-Whitley, H. Wethington, J. Lowry, A. Liberman, and others. 2007. "The Effectiveness of Universal School-Based Programs to Prevent Violent and Aggressive Behavior: A Systematic Review." *American Journal of Preventive Medicine* 33 (Suppl 2): S114–29.

Haider, R. 2006. *Adolescent Nutrition: A Review of the Situation in Selected South-East Asian Countries.* New Delhi: WHO, Regional Office for South-East Asia.

Harden, A., G. Brunton, A. Fletcher, and A. Oakley. 2009. "Teenage Pregnancy and Social Disadvantage: Systematic Review Integrating Controlled Trials and Qualitative Studies." *BMJ* 339 (November 12): b4254.

Hawton, K., D. Zahl, and R. Weatherall. 2003. "Suicide Following Deliberate Self-Harm: Long-Term Follow-Up of Patients Who Presented to a General Hospital." *British Journal of Psychiatry* 182 (June): 537–42.

Hazell, P. 1993. "Adolescent Suicide Clusters: Evidence, Mechanisms, and Prevention." *Australian and New Zealand Journal of Psychiatry* 27 (4): 653–65.

Jamison, D. T., L. H. Summers, G. Alleyne, K. J. Arrow, S. Berkley, and others. 2013. "Global Health 2035: A World Converging within a Generation." *The Lancet* 382 (9908): 1898–955. doi:10.1016/S0140-6736(13)62105-4.

Jensen, C. D., C. C. Cushing, B. S. Aylward, J. T. Craig, D. M. Sorell, and others. 2011. "Effectiveness of Motivational Interviewing Interventions for Adolescent Substance Use Behavior Change: A Meta-Analytic Review." *Journal of Consulting and Clinical Psychology* 79 (4): 433–40. doi:10.1037/a0023992.

Jordan, A. B., E. K. Kramer-Golinkoff, and V. C. Strasburger. 2008. "Does Adolescent Media Use Cause Obesity and Eating Disorders?" *Adolescent Medicine State of the Art Review* 19 (3): 431–49.

Jorm, A. F. 2015. "How Effective Are 'Headspace' Youth Mental Health Services?" *Australian and New Zealand Journal of Psychiatry* 49 (10): 861–62.

Katz, C., S. L. Bolton, L. Y. Katz, C. Isaak, T. Tilston-Jones, and others. 2013. "A Systematic Review of School-Based Suicide Prevention Programs." *Depression and Anxiety* 30 (10): 1030–45. doi:10.1002/da.22114.

Kessler, R. C., P. Berglund, O. Dernier, R. Jin, K. R. Merikangas, and others. 2005. "Lifetime Prevalence and Age-of-Onset Distributions of DSM-IV Disorders in the National Comorbidity Survey Replication." *Archives of General Psychiatry* 62 (6): 593–602.

King, J. C. 2003. "The Risk of Maternal Nutritional Depletion and Poor Outcomes Increases in Early or Closely Spaced Pregnancies." *Journal of Nutrition* 133 (5): 1732S–36.

Klimes-Dougan, B., D. A. Klingbeil, and S. J. Meller. 2013. "The Impact of Universal Suicide-Prevention Programs on the Help-Seeking Attitudes and Behaviors of Youths." *Crisis* 34 (2): 82–97. doi:10.1027/0227-5910/a000178.

Krug, E. G., L. L. Dahlberg, J. A. Mercy, A. B. Zwi, and R. Lozano. 2002. *World Report on Violence and Health.* Geneva: WHO.

Kumpfer, K. L., R. Alvarado, and H. O. Whiteside. 2003. "Family-Based Interventions for Substance Use and Misuse Prevention." *Substance Use and Misuse* 38 (11–13): 1759–87.

Lalloo, D. G., P. Olukoya, and P. Olliaro. 2006. "Malaria in Adolescence: Burden of Disease, Consequences, and Opportunities for Intervention." *The Lancet Infectious Diseases* 6 (12): 780–93. doi:10.1016/S1473-3099(06)70655-7.

Langford, R., C. P. Bonell, H. E. Jones, T. Pouliou, S. M. Murphy, and others. 2014. "The WHO Health Promoting School Framework for Improving the Health and Well-Being of Students and Their Academic Achievement." *Cochrane Database of Systematic Reviews* 4: CD008958. doi:10.1002/14651858.CD008958.pub2.

Laska, M. N., J. E. Pelletier, N. I. Larson, and M. Story. 2012. "Interventions for Weight Gain Prevention during the Transition to Young Adulthood: A Review of the Literature." *Journal of Adolescent Health* 50 (4): 324–33. doi:10.1016/j.jadohealth.2012.01.016.

Limbos, M. A., L. S. Chan, C. Warf, A. Schneir, E. Iverson, and others. 2007. "Effectiveness of Interventions to Prevent Youth Violence: A Systematic Review." *American Journal of Preventive Medicine* 33 (1): 65–74.

Lundgren, R., and A. Amin. 2015. "Addressing Intimate Partner Violence and Sexual Violence among Adolescents: Emerging Evidence of Effectiveness." *Journal of Adolescent Health* 56 (Suppl 1): S42–50. doi:10.1016/j.jadohealth.2014.08.012.

Mann, J. J., A. Apter, J. Bertolote, A. Beautrais, D. Currier, and others. 2005. "Suicide Prevention Strategies: A Systematic Review." *Journal of the American Medical Association* 294 (16): 2064–74. doi:10.1001/jama.294.16.2064.

Martineau, F., E. Tyner, T. Lorenc, M. Petticrew, and K. Lock. 2013. "Population-Level Interventions to Reduce Alcohol-Related Harm: An Overview of Systematic Reviews." *Preventive Medicine* 57 (4): 278–96. doi:10.1016/j.ypmed.2013.06.019.

Masset, E., L. Haddad, A. Cornelius, and J. Isaza-Castro. 2011. *A Systematic Review of Agricultural Interventions That Aim to Improve the Nutritional Status of Children.* London: EPPI-Centre, Social Science Research Unit, Institute of Education, University of London.

Mavedzenge, S. N., E. Luecke, and D. A. Ross. 2014. "Effective Approaches for Programming to Reduce Adolescent Vulnerability to HIV Infection, HIV Risk, and HIV-Related Morbidity and Mortality: A Systematic Review of Systematic Reviews." *Journal of Acquired Immune Deficiency Syndromes* 66 (Suppl 2): S154–69. doi:10.1097/QAI.0000000000000178.

McGorry, P., T. Bates, and M. Birchwood. 2013. "Designing Youth Mental Health Services for the 21st Century: Examples from Australia, Ireland, and the UK." *British Journal of Psychiatry* (Suppl 54): S30–35. doi:10.1192/bjp.bp.112.119214.

Medina-Mora, M. E., M. Monteiro, R. Room, J. Rehm, D. Jernigan, and others. 2015. "Alcohol Use and Alcohol Use Disorders." In *Disease Control Priorities* (third edition): Volume 4, *Mental, Neurological, and Substance Use Disorders*, edited by V. Patel, D. Chisholm, T. Dua, R. Laxminarayan, and M. E. Medina-Mora. Washington, DC: World Bank.

Milat, A. J., L. King, A. E. Bauman, and S. Redman. 2013. "The Concept of Scalability: Increasing the Scale and Potential Adoption of Health Promotion Interventions into Policy and Practice." *Health Promotion International* 28 (3): 285–98. doi:10.1093/heapro/dar097.

Miller, D. N., T. L. Eckert, and J. J. Mazza. 2009. "Suicide Prevention Programs in the Schools: A Review and Public Health Perspective." *School Psychology Review* 38 (2): 168–88.

Murillo Pardo, B., G. Bengoechea, G. Lanaspa, P. L. Bush, Z. Casterad, and others. 2013. "Promising School-Based Strategies and Intervention Guidelines to Increase Physical Activity of Adolescents." *Health Education Research* 28 (3): 523–38.

Mytton, J. A., C. DiGuiseppi, D. Gough, R. Taylor, and S. Logan. 2006. "School-Based Secondary Prevention Programmes for Preventing Violence." *Cochrane Database of Systematic Reviews* 3: CD004606.

Nesi, J., and M. J. Prinstein. 2015. "Using Social Media for Social Comparison and Feedback-Seeking: Gender and Popularity Moderate Associations with Depressive Symptoms." *Journal of Abnormal Child Psychology* 43 (8): 1427–38.

Ng, M., T. Fleming, M. Robinson, B. Thomson, N. Graetz, and others. 2014. "Global, Regional, and National Prevalence of Overweight and Obesity in Children and Adults during 1980-2013: A Systematic Analysis for the Global Burden of Disease Study 2013." *The Lancet* 384 (9945): 766–81. doi:10.1016/S0140-6736(14)60460-8.

Niemeier, H. M., H. A. Raynor, E. E. Lloyd-Richardson, M. L. Rogers, and R. R. Wing. 2006. "Fast Food Consumption and Breakfast Skipping: Predictors of Weight Gain from Adolescence to Adulthood in a Nationally Representative Sample." *Journal of Adolescent Health* 39 (6): 842–49. doi:10.1016/j.jadohealth.2006.07.001.

Norton, R., A. A. Hyder, D. Bishai, and M. Peden. 2006. "Unintentional Injuries." In *Disease Control Priorities in Developing Countries* (second edition), edited by D. T. Jamison, J. G. Breman, A. R. Measham, G. Alleyne, M. Claeson, D. B. Evans, P. Jha, A. Mills, and P. Musgrove. Washington, DC: World Bank and Oxford University Press.

NRC (National Research Council) and IOM (Institute of Medicine). 2005. "Growing Up Global: The Changing Transitions to Adulthood in Developing Countries." In *Panel on Transitions to Adulthood in Developing Countries*, edited by C. B. Lloyd. Washington, DC: National Academies Press.

O'Neill, J., H. Tabish, V. Welch, M. Petticrew, K. Pottie, and others. 2014. "Applying an Equity Lens to Interventions: Using PROGRESS Ensures Consideration of Socially Stratifying Factors to Illuminate Inequities in Health." *Journal of Clinical Epidemiology* 67 (1): 56–64. doi:10.1016/j.jclinepi.2013.08.005.

Oringanje, C., M. M. Meremikwu, H. Eko, E. Esu, A. Meremikwu, and others. 2009. "Interventions for Preventing Unintended Pregnancies among Adolescents." *Cochrane Database of Systematic Reviews* 4: CD005215. doi:10.1002/14651858.CD005215.pub2.

Park-Higgerson, H.-K., S. E. Perumean-Chaney, A. A. Bartolucci, D. M. Grimley, and K. P. Singh. 2008. "The Evaluation of School-Based Violence Prevention Programs: A Meta-Analysis." *Journal of School Health* 78 (9): 465–79. doi:10.1111/j.1746-1561.2008.00332.x.

Patton, G. C., P. Azzopardi, E. Kennedy, and C. Coffey. 2017. "Global Measures of Health Risks and Disease Burden in Adolescents." In *Disease Control Priorities* (third edition): Volume 8, *Child and Adolescent Health and Development*, edited by D. A. P. Bundy, N. de Silva, S. Horton, D. T. Jamison, and G. C. Patton. Washington, DC: World Bank.

Patton, G. C., C. Coffey, H. Romaniuk, A. MacKinnon, J. B. Carlin, and others. 2014. "The Prognosis of Common Mental Disorders in Adolescents: A 14-Year Prospective Cohort Study." *The Lancet* 383 (9926): 1404–11.

Patton, G. C., C. Coffey, S. M. Sawyer, R. M. Viner, D. M. Haller, and others. 2009. "Global Patterns of Mortality in Young People: A Systematic Analysis of Population Health Data." *The Lancet* 374 (9693): 881–92. doi:10.1016/S0140-6736(09)60741-8.

Patton, G. C., S. M. Sawyer, J. S. Santelli, D. A. Ross, R. Afifi, and others. 2016. "Our Future: A *Lancet* Commission on Adolescent Health and Wellbeing." *The Lancet* 387 (10036): 2423–78. doi:10.1016/S0140-6736(16)00579-1.

Pearson, N., R. Braithwaite, and S. J. Biddle. 2015. "The Effectiveness of Interventions to Increase Physical Activity among Adolescent Girls: A Meta-Analysis." *Academic Pediatrics* 15 (1): 9–18. doi:10.1016/j.acap.2014.08.009.

Peden, M., R. Scurfield, D. Sleet, D. Mohan, A. A. Hyder, and others, eds. 2004. *World Report on Road Traffic Injury Prevention*. Geneva: WHO.

Porchia, B. R., A. Baldasseroni, C. Dellisanti, C. Lorini, and G. Bonaccorsi. 2014. "Effectiveness of Two Interventions in Preventing Traffic Accidents: A Systematic Review." *Annali di Igiene: Medicina Preventiva e di Comunità* 26 (1): 63–75. doi:10.7416/ai.2014.1959.

Prentice, A. M., K. A. Ward, G. R. Goldberg, L. M. Jariou, S. E. Moore, and others. 2013. "Critical Windows for Nutritional Interventions against Stunting." *American Journal of Clinical Nutrition* 97 (5): 911–18.

Rees, R., J. Kavanagh, A. Harden, J. Shepherd, G. Brunton, and others. 2006. "Young People and Physical Activity: A Systematic Review Matching their Views to Effective Interventions." *Health Education Research* 21 (6): 806–25.

Reinhardt, K., and J. Fanzo. 2014. "Addressing Chronic Malnutrition through Multi-Sectoral, Sustainable Approaches: A Review of the Causes and Consequences." *Frontiers in Nutrition* 1 (August 15): 13.

Retting, R. A., S. A. Ferguson, and A. T. McCartt. 2003. "A Review of Evidence-Based Traffic Engineering Measures Designed to Reduce Pedestrian-Motor Vehicle Crashes." *American Journal of Public Health* 93 (9): 1456–63.

Roberts, I. G., and I. Kwan. 2001. "School-Based Driver Education for the Prevention of Traffic Crashes." *Cochrane Database of Systematic Reviews* 3: CD003201.

Robinson, J., G. Cox, A. Maline, M. Williamson, G. Baldwin, and others. 2013. "A Systematic Review of School-Based Interventions Aimed at Preventing, Treating, and Responding to Suicide-Related Behavior in Young People." *Crisis* 34 (3): 164–82. doi:10.1027/0227-5910/a000168.

Robinson, J., S. E. Hetrick, and C. Martin. 2011. "Preventing Suicide in Young People: Systematic Review." *Australia and New Zealand Journal of Psychiatry* 45 (1): 3–26. doi:10.3109/00048674.2010.511147.

Ruager-Martin, R., M. J. Hyde, and N. Modi. 2010. "Maternal Obesity and Infant Outcomes." *Early Human Development* 86 (11): 715–22. doi:10.1016/j.earlhumdev.2010.08.007.

Sawyer, S. M., R. A. Afifi, L. H. Bearinger, S. J. Blakemore, B. Dick, and others. 2012. "Adolescence: A Foundation for Future Health." *The Lancet* 379 (9826): 1630–40. doi:10.1016/s0140-6736(12)60072-5.

Sawyer, S. M., N. Reavley, C. Bonell, and G. C. Patton. 2017. "Platforms for Delivering Adolescent Health Actions." In *Disease Control Priorities* (third edition): Volume 8, *Child and Adolescent Health and Development*, edited by D. A. P. Bundy, N. de Silva, S. Horton, D. T. Jamison, and G. C. Patton. Washington, DC: World Bank.

Seo, D. C., and J. Sa. 2010. "A Meta-Analysis of Obesity Interventions among U.S. Minority Children." *Journal of Adolescent Health* 46 (4): 309–23. doi:10.1016/j.jadohealth.2009.11.202.

Sethi, D., K. Hughes, M. Bellis, F. Mitis, and F. Racioppi, eds. 2010. *European Report on Preventing Violence and Knife Crime among Young People*. Geneva: WHO.

Simpson, H. M. 2003. "The Evolution and Effectiveness of Graduated Licensing." *Journal of Safety Research* 34 (1): 25–34.

Smit, E., J. Verdumen, K. Monshouwer, and F. Smit. 2008. "Family Interventions and Their Effect on Adolescent Alcohol Use in General Populations; A Meta-Analysis of Randomized Controlled Trials." *Drug and Alcohol Dependence* 97 (3): 195–206.

Snow, K., L. Nelson, C. Sismanidis, S. M. Sawyer, and S. Graham. 2015. "Incidence and Prevalence of Active Tuberculosis among Adolescents and Young Adults: A Systematic Review." Unpublished.

Steinberg, L. 2008. "A Social Neuroscience Perspective on Adolescent Risk-Taking." *Developmental Review* 28 (1): 78–106. doi:10.1016/j.dr.2007.08.002.

Stice, E., H. Shaw, and C. N. Marti. 2006. "A Meta-Analytic Review of Obesity Prevention Programs for Children and Adolescents: The Skinny on Interventions That Work." *Psychological Bulletin* 132 (5): 667–91.

Stockings, E. A., L. Degenhardt, T. Dobbins, Y. Y. Lee, H. E. Erskine, and others. 2016. "Preventing Depression and Anxiety in Young People: A Review of the Joint Efficacy of Universal, Selective and Indicated Prevention." *Psychological Medicine* 46 (1): 11–26. doi:10.1017/S0033291715001725.

Strang, J., T. Babor, J. Caulkins, B. Fischer, D. Foxcroft, and others. 2012. "Drug Policy and the Public Good: Evidence for Effective Interventions." *The Lancet* 379 (9810): 71–83. doi:10.1016/S0140-6736(11)61674-7.

Thomas, R. E., P. R. Baker, B. V. Thomas, and D. L. Lorenzetti. 2015. "Family-Based Programmes for Preventing Smoking by Children and Adolescents." *Cochrane Database of Systematic Reviews* 2: CD004493. doi:10.1002/14651858.CD004493.pub3.

Thomas, R. E., J. McLellan, and R. Perera. 2013. "School-Based Programmes for Preventing Smoking." *Cochrane Database of Systematic Reviews* 4:Cd001293. doi:10.1002/14651858.CD001293.pub3.

Toroyan, T., and M. Peden. 2007. *Youth and Road Safety*. Geneva: WHO.

Udonwa, N. E., A. N. Gyuse, and A. S. J. Etokidem. 2010. "Malaria: Knowledge and Prevention Practices among School Adolescents in a Coastal Community in Calabar, Nigeria." *African Journal of Primary Health Care and Family Medicine* 2 (1): 103.

van Sluijs, E. M., A. M. McMinn, and S. J. Griffin. 2008. "Effectiveness of Interventions to Promote Physical Activity in Children and Adolescents: Systematic Review of Controlled Trials." *British Journal of Sports Medicine* 42 (8): 653–57.

Vijayakumar, L., M. R. Phillips, M. M. Silverman, D. Gunnell, and V. Carli. 2015. "Suicide." In *Disease Control Priorities* (third edition): Volume 4, *Mental, Neurological, and Substance Use Disorders*, edited by V. Patel, D. Chisholm, T. Dua, R. Laxminarayan, and M. E. Medina-Mora. Washington, DC: World Bank.

Viner, R. M., E. M. Ozer, S. Denny, M. Marmot, M. Resnick, and others. 2012. "Adolescence and the Social Determinants of Health." *The Lancet* 379 (9826): 1641–52. doi:10.1016/s0140-6736(12)60149-4.

Wakefield, M., and F. Chaloupka. 2000. "Effectiveness of Comprehensive Tobacco Control Programmes in Reducing Teenage Smoking in the USA." *Tobacco Control* 9 (2): 177–86.

Warren, C. W., V. Lea, J. Lee, N. R. Jones, S. Asma, and others. 2009. "Change in Tobacco Use among 13–15 Year Olds between 1999 and 2008: Findings from the Global Youth Tobacco Survey." *Global Health Promotion* 16 (Suppl 2): 38–90. doi:10.1177/1757975909342192.

Whitaker, D. J., S. Momson, C. Lindquist, S. R. Hawkins, J. A. O'Neill, and others. 2006. "A Critical Review of Interventions for the Primary Prevention of Perpetration of Partner Violence." *Aggression and Violent Behavior* 11 (2): 151–66.

Whitaker, R. C., J. A. Wright, M. S. Pepe, K. D. Seidel, and W. H. Dietz. 1997. "Predicting Obesity in Young Adulthood from Childhood and Parental Obesity." *New England Journal of Medicine* 337 (13): 869–73. doi:10.1056/NEJM199709253371301.

WHO (World Health Organization). 2010a. *Violence Prevention: The Evidence*. Geneva: WHO.

———. 2010b. *Global Strategy to Reduce the Harmful Use of Alcohol*. Geneva: WHO.

WHO and ExpandNet. 2010. *Nine Steps for Developing a Scaling-Up Strategy*. Geneva: WHO.

———. 2011. *Global Health Sector Strategy on HIV/AIDS 2011–2015*. Geneva: WHO.

———. 2013. *Global Status Report on Road Safety 2013: Supporting a Decade of Action*. Geneva: WHO.

Williams, A. F. 2006. "Young Driver Risk Factors: Successful and Unsuccessful Approaches for Dealing with Them and an Agenda for the Future." *Injury Prevention* 12 (Suppl 1): i4–8. doi:10.1136/ip.2006.011783.

Wood, S. K., L. Eckley, K. E. Hughes, and L. Voorham. 2014. "Computer-Based Programmes for the Prevention and Management of Illicit Recreational Drug Use: A Systematic Review." *Addictive Behaviors* 39 (1): 30–38. doi:10.1016/j.addbeh.2013.09.010.

Woolfenden, S. R., K. Williams, and J. K. Peat. 2002. "Family and Parenting Interventions for Conduct Disorder and Delinquency: A Meta-Analysis of Randomised Controlled Trials." *Archives of Disease in Childhood* 86 (4): 251–56.

Platforms to Reach Children in Early Childhood

Maureen M. Black, Amber Gove, and Katherine A. Merseth

INTRODUCTION

This chapter reports on platforms that promote early child development. The economics of early child development programs and packages are covered in chapter 24 in this volume (Horton and Black 2017). Early child development research, programs, and policies have advanced significantly in low- and middle-income countries (LMICs) during the past two decades (Black, Walker, and others 2016), spearheaded by three prominent advances.

The first advance is the recognition that the foundations of adult health and well-being are based on prenatal and early-life genetic-environmental interactions that affect brain development. This recognition has created a strong emphasis on strategies to ensure that young children reach their developmental potential (Shonkoff and others 2012).

The second advance is the urgent call for strategies to promote early child development, following estimates that more than 200 million children younger than age five years in LMICs are at risk of not reaching their developmental potential (Grantham-McGregor and others 2007), largely due to nutritional deficiencies and a lack of responsive caregiving. Recent estimates report that although the prevalence of at-risk children has declined, more than 43 percent of children in LMICs are at risk for poor development (Lu, Black, and Richter 2016). Initiatives during the first 1,000 days of life—the period from conception through age 24 months, when nutritional requirements are high and brain development is rapid—have focused attention on the need to ensure that children receive the interventions necessary to achieve their developmental potential.

Finally, global economic growth in the 1990s and the success of the Millennium Development Goals in reducing poverty and stunting and in increasing child survival have brought optimism to efforts to promote child health and development. The evidence that interventions early in life are effective in promoting early child development (Engle and others 2007; Engle and others 2011; Nores and Barnett 2010) supports the implementation of such programs at scale.

Calls from global leaders have emphasized increased investment, programs, and policies for early child development (Lake and Chan 2015) and have brought about the inclusion of early child development in the United Nations' Sustainable Development Goals (SDGs) (UN 2015). This chapter reviews the definition of early child development; risks and protective factors related to early child development; early child development systems (rights and equity, integrated interventions and multisectoral coordination, governance, and quality improvement and accountability); and platforms needed to implement early child development programs that address children's changing developmental skills across the continuum from infancy through early primary school. Definitions of age groupings and age-specific terminology used in this volume can be found in chapter 1 (Bundy and others 2017).

Corresponding author: Maureen M. Black, Distinguished Fellow, RTI International; and Department of Pediatrics, University of Maryland School of Medicine, Baltimore, Maryland, United States; maureenblack@rti.org.

EARLY CHILD DEVELOPMENT

Early child development refers to the developmental progression of perceptual, motor, cognitive, language, socioemotional, and self-regulation skills through the first eight years of life. Within the grounding of social ecological theory (Bronfenbrenner and Morris 2007), children's early development is influenced by family, community, and environmental interactions. Families and caregivers provide proximal care for children and mediate distal influences from neighborhoods, communities, and the larger environments, including legal, safety, and cultural factors. Because children influence caregivers' interactions through their characteristics and behavior, and in turn, are influenced by caregivers (Bergmeier and others 2014), children participate in their own development through a transactional process. As children grow older, their direct interactions outside their family increase, through contact with friends, care providers, teachers, and other community members.

Children reach their developmental potential with the acquisition of competencies in academic, behavioral, socioemotional, and economic areas. Theories of child development take a life-course perspective, emphasizing that the skills acquired throughout childhood, adolescence, and adulthood build on the capacities established prenatally and early in life. Criteria for the proximal home environment, referred to as *nurturing care* (Black,

Walker, and others 2016), include a home environment that is sensitive to children's health and nutritional needs, responsive, emotionally supportive, and developmentally stimulating and appropriate, with opportunities for play and early learning, and protection from adversities (Black and Aboud 2011; Bradley and Putnick 2012). Nurturing care occurs through caregiver-child interactions and promotes children's developmental potential in multiple areas, including health, nutrition, security and safety, responsive caregiving, and early learning (figure 19.1).

Research into interventions has shown that in keeping with theories of early child development (Bronfenbrenner and Morris 2007), nurturing care extends beyond families to include community child care providers, teachers in early education, and community support to families (Farnsworth and others 2014). A family's capacity to provide nurturing care is enabled proximally by household characteristics and resources, and distally by community resources and exposures, policies, laws, and cultural variations. Recent evidence has shown that nurturing care during early childhood attenuates the detrimental effects of various risks on brain development (Hanson and others 2015; Noble, Houston, and others 2015) and on early growth (Black, Tilton, and others 2016) and helps children build healthy habits that promote development.

Figure 19.1 Domains of Nurturing Care Necessary for Children to Reach Their Developmental Potential

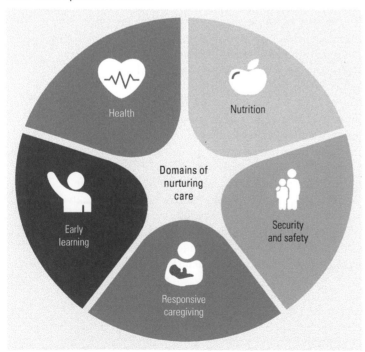

RISK AND PROTECTIVE FACTORS FOR EARLY CHILD DEVELOPMENT

Risks to children's development begin before conception and are often associated with poverty, nutritional deficiencies, and maternal stress; they can result in lifelong physical and mental health consequences that are thought to operate through epigenetic processes (Boersma and others 2014; Hanson and others 2012). The concept of biological embedding theorizes that the burden of many adult diseases is partially caused by early adversity, particularly socioeconomic stress factors, through a combination of latent effects, pathway effects, and accumulation of disadvantage (Hertzman 1999, 2013). Associations have been documented between adverse childhood experiences and later health outcomes (Brown and others 2010), including epigenetic signatures of the human genome (Bick and others 2012). These findings have led to the conclusion that the origins of adult disease are often found among developmental and biological disruptions occurring early in life (Shonkoff, Boyce, and McEwen 2009). Although there is increasing recognition that the early years serve as an entry point for reducing the burden of disease and improving population health, policies and programs that promote early development are only beginning to emerge (Hertzman 2013).

Children in LMICs face multiple threats from infectious diseases, such as HIV/AIDS (human immunodeficiency virus/acquired immune deficiency syndrome), diarrhea, malaria, and pneumonia, which can negatively affect their development, particularly when they occur in the context of malnutrition. In addition, diagnostic and treatment services for children with developmental disabilities are limited in these settings (Engle and others 2011).

Poverty

Early life poverty is a well-documented risk to children's early development. Not only can poverty contribute to caregiver stress, but the effects are evident in children's brain development. Children raised in low-income families are at risk for smaller hippocampal gray matter volume (Hanson and others 2015; Noble, Engelhardt, and others 2015) and low frontal and temporal lobe volume—brain areas associated with cognitive and academic performance (Hair and others 2015). The impact of poverty is evident in children's growth and development in the first year of life (Black, Tilton, and others 2016; Hamadani and others 2014) and in language processing and vocabulary by age 18 months (Fernald, Marchman, and Weisleder 2013). Disparities increase throughout childhood; the effects of being raised in poverty extend to adulthood and result in low task-related activation of the brain regions that support language, cognitive control, and memory skills, and high activation of regions associated with emotional reactivity (Liberzon and others 2015; Pavlakis and others 2015).

Maternal education is one pathway out of the poverty trap. Maternal education has been positively related to children's health and development in LMICs (Black, Tilton, and others 2016; Walker, Wachs, and others 2011). Better-educated mothers are able to manage household resources and provide the protection, nurturance, and early learning opportunities that promote children's healthy growth and development (Bornstein and Putnick 2012). An increase in maternal education has been credited with the significant reduction in mortality in children under age five years in 175 countries from 1970 to 1990 (controlling for per capita income) (Gakidou and others 2010). This finding has been replicated in other cross-national studies as well as national studies in both low-income and high-income countries (HICs). For example, an inverse association between infant mortality and maternal education within families of equal poverty levels has been shown in Nicaragua (Peña, Wall, and Persson 2000), replicating findings from an early study in Brazil (Victoria and others 1992); an inverse association between zinc deficiency, preschooler stress, and maternal education has been found in Vancouver (Vaghri and others 2011).

Nutritional Deficiencies

Children have specific nutritional requirements early in life to support their rapid physical growth and brain development. Many aspects of brain development are activated either prenatally or in the first months of life (Fox, Levitt, and Nelson 2010). Stunting (length-for-age greater than two standard deviations below the median) and micronutrient deficiencies during this period increase the risk of subsequent cognitive, motor, and academic problems (Black 2003; Sudfeld and others 2015). Although the first 1,000 days are sensitive for nutritional adequacy, the timing of early brain development—with regions developing and maturing at different points—and the plasticity of early brain development suggest that the window of opportunity for early child development interventions extends through the second 1,000 days, up to age five years (Wachs and others 2014).

Maternal Stress

Stress, depression, and anxiety during pregnancy can affect fetal development, leading to low birth weight and increased risk of anxiety and metabolic dysregulation (Wachs and others 2014). Postnatal stress can interfere with parenting and early caregiver-child interactions, with long-term effects on child brain structure and function (Glover 2011). Recent evidence has also shown associations between maternal-reported stress and children's neuroendocrine-immune functioning (measured through saliva), suggesting that children of stressed mothers may be desensitized to inflammatory immune processes and therefore at risk for inflammatory diseases (Riis and others 2016). These findings occurred regardless of socioeconomic status in a sample of children age five years whose families were of high and low socioeconomic status, and suggest that interventions to reduce maternal stress may have additional benefits for children's health and development.

Accumulated Risks

Risks often co-occur, with accumulated risks more likely to undermine children's developmental potential than single risks, particularly when they co-occur early in life (Wachs and others 2014). The focus on risks to child development has often led to a harm-reduction perspective, with delivery strategies targeting children at greatest risk. Although programs to alleviate single risks may be effective, evidence suggests that programs addressing multiple risks, such as both nutrition and early child development, have greater likelihood of producing sustainable results (Nores and Barnett 2010; Rao and others 2014). The co-occurrence of multiple risks has spurred recommendations for integrated interventions that address multiple risks (Black and Dewey 2014).

EARLY CHILD DEVELOPMENT SYSTEMS

Successful early child development programs are grounded in solid policy frameworks and systems. Vargas-Barón (2013) has identified eight domains that characterize strong and sustainable early child development systems. Five domains are particularly relevant to this chapter: equity and rights, integration and coordination, governance, quality improvement, and accountability.

Equity and Rights

Equity and rights can refer to the availability of early child development services. Delivery strategies for early child development programs are categorized as follows:

- *Universal*, when they are available to all
- *Selective*, when targeted to subpopulations at risk
- *Indicated*, when available to children identified by screening (Gordon 1983).

Public educational programs are universal and incorporated into the governance structure of the education sector. Making early child development programs universal can improve equity by ensuring that all children are able to acquire the skills to reach their developmental potential (Irwin, Siddiqi, and Hertzman 2007). However, universal approaches may not reach all children in low socioeconomic status households because of barriers to access, such as inability to pay fees, lack of transportation, and multiple languages (Carey, Crammond, and De Leeuw 2015). Early child development programs are often selective and available in regions or areas where large segments of the population experience extreme poverty, malnutrition, or other conditions that put them at risk of not reaching their developmental potential. The drawback of selective approaches is that they may be inequitable because they miss children in the middle socioeconomic status range, where most vulnerable children are found (Carey, Crammond, and De Leeuw 2015; Marmot and others

2010). The limitations of the traditional universal and selective approaches have led program personnel to seek an alternative that reaches all children by addressing the barriers that prevent children most in need from accessing services. The concept of proportionate universality, a universal service with scale and intensity proportionate to the level of disadvantage, is a promising approach to reducing inequity in areas with a social gradient in child development (Marmot and others 2010).

Integrated Interventions and Multisectoral Coordination

The concept of integrated interventions refers to services that address multiple issues with shared messages, the use of shared or existing platforms, and opportunities for synergy (Black, Perez-Escamilla, and Fernandez Rao 2015). Multisectoral coordination refers to coordinated services across sectors, with either sector-specific or unifying policies (Vargas-Barón 2013). Although multiple calls for integrated services have been made on theoretical and practical grounds (Black and Dewey 2014), few evaluations have been conducted (Grantham-McGregor and others 2014). The international community and development agencies have incorporated early child development into high-profile documents such as the World Health Organization's (WHO) *Report of the World Health Organization Commission on Social Determinants of Health* (WHO 2009), the World Bank's World Declaration on Education for All (UNESCO 1990), and the United Nations Educational, Scientific and Cultural Organization's Dakar Framework for Action (UNESCO 2000), and the SDGs. A critical role of these agencies is to support the governments of LMICs in the establishment of national early child development policies and structures, such as a national commission to coordinate early child development programs across ministries and sectors. Successful integrated programs and coordinated multisectoral processes can be sustainable and scaled up when they stand on solid policy ground (Vargas-Barón 2013). Very few LMICs have well-defined national early child development frameworks or policies. An early child development agenda within LMICs can benefit greatly from policies that are strong and comprehensive and result in enforceable mandates (Shonkoff and others 2012).

Table 19.1 lists considerations regarding integrated programs and multisectoral coordination related to early child development, highlighting both benefits and cautions. Integrated programs address the interdependencies among young children's basic needs, often building strength and learning through play (Woodhead and others 2014).

Table 19.1 Integrated Programs and Multisectoral Coordination for Nutrition and Child Development Interventions

Issue	Benefit	Cautionary note
Scientific basis	Children require support for health, nutrition, security and safety, responsive caregiving, and early learning. Single components are not sufficient.	Avoid overwhelming or confusing caregivers with multiple messages across domains.
Impact of integrated intervention may be stronger than single-sector models	Impact of nutrition intervention is strongest in the first 1,000 days.	Impact of child development interventions continues beyond the first 1,000 days.
Economy of effort	One community worker may be able to deliver multiple messages.	Additional time per visit may be required to deliver multiple messages.
Financial support	Sharing community workers across sectors may be economical.	Clarity is needed in balancing financial investment and administrative coordination across sectors.
Comprehensive approach	Integrated nutrition and child development intervention can address children's needs and may result in synergy.	Avoid overwhelming caregivers with multiple messages.
Promotion of integrated multisectoral policies by international organizations	Strong policies may result in more and better-quality programs that address the comprehensive needs of children.	Policy support from international agencies requires program, training, and evaluation support.
Existing delivery platform	Delivery platforms may vary across sectors, providing additional opportunities to reach participants.	Limited data exist on the impact of varying platforms (such as individual versus group).
Evaluation	Conducting evaluation across multiple domains may be efficient.	Evaluation demands from two sectors may occur.
Governance	Governance structure may facilitate cross-sector coordination.	Sectors have separate budgets, priorities, and management targets.
Training and supervision	Training and supervision could be coordinated across sectors to develop comprehensive, integrated messages.	Specialized training and supervision may be necessary to adequately meet the needs of differing domain and sector priorities.
Feasibility	Information on feasibility and lessons learned could enhance program development.	Additional costs may be incurred to evaluate feasibility across two sectors.
Costing	Cost analyses can be helpful to evaluate cost-benefit ratio of services.	Additional expenses may be incurred to build costing into services across two sectors.
Implementation science	Principles of implementation science, including stakeholder involvement, can assist with program sustainability and scaling.	Additional costs may be incurred to apply principles of implementation science across two sectors.

A meta-analysis of the impact of preschool programs concluded that integrated programs, which typically are government funded, had the largest effect on children's cognitive development (Rao and others 2014). The analysis, which included 115 interventions from 70 studies in 30 LMICs, also found that the most effective programs were provided by well-qualified personnel working with both parents and children.

In 1975, India established the Integrated Child Development Services, a government-sponsored nutrition and child development program for pregnant women and for children up to age six years (Rao 2005). The program is administered through the Ministry of Women and Child Development, and includes preschools (Anganwadi Centers) in local communities throughout the country. Evaluations of the centers have demonstrated that they increase children's nutrition and development, although also showing variability in the quality of staff training and implementation and in the benefits to children (Chudasama and others 2014; Malik and others 2015; Rao 2010). With support from the World Bank and other organizations, the Indian government has launched the Integrated Child Development Services Systems Strengthening and Nutrition Improvement Program to promote children's nutrition and to raise the quality of the program by strengthening the policy framework, facilitating community engagement, and increasing the focus on children under age three years.

Governance

Implementation of early child development programs is often fragmented, particularly for children under age five years, with limited regulatory systems or government oversight. Indicated approaches are generally reserved for children with specialized needs. The governance structure needs to be considered in making decisions regarding integrated services and coordination across sectors. Integrated services require governance structures that support integrated policies and programming, with attention to training, supervision, and monitoring.

Services that are incorporated into governance structures benefit from being able to call on infrastructure, public financing, and planning and coordination with other government services. Health and education are well-established government sectors, and both relate to early child development. However, the locus of early child development services varies widely across governance systems and often operates through nongovernmental organizations with limited state oversight (Britto and others 2014).

Health Sector

Young children with adequate health and nutrition from conception through age 24 months have the best chance of thriving and reaching their developmental potential (Black and others 2013). Growth during this sensitive period is associated with subsequent cognition and school attainment (Martorell and others 2010); associations between growth and cognition or school attainment after 24 months are less strong (Hoddinott and others 2008). The timing of adequate nutrition is critical in health and nutritional interventions (Wachs and others 2014). For example, stunting before age 24 months is related to poor child development; increases in length-for-age before age 24 months are associated with increases in school-age cognitive performance (Sudfeld and others 2015). Although increases in height-for-age after 24 months have been associated with subsequent cognitive performance, the findings are relatively modest (Black, Perez-Escamilla, and Fernandez Rao 2015; Crookston and others 2013).

Similarly, micronutrient deficiencies are prevalent among young children, particularly during the first 1,000 days when rates of growth are high and children are moving from a milk-based to a food-based diet. Evidence on the impact of micronutrient supplementation among children younger than age 24 months is emerging, with indications of benefits to children's motor and socioemotional development (Ramakrishnan, Goldenberg, and Allen 2011). The timing imperative of children's early health and nutrition is often addressed by the health sector through close involvement with women before delivery and with children through the first 24 months. After age 24 months, fewer routine health visits take place, and health sector services are dominated by acute care. The health sector plays an important role in providing anticipatory guidance, screening for developmental delays, and referring children for services, but there are few links with the education sector.

Education Sector

Early child development interventions have focused strongly on primary school education, with estimates from 2015 that 91 percent of eligible children are enrolled in primary school (UNESCO 2015). Historically, governments in LMICs provided a basic cycle of primary school beginning with grade 1 (usually from age six years, with some variation across countries), with no public educational services available before that.

Early child development was included in the initial Education for All documents of the United Nations (UNESCO 1990, 2000). Although preprimary education has since been incorporated into the educational sector in many LMICs, its structure and quality are variable. Primary school performance is enhanced by preprimary attendance (Berlinski, Galiani, and Gertler 2009), especially when the quality of preprimary education is high and the transition to primary school is well coordinated. High-quality preprimary education refers to both structural characteristics, such as environmental safety and hygiene, and teaching and learning characteristics, such as staff-child interaction and opportunities for play, exploration, and early learning.

Although healthy development depends on the complex and carefully timed interplay of nutritional, health, and educational inputs throughout children's first eight years, there is extremely limited coordination between the health and education sectors and a notable lack of purposeful investment. As a result, there is a gap between the end of regular health services at approximately age two years and the initiation of formal education at age five or six years (figure 19.2). This gap occurs at a very sensitive time in children's physical, cognitive, and socioemotional development. The impact of missed opportunities to intervene in support of healthy development for the most vulnerable may have lasting consequences for children and societies.

Figure 19.2 Age Gap in Early Child Development Services between Health and Education Sectors

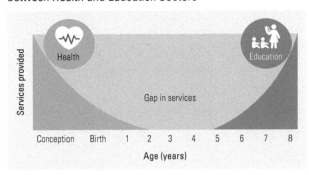

Quality Improvement and Accountability

Quality assurance is a critical component of early child development programs, guided by strong monitoring and evaluation procedures (Berlinski and Schady 2015). A major challenge to early child development has been the lack of population-level indicators, such as stunting is for nutrition. Individual-level assessments provide information on the development of individual children, but require too much time and technical expertise to evaluate programs administered at scale. Population-level indicators are needed that are easy to administer and interpret; are reactive to program changes; and have strong psychometric properties, including reliability and validity (McCoy and others 2016; Raikes, Dua, and Britto 2015).

PLATFORMS TO IMPLEMENT EARLY CHILD DEVELOPMENT ACROSS A DEVELOPMENTAL CONTINUUM

The fragmentation in early child development services is partially associated with the rapidly changing societal and economic structure surrounding families. Historically, families have cared for young children with support from the health sector, through services such as monitoring growth and development, preventing infectious diseases with vaccines, treating childhood illnesses, and promoting breastfeeding and complementary feeding. Although families have succeeded in promoting their children's growth and development, particularly when mothers are well educated (Walker, Wachs, and others 2011), changes in social and economic structures in which mothers are employed, either inside or outside of the home, have led to heightened demand for alternative sources of care. Based on children's changing developmental needs, government and nongovernment platforms have emerged to provide care (table 19.2), although they vary in how well they enable children to meet their developmental potential.

Preconception and Pregnancy

Recent evidence has shown that adequate health, nutritional status, and psychological well-being before conception provide the best chance of a healthy pregnancy and healthy fetal and infant development (Boersma and others 2014). Although few systematic preparation programs for childbearing have been established, recent calls focus on ensuring that adolescents are prepared for pregnancy, particularly in areas where there are nutritional deficiencies among women of childbearing age (Thurnham 2013). Both the health and the education sectors could be engaged in preconception preparation for adolescents that includes reproductive health education to avoid unplanned early pregnancies and that also includes empowerment, stress alleviation strategies, and preparation for adulthood and parenting.

Birth to Age 24 Months: Clinic Services, Home Visiting, and Community Services

Although significant advances in maternal, newborn, and child health have been made, evidenced by declines in neonatal, under-five, and maternal mortality, rates of mortality remain high, especially in LMICs (Lassi, Kumar, and Bhutta 2016). In addition to poverty, mortality is associated with low maternal education, poor nutrition, comorbid health conditions, and lack of access to skilled care. Interventions to alleviate many of the causes of mortality are available through community-based care. Platforms to promote child development during infancy are also available through community-based care and include individual or group sessions in health clinics, home visiting, and community groups.

Care for Child Development is a comprehensive program developed by the World Health Organization (WHO) and United Nations Children's Fund (UNICEF) to promote early growth and development in the context of health care contacts, either in clinics or homes (WHO and UNICEF 2012). The program is delivered through health care providers in Turkey, where there were benefits in the home environment (Ertem and others 2006), and through community home visitors in China and Pakistan (Jin and others 2007; Yousafzai and others 2014), with benefits to children's development. In a follow-up of children at age four years who participated in a randomized trial of home intervention from birth through two years, the children who received responsive caregiving had sustained effects in IQ, executive functioning, preacademic skills, and prosocial behaviors, and the mothers had benefits in responsive caregiving behaviors (Yousafzai and others 2016).

Table 19.2 Early Child Development Platforms by Age of Child

Sector	Platform	Preconception and prenatal	Ages 0–24 months	Ages 2–4 years	Age 5 years	Ages 6–8 years
Health sector	Clinic: individual or group sessions	X	X			
	Home visiting	X	X			
Nongovernmental organization, health and education sectors	Home visiting		X	X	X	
	Community groups		X	X	X	
	Media		X	X	X	
	Child care			X	X	
Education sector	Preprimary school				X	
	Primary school					X

Home visiting programs are often conducted by community health workers linked to health or social sectors and deliver interventions related to health and nutrition (Yousafzai and others 2014), maternal mental health (Rahman, Patel, and Maselko 2008), and child development (Walker, Chang, and others 2011). The long-term effects of early home visits can be seen in the Jamaica trial, a two-year randomized controlled assessment of home-based intervention promoting opportunities for play and early learning through homemade toys and materials, delivered to low-income families of stunted toddlers (Grantham-McGregor and others 1991). By age two years, no differences in performance were seen in standardized developmental assessments between stunted children who received the home visiting intervention and a comparison sample of healthy nonstunted children. The children received no further intervention and entered the Jamaican educational system. At ages 17–18 years, the stunted children in the early home visiting group did better in 11 of 12 measures of cognitive and educational performance, and they had better mental health indicators (lower rates of depression and anxiety, and higher self-esteem) and fewer attentional problems than stunted children in the control group (Walker and others 2005; Walker and others 2006). In early adulthood, those who had been randomized to the intervention group were less likely to exhibit serious violent behavior, and they had higher IQ scores, higher educational attainment, fewer symptoms of depression (Walker, Chang, and others 2011), and earnings of 25 percent more than young adults in the control group (Gertler and others 2014). Jamaica has a strong history of universal preschool education, suggesting that the continuity of home visiting with preschool and primary school may have contributed to the long-term success.

With support from the Saving Brains program of Grand Challenges Canada and the Inter-American Development Bank, the Jamaican program is being scaled up to other LMICs, as Reach Up and Learn.[1] Reviews of other home visiting programs have also demonstrated success in promoting developmental skills (Aboud and Yousafzai 2015), although there have been few long-term follow-ups.

Community programs to promote early child development are often organized by nonprofit organizations and provide general information on strategies to promote early child development. In a recent example from Uganda sponsored by Plan International, trained male and female community volunteers provided 12 family-oriented sessions that addressed child care (play, talk, diet, hygiene, and love and respect) and maternal well-being (for example, increasing father involvement) among families with children ages 12–36 months (Singla, Kumbakumba, and Aboud 2015). Most sessions were directed to both parents, with two exclusively for mothers and two for fathers. Sessions based on principles of social cognitive learning theory included messages, games, role plays, parent-child interaction, group problem solving, homework, and activity booklets with activities that parents were encouraged to practice with their child at home. The impact of the program on the home environment, maternal mental health symptoms, and children's development suggests that the group sessions were effective in altering the behavior of families and in promoting child development.

Ages Two to Four Years: Child Care

The period that encompasses ages two to four years presents a major gap (figure 19.2) in LMICs; neither the health sector nor the educational sector is sufficiently responding to the needs of this group. Few government-supported programs are available, and child care is often provided by private, nongovernmental organizations with little regulation or oversight.

The number of child care programs has increased globally, often in response to the need for mothers of young children to work. However, there is little evidence regarding the impact on children. Cochrane reviews of the effects of child care programs on children's development and well-being were conducted in LMICs (Brown and others 2014) and in HICs (van Urk and others 2014). Both reviews yielded only a single controlled study. Child care enrollment has increased substantially, especially in Latin America (Berlinski and Schady 2015). A recent review of programs in LMICs, all from Latin America, reported large positive effects on children's development, with no evidence of either positive or negative effects on children's health and nutrition (Leroy, Gadsden, and Guijarro 2012). Regulatory guidelines for child care are emerging, but their quality varies substantially. The effects of child care on development vary by quality of child care, with stronger effects among programs that deliver opportunities for play and exploration along with safety and hygiene (Berlinski and Schady 2015).

Child care programs range from custodial care, often tied to maternal employment, to the provision of developmentally oriented, early learning opportunities. Much of the research into child care has been conducted in HICs. One of the most striking studies of the impact of a developmentally oriented, early learning program is the Abecedarian Project, a randomized controlled trial of a high-quality program for disadvantaged children from North Carolina, with long-term adult follow-up (Campbell and others 2012; Campbell and others 2014). The program, initiated in the 1970s, included all-day care from shortly after birth through age five years, with planned opportunities for learning, activities that promote social-emotional development, healthy nutrition, and access to health care. Follow-up when participants were in their thirties found the intervention produced beneficial effects on years of schooling (Campbell and others 2012) and on the risk factors for cardiovascular and metabolic diseases (Campbell and others 2014); effects on economic indicators were mixed, and few differences on social adjustment were observed.

The Abecedarian study, together with the Jamaican study (Gertler and others 2014), provide evidence that early intervention can have long-term effects on many aspects of children's health and development. Additional long-term systematic studies are needed to understand the impact of child care on children's health and development.

Age Five Years: Preprimary School

Access to preprimary education has been a central objective of the Education for All initiative. Preschool has benefits for subsequent performance in primary school (Berlinski and Schady 2015), especially when programs include education (UNESCO 2015) and nutrition (Nores and Barnett 2010). Global preprimary enrollment increased by nearly two-thirds from 1999 to 2012, especially in Latin America and the Caribbean (UNESCO 2015). Despite that impressive increase, preprimary coverage ranges from 19 percent for low-income countries to 86 percent for HICs; the largest enrollment is among children from the highest wealth quintiles and in urban centers (UNESCO 2015). These trends are consistent with caregiver reports of early childhood care attendance from UNICEF's Multiple Indicator Cluster Survey. Based on data from 164,900 children across 58 LMICs, 31.4 percent of all children ages 36–59 months in the sample had access to early education programs; preprimary enrollment rates were nearly twice as high among children from the top wealth quintile (47.3 percent) than from the lowest quintile (19.7 percent).

Preprimary access and coverage are variable; 40 of the 58 LMICs in the Multiple Indicator Cluster Survey provide compulsory preprimary education. The recently adopted SDG pledge to ensure "all girls and boys have access to quality early childhood development, care, and preprimary education so that they are ready for primary education" marks the first time the global goal regime has made explicit the link between early childhood development and primary school readiness.

The body of rigorous evaluation of preprimary programs in LMICs in general, and in Sub-Saharan Africa in particular, is growing. Several recent studies serve as examples for the examination of the effect of preprimary attendance on children's cognitive development. A study of 423 preprimary-age children in Kenya; Zanzibar, Tanzania; and Uganda found that children who attended preprimary programs performed better on measures of cognitive development 18 months after enrollment, compared with children who did not attend (Mwaura, Sylva, and Malmberg 2008). A follow-up cross-sequential study found a positive curvilinear effect of preprimary programs on children's cognitive development (Malmberg, Mwaura, and Sylva 2011). Similar cognitive gains, as well as improvement in other developmental domains, have been documented in Mozambique in a randomized controlled trial of a community preprimary program sponsored by Save the Children (Martinez, Naudeau, and Pereira 2012).

Children who attended this program demonstrated improved cognitive, fine motor, and socioemotional skills, as well as increased primary school enrollment at the appropriate age. The preprimary program also produced positive impacts on the primary school enrollment of older siblings and increased the labor supply of primary caregivers, suggesting that the benefits of preprimary attendance extend beyond the enrolled children to their families. The researchers estimated the cost of the program to be US$2.17 per student per month.

Evaluations of preprimary education elsewhere have also concluded that preprimary attendance is associated with better academic and preacademic performance. An assessment of 880 Cambodian children age five years showed children who had attended any type of preprimary school performed better than those who had not, although children in state-supported preprimary schools had significantly higher scores than children in community or home-based schools (Rao and others 2012).

Other efforts are underway to reach young children with educational content through media. Radio, television, and other media can increase home access to early child development programming aimed at either children or parents. Local versions of *Sesame Street* reach children in more than 150 countries (Cole, Richman, and McCann Brown 2001). In Bangladesh, almost 50 percent of a sample of preschoolers watched television daily (Khan and others 2007); among television watchers, 83 percent of urban and 58 percent of rural children watched *Sesame Street*. A meta-analysis representing more than 10,000 young children from 15 countries found significant benefits from *Sesame Street* in literacy and numeracy, in health and safety, and in social reasoning and attitudes toward others (Mares and Pan 2013).

As children approach school age, limited attention is often paid to the impact of health and nutrition on learning and well-being. However, nutritional deficiencies, infection, and inflammation are major contributors to impaired child neurodevelopment during early and middle childhood and can adversely affect children's academic performance and social-emotional development (John, Black, and Nelson 2016).

Ages Six to Eight Years: Primary School

The past 25 years have seen an enormous expansion of access to primary school, with the largest growth in LMICs (UNESCO 2015). The enrollment gap between HICs and LMICs has closed considerably, driven in part by the commitments to Education for All that were made in Jomtien, Thailand, in 1990 (UNESCO 1990) and affirmed in Dakar, Senegal, in 2000 (UNESCO 2000).

By 2008, the average LMIC was enrolling students in primary school at nearly the same rate as the average HIC (Gove and Cvelich 2011). However, access to primary school continues to be a global concern. The 2015 *Global Monitoring Report* estimates that 58 million children of primary school age were out of school in 2015. The main contributors to persistently large numbers of out-of-school children include crisis and conflict, challenging economic conditions, distance to school, and denial of access for girls and for children with disabilities (UNESCO 2015).

Although substantial gains in primary school enrollment have been achieved, by the 2015 Education for All deadline, one in six children in LMICs—more than 100 million—did not complete primary school (UNESCO 2015). Not only are children in LMICs less likely to complete primary education than children in HICs, they are learning less while in school. Estimates from large-scale international assessments of literacy and numeracy conducted in fourth grade show that the average student in low-income countries is performing at the third percentile of students in HICs (Crouch and Gove 2011).

Although raising the quality of learning is central to global goals, much of government and donor efforts have focused on expanding access to education. The goals of universal primary enrollment and completion are clear and reasonably easy to measure, and can readily be compared across countries with common methods developed and publicized by the UNESCO Institute for Statistics. In contrast, systematic approaches to student learning measurements that can be reported at the global level are lacking. While international large-scale assessments—such as the Progress in International Reading Literacy Study and the Trends in International Mathematics and Science Study—contribute to cross-country learning comparisons, their coverage is largely restricted to the global north. The few LMIC participants scored quite poorly on these assessments, with the overall results deemed to be unreliable in some cases. Regional assessments, such as the Second Regional Comparative and Explanatory Study from Latin America and the Caribbean, the Southern and Eastern Africa Consortium for Monitoring Educational Quality, and the CONFEMEN Programme for the Analysis of Education Systems in West Africa, have been slow to expand, and LMICs continue to struggle with how to conduct and use student assessment results to improve learning in their classrooms (Gove and others 2015).

The U.S. Agency for International Development (USAID) commissioned development of the Early Grade Reading Assessment (EGRA) to help LMICs rapidly diagnose and improve learning outcomes while also informing the global community. The EGRA was formulated in 2006, guided by research on the development of early reading skills, and relies on individual oral assessment of children to understand the reading process in achieving and struggling readers. The EGRA has been adapted for use in more than 75 countries and in more than 120 languages. Open-source versions are available, with guidance for adaptation based on the characteristics of a given language and country (RTI International 2016). Its widespread use has delivered a shared language for describing results and monitoring educational system changes, while enabling countries to incorporate their unique contexts and cultures (Dubeck and Gove 2015).

More than a dozen countries have used the EGRA data to develop benchmarks and standards for achievement across different grades. The EGRA has been used for program monitoring and evaluation and for development of reports reflecting educational systems within countries and at the country-level[2] and consolidated information across contexts (Gove and Cvelich 2011). Using these benchmarks, countries can estimate the proportion of children in grades 2–3 meeting minimum proficiency in reading, an indicator that could be reported globally, as required by the SDGs (specifically SDG 4.1). Enabling LMICs to monitor and improve learning outcomes in the early grades is likely to promote attendance and academic success and to improve the quality of the education system.

The expansion of primary schools and the elimination or reduction of school fees have boosted primary school enrollment. However, quality in many primary schools in LMICs is low, particularly in Sub-Saharan Africa (UNESCO 2012). Assessment strategies, such as the EGRA, India's Annual Status of Education Report, and East Africa's Uwezo initiative, have helped focus attention on the low learning levels in many primary schools in LMICs (UNESCO Institute for Statistics 2016). Children who do not acquire basic literacy and numeracy skills early in their academic careers have difficulty with subsequent subjects and are at risk of dropping out, which would limit their economic opportunities and those of entire societies.

Early academic success depends on strong teacher training and a curriculum and materials that support learning. With the global shift in focus from access to learning, governments and donors are experimenting with classroom-level interventions, such as the Primary Mathematics and Reading Initiative (PRIMR) (Piper, Zuilkowski, and Mugenda 2014). A randomized controlled trial of the approach in more than 400 schools in Kenya found that the intervention significantly improved oral reading fluency in grades 1 and 2 for both English and Kiswahili, with PRIMR students two to three times more likely to read and comprehend than control students (Piper, Zuilkowski, and Mugenda 2014).

Based on the success of PRIMR, the Kenyan government extended the collaboration to develop the Tusome Early Grade Reading Activity. Tusome means "let's read" in Kiswahili and is designed to promote early literacy in English and Kiswahili through the provision of structured teaching and learning materials and extra training for grade 1 and 2 teachers through tutors and coaching. Tusome has been scaled up into more than 23,500 public and alternative education institutions nationwide, and by 2018 it will reach 5.4 million Kenyan children in grades 1 and 2 (USAID 2016). Kenya's experience and similar efforts supported by USAID and other donors have highlighted the need for additional evidence on how to take pilot programs to scale. While there have been several reviews of evaluations of learning improvement efforts in LMICs (Evans and Popova 2015; McEwan 2015), few programs have been able to scale up and sustain the level of improvement observed in the pilot.

CONCLUSIONS

The field of global early child development is emerging, stimulated by promising findings from the impact of ensuring adequate development early in life and by encouragement from international leaders through the SDGs. Significant gaps exist in programming and investment that may interfere with future success, particularly for children under age five years. Limited attention to workforce development and support, program standards and materials, best practices, and quality are concerns (Yousafzai and Aboud 2014). Although initial efforts to estimate cost-effectiveness suggest that interventions that include responsive stimulation are more cost-effective than nutrition interventions alone in promoting children's early development (Gowani and others 2014), there have been few attempts to estimate costs (Horton and Black 2017). Population-based indicators are needed for early child development, along with national databases to enable countries to plan and evaluate intervention programs for young children.

These actions are meant to continue the advances that have been made in early child development policies, programs, and research in recent decades. Government commitments through education ministries to provide schools, teacher training, learning materials, and supplementary support to enable young children to attend primary school—such as the elimination of school fees and the provision of school meals—have helped increase primary school access. LMICs, with the support of international donors, have developed and evaluated curricula designed to promote early grade reading and mathematics, as well as systematic methods to measure progress. Children who acquire these skills in the first years of primary school are likely to remain in school, to learn, and to acquire the skills needed for sustainable development.

Policies and programs for children up to age five years are less well developed than those for primary schools. From a positive perspective, preprimary education has been endorsed globally by Education for All and incorporated into the SDGs, the number of programs has increased, and the evidence demonstrates that many preprimary programs prepare children well for primary school. However, standards for preprimary vary, and the exclusion of many children increases inequities. Recommendations for preprimary include stronger attention to quality, to preprimary curricula and standards, to learning materials, and to teacher training and support.

The gap between the health and education sectors for children up to age five years is a major concern that may impede children's early development. Although the number of child care programs has been increasing, often to support employment of mothers, few organized platforms are available; many programs are fragmented, with limited attention to developmentally oriented early learning activities, little oversight, and few evaluations.

The health and nutrition sectors focus on children during the first 1,000 days, with primary emphasis on the first year of life. Although they promote breastfeeding, complementary feeding, and other health- and nutrition-related care, other aspects of nurturing, including responsive caregiving and early learning, are often minimal or absent. Integrated programs that combine health and nutrition with early child development, and coordinated programs across multiple sectors, have been recommended. Examples are emerging, and the logistical and workforce issues are being clarified. In particular, platforms that support families, such as home visiting, have shown long-term success in enabling children to reach their developmental potential.

Early experiences, both positive and negative, are the foundation of life-course trajectories that affect adult health and well-being. Investing in effective policies and programs and ensuring that they are part of an organizational structure that pays attention to quality will enhance early child development. This will enable children to build the health, intelligence, innovativeness, and dedication necessary to become healthy and productive adults.

NOTES

World Bank Income Classifications as of July 2014 are as follows, based on estimates of gross national income (GNI) per capita for 2013:

- Low-income countries (LICs) = US$1,045 or less
- Middle-income countries (MICs) are subdivided:
  a) lower-middle-income = US$1,046 to US$4,125
  b) upper-middle-income (UMICs) = US$4,126 to US$12,745
- High-income countries (HICs) = US$12,746 or more.

1. For more information, see http://www.reachupandlearn.com/.
2. For more information, see the websites http://www.eddataglobal.org and http://www.earlygradereadingbarometer.org.

REFERENCES

Aboud, F. E., and A. K. Yousafzai. 2015. "Global Health and Development in Early Childhood." *Annual Review of Psychology* 66: 433–57. doi:10.1146/annurev-psych-010814-015128.

Bergmeier, H., H. Skouteris, S. Horwood, M. Hooley, and B. Richardson. 2014. "Child Temperament and Maternal Predictors of Preschool Children's Eating and Body Mass Index: A Prospective Study." *Appetite* 74: 125–32.

Berlinski, S., S. Galiani, and P. Gertler. 2009. "The Effect of Pre-Primary Education on Primary School Performance." *Journal of Public Economics* 93 (1): 219–34.

Berlinski, S., and N. Schady. 2015. *The Early Years: Child Well-Being and the Role of Public Policy.* Development in the Americas Series. New York: Macmillan.

Bick, J., O. Naumova, S. Hunter, B. Barbot, M. Lee, and others. 2012. "Childhood Adversity and DNA Methylation of Genes Involved in the Hypothalamus-Pituitary-Adrenal Axis and Immune System: Whole-Genome and Candidate-Gene Associations." *Development and Psychopathology* 24 (4): 1417–25.

Black, M. M. 2003. "Micronutrient Deficiencies and Cognitive Functioning." *Journal of Nutrition* 133 (11): 3927S–31S.

Black, M. M., and F. E. Aboud. 2011. "Responsive Feeding Is Embedded in a Theoretical Framework of Responsive Parenting." *Journal of Nutrition* 141 (3): 490–94.

Black, M. M., and K. G. Dewey. 2014. "Promoting Equity through Integrated Early Child Development and Nutrition Interventions." *Annals of the New York Academy of Sciences* 1308 (1): 1–10. doi:10.1111/nyas.12351.

Black, M. M., R. Perez-Escamilla, and S. Fernandez Rao. 2015. "Integrating Nutrition and Child Development Interventions: Scientific Basis, Evidence of Impact, and Implementation Considerations." *Advances in Nutrition* 6: 852–59. doi:10.3945/An.115.010348.

Black, M. M., N. A. Tilton, K. Harding, S. Fernandez-Rao, K. M. Hurley, and others. 2016. "Growth and Development among Infants and Preschoolers in Rural India: Economic Inequities and Caregiver Protective/Promotive Factors."

International Journal of Behavioral Development. doi: 10.1177/0165025416644690.

Black, R. E., C. G. Victora, S. P. Walker, Z. A. Bhutta, P. Christian, and others. 2013. "Maternal and Child Undernutrition and Overweight in Low-Income and Middle-Income Countries." *The Lancet* 382 (9890): 427–51.

Black, M. M., S. P. Walker, L. C. H. Fernald, C. T. Anderson, A. Digirolamo, and others. 2016. "Early Child Development Coming of Age: Science Through the Life-Course." *The Lancet.* http://www.sciencedirect.com/science/article/pii /S0140673616313897.

Boersma, G. J., T. L. Bale, P. Casanello, H. E. Lara, A. B. Lucion, and others. 2014. "Long-Term Impact of Early Life Events on Physiology and Behaviour." *Journal of Neuroendocrinology* 26 (9): 587–602.

Bornstein, M. H., and D. L. Putnick. 2012. "Cognitive and Socioemotional Caregiving in Developing Countries." *Child Development* 83 (1): 46–61.

Bradley, R. H., and D. L. Putnick. 2012. "Housing Quality and Access to Material and Learning Resources within the Home Environment in Developing Countries." *Child Development* 83 (1): 76–91. doi:10.1111/J.1467-8624.2011.01674.X.

Britto, P. R., H. Yoshikawa, J. Van Ravens, L. A. Ponguta, M. Reyes, and others. 2014. "Strengthening Systems for Integrated Early Childhood Development Services: A Cross-National Analysis of Governance." *Annals of the New York Academy of Sciences* 1308 (1): 245–55. doi:10.1111 /nyas.12365.

Bronfenbrenner, U., and P. A. Morris. 2007. "The Bioecological Model of Human Development." In *Handbook of Child Psychology* (sixth edition): Volume 1, *Theoretical Models of Human Development*, edited by R. M. Lerner, 793–828. Hoboken, NJ: John Wiley & Sons, Inc.

Brown, D. W., R. F. Anda, V. J. Felitti, V. J. Edwards, A. M. Malarcher, and others. 2010. "Adverse Childhood Experiences Are Associated with the Risk of Lung Cancer: A Prospective Cohort Study." *BioMed Central Public Health* 10 (1): 1.

Brown, T. W., F. C. Van Urk, R. Waller, and E. Mayo-Wilson. 2014. "Centre-Based Day Care for Children Younger than Five Years of Age in Low- and Middle-Income Countries." *Cochrane Database of Systematic Reviews* (9): CD010544. doi:10.1002/14651858.CD010543.pub2.

Bundy, D. A. P., N. de Silva, S. Horton, G. C. Patton, L. Schultz, and D. T. Jamison. 2017. "Child and Adolescent Health and Development: Realizing Neglected Potential." In *Disease Control Priorities* (third edition): Volume 8, *Child and Adolescent Health and Development*, edited by D. A. P. Bundy, N. de Silva, S. Horton, D. T. Jamison, and G. C. Patton. Washington, DC: World Bank.

Campbell, F. A., G. Conti, J. J. Heckman, S. H. Moon, R. Pinto, and others. 2014. "Early Childhood Investments Substantially Boost Adult Health." *Science* 343 (6178): 1478–85.

Campbell, F. A., E. P. Pungello, M. Burchinal, K. Kainz, Y. Pan, and others. 2012. "Adult Outcomes as a Function of an Early Childhood Educational Program: An Abecedarian Project Follow-Up." *Developmental Psychology* 48 (4): 1033–43. doi:10.1037/a0026644.

Carey, G., B. Crammond, and E. De Leeuw. 2015. "Towards Health Equity: A Framework for the Application of Proportionate Universalism." *International Journal for Equity in Health* 14 (1): 81. doi:10.1186/s12939-015-0207-6.

Chudasama, R. K., A. M. Kadri, P. B. Verma, U. V. Patel, N. Joshi, and others. 2014. "Evaluation of Integrated Child Development Services Program in Gujarat, India." *Indian Pediatrics* 51 (9): 707–11.

Cole, C. F., B. A. Richman, and S. A. McCann Brown. 2001. "The World of Sesame Street Research." In *"G" Is for Growing: Thirty Years of Research on Children and Sesame Street*, edited by S. M. Fisch and R. T. Truglio, 147–79. Mahwah, NJ: Lawrence Erlbaum.

Crookston, B. T., W. Schott, S. Cueto, K. A. Dearden, P. Engle, and others. 2013. "Postinfancy Growth, Schooling, and Cognitive Achievement: Young Lives." *American Journal of Clinical Nutrition* 98 (6): 1555–63. doi:10.3945/ajcn.113.067561.

Crouch, L., and A. K. Gove. 2011. "Leaps or One Step at a Time: Skirting or Helping Engage the Debate? The Case of Reading." In *Policy Debates in Comparative, International, and Development Education*, edited by W. Jacob and J. Hawkins, 155–74. New York: Palgrave Macmillan.

Dubeck, M. M., and A. Gove. 2015. "The Early Grade Reading Assessment (EGRA): Its Theoretical Foundation, Purpose, and Limitations." *International Journal of Educational Development* 40: 315–22.

Engle, P. L., M. M. Black, J. R. Behrman, M. Cabral de Mello, P. J. Gertler, and others. 2007. "Strategies to Avoid the Loss of Developmental Potential among Over 200 Million Children in the Developing World." *The Lancet* 369 (9557): 230–42.

Engle, P. L., L. C. Fernald, H. Alderman, J. Behrman, C. O'Gara, and others. 2011. "Strategies for Reducing Inequalities and Improving Developmental Outcomes for Young Children in Low-Income and Middle-Income Countries." *The Lancet* 378 (9799): 1339–53. doi:10.1016 /S0140-6736(11)60889-1.

Ertem, I. O., G. Atay, B. E. Bingoler, D. G. Dogan, A. Bayhan, and others. 2006. "Promoting Child Development at Sick-Child Visits: A Controlled Trial." *Pediatrics* 118 (1): e124–31.

Evans, D. K., and A. Popova. 2015. "What Really Works to Improve Learning in Developing Countries? An Analysis of Divergent Findings in Systematic Reviews." Policy Research Working Paper 7203, World Bank, Washington, DC.

Farnsworth, S. K., K. Böse, O. Fajobi, P. P. Souza, A. Peniston, and others. 2014. "Community Engagement to Enhance Child Survival and Early Development in Low- and Middle-Income Countries: An Evidence Review." *Journal of Health Communication* 19 (Suppl 1): 67–88.

Fernald, A., V. A. Marchman, and A. Weisleder. 2013. "SES Differences in Language Processing Skill and Vocabulary Are Evident at 18 Months." *Developmental Science* 16 (2): 234–48.

Fox, S. E., P. Levitt, and C. A. Nelson III. 2010. "How the Timing and Quality of Early Experiences Influence the Development of Brain Architecture." *Child Development* 81 (1): 28–40.

Gakidou, E., K. Cowling, R. Lozano, and C. J. L. Murray. 2010. "Increased Educational Attainment and Its Effect on Child

Mortality in 175 Countries between 1970 and 2009: A Systematic Analysis." *The Lancet* 376 (9745): 959–74.

Gertler, P., J. Heckman, R. Pinto, A. Zanolini, C. Vermeersch, and others. 2014. "Labor Market Returns to an Early Childhood Stimulation Intervention in Jamaica." *Science* 344 (6187): 998–1001. doi:10.1126/Science.1251178.

Glover, V. 2011. "Annual Research Review: Prenatal Stress and the Origins of Psychopathology: An Evolutionary Perspective." *Journal of Child Psychology and Psychiatry* 52 (4): 356–67.

Gordon, R. S. 1983. "An Operational Classification of Disease Prevention." *Public Health Reports* 98 (2): 107–9.

Gove, A., C. Chabbott, A. Dick, J. Destefano, S. King, and others. 2015. "Early Learning Assessments: A Retrospective." Background Paper for Education for All Global Monitoring Report, United Nations Educational, Cultural and Scientific Organization, Paris. http://unesdoc.unesco.org/images/0023/002324/232419e.pdf.

Gove, A., and P. Cvelich. 2011. "Early Reading: Igniting Education for All. A Report by the Early Grade Learning Community of Practice." RTI International, Research Triangle Park, NC.

Gowani, S., A. K. Yousafzai, R. Armstrong, and Z. A. Bhutta. 2014. "Cost Effectiveness of Responsive Stimulation and Nutrition Interventions on Early Child Development Outcomes in Pakistan." *Annals of the New York Academy of Sciences* 1308 (1): 149161.

Grantham-McGregor, S. M., Y. B. Cheung, S. Cueto, P. Glewwe, L. Richter, and others. 2007. "Developmental Potential in the First 5 Years for Children in Developing Countries." *The Lancet* 369 (9555): 60–70. doi:10.1016/S0140-6736(07)60032-4.

Grantham-McGregor, S. M., L. C. Fernald, R. M. Kagawa, and S. Walker. 2014. "Effects of Integrated Child Development and Nutrition Interventions on Child Development and Nutritional Status." *Annals of the New York Academy of Sciences* 1308: 11–32. doi:10.1111/nyas.12284.

Grantham-McGregor, S. M., C. A. Powell, S. P. Walker, and J. H. Himes. 1991. "Nutritional Supplementation, Psychosocial Stimulation, and Mental Development of Stunted Children: The Jamaican Study." *The Lancet* 338 (8758): 1–5. doi:10.1016/0140-6736(91)90001-6.

Hair, N. L., J. L. Hanson, B. L. Wolfe, and S. D. Pollak. 2015. "Association of Child Poverty, Brain Development, and Academic Achievement." *Journal of the American Medical Association* 169 (9): 822–29. doi:10.1001/Jamapediatrics.2015.1475.

Hamadani, J. D., F. Tofail, S. N. Huda, D. S. Alam, D. A. Ridout, and others. 2014. "Cognitive Deficit and Poverty in the First 5 Years of Childhood in Bangladesh." *Pediatrics* 134 (4): E1001–08. doi:10.1542/Peds.2014-0694.

Hanson, J. L., B. M. Nacewicz, M. J. Sutterer, A. A. Cayo, S. M. Schaefer, and others. 2015. "Behavioral Problems after Early Life Stress: Contributions of the Hippocampus and Amygdala." *Biological Psychiatry* 77 (4): 314–23. doi:10.1016/J.Biopsych.2014.04.020.

Hanson, M. A., P. D. Gluckman, R. C. W. Ma, P. Matzen, and R. G. Biesma. 2012. "Early Life Opportunities for Prevention of Diabetes in Low and Middle Income Countries." *BioMed Central Public Health* 12: 1025.

Hertzman, C. 1999. "The Biological Embedding of Early Experience and Its Effects on Health in Adulthood." *Annals of the New York Academy of Sciences* 896 (1): 85–95.

———. 2013. "The Significance of Early Childhood Adversity." *Paediatrics and Child Health* 18 (3): 127.

Hoddinott, J., J. A. Maluccio, J. R. Behrman, R. Flores, and R. Martorell. 2008. "Effect of a Nutrition Intervention during Early Childhood on Economic Productivity in Guatemalan Adults." *The Lancet* 371 (9610): 411–16. doi:10.1016/S0140-6736(08)60205-6.

Horton, S., and M. M. Black. 2017. "Identifying an Essential Package for Early Childhood Development: Economic Analysis." In *Disease Control Priorities* (third edition): Volume 8, *Child and Adolescent Health and Development,* edited by D. A. P. Bundy, N. de Silva, S. Horton, D. T. Jamison, and G. C. Patton. Washington, DC: World Bank.

Irwin, L. G., A. Siddiqi, and C. Hertzman. 2007. *Early Child Development: A Powerful Equalizer.* Final Report to the World Health Organization Commission on Social Determinants of Health. Geneva: World Health Organization.

Jin, X., Y. Sun, F. Jiang, J. Ma, C. Morgan, and others. 2007. "Care for Development Intervention in Rural China: A Prospective Follow-Up Study." *Journal of Developmental and Behavioral Pediatrics* 28 (3): 213–18.

John, C. C., M. M. Black, and C. A. Nelson. 2016. "Neurodevelopment: The Impact of Nutrition and Inflammation during Early to Middle Childhood." *Pediatrics.* Under review.

Khan, M. S. H., N. Chakraborty, A. P. M. Rahman, and T. Nasrin. 2007. "2007 Follow-Up (Wave II) Evaluation of the Reach and Impact of Sisimpur: A Technical Report." Associates for Community and Population Research, Dhaka, Bangladesh.

Lake, A., and M. Chan. 2015. "Putting Science into Practice for Early Child Development." *The Lancet* 385 (9980): 1816–17. doi:10.1016/S0140-6736(14)61680-9.

Lassi, Z. S., R. Kumar, and Z. A. Bhutta. 2016. "Community-Based Care to Improve Maternal, Newborn, and Child Health." In *Disease Control Priorities* (third edition): Volume 2, *Reproductive, Maternal, Newborn, and Child Health,* edited by R. Black, R. Laxminarayan, M. Temmerman, and N. Walker, 263–84. Washington, DC: World Bank.

Leroy, J. L., P. Gadsden, and M. Guijarro. 2012. "The Impact of Daycare Programmes on Child Health, Nutrition and Development in Developing Countries: A Systematic Review." *Journal of Development Effectiveness* 4 (3): 472–96. doi:10.1080/19439342.2011.639457.

Liberzon, I., S. T. Ma, G. Okada, S. Shaun Ho, J. E. Swain, and others. 2015. "Childhood Poverty and Recruitment of Adult Emotion Regulatory Neurocircuitry." *Social Cognitive Affective Neuroscience* 10 (11): 1596–606. doi:10.1093/Scan/Nsv045.

Lu, C., M. M. Black, and L. M. Richter. 2016. "Risk of Poor development in Young Children in Low-Income and Middle-Income Countries: An Estimation and Analysis at the Global, Regional, and Country Level." *Lancet Global Health.* Epub ahead of print. https://www.ncbi.nlm.nih.gov/pubmed/27717632.

Malik, A., M. Bhilwar, N. Rustagi, and D. K. Taneja. 2015. "An Assessment of Facilities and Services at Anganwadi Centers under the Integrated Child Development Service Scheme in Northeast District of Delhi, India." *International Journal for Quality in Health Care* 27 (3): 201–6. doi:10.1093/Intqhc/Mzv028.

Malmberg, L.-E., P. Mwaura, and K. Sylva. 2011. "Effects of a Preschool Intervention on Cognitive Development among East-African Preschool Children: A Flexibly Time-Coded Growth Model." *Early Childhood Research Quarterly* 26 (1): 124–33.

Mares, M.-L., and Z. Pan. 2013. "Effects of Sesame Street: A Meta-Analysis of Children's Learning in 15 Countries." *Journal of Applied Developmental Psychology* 34 (3): 140–51.

Marmot, M. G., J. Allen, P. Goldblatt, T. Boyce, D. McNeish, and others. 2010. *Fair Society, Healthy Lives: The Marmot Review*. London: The Marmot Review.

Martinez, S., S. Naudeau, and V. Pereira. 2012. "The Promise of Preschool in Africa: A Randomized Impact Evaluation of Early Child Development in Rural Mozambique." World Bank and Save the Children, Washington, DC. http://www.Savethechildren.Org/Atf/Cf/%7b9def2ebe-10ae-432c-9bd0-Df91d2eba74a%7D/MARTINEZ_NAUDEAU_PEREIRA.MOZ_ECD_REPORT-FEB_7_2012.PDF.

Martorell, R., B. L. Horta, L. S. Adair, A. D. Stein, L. Richter, and others. 2010. "Weight Gain in the First Two Years of Life Is an Important Predictor of Schooling Outcomes in Pooled Analyses from Five Birth Cohorts from Low- and Middle-Income Countries." *Journal of Nutrition* 140 (2): 348–54. doi:10.3945/Jn.109.112300.

McCoy, D. C., M. Black, B. Daelmans, and T. Dua. 2016. "Measuring Development in Children from Birth to Age 3 at Population Level." *Early Childhood Matters* 125: 34–39. https://bernardvanleer.org/app/uploads/2016/07/Early-Childhood-Matters-2016_6.pdf.

McEwan, P. J. 2015. "Improving Learning in Primary Schools of Developing Countries: A Meta-Analysis of Randomized Experiments." *Review of Educational Research* 85 (3): 353–94.

Mwaura, P. A. M., K. Sylva, and L.-E. Malmberg. 2008. "Evaluating the Madrasa Preschool Programme in East Africa: A Quasi-Experimental Study." *International Journal of Early Years Education* 16 (3): 237–55.

Noble, K. G., L. E. Engelhardt, N. H. Brito, L. J. Mack, E. J. Nail, and others. 2015. "Socioeconomic Disparities in Neurocognitive Development in the First Two Years of Life." *Developmental Psychobiology* 57 (5): 535–51.

Noble, K. G., S. M. Houston, N. H. Brito, H. Bartsch, E. Kan, and others. 2015. "Family Income, Parental Education and Brain Structure in Children and Adolescents." *Nature Neuroscience* 18 (5): 773–78. doi:10.1038/Nn.3983.

Nores, M., and W. S. Barnett. 2010. "Benefits of Early Childhood Interventions across the World: (Under) Investing in the Very Young." *Economics of Education Review* 29 (2): 271–82.

Pavlakis, A. E., K. Noble, S. G. Pavlakis, N. Ali, and Y. Frank. 2015. "Brain Imaging and Electrophysiology Biomarkers: Is There a Role in Poverty and Education Outcome Research?" *Pediatric Neurology* 52 (4): 383–88. doi:http://dx.doi.org/10.1016/J.Pediatrneurol.2014.11.005.

Peña, R., S. Wall, and L.-A. Persson. 2000. "The Effect of Poverty, Social Inequity, and Maternal Education on Infant Mortality in Nicaragua, 1988–1993." *American Journal of Public Health* 90 (1): 64.

Piper, B., S. S. Zuilkowski, and A. Mugenda. 2014. "Improving Reading Outcomes in Kenya: First-Year Effects of the PRIMR Initiative." *International Journal of Educational Development* 37: 11–21.

Rahman, A., V. Patel, and J. Maselko. 2008. "Maternal Depressive Symptoms at 2 to 4 Months Post Partum and Early Parenting Practices." *Archive of General Psychiatry* 160: 279–84.

Raikes, A., T. Dua, and P. R. Britto. 2015. "Measuring Early Childhood Development: Priorities for Post-2015." *Early Childhood Matters* 124: 74–77.

Ramakrishnan, U., T. Goldenberg, and L. H. Allen. 2011. "Do Multiple Micronutrient Interventions Improve Child Health, Growth, and Development?" *Journal of Nutrition* 141: 2066–75.

Rao, N. 2005. "Children's Rights to Survival, Development, and Early Education in India: The Critical Role of the Integrated Child Development Services Program." *International Journal of Early Childhood* 37 (3): 15–31.

———. 2010. "Preschool Quality and the Development of Children from Economically Disadvantaged Families in India." *Early Education and Development* 21 (2): 167–85.

Rao, N., J. Sun, V. Pearson, E. Pearson, H. Liu, and others. 2012. "Is Something Better than Nothing? An Evaluation of Early Childhood Programs in Cambodia." *Child Development* 83 (3): 864–76. doi:10.1111/j.1467-8624.2012.01746.x.

Rao, N., J. Sun, J. M. S. Wong, B. S. Weekes, P. Ip, and others. 2014. "Early Childhood Development and Cognitive Development in Developing Countries: A Rigorous Literature Review." U.K. Department for International Development, London.

Riis, J. L., D. A. Granger, C. S. Minkovitz, K. Bandeen-Roche, J. A. Dipietro, and others. 2016. "Maternal Distress and Child Neuroendocrine and Immune Regulation." *Social Science and Medicine* 151: 206–14.

RTI International. 2016. *Early Grade Reading Assessment Toolkit*. 2nd ed. https://www.Eddataglobal.Org/Reading/Index.Cfm?Fuseaction=Pubdetail&ID=929.

Shonkoff, J. P., W. T. Boyce, and B. S. McEwen. 2009. "Neuroscience, Molecular Biology, and the Childhood Roots of Health Disparities: Building a New Framework for Health Promotion and Disease Prevention." *Journal of the American Medical Association* 301 (21): 2252–59.

Shonkoff, J. P., L. Richter, J. Van Der Gaag, and Z. A. Bhutta. 2012. "An Integrated Scientific Framework for Child Survival and Early Childhood Development." *Pediatrics* 129 (2): E460–72. doi:10.1542/Peds.2011-0366.

Singla, D. R., E. Kumbakumba, and F. E. Aboud. 2015. "Effects of a Parenting Intervention to Address Both Maternal

Psychological Wellbeing and Child Development and Growth in Rural Uganda: A Community-Based, Cluster Randomised Trial." *The Lancet Global Health* 3 (8): E458–69. doi:10.1016/S2214-109x(15)00099-6.

Sudfeld, C. R., D. C. McCoy, G. Danaei, G. Fink, M. Ezzati, and others. 2015. "Linear Growth and Child Development in Low- and Middle-Income Countries: A Meta-Analysis." *Pediatrics* 135 (5): E1266–75. doi:10.1542/Peds.2014-3111.

Thurnham, D. I. 2013. "Nutrition of Adolescent Girls in Low- and Middle-Income Countries." *Sight Life* 27: 26–37.

UN (United Nations). 2015. *Transforming Our World: The 2030 Agenda for Sustainable Development*. New York: United Nations General Assembly. http://www.un.org/ga/search/view_doc.asp?symbol=A/RES/70/1&Lang=E.

UNESCO (United Nations Educational, Scientific and Cultural Organization). 1990. *Meeting Basic Learning Needs: A Vision for the 1990s*. Jomtien, Thailand: UNESCO. http://Unesdoc.Unesco.Org/Images/0009/000975/097552e.pdf.

———. 2000. *The Dakar Framework for Action: Education for All Meeting Our Collective Commitments*. Paris: UNESCO.

———. 2012. *Adult and Youth Literacy 1990–2015: Analysis of Data for 41 Selected Countries*. Montreal: UNESCO Institute for Statistics. http://www.uis.unesco.org/literacy/documents/uis-literacy-statistics-1990-2015-en.pdf.

———. 2015. *EFA Global Monitoring Report 2015*. Paris: UNESCO. http://Unesdoc.Unesco.Org/Images/0023/002322/232205e.Pdf.

UNESCO Institute for Statistics. 2016. *Understanding What Works in Oral Reading Assessments*. Recommendations from Donors, Implementers and Practitioners. Montreal: UNESCO Institute for Statistics. http://www.uis.unesco.org/Education/Documents/what-works-oral-reading-assessments.pdf.

USAID (U.S. Agency for International Development). 2016. "Kenya and East Africa: Tusome Early Grade Reading Activity." USAID, Washington, DC. https://www.usaid.gov/sites/default/files/documents/1860/Tusome%20%20Factsheet%202016.pdf.

Vaghri, Z., H. Wong, S. I. Barr, G. E. Chapman, and C. Hertzman. 2011. "Associations of Socio-Demographic and Behavioral Variables with Hair Zinc of Vancouver Preschoolers." *Biological Trace Element Research* 143 (3): 1398–412.

van Urk, F. C., T. W. Brown, R. Waller, and E. Mayo-Wilson. 2014. "Centre-Based Day Care for Children Younger than Five Years of Age in High-Income Countries." *Cochrane Database of Systematic Reviews* (9): CD010544. doi:10.1002/14651858.CD010544.pub2.

Vargas-Barón, E. 2013. "Building and Strengthening National Systems for Early Childhood Development." In *Handbook of Early Childhood Development Research and Its Impact on Global Policy*, edited by P. E. Engle, P. R. Britto, and C. S. Super, 443–66. New York: Oxford University Press.

Victoria, C. G., S. R. A. Huttly, F. C. Barros, C. Lombardi, and J. P. Vaughan. 1992. "Maternal Education in Relation to Early and Late Child Health Outcomes: Findings from a Brazilian Cohort Study." *Social Science and Medicine* 34 (8): 899–905.

Wachs, T. D., M. Georgieff, S. Cusick, and B. S. McEwen. 2014. "Issues in the Timing of Integrated Early Interventions: Contributions from Nutrition, Neuroscience, and Psychological Research." *Annals of the New York Academy of Sciences* 1308: 89–106. doi:10.1111/Nyas.12314.

Walker, S. P., S. M. Chang, C. A. Powell, and S. M. Grantham-McGregor. 2005. "Effects of Early Childhood Psychosocial Stimulation and Nutritional Supplementation on Cognition and Education in Growth-Stunted Jamaican Children: Prospective Cohort Study." *The Lancet* 366 (9499): 1804–7. doi:10.1016/S0140-6736(05)67574-5.

Walker, S. P., S. M. Chang, C. A. Powell, E. Simonoff, and S. M. Grantham-McGregor. 2006. "Effects of Psychosocial Stimulation and Dietary Supplementation in Early Childhood on Psychosocial Functioning in Late Adolescence: Follow-Up of Randomised Controlled Trial." *BMJ* 333 (7566): 472.

Walker, S. P., S. M. Chang, M. Vera-Hernandez, and S. Grantham-McGregor. 2011. "Early Childhood Stimulation Benefits Adult Competence and Reduces Violent Behavior." *Pediatrics* 127 (5): 849–57. doi:10.1542/Peds.2010-2231.

Walker, S. P., T. D. Wachs, S. Grantham-McGregor, M. M. Black, C. A. Nelson, and others. 2011. "Inequality in Early Childhood: Risk and Protective Factors for Early Child Development." *The Lancet* 378 (9799): 1325–38. doi:http://dx.doi.org/10.1016/S0140-6736(11)60555-2.

WHO (World Health Organization). 2009. *Closing the Gap in a Generation: Health Equity through Action on the Social Determinants of Health*. Final Report of the Commission on Social Determinants of Health. Geneva: WHO. http://www.who.int/social_determinants/thecommission/finalreport/en/.

WHO (World Health Organization) and UNICEF (United Nations Children's Fund). 2012. *Care for Child Development: Improving the Care of Young Children*. Geneva: WHO.

Woodhead, M., I. Feathersone, L. Bolton, and P. Robertson. 2014. *Early Childhood Development: Delivering Inter-Sectoral Policies, Programmes and Services in Low-Resource Settings*. Oxford: Health and Education Advice and Resource Team.

Yousafzai, A. K., and F. Aboud. 2014. "Review of Implementation Processes for Integrated Nutrition and Psychosocial Stimulation Interventions." *Annals of the New York Academy of Sciences* 1308 (1): 33–45.

Yousafzai, A. K., J. Obradovic, M. A. Rasheed, A. Rizvi, and X. A. Portilla. 2016. "The Effects of Responsive Stimulation and Nutrition Intervention on Children's Development and Growth at 4 Years in a Disadvantaged Population in Pakistan: Longitudinal Follow-Up of a Cluster-Randomized Effectiveness Trial." *The Lancet Global Health* 4 (8): E548–58.

Yousafzai, A. K., M. A. Rasheed, A. Rizvi, R. Armstrong, and Z. A. Bhutta. 2014. "Effect of Integrated Responsive Stimulation and Nutrition Interventions in the Lady Health Worker Programme in Pakistan on Child Development, Growth, and Health Outcomes: A Cluster-Randomised Factorial Effectiveness Trial." *The Lancet* 384 (9950): 1282–93.

Chapter 20

The School as a Platform for Addressing Health in Middle Childhood and Adolescence

Donald A. P. Bundy, Linda Schultz, Bachir Sarr, Louise Banham, Peter Colenso, and Lesley Drake

INTRODUCTION

Health and nutrition programs targeted at school-age children are among the most ubiquitous of all public health programs worldwide. Since the inclusion of school health and nutrition (SHN) in the launch of the call for Education for All (EFA) in 2000, it has been difficult to find a country that is not attempting at some level to provide SHN services (Sarr and others 2017). It is estimated that more than 368 million schoolchildren are provided with school meals every day (World Food Programme 2016), and according to the World Health Organization (WHO) statistics (WHO 2015), 416 million school-age children were dewormed in 2015, which equals 63.2 percent of the target population of children in endemic areas; see chapter 29 in this volume (Ahuja and others 2017). These largely public efforts are variable in quality, and coverage is greatest in the richer countries, but the scale indicates public recognition of the willingness to invest in middle childhood and adolescence.

Health status affects cognitive ability, educational attainment, quality of life, and the ability to contribute to society. Some of the most common health conditions of childhood have consequences for education. SHN interventions can support vulnerable children throughout key stages of their development in middle childhood and adolescence. A set of priority school-based interventions, selected on the basis of cost-effectiveness, benefit-cost analysis, and rate of return, is described in chapter 25 in this volume (Fernandes and Aurino 2017).

Schools are a cost-effective platform for providing simple, safe, and effective health interventions to school-age children and adolescents (Horton and others 2017). Many of the health conditions that are most prevalent among poor students have important effects on education—causing absenteeism, leading to grade repetition or dropout, and adversely affecting student achievement—and yet are easily preventable or treatable. With gains in enrollment achieved by the Millennium Development Goals, SHN interventions are important cross-sectoral collaborations between Ministries of Health and Education to promote health, cognition, and physical growth across the life course.

The education system is particularly well situated to promoting health among children and adolescents in poor communities without effective health systems who otherwise might not receive health interventions. There are typically more schools than health facilities in all income settings, and rural and poor areas are significantly more likely to have schools than health centers. The economies of scale, coupled with the efficiencies of using existing infrastructure and the potential to administer additional interventions through the same delivery mechanism, make SHN interventions

Corresponding authors: Linda Schultz, World Bank, Washington, DC, United States; lschultz@worldbank.org.

particularly cost-effective. As a result, schools can reach an unprecedented number of children and adolescents and play a key role in national development efforts by improving both child health and education. Because schools are at the heart of all communities, we have an opportunity to use the school as a sustainable, scalable option for simple health service delivery.

This chapter explores the developmental rationale for improving the health of school-age children and the economic rationale for administering health interventions to school-age children (typically from ages 5 to 14 years) through existing educational systems as compared with the health system. Definitions of age groupings and age-specific terminology used in this volume can be found in chapter 1 (Bundy, de Silva, and others 2017).

SCHOOL HEALTH AND NUTRITION

SHN describes a wide range of interventions delivered through schools to improve education and health outcomes by enhancing nutrition, alleviating hunger, and preventing disease. SHN interventions can target the most common local health conditions that affect school-age children and can be delivered by teachers and other proxies for the health system. Delivery of health interventions through schools enables children to take advantage of investments made in the education sector and improves country competitiveness, given that each increased year of schooling is associated with greater earning capacity and lower levels of mortality, illness, and health risks. As more children survive and thrive (figure 20.1), the role of schools becomes increasingly important.

These programs have a long history. At the turn of the twentieth century, school feeding[1] initiatives were among the first social welfare programs to emerge in high-income countries (Atkins 2007). Recognition that SHN benefits learning had been clear from the 1920s, when school-based deworming programs were instituted across the southern United States specifically to promote education and reduce poverty (Ettling 1981). By the 1980s, SHN programs had become ubiquitous in upper-middle-income countries and high-income countries. Change also began in the 1980s in low- and middle-income countries (LMICs) with a shift away from the traditional complex, medical-based approach, usually targeted to elite urban or boarding schools, and toward interventions targeted to the poorest schools.

Both the health and education communities have championed SHN in LMICs. The WHO's Ottawa Charter for Health Promotion, launched in 1986, provided momentum for global recognition of the importance of addressing health in the educational context (WHO 1986). This recognition was further propelled by the work of the WHO Expert Committee on Comprehensive School Health and Nutrition Education and Promotion in the mid-1990s. The WHO's Information Series on School Health and Nutrition, together with the United Nations Educational, Scientific and Cultural Organization (UNESCO) and Education Development Center, commenced in the late 1990s (WHO 1997). There was also an attempt to promote thinking around SHN at the 1990 World Education Forum in Jomtien, Thailand, but it was not until 10 years later that the concept gained traction in the global commitment to achieve EFA launched at the World Education Forum in Dakar, Senegal, in 2000. To strengthen the focus on SHN, several organizations, including UNESCO, the United Nations Children's Fund (UNICEF), the WHO, and the World Bank, used the Dakar Forum to launch an organizing framework entitled Focusing Resources on Effective School Health and Nutrition (FRESH). Since then, an increasing number of low- and lower-middle-income countries have adopted more comprehensive SHN policies with the specific aims of achieving EFA along with the education-specific Millennium Development Goals of universal basic education and gender equality in educational access (Bundy 2011). In Sub-Saharan Africa, the percentage of countries implementing programs that meet the minimum WHO Health Promoting School criteria of equity and effectiveness rose from 10 percent in 2000 to more than 80 percent in 2014 (Drake, Maier, and de Lind van Wijngaarden 2007) (figure 20.2). In Sub-Saharan Africa, the percentage of reproductive health service–supported programs rose from 10 percent to more than 70 percent, with an estimate of 80 percent in 2014.

Figure 20.1 Rate of Survival beyond Age Five Years

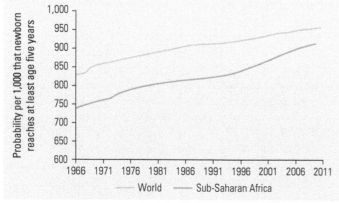

Source: World Bank 2016.
Note: Survival rate is the inverse of the under-five year mortality rate, which is the probability per 1,000 that a newborn will die before reaching age five years, subject to age-specific mortality rates for the specified year.

Figure 20.2 Expansion of School Health and Nutrition in Sub-Saharan Africa

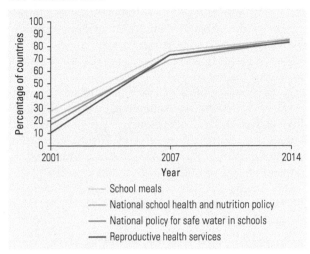

Source: Adapted from Drake, Maier, and de Lind van Wijngaarden 2007.

HEALTHY CHILDREN, BETTER LEARNING

SHN programming is increasingly recognized as a critical element for achieving universal access to education. Access to a school, provision of quality teaching and learning materials, and availability of trained teachers are necessary, but insufficient, to achieve good learning outcomes. Children also need to be healthy and regularly attending school to be able to benefit fully from the learning opportunities. Ill health can be the catalyst for extended absence or dropping out of school completely; malaria and worm infections can reduce enrollment; anemia can affect cognition, attention span, and learning; and the pain associated with tooth decay can affect both attendance and learning (chapters 11–16 of this volume; Benzian and others 2017; Brooker and others 2017; Bundy, Appleby, and others 2017; Drake, Fernandes, and others 2017; LaMontagne and others 2017; Lassi, Moin, and Bhutta 2017). The potential for school health interventions to shape physical and psychosocial health as well as education outcomes for youth has been explored to a

greater extent in high-income countries, especially in the United States (Durlak, Weissberg, and Dymnicki 2011; Murray and others 2007; Shackleton and others 2016).

Some of the most prevalent health conditions of school-age children affect children's education participation and learning outcomes significantly (table 20.1). Typical interventions and their target conditions include the following: deworming and worm infection; bednets and malaria; handwashing and bacterial infections; toothbrushing and dental caries; spectacles and refractive error; micronutrients and micronutrient deficiency; and food and hunger. Research has shown that the average IQ loss for children with these conditions can range from 3.7 IQ points per child with untreated worm infections to 6.0 IQ points for children with anemia. Together, these prevalent conditions are estimated to translate into the equivalent of between 200 million and 500 million years of school lost due to ill health in LMICs each year (Bundy 2011).

Interventions for these common health conditions can have long-term economic benefits. Estimates show that poor students in areas where these conditions are prevalent would gain the equivalent of 0.5–2.5 extra years of schooling if their health benefited from appropriate interventions. Sustaining the benefits across multiple years of schooling could improve cognitive abilities by 0.25 standard deviations, on average; extrapolating the benefits of improved accumulation in human capital could translate to roughly a 5 percent increase in earning capacity over the life course; see chapter 29 in this volume (Ahuja and others 2017).

SHN interventions can enhance equity by supporting student participation and contributing to a reduction in the education achievement gap between well-performing and underperforming students. A study in South Africa found that children who score 0.25 standard deviations above the mean on grade 2 examinations were significantly more likely to complete grade 7 (figure 20.3). If schools that delivered health and nutrition interventions could raise examination scores, they may experience higher student retention, compared with schools without health programs.

Although better health alone cannot compensate for missed learning opportunities, it can provide children with the potential to take advantage of learning

Table 20.1 Estimates of the Global Cognitive Impact of Common Diseases of School-Age Children in LMICs

Common diseases	Prevalence (%)	Total cases (millions)	IQ points lost per child	Additional cases of IQ <70 (millions)	Lost years of schooling (millions)
Worms	30	169	3.75	15.8	201
Stunting	52	292	3	21.6	284
Anemia	53	298	6	45.6	524

Source: Bundy 2011.
Note: IQ = intelligence quotient; LMICs = low- and middle-income countries.

Figure 20.3 Estimated School Dropout Rates, with and without School Health and Nutrition Interventions, in South Africa

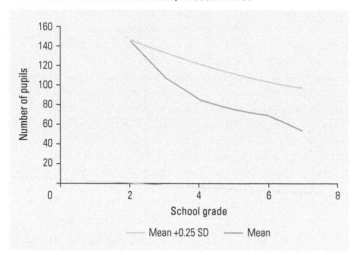

Source: Liddell and Rae 2001.

Note: SD = standard deviation. Students who score 0.25 SD higher on exams in grade 2 are more likely to complete grade 7. If schools that delivered health and nutrition interventions could raise examination scores, they may experience higher student retention compared with schools without health programs.

opportunities (Grigorenko and others 2006). Children are more ready to learn after treatment; they may be able to catch up with better-off peers if their improved learning potential can be used effectively in the classroom. The education sector is responsible for the quality of education delivered and for leveraging the investment it has already made.

A key message of this volume is that different types of health interventions are required at different stages in child and adolescent development. The accumulating evidence on the benefits of targeted interventions from middle childhood to late adolescence is summarized in chapter 6 in this volume (Bundy and Horton 2017); the potential impact of targeted intervention in school-age children is discussed in chapter 8 of this volume (Watkins and others 2017).

SHN and school feeding interventions build on the foundation of early child development interventions and exploit the accessibility of children in schools. Figure 20.4 demonstrates how the World Bank characterized the varied opportunities for health interventions at different life

Figure 20.4 Learning as a Lifelong Process

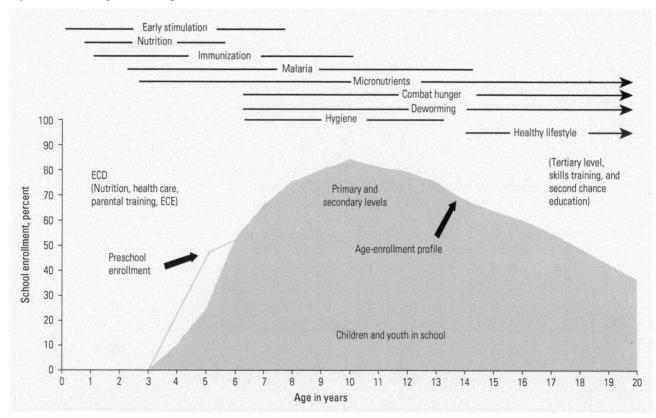

Source: Adapted from World Bank 2011, updated to include preschool enrollment; World Bank 2016.

Note: ECD = early child development; ECE = early childhood education. Rates of preschool enrollment by country group: 18.05 (low income), 49.56 (lower-middle income; reflects reported rate from 2012), 58.39 (middle income). The rates indicate the total enrollment in preprimary education, regardless of age, expressed as a percentage of the total population of official preprimary education age.

stages as part of an education strategy. The figure indicates schematically when interventions might be particularly helpful. For example, early stimulation can help ensure school readiness; malaria prevention and education on bednet use, school feeding, and deworming treatments can help keep children in school by enhancing attendance and reducing dropout rates; and vision correction and skills-based health education, along with school feeding, might help improve learning by enhancing cognition and educational achievement (World Bank 2012).

SCHOOLS AS ENTRY POINTS FOR HEALTH INTERVENTIONS

Schools are one of the few institutions in poor communities that provide access to trained human resources. In contrast, the health systems in many LMICs experience multiple barriers, especially in costs and human resources, that limit their ability to reach beyond health facilities. Schools cannot replace health systems, which remain the formal avenue for health delivery, but education systems can complement health delivery mechanisms by providing outreach opportunities through schools. Even in LMICs, school-based interventions can be widely implemented by the education sector, with the health sector ensuring proper oversight and training of school staff (Bundy 2011).

School-based health programs have the potential to reach an estimated 575 million school-age children in low-income countries (UNESCO 2008). This opportunity is particularly relevant to Sub-Saharan Africa. Young people constitute the greatest proportion of the population, and this is the only region in which the number of young people continues to grow substantially (UNFPA 2012). It is also important that this is now a region in which most children attend school. As shown in figure 20.5, the percentage of the population that has enrolled in school, completed primary education, and moved on to secondary school has increased considerably during the past four decades, so that the proportion of school-going children and adolescents in Sub-Saharan Africa today approaches that of South Asia. Despite the increasing number of children in school, Sub-Saharan Africa has low enrollment rates compared with the rest of the world. Looking ahead, an unprecedented number of children are anticipated to be in school in this region as enrollment rates improve. Because most countries have SHN programs, opportunities exist to scale up the scope of services and tailor specific types of programs to local contexts. It is important to note that the high pupil-to-teacher ratio in many schools may discourage educators and the education sector from adding extra

Figure 20.5 Percentage of Population Enrolled in Primary School and Who Move on to Secondary School in South Asia and Sub-Saharan Africa, 1970 and 2015

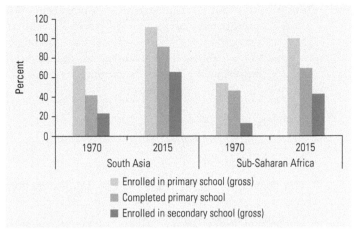

Source: World Bank 2016.
Note: Total enrollment, regardless of age, expressed as a percentage of the population of official primary or secondary education age. Gross enrollment rate can exceed 100 percent as a result of the inclusion of over-age and under-age students because of early or late school entrance and grade repetition.

Figure 20.6 Ratio of Primary School Teachers to Community Health Workers in 13 Low- and Lower-Middle-Income Countries, by GDP per Capita

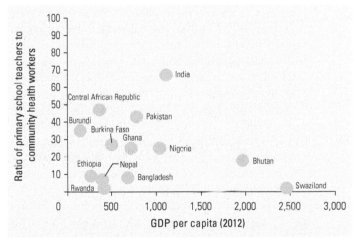

Sources: Data on the number of primary school teachers are from UNESCO Institute for Statistics (http://stats.uis.unesco.org); data on the number of community health workers are from the WHO Global Health Observatory Data Repository (http://apps.who.int/ghodata/); and GDP data are from World Bank 2016.
Note: GDP = gross domestic product.

responsibilities that accompany SHN programming. Preservice sensitization and training can help educators recognize that healthy children learn better.

SHN systems build on existing infrastructure, curriculum opportunities, and teacher networks to accelerate implementation and reduce costs. There are more teachers than nurses and more schools than clinics, often by an order of magnitude. Figure 20.6 shows that the ratio of primary teachers to community health workers in several countries is in the range of 20:1 to 65:1; this relationship is only loosely related to gross domestic product (GDP). Including teachers—as the largest segment of the workforce and often community leaders—in public health activities can also broaden awareness of, and community commitment to, public health interventions.

SCHOOL HEALTH AND NUTRITION PROGRAMS: PRO-POOR AND PRO-GIRL INTERVENTIONS

SHN programs can help level the playing field for the most vulnerable students: the poor, the sick, and the malnourished. These are the children who require the greatest support throughout their schooling to minimize the risk of absenteeism and dropping out, but who generally have the least access to care and support (World Bank 2012). SHN and nutrition programs are pro-poor because the greatest benefits accrue to those children who are most affected at the outset (Bundy 2011). This pro-poor focus has also been increasingly emphasized in WHO SHN policies and practices (Tang and others 2009).

Poverty is a key consideration in the design of SHN and school feeding programs. The negative correlations between ill health, malnutrition, and income level are clearly demonstrated in both cross-country comparisons and individual country analyses (de Silva and others 2003), partly because low income and poverty promote disease and inadequate diets. Paradoxically, SHN programs are often most equitable when they are universal; mass delivery can help ensure that the interventions reach those poorest children who are more often systematically overlooked, especially by intervention programs that operate through diagnoses at health facilities.

However, the equity value of universal access within schools does not imply that there is no value in targeting poor communities. With few exceptions, the diseases that affect children and their education are most prevalent in poor countries, particularly in the poorest communities within those countries. As a result, targeting interventions to those communities most likely to benefit is cost-effective and a common characteristic of strong SHN programs. The benefits of targeting school feeding interventions is discussed in depth in chapter 12 in this volume (Drake, Fernandes, and others 2017). Lessons gleaned from country case studies can illustrate the strengths of different school feeding approaches in both program design and service delivery (Drake, Woolnough, and others 2016).

Girls and young women benefit particularly from SHN and school feeding programs because some of the most common health conditions affecting education are more prevalent in girls, and because gender-based vulnerability and exclusion can place girls at greater risk of ill health, neglect, and hunger (Bundy 2011). Deworming and iron supplementation offer particular benefits to girls because women and girls are, for physiological reasons, more likely to experience high rates of anemia. SHN programs draw children—especially girls—into schools and encourage them to stay (Gelli, Meir, and Espejo 2007). This dynamic is particularly relevant to achieving EFA; marginalized children, among whom girls are overrepresented, account for the majority of out-of-school children (UNESCO 2011). Moreover, improved health and increased educational attainment for young women can help delay age at first birth, which is associated with improved financial risk protection and enhanced intergenerational health outcomes; see chapter 28 in this volume (Verguet and others 2017).

Girls can benefit greatly from health promotion and life-skills lessons offered in schools. This benefit is exemplified with human immunodeficiency virus/ acquired immune deficiency syndrome (HIV/AIDS) education, particularly because young women in Sub-Saharan Africa are estimated to be two to seven times more likely to be infected with HIV than young men (MacPhail, Williams, and Campbell 2002). Health responses are more sustainable and have a greater reach when integrated into an existing framework, such as through a wider curriculum of health promotion (Jukes, Simmons, and Bundy 2008). Research shows that the most trusted source for young people to learn about HIV/AIDS is through schools and teachers (Boler 2003). A wide range of life skills and health promotion curriculum design, content, and implementation is available (Hargreaves and Boler 2006). Relatively simple lessons on skills-based health education can usefully address stigma and discrimination, and an integrated curriculum at a higher level of complexity can usefully influence protective health behaviors. Data show that for every extra year children remain in school HIV/AIDS rates are reduced (World Bank 2002). The years of school attended may not equate to greater attainment of skills-based health education because curriculum quality and extent of integration into the larger school framework vary widely (Hargreaves and others 2008; Jukes, Simmons, and Bundy 2008).

SHN programs may also work synergistically with conditional and unconditional social transfer programs; see chapter 7 in this volume (Alderman and others 2017) and chapter 12 in this volume (Drake, Fernandes, and others 2017). Take-home rations and conditional cash transfers can encourage girls to go to school; bursaries, which give rations directly to girl students, can encourage girls to stay in school (Chapman 2006). The broader value of these programs is discussed in chapter 23 in this volume (de Walque and others 2017).

Schools are an increasingly attractive and effective platform for reaching girls given that the gender gap in enrollment is closing in most countries. Figure 20.7 illustrates decreasing out-of-school rates between 1970 and 2010. The trend for girls is especially clear: between 1970 and 2010 the significant gap in enrollment of boys and girls was dramatically reduced, although a substantial number of children—more or less equally boys and girls—never enroll in school. Figures 20.8 and 20.9 provide a more nuanced look at the narrowing gender disparities in out-of-school children in South Asia and Sub-Saharan Africa, showing that greater change in enrollment among girls has occurred in South Asia.

Significant cross-country differences exist in gender disparities in enrollment rates based on historical experience and government policies. Data from five Sub-Saharan African countries are presented in figure 20.10. In Mozambique, the number of out-of-school children decreased significantly from 2000 to 2014, while gender gaps remained substantial. In contrast, the gender gap remained small in Ghana, while the trend was downward; in Niger, the number of out-of-school children remained relatively constant over the period, while the gender gap widened.

In some Sub-Saharan African countries, the numbers of out-of-school children have proved difficult to reduce; as a result, the observation that SHN programs can benefit out-of-school children becomes increasingly important. As documented in Guinea and Madagascar, many out-of-school children will take advantage of simple health services provided in schools, for example, deworming and micronutrient supplements; school feeding programs, especially take-home rations, have been shown to benefit siblings at home (Adelman and others 2008; Bundy and others 2009; Del Rosso and Marek 1996). Deworming programs in schools have been found to reach out-of-school children at scale (Drake and others 2015) and reduce disease transmission in the community as a whole (Bundy and others 1990; Miguel and Kremer 2004). Although the benefits of SHN programs can extend beyond those who attend school, SHN programs are best considered in conjunction with other approaches to encouraging enrollment and attendance.

Figure 20.7 Global Out-of-School Children of Primary School Age, by Gender, 1970–2010

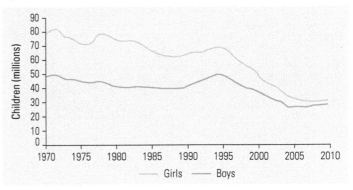

Source: World Bank 2016.
Note: The total number of boys and girls of primary school age who are not enrolled in either primary or secondary schools.

Figure 20.8 Out-of-School Children of Primary School Age in South Asia, 1975–2013

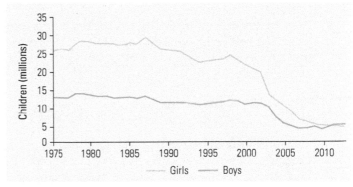

Source: World Bank 2016.
Note: The total number of boys and girls of primary school age who are not enrolled in either primary or secondary schools.

Figure 20.9 Out-of-School Children of Primary School Age in Sub-Saharan Africa, 1975–2013

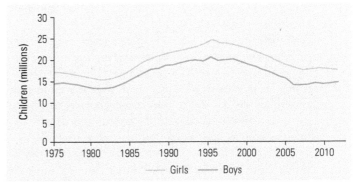

Source: World Bank 2016.
Note: The total number of boys and girls of primary school age who are not enrolled in either primary or secondary schools.

Figure 20.10 Out-of-School Children of Primary School Age, in Five Countries, by Gender, 2000–14

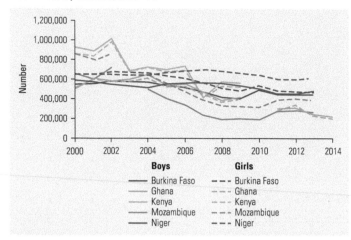

Source: World Bank 2016.
Note: Out-of-school children of primary school age for specific countries. Figure shows the total number of boys and girls of primary school age who are not enrolled in primary or secondary schools. Gaps in the graphs are due to lack of data for those years.

It is important that out-of-school children have access to skills-based health education and life-skills development to prevent illnesses such as HIV/AIDS (Hargreaves and others 2008).

DEFINING SECTOR ROLES

The implementation, funding, and oversight of SHN programs do not fall squarely within either the education or the health sector. Rather, many approaches, stakeholders, and collaborations are involved in the delivery of health and nutrition services in schools. Diverse experiences suggest that existing programs highlight certain consistent roles played by government and nongovernmental agencies and other partners and stakeholders. It is clear that program success depends on the effective participation and support of strategic partnerships, especially with the beneficiaries and their parents or guardians (table 20.2).

In nearly every national SHN program, the Ministry of Education is the lead implementing agency, reflecting both the goal of SHN programs to improve educational achievement and the fact that the education system often provides the most complete existing infrastructure to reach school-age children. In successful programs this responsibility has been shared between the Ministry of Education and the Ministry of Health, particularly since the latter has the ultimate responsibility for the health of all children. However, collaboration across sectors is not easy, particularly given different institutional structures, operational

mechanisms, and working cultures between different line ministries. Each sector needs to identify its respective role and responsibilities and present a coordinated plan of action to improve the health and education outcomes of children. Beyond the education and health ministries and nonstate actors, intersectoral collaboration is more complex. The starting point is usually the establishment of cross-sectoral working groups or steering committees at national, district, and local levels to coordinate actions and decision making (FRESH 2014). The understanding and recognition by the education and health sectors of each other's core business and priorities are also essential; the stronger and more explicit focus that the WHO places on achieving both health and education outcomes can facilitate collaboration between health promotion practitioners and teachers.

Successful multisector school-based health service delivery includes referral and treatment opportunities that extend beyond the school platform. School-based responses to the various diseases affecting school-age children vary depending on the nature of the treatment required. For example, there is a clear policy context for integrating the identification and referral of refractive error into wider SHN programs. It is essential that school-based vision screening programs include screening and referral at the primary level; refraction and optical dispensing at the district level; and supported advanced care, including pediatric and contact lens services, at the tertiary health care level, although the costs increase and feasibility decreases with each step away from the primary level (World Bank 2012). See chapter 17 in this volume (Graham and others 2017) for a more detailed look at school-based vision programming.

SHN programs offer a compelling case for public sector investment and interventions. First, these interventions may create externalities whereby external benefits accrue to people other than treated individuals. For example, deworming programs reduce the intensity of infection in untreated children in schools, in neighboring schools, and in siblings of those treated at schools (Miguel and Kremer 2004). Second, some health interventions are pure public goods—all school-age children are eligible to access these services and there is typically little private demand for general preventive measures. Accordingly, the private sector is unlikely to compete to deliver these goods and services. SHN programs are most likely to achieve universal coverage and be sustainable when they are under the jurisdiction of the public sector and integrated into national education sector plans (ESPs).

Table 20.2 Comparison of Roles Played by Government Agencies, Partners, and Stakeholders in School Health and Nutrition Programs

Partner	Roles	Comments
Ministry of Education	• Lead implementing agency • Lead financial resource • Education sector policy	• Health and nutrition of schoolchildren is a priority for EFA. • Education policy defines school environment, curriculum, duties of teachers. • Education system has a pervasive infrastructure for reaching teachers and school-age children.
Ministry of Health	• Lead technical agency • Health sector policy	• Health of school-age children has lower priority than clinical services and infant health. • Health policy defines role of teachers in service delivery and how health materials are procured.
Other public sector agencies (for example, ministries of welfare, social affairs, local government, agriculture)	• Support education and health systems • Fund holders	• Ministries of local government are often fund holders for teachers and schools, as well as for clinics and health agents. • Ministries of welfare and social affairs provide mechanisms for the provision of social funds.
Private sector (for example, health services, pharmaceuticals, publications)	• Specialist service delivery • Materials provision	• Major role in drug procurement and production of training materials. • Specialist roles in health diagnostics.
Civil society (for example, NGOs, FBOs, PTAs)	• Training and supervision • Local resource provision	• At the local level, serve as gatekeepers and fund holders; may also target implementation. • Offer additional resource streams, particularly through INGOs.
Teachers associations, local community (for example, children, teachers, parents)	• Define teachers' roles • Partners in implementation • Define acceptability of curriculum • Supplement resources	• School health programs demand an expanded role for teachers. • Gatekeepers for both the content of health education (especially moral and sexual content) and the role of nonhealth agents (especially teachers) in health service delivery. Pupils are active participants in all aspects of the process at the school level. • Communities supplement program finances at the margins.

Source: Jukes, Drake, and Bundy 2008.
Note. EFA = Education for All; FBO = faith-based organization; INGO = international nongovernmental organization; NGO = nongovernmental organization; PTA = parent-teacher association.

ECONOMIC RATIONALE FOR SCHOOL-BASED HEALTH INTERVENTIONS

In the complex set of conditions required for children to learn well, improved health can be one of the simplest and cheapest conditions to achieve (World Bank 2012). The focus of this economic rationale is on conditions for which there are existing interventions that are sufficiently safe, simple, and well evaluated to be appropriate for education sector implementation through schools, typically with health sector supervision.

Several factors support the economic rationale for schools as a platform for the delivery of health interventions. One of the main factors is the potential savings offered by school systems, rather than health systems, as the delivery mechanism. From this perspective, schools provide a preexisting mechanism, so costs are marginal; they also provide a system that as part of its primary educational purpose aims to be sustainable and pervasive, reach disadvantaged children, and promote social equity. Tailoring and targeting the types of interventions to local contexts lies at the heart of practical success. Targeting reduces costs and facilitates management; it may optimize outcomes.

Education sector spending exceeds public health spending in most LMICs. In Ghana, Mozambique, and Niger, for example, public expenditures for education are more than double those for public health (figure 20.11). The higher investment in the education sector relative to the health sector is reflected in the greater number of schools and teachers versus health centers and health workers in communities (see figure 20.6).

Figure 20.11 Expenditures on Education versus Health as a Proportion of GDP, 2013

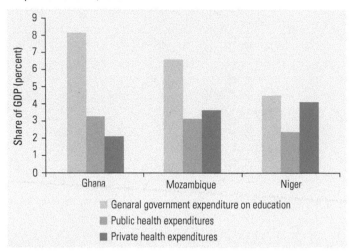

Source: World Bank 2016.

Note: GDP = gross domestic product. Total health expenditure is the sum of public and private health expenditure. It covers the provision of preventive and curative health services, family planning activities, nutrition activities, and emergency aid designated for health; it does not include provision of water and sanitation. General government expenditure on education (current, capital, and transfers) is expressed as a percentage of GDP. It includes expenditure funded by transfers from international sources to government. General government usually refers to local, regional, and central governments. Data are more readily available (as are world and regional estimates) for health than for education.

The large share of the population that school-age children represent and the high percentage of children that attend school imply significant economies of scale in the cost of delivering school-based health interventions. The economies of scale can be expected to be larger for interventions with small variable or marginal costs, that is, the cost of treating an additional child. School-based health interventions may also have fixed costs for establishing infrastructure, staffing, government capacity, intersectoral policies, and monitoring systems.

The rationale for school-based health interventions is also stronger for interventions that address prevalent conditions in populations (see table 20.1). In this case, the expected benefits are higher per dollar invested. Targeting school-based health interventions to children at greater risk may lead to greater benefits, but it may also lead to higher costs, depending on how the targeting is achieved.

COMPARATIVE COST-EFFECTIVENESS OF DELIVERING HEALTH INTERVENTIONS THROUGH SCHOOLS

Schools offer advantages over community and primary health center platforms. Chapter 25 in this volume presents an essential package of low-cost health interventions that can be delivered effectively in LMICs

through schools (Fernandes and Aurino 2017). The analysis suggests that the economic benefits as measured by the returns to health and education outweigh the costs, while remaining affordable within government budget constraints. The essential package includes targeted school meals with micronutrient fortification, education on malaria prevention and oral hygiene, deworming treatment, screening for refractive error, and appropriate immunization.

The cost savings of delivering simple and safe interventions through schools can be illustrated in deworming and screening for refractive error. For example, delivery of mass administration of deworming treatment through schools (not including the cost of treatment because it is currently donated for schoolchildren) is estimated to cost US$0.03–US$0.04 per child per year, compared with US$0.21–US$0.51 through mobile health teams coordinated by primary health centers (Guyatt 2003). Screening costs for refractive error and provision of glasses through area hospitals were estimated to be US$8.17, but the cost drops to US$2–US$3 if the screening is provided by mobile teams dispatched to schools following screening by teachers (Baltussen, Naus, and Limburg 2009; Graham and others 2017) (table 20.3). With minimal training combined with access to periodic supervision and support, school teachers can safely administer pills or screen children for health conditions of interest, limiting the time requirement and cost of access to skilled health personnel.

The presence of children at school obviates the need to draw children to another point of service at regular intervals or for mobile health teams to travel to reach them. Furthermore, the implementation of multiple interventions through the same delivery system allows for shared costs and efficiencies, for example, for teacher training. The effectiveness of primary health centers is contingent on the target population coming to clinics to receive the interventions, which can be a significant time

Table 20.3 Essential Package of School-Based Health Interventions, 2012 U.S. dollars

	Annual cost per child per year ($)
School meals	44
MNP supplementation	3
Malaria	2–3
Refractive error screening	2–3
Toothbrush provision	0.50
HPV vaccine	2
Tetanus toxoid vaccine	0.40

Source: Fernandes and Aurino 2017.
Note: HPV = human papillomavirus; MNP = micronutrient powder.

and cost burden on poorer families and especially challenging for interventions with multiple dosages, such as the human papillomavirus (HPV) vaccine, and for the school-age population; see chapter 15 in this volume (LaMontagne and others 2017). The economic analysis of the effect of health interventions on improved education attainment is discussed in chapter 22 in this volume (Plaut and others 2017).

CONTEXT FRAMING AND POLICY FRAMEWORK

Creating and refining an SHN program involves a series of policy decisions, especially how to work effectively across sectors and how to select interventions to include. Fortunately, two policy tools track some of the decisions that countries made in developing their SHN programs.

- The FRESH framework was introduced at the beginning of LMIC programming in this area and is still widely used. Its primary purpose was to provide a policy framework to support the start-up of new programs or the strengthening of existing programs.
- The Systems Approach for Better Education Results (SABER) was introduced more than a decade later as a mechanism for refining the policy environment of existing programs. The emergence of this tool reflects the need created by the remarkable proliferation of new school health and school feeding programs in LMICs.

FRESH

The use of schools as a platform for delivering SHN interventions was accelerated by the launch of the FRESH framework at the World Education Forum in 2000, by a multi-agency partnership that included UNESCO, UNICEF, the WHO, the World Food Programme, and the World Bank (Sarr and others 2017).

FRESH is a comprehensive, evidence-based framework that promotes better education through health interventions delivered by schools and is supported by an international consensus among partners and stakeholders. The FRESH framework offers strategic guidance to ensure that program implementation is standardized and evidence based (World Bank 2012). It lays the foundation for effective and equitable SHN programs and consists conceptually of four mutually reinforcing pillars (FRESH 2014):

- *Pillar 1: Health-related school policies.* Health- and nutrition-related school policies that are nondiscriminatory, protective, inclusive, and gender sensitive to promote the physical and psychosocial health of children, teachers, and school staff
- *Pillar 2: Safe learning environment.* Access to safe water and provision of separate sanitation facilities for girls, boys, and teachers; a safe, healthy, clean, and emotionally supportive environment that fosters children's ability to attend school, pay attention, and learn
- *Pillar 3: Skill-based health education.* Life-skills education that addresses health, nutrition, and hygiene issues with knowledge, attitudes, and skills to promote positive behaviors
- *Pillar 4: School-based health and nutrition services.* Simple, safe, and familiar health and nutrition services that can be delivered cost-effectively in schools, and increased access to youth-friendly clinics

All four of these components are necessary for a successful program. They can be implemented effectively only if they are supported by strategic partnerships between (1) the health and education sectors, especially teachers and health workers; (2) schools and their respective communities; and (3) pupils' awareness and participation. Figure 20.12 provides an illustrative example of the mutually reinforcing nature of the four FRESH pillars.

Governments that sought EFA outcomes also sought to mainstream programs based on these pillars into their national ESPs. Typically, ESPs reflect both expected budgetary and capacity needs, and are developed in consultation with key external and national stakeholders and partners. Analysis of the country ESPs provides insight into the relevance and prioritization of specific SHN issues by national governments. A comparison between the content of ESPs that were developed immediately following the launch of FRESH and those developed 15 years later provides an indication of how SHN programs have been mainstreamed into education systems. Figure 20.13 illustrates the proportion of countries seeking financing for each of the four pillars of FRESH at the two time points for a set of 25 countries in Sub-Saharan Africa. Countries include Benin, Burkina Faso, Burundi, Cameroon, the Central African Republic, Chad, Eritrea, Ethiopia, The Gambia, Ghana, Guinea, Guinea Bissau, Kenya, Liberia, Madagascar, Mali, Mauritania, Mozambique, the Democratic Republic of Congo, Rwanda, Senegal, Togo, Uganda, Zambia, and Zimbabwe.

The share of ESPs seeking financing for policy pillar 1 is low at both times, reflecting the long-term nature of the policy planning cycle and the typically fixed, nonrecurrent cost of implementing policy change.

Figure 20.12 FRESH Components Supported by the Strategic Partnerships

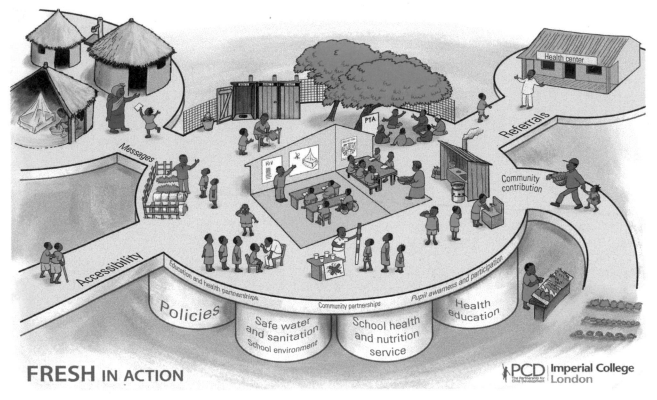

Figure 20.13 Reflection of Funding Prioritized for FRESH Pillars in Education Sector Plans from 25 Countries in Sub-Saharan Africa, 2001–15

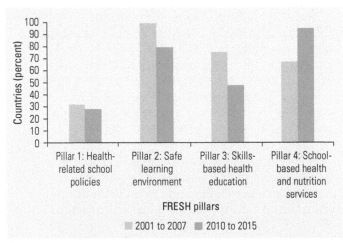

In contrast, infrastructure and service costs, reflected under pillars 2 and 4, respectively, have a substantial recurrent component, which is reflected in the large proportion of countries seeking financing for these pillars at both times. Pillar 2 also reflects the focus on building new schools to support EFA, hence its inclusion in the ESPs for all countries in the earlier period and to a lesser degree in the later period, perhaps reflecting investment in additional water and sanitation facilities and a new focus on menstrual hygiene management. Pillar 3 in the 2000s in Sub-Saharan Africa was focused on HIV/AIDS prevention education. In the early period, this intervention was given special emphasis by the regional Accelerate initiative, in which most countries participated. As the HIV/AIDS epidemic waned, financing for pillar 3 declined (Sarr and others 2017).

Perhaps the most important consequence of FRESH has been to offer a common point of entry for new efforts to improve health in schools. This is important because over time SHN programs can address issues that both the education and health sectors are unfamiliar with and that are intrinsically multisectoral.

The FRESH framework remains a driver of new SHN programming and has provided a common platform upon which to build agency-specific programs. Chapter 17 in this volume (Graham and others 2017) discusses how countries have used the FRESH framework to guide education that is inclusive for children with disabilities.

SABER

The degree to which SHN in practice is embedded in the education sector can be benchmarked with the SABER tool. The SABER tool was developed by a partnership led by the World Bank (2012) and was based on the FRESH framework. The tool consists of a structured questionnaire whose responses are determined based on consultation with representatives from relevant ministries, including Ministries of Education, Health, and Social Protection. One of the domains developed for SABER is SHN programming, with a large subcomponent for analysis of school feeding programs.

The SABER School Health and Nutrition and School Feeding diagnostic tools provide a snapshot of the development status of their related policies in countries. Specifically, SABER assists governments in assessing the quality of their SHN and school feeding programs and progress in implementing each indicator, and it benchmarks them against other programs and education domains. As such, SABER inspires and supports policy dialogue and reform, and lays the groundwork for a deeper analysis of the implementation of these frameworks. The SABER School Health and Nutrition and School Feeding rubric frameworks help ensure that when possible, schools can serve as entry points for health care for school-age children (World Bank 2012).

Figure 20.14 presents findings from an analysis of select indicators from SABER SHN reports from 16 LMICs published between 2011 and 2013, using the four pillars of FRESH as the guiding principle.

The results indicate that 13 of the 16 countries have national SHN policies; more than 50 percent have water, sanitation, and handwashing standards in place; 12 of the 16 countries implementing SHN services had specific recurrent budget lines to support delivery. In addition, gender-responsive policies, skills, and services were highlighted in SABER reports from 10 of the 16 countries.

Approaches to school feeding and SHN, as well as different routes to educational success, can be very diverse. No single set of policy options will be relevant to all countries. In developing national and subnational policies—and there are always trade-offs in the choices

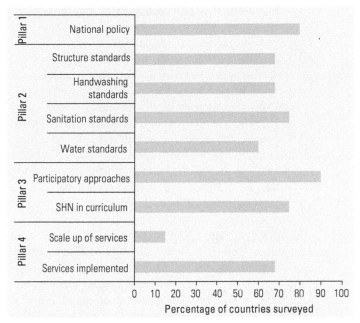

Figure 20.14 Reflection of FRESH Pillars in School Health and Nutrition Practices in 16 Countries

Source: Sarr and others 2017.
Note: FRESH = Focusing Resources on Effective School Health; SABER = Systems Approach for Better Education Results; SHN = school health and nutrition. Indicators from SABER School Health and Nutrition report from 16 countries conducted between 2011 and 2013. Countries comprise Benin, Cape Verde, Côte d'Ivoire, Ethiopia, Ghana, Kenya, Madagascar, Malawi, Mali, Niger, Nigeria, Rwanda, Senegal, Tanzania, Uganda, and Zanzibar.

made—SABER helps identify common policy and institutional threads that run through most of the more successful experiences, such as the following:

- Focus on education outcomes
- Multisectoral policy and a memorandum of understanding between health and education sectors, backed by strong senior leadership from politicians and senior officials
- Information dissemination and consultation with local communities (World Bank 2012)

Other School Health and Nutrition Policy Tools

Other tools for policy making on SHN programs are available, in addition to FRESH and SABER. The School Health Policies and Practices Survey, the Global School-based Student Health Survey (GSHS), and the Health Behavior in School-aged Children Survey (HBSC) are three such tools.

The School Health Policies and Practices Survey was developed by the WHO in collaboration with the U.S. Centers for Disease Control and Prevention (WHO and

CDC, n.d.). The survey aims to assess the status of school health policies and practices in primary and secondary schools. It is administered through a questionnaire for school principals or head teachers. There are 150 questions divided into six content areas: general school information, healthy and safe school environment, health services, nutrition services, health education, and physical education.

The self-administered GSHS, similarly developed by the WHO and the U.S. CDC, is designed to help countries measure and assess the behavioral risk and protective factors among students ages 13–15 years. The data collected through the survey help set priorities, establish programs, advocate for resources, and allow for comparison across countries. It is a school-based questionnaire survey, managed by a survey coordinator who is appointed through the Ministries of Health and Education. Ten key topics covered include alcohol use, dietary behaviors, drug use, hygiene, mental health, physical activity, protective factors, sexual behaviors, tobacco use, and violence and unintended injury. To date, some 110 countries in all six WHO regions have either implemented the GSHS or are in the process of doing so (WHO 2016a). Of the 110 countries, only 3 are in Europe.

The HBSC is the primary behavioral survey administered in the WHO European Region for this target population. HBSC collects data every four years on the health and well-being, social environments, and health behaviors of boys and girls ages 11, 13, and 15 years through self-administered questionnaires in classrooms. The key content areas covered by the GSHS and HBSC surveys are similar, while the HBSC survey also includes a focus on social and economic determinants. To date, 44 countries and regions across Europe and North America have been involved in the HBSC survey (WHO 2016b).

CONCLUSIONS

The school system offers a number of advantages as a health delivery system in low-income countries. Building on an existing and pervasive infrastructure can reduce start-up costs, accelerate program implementation, and reduce programmatic costs, while optimizing the benefits for education, increasing access to care for the most marginalized, and encouraging girls to attend and stay in school.

Sustainable national school health programs depend on mainstreaming these programs into national policies and plans, as well as increasing national financing for SHN and strengthening cross-sectoral institutional implementation capacity. Existing resources, such as SABER and FRESH, can help the education sector

identify policy gaps and opportunities, improve implementation, and scale up. HSBC and GSHS provide similar tools for guiding the school health policy decisions of the health sector.

This approach is most effective if the health sector retains responsibility for the health of children and the education sector retains responsibility for implementation. By working together, Ministries of Education and Health can promote better health and education through multisector SHN interventions.

ACKNOWLEDGMENTS

The author team would like to recognize Kwok-Cho Tang, formerly with the World Health Organization, and Meena Fernandes, Partnership for Child Development, for their important contributions to the chapter.

NOTES

World Bank Income Classifications as of July 2014 are as follows, based on estimates of gross national income (GNI) per capita for 2013:

- Low-income countries (LICs) = US$1,045 or less
- Middle-income countries (MICs) are subdivided:
  a) lower-middle-income = US$1,046 to US$4,125
  b) upper-middle-income (UMICs) = US$4,126 to US$12,745
- High-income countries (HICs) = US$12,746 or more.

1. When an intervention involves the provision of food, the term *school feeding* is used. The term includes at least two modalities: in-school feeding, where children are fed in school; and take-home rations, where families are given food if their children attend school regularly. *Nutrition* is properly reserved for when a specific nutrition outcome is sought, such as correcting a micronutrient deficiency.

REFERENCES

Adelman, S., H. Alderman, D. O. Gilligan, and K. Lehrer. 2008. "The Impact of Alternative Food for Education Programs on Learning Achievement and Cognitive Development in Northern Uganda." International Food Policy Research Institute, Washington, DC.

Ahuja, A., S. Baird, J. Hamory Hicks, M. Kremer, and E. Miguel. 2017. "Economics of Mass Deworming Programs." In *Disease Control Priorities* (third edition): Volume 8, *Child and Adolescent Health and Development*, edited by D. A. P. Bundy, N. de Silva, S. Horton, D. T. Jamison, and G. C. Patton. Washington, DC: World Bank.

Alderman, H., J. R. Behrman, P. Glewwe, L. Fernald, and S. Walker. 2017. "Evidence of Impact of Interventions on Growth and Development during Early and Middle Childhood." In *Disease Control Priorities* (third edition): Volume 8, *Child and Adolescent Health and Development*, edited by D. A. P. Bundy, N. de Silva, S. Horton, D. T. Jamison, and G. C. Patton. Washington, DC: World Bank.

Atkins, P. 2007. "School Milk in Britain, 1900–1934." *Journal of Policy History* 19 (4): 395–427.

Baltussen, R., J. Naus, and H. Limburg. 2009. "Cost-Effectiveness of Screening and Correcting Refractive Errors in School Children in Africa, Asia, America, and Europe." *Health Policy* 89 (2): 201–15.

Benzian, H., B. Varenne, N. Stauf, R. Garg, and B. Monse. 2017. "Promoting Oral Health through Programs in Middle Childhood and Adolescence." In *Disease Control Priorities* (third edition): Volume 8, *Child and Adolescent Health and Development*, edited by D. A. P. Bundy, N. de Silva, S. Horton, D. T. Jamison, and G. C. Patton. Washington, DC: World Bank.

Boler, T. 2003. *The Sound of Silence*. London: ActionAid.

Brooker, S., S. Clarke, D. Fernando, C. Gitonga, J. Nankabirwa, and others. 2017. "Malaria in Middle Childhood and Adolescence." In *Disease Control Priorities* (third edition): Volume 8, *Child and Adolescent Health and Development*, edited by D. A. P. Bundy, N. de Silva, S. Horton, D. T. Jamison, and G. C. Patton. Washington, DC: World Bank.

Bundy, D. A. P. 2011. *Rethinking School Health: A Key Component of Education for All*. Directions in Development. Washington, DC: World Bank. doi:10.1596/978-0-8213-7907-3.

Bundy, D. A. P., L. J. Appleby, M. Bradley, K. Croke, T. D. Hollingsworth, and others. 2017. "Mass Deworming Programs in Middle Childhood and Adolescence." In *Disease Control Priorities* (third edition): Volume 8, *Child and Adolescent Health and Development*, edited by D. A. P. Bundy, N. de Silva, S. Horton, D. T. Jamison, and G. C. Patton. Washington, DC: World Bank.

Bundy, D. A. P., C. Burbano, M. Grosh, A. Gelli, M. C. H. Jukes, and others. 2009. *Rethinking School Feeding: Social Safety Nets, Child Development, and the Education Sector*. Directions in Development Series. Washington, DC: World Bank. doi:10.1596/978-0-8213-7974-5.

Bundy, D. A. P., N. de Silva, S. Horton, G. C. Patton, L. Schultz, and D. T. Jamison. 2017. "Child and Adolescent Health and Development: Realizing Neglected Potential." In *Disease Control Priorities* (third edition): Volume 8, *Child and Adolescent Health and Development*, edited by D. A. P. Bundy, N. de Silva, S. Horton, D. T. Jamison, and G. C. Patton. Washington, DC: World Bank.

Bundy, D. A. P., and S. Horton. 2017. "Impact of Interventions on Health and Development during Childhood and Adolescence: A Conceptual Framework." In *Disease Control Priorities* (third edition): Volume 8, *Child and Adolescent Health and Development*, edited by D. A. P. Bundy, N. de Silva, S. Horton, D. T. Jamison, and G. C. Patton. Washington, DC: World Bank.

Bundy, D. A. P., M. S. Wong, L. L. Lewis, and J. Horton. 1990. "Control of Geohelminths by Delivery of Targeted Chemotherapy through Schools." *Transactions of the Royal Society of Tropical Medicine and Hygiene* 84 (1): 115–20.

Chapman, K. 2006. "Using Social Transfers to Scale Up Equitable Access to Education and Health Services." Background paper, Scaling Up Services Team, DFID Policy Division. https://www.ids.ac.uk/files/dmfile/socialtransfersback.pdf.

Del Rosso, J. M., and T. Marek. 1996. *Class Action: Improving School Performance in the Developing World through Better Health and Nutrition*. Washington, DC: World Bank.

de Silva, N., S. Brooker, P. J. Hotez, A. Montresor, D. Engels, and others. 2003. "Soil-Transmitted Helminth Infections: Updating the Global Picture." *Trends in Parasitology* 19 (12): 547–51.

de Walque, D., L. Fernald, P. Gertler, and M. Hidrobo. 2017. "Cash Transfers and Child and Adolescent Development." In *Disease Control Priorities* (third edition): Volume 8, *Child and Adolescent Health and Development*, edited by D. A. P. Bundy, N. de Silva, S. Horton, D. T. Jamison, and G. C. Patton. Washington, DC: World Bank.

Drake, L., M. Fernandes, E. Aurino, J. Kiamba, B. Giyosa, and others. 2017. "School Feeding Programs in Middle Childhood and Adolescence." In *Disease Control Priorities* (third edition): Volume 8, *Child and Adolescent Health and Development*, edited by D. A. P. Bundy, N. de Silva, S. Horton, D. T. Jamison, and G. C. Patton. Washington, DC: World Bank.

Drake, L., C. Maier, and J. W. L. de Lind van Wijngaarden. 2007. *Directory of Support to School-Based Health and Nutrition Programmes*. London: Partnership for Child Development.

Drake, L., S. Singh, C. K. Mishra, A. Sinha, S. Kumar, and others. 2015. "Bihar's Pioneering School-Based Deworming Programme: Lessons Learned in Deworming over 17 Million Indian School-Age Children in One Sustainable Campaign." *PLoS Neglected Tropical Diseases* 9 (11): e0004106. doi:10.1371/journal.pntd.0004106.

Drake, L., A. Woolnough, C. Burbano, and D. A. P. Bundy. 2016. *Global School Feeding Sourcebook: Lessons from 14 Countries*. London: Imperial College Press.

Durlak, J. A., R. P. Weissberg, and A. B. Dymnicki. 2011. "The Impact of Enhancing Students' Social and Emotional Learning: A Meta-Analysis of School-Based Universal Interventions." *Child Development* 82 (1): 405–32.

Ettling, J. 1981. *The Germ of Laziness: Rockefeller Philanthropy and Public Health in the New South*. Cambridge, MA: Harvard University Press.

Fernandes, M., and E. Aurino. 2017. "Identifying an Essential Package for School-Age Child Health: Economic Analysis." In *Disease Control Priorities* (third edition): Volume 8, *Child and Adolescent Health and Development*, edited by D. A. P. Bundy, N. de Silva, S. Horton, D. T. Jamison, and G. C. Patton. Washington, DC: World Bank.

FRESH (Focusing Resources on Effective School Health). 2014. "Monitoring and Evaluation Guidance for School Health Programs: Eight Core Indicators to Support FRESH." http://www.unesco.org/new/en/education/themes /leading-the-international-agenda/health-education/fresh /me-indicators.

Gelli, A., U. Meir, and F. Espejo. 2007. "Does Provision of Food in School Increase Girls' Enrollment? Evidence from

Schools in Sub-Saharan Africa." *Food and Nutrition Bulletin* 28 (2): 149–55.

Graham, N., L. Schultz, S. Mitra, and D. Mont. 2017. "Disability in Middle Childhood and Adolescence." In *Disease Control Priorities* (third edition): Volume 8, *Child and Adolescent Health and Development*, edited by D. A. P. Bundy, N. de Silva, S. Horton, D. T. Jamison, and G. C. Patton. Washington, DC: World Bank.

Grigorenko, E. L., R. J. Sternberg, M. Jukes, K. Alcock, J. Lambo, and others. 2006. "Effects of Antiparasitic Treatment on Dynamically and Statically Tested Cognitive Skills over Time." *Journal of Applied Developmental Psychology* 27 (6): 499–526.

Guyatt, H. 2003. "The Cost of Delivering and Sustaining a Control Programme for Schistosomiasis and Soil-Transmitted Helminthiasis." *Acta Tropica* 86 (2–3): 267–74.

Hargreaves, G. C., and T. Boler. 2006. "Girl Power: The Impact of Girls' Education on HIV and Sexual Behaviour." Education and HIV Series 01, ActionAid International.

Hargreaves, J. R., C. P. Bonell, T. Boler, D. Boccia, I. Birdthistle, and others. 2008. "Systematic Review Exploring Time Trends in the Association between Educational Attainment and Risk of HIV Infection in Sub-Saharan Africa." *AIDS* 22: 403–14.

Horton, S., J. Waldfogel, E. De la Cruz Toledo, J. Mahon, and J. Santelli. 2017. "Identifying an Essential Package for Adolescent Health: Economic Analysis." In *Disease Control Priorities* (third edition): Volume 8, *Child and Adolescent Health and Development*, edited by Bundy, D. A. P., N. de Silva, S. Horton, D. T. Jamison, and G. C. Patton. Washington, DC: World Bank.

Jukes, M. C. H., L. Drake, and D. A. P. Bundy. 2008. *School Health, Nutrition and Education for All: Levelling the Playing Field*. Wallingford, U.K.: CABI Publishing.

Jukes, M. C. H., S. Simmons, and D. A. P. Bundy. 2008. "Education and Vulnerability: The Role of Schools in Protecting Young Women and Girls from HIV in Southern Africa." *AIDS* 22 (4): S41–S56.

LaMontagne, D. S., T. Cernuschi, A. Yabuku, P. Bloem, D. Watson-Jones, and others. 2017. "School-Based Delivery of Vaccines to 5 to 19 Year Olds." In *Disease Control Priorities* (third edition): Volume 8, *Child and Adolescent Health and Development*, edited by D. A. P. Bundy, N. de Silva, S. Horton, D. T. Jamison, and G. C. Patton. Washington, DC: World Bank.

Lassi, Z., A. Moin, and Z. Bhutta. 2017. "Nutrition in Middle Childhood and Adolescence." In *Disease Control Priorities* (third edition): Volume 8, *Child and Adolescent Health and Development*, edited by D. A. P. Bundy, N. de Silva, S. Horton, D. T. Jamison, and G. C. Patton. Washington, DC: World Bank.

Liddell, C., and G. Rae. 2001. "Predicting Early Grade Retention: A Longitudinal Investigation of Primary School Progress in a Sample of Rural South African Children." *British Journal of Educational Psychology* 71 (3): 413–28.

MacPhail, C., B. Williams, and C. Campbell. 2002. "Relative Risk of HIV Infection among Young Men and Women in a South African Township." *International Journal of STD and AIDS* 13 (5): 331–42.

Miguel, E., and M. Kremer. 2004. "Worms: Identifying Impacts on Education and Health in the Presence of Treatment Externalities." *Econometrica* 72 (1): 159–217.

Murray N. G., B. J. Low, C. Hollis, A. W. Cross, and S. M. Davis. 2007. "Coordinated School Health Programs and Academic Achievement: A Systematic Review of the Literature." *Journal of School Health* 77: 589–600.

Plaut, D., T. Hill, M. Thomas, J. Worthington, M. Fernandes, and others. 2017. "Getting to Education Outcomes: Reviewing Evidence from Health and Education Interventions." In *Disease Control Priorities* (third edition): Volume 8, *Child and Adolescent Health and Development*, edited by D. A. P. Bundy, N. de Silva, S. Horton, D. T. Jamison, and G. C. Patton. Washington, DC: World Bank.

Sarr, B., M. Fernandes, L. Banham, D. A. P. Bundy, A. Gillespie, and others. 2017. "The Evolution of School Health and Nutrition in the Education Sector 2000–2015." *Frontiers in Public Health*. https://doi.org/10.3389/fpubh.2016.00271.

Shackleton N, F. Jamal, R. M. Viner, K. Dickson, G. C. Patton, and C. Bonell. 2016. "School-Level Interventions to Promote Adolescent Health: Systematic Review of Reviews." *Journal of Adolescent Health* 58 (4): 382–96.

Tang, K. C., D. Nutbeam, C. Aldinger, L. St. Leger, D. A. P. Bundy, and others. 2009. "Schools for Health, Education and Development: A Call for Action." *Health Promotion International* 24 (1): 68–77.

UNESCO (United Nations Educational, Scientific and Cultural Organization). 2008. "EDUCAIDS Overviews of Practical Resources." http://portal.unesco.org/en/ev.phpURL_ID=36412 &URL_DO=DO_TOPIC&URL_SECTION=201.html.

———. 2011. *EFA Global Monitoring Report 2011: The Hidden Crisis: Armed Conflict and Education*. Paris: UNESCO.

UNFPA (United Nations Population Fund). 2012. *Status Report: Adolescents and Young People in Sub-Saharan Africa*. Johannesburg: UNFPA http://www.prb.org/pdf12 /status-report-youth-subsaharan-Africa.pdf.

Verguet, S., A. Nandi, V. Filippi, and D. A. P. Bundy. 2017. "Postponing Adolescent Parity in Developing Countries through Education: An Extended Cost-Effectiveness Analysis." In *Disease Control Priorities* (third edition): Volume 8, *Child and Adolescent Health and Development*, edited by D. A. P. Bundy, N. de Silva, S. Horton, D. T. Jamison, and G. C. Patton. Washington, DC: World Bank.

Watkins, K., D. A. P. Bundy, D. T. Jamison, F. Guenther, and A. Georgiadis. 2017. "Evidence of Impact of Interventions on Health and Development during Middle Childhood and School Age." In *Disease Control Priorities* (third edition): Volume 8, *Child and Adolescent Health and Development*, edited by D. A. P. Bundy, N. de Silva, S. Horton, D. T. Jamison, and G. C. Patton. Washington, DC: World Bank.

WHO (World Health Organization). 1986. *Ottawa Charter*. Geneva: WHO.

———. 1997. *Promoting Health through Schools: Report of a WHO Expert Committee on Comprehensive School Health Education and Promotion*. WHO Technical Report Series 870.

———. 2015. "Summary of Global Update on Preventative Chemotherapy Implementation in 2015." *Weekly Epidemiological Record* 90 (49): 661–74.

———. 2016a. "Global School-Based Student Health Survey." http://www.who.int/chp/gshs/en/.

———. 2016b. "Health Behavior in School-Age Children." http://www.euro.who.int/en/health-topics/Life-stages /child-and-adolescent-health/child-and-adolescent-health2 /youth-friendly-services/health-behaviour-in-school -aged-children-hbsc2.-who-collaborative-cross-national -study-of-children-aged-1115.

WHO and CDC (U.S. Centers for Disease Control and Prevention). Not dated. "Global School Health Policies and Practices Surveys: Survey Implementation Workshop." WHO, Geneva, and CDC, Washington, DC. http://www .searo.who.int/entity/noncommunicable_diseases/events /global-shpps-survey-implementation-slides.pdf.

World Bank. 2002. *Education and HIV/AIDS: Windows of Hope.* Washington, DC: World Bank.

———. 2011. "World Bank Education Sector Strategy 2020: Learning for All." World Bank, Washington, DC. http:// siteresources.worldbank.org/EDUCATION/Resources /ESSU/Education_Strategy_4_12_2011.pdf.

———. 2012. "What Matters Most for School Health and School Feeding: A Framework Paper." SABER Working Paper No. 3, World Bank, Washington, DC. http://wbgfiles .worldbank.org/documents/hdn/ed/saber/supporting_doc /Background/SHN/Framework_SABER-School_Health.pdf.

———. 2016. "World Development Indicators." Education Statistics. World Bank, Washington, DC. http://databank .worldbank.org/data/reports.aspx?source=education -statistics-~-all-indicators.

World Food Programme. 2016. "School Meals." World Food Programme, Rome. https://www.wfp.org/school-meals.

Chapter 21

Platforms for Delivering Adolescent Health Actions

Susan M. Sawyer, Nicola Reavley, Chris Bonell, and George C. Patton

INTRODUCTION

Adolescent health has been gaining attention in the past decade (Levine and others 2008; UNICEF 2011; WHO 2014; World Bank 2007). As described by the *Lancet* Commission on Adolescent Health and Wellbeing (Patton, Sawyer, and others 2016), the adolescent years are crucial for the development of human capital. During adolescence, neurocognitive and pubertal maturation interact with the social determinants of health, creating a highly dynamic profile of health as individuals pass from childhood through adolescence and into adulthood (Sawyer and others 2012).

During these years, the burden of disease rises, including the burden of human immunodeficiency virus/acquired immune deficiency syndrome (HIV/AIDS), mental disorders, and injuries. At the same time, new health risks emerge in response to biological maturation (sexual behaviors); marketing of unhealthy products (tobacco; alcohol; foods high in sugar, salt, and fats); and community attitudes, traditions, and values (female genital mutilation, lack of access to secondary education, support for too early marriage, unsafe work practices). Due to the extent of neurocognitive maturation, increasing participation in education and changing social contexts, adolescence is also a time when interventions to improve adolescent health outcomes can expand beyond families or health services to the wider

settings in which adolescents learn, participate, and engage. Actions to improve adolescent health are most effective when embedded in contemporary understanding of adolescent development and prevention science (Catalano and others 2012), which underscores the importance of engaging with young people themselves as they become more active agents in their own lives (Patton, Sawyer, and others 2016).

Patterns of disease burden and health risk vary widely between countries as they progress through the epidemiological transition. As undernutrition, infectious and vaccine-preventable diseases, HIV/AIDS, and reproductive health needs are brought under control, the burden of road traffic injuries, violence, chronic physical disorders, mental disorders, and substance use becomes more prominent (Patton, Sawyer, and others 2016). Actions to improve health in adolescence need to include a wider range of health concerns in addition to sexual and reproductive health, and they also need to extend beyond treating disorders to addressing their root causes, including poverty and homelessness, lack of education, disability, minority sexual identity, indigenous status, and other causes of social marginalization in adolescents.

Following a brief review of the developmental context of adolescent health, this chapter categorizes countries according to their excess burden of disease and then describes six platforms that can be used to deliver health

Corresponding author: Susan M. Sawyer, Department of Paediatrics, the University of Melbourne, Parkville, Victoria, Australia; susan.sawyer@rch.org.au.

actions to adolescents (ages 10–19 years): health services, schools, media and social marketing, community, mobile health (m-health), and structural actions. The chapter discusses the rationale of these platforms for delivering health treatments for established health issues, for responding to emerging needs, and for preventing future health problems. It also emphasizes the importance of matching actions to health needs, responding to differences between and within countries, and aligning actions across platforms spanning different sectors, including health and education.

A key message relates to how knowledge of adolescent development promotes understanding of why different platforms are needed to deliver actions for adolescent health. While the term "action" is used interchangeably with the term "intervention," action is preferred when describing the need for multicomponent interventions that require more than one platform and interventions that are more distal to the individual. The term "platform" is used to describe the mechanism or infrastructure that is required to deliver actions or interventions (health services, schools, laws). In reading the text, it is important to remember that nearly all of the data and evidence come from studies of programs in high-income countries (HICs). We cannot say with any certainty the extent to which the results presented here apply to low- and middle-income countries (LMICs). This limitation is a particular challenge in planning and selecting interventions for this age group and emphasizes the need for much more research into the health of adolescents in LMICs. Definitions of age groupings and age-specific terminology used in this volume can be found in chapter 1 (Bundy, de Silva, and others 2017).

THE DEVELOPMENTAL CONTEXT OF ADOLESCENT HEALTH

During adolescence, neurodevelopment drives adolescents to engage with and challenge their social environments and requires parents to balance their protective role with one that enables adolescents to engage safely with their communities and the wider world. Beyond family, the social context in which young people mature profoundly influences their health and well-being. At this time, adolescents become more sensitive to social standing and engagement with their peers (Crone and Dahl 2012). Bullying and peer victimization become more common in adolescence, increasing the feeling of social exclusion and the odds of mental disorders, especially in girls (Bond and others 2007). Indeed, adolescents are at heightened risk for the onset of mental disorders. Schools become the main context of peer relationships,

and teachers become important adult figures in addition to parents and other family members. Social media becomes an important space for peer relationships, which also shape identity, health, and well-being.

Poverty and homelessness contribute to social marginalization and poor health at all ages, but pose additional risks in the context of adolescent development. The biological amplification of sexual attraction during adolescence increases the risk of too early pregnancy and sexually transmitted infections (STIs). For girls, too early pregnancy, whether within or outside of marriage, results in premature completion of education, which compromises their future employment and financial independence, with accompanying risks to their health and that of their children. For persons who are lesbian, gay, bisexual, or transgender, minority sexual status increases the risk of social marginalization, which makes them vulnerable to violence and stigma. Health outcomes in adolescence (for example, HIV/AIDS, mental disorders, disability) can themselves be a risk for social exclusion and a source of inequality.

As a consequence of age and development, young people lack life experience, have poor health literacy (Manganello and others 2015), are sensitive to stigma and shame, have a strong desire for confidentiality (Ford and others 1997), have poorly developed organizational skills, and lack financial resources. They often depend on their parents or caregivers to transport them to, consent to, and pay for health care. They can have difficulty understanding and regulating their emotional states, which affects their decision making. For example, they may know how to prevent unplanned pregnancies and STIs, but may not use such measures when they are in the midst of powerful emotions or "hot cognitions." Young people tend to be less influenced than adults by concerns about long-term risks, but are more vulnerable than adults to advertising and marketing of unhealthy products that provide social status. All of these attributes make young people vulnerable to unhealthy behaviors and make it difficult for them to seek and access health care and sustain healthy behaviors.

However, just as the developmental context of adolescence informs the pattern of health risks and outcomes experienced at this time, it also creates opportunities for improving future health and well-being. For example, children who do not smoke during adolescence are unlikely to smoke as adults. Thus, primary prevention (actions to keep adolescents from starting to smoke) is far better at improving health across the life course than secondary prevention (actions to encourage older adults to stop smoking), at less cost.

Some actions are universally applicable to a population but are adolescent-sensitive. For example, tobacco taxation is a universal action that is adolescent-sensitive, as adolescents are more sensitive to price than adults (Jha and Peto 2014). Other actions are adolescent-specific. For example, school-based actions to raise awareness of the harmful effects of tobacco are adolescent-specific because they only target students. Certain sexual and reproductive health laws are also adolescent-sensitive due to their disproportionate impact on adolescents. Thus, while access to legal abortion is universally relevant for sexually active women, it disproportionately affects adolescents due to their higher unmet need for contraception, the relative impact of unplanned pregnancy on girls' education, and their disproportionate use of unsafe abortion services (Woog and others 2015). Other sexual and reproductive health laws are adolescent-specific (for example, laws that restrict the access of unmarried adolescents to contraception, laws about the age of legal majority, and the minimum legal age for sexual intercourse).

With the exception of schools, platforms to deliver adolescent health actions are universal platforms that can be used to deliver adolescent-specific actions. For example, the universal platform of health services includes adolescent-specific components such as adolescent sexual and reproductive health clinics and school-based clinics.

Many actions and interventions that are effective in younger children (for example, community-based immunization clinics) or older adults (for example, population approaches to HIV/AIDS prevention) do not gain the same traction in adolescents. Legal barriers may prevent unmarried girls from accessing contraception, financial barriers may make it difficult for adolescents to pay for health care without the consent of their parent or spouse, and community immunization clinics may not be convenient for adolescents at school. Adolescent-sensitive and adolescent-specific interventions are most effective when they build on a solid understanding of adolescent development, including how adolescents engage with and pay for health care, and when they empower adolescents to become active protagonists in their own lives.

MATCHING HEALTH ACTIONS TO HEALTH NEEDS

To begin to understand how needs change as countries pass through the epidemiological transition, the *Lancet* Commission on Adolescent Health and Wellbeing grouped 236 causes of disability-adjusted life years (DALYs) and deaths into nine categories of disease (Patton, Sawyer, and others 2016) and classified countries into three broad categories according to their excess burden of disease (figure 21.1). Within this

Figure 21.1 Country Categorization Based on Adolescent Burden of Disease

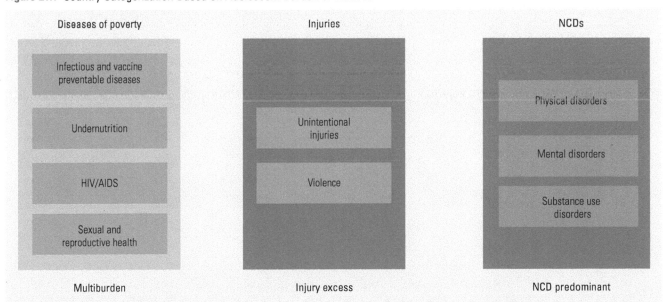

Source: Reprinted from *The Lancet* 387 (10036): G. C. Patton, S. M. Sawyer, J. S. Santelli, D. A. Ross, R. Afifi, and others, "Our Future: A Lancet Commission on Adolescent Health and Wellbeing," 2423–78, © 2016, with permission from Elsevier.
Note: HIV/AIDS = human immunodeficiency virus/acquired immune deficiency syndrome; NCD = noncommunicable disease. Countries are categorized according to adolescent burden of disease (per 100,000 people), reflecting their passage through the epidemiological transition. Multiburden countries are defined as having 2,500 or more disability-adjusted life years (DALYs) per 100,000 population per year due to diseases of poverty. Injury-excess countries are defined as having 2,500 or more DALYs per 100,000 population per year due to injury and less than 2,500 due to diseases of poverty. NCD-predominant countries are defined as having less than 2,500 DALYs per 100,000 population due to injury and less than 2,500 due to diseases of poverty.

Figure 21.2 Patterns of Disease Burden by Age and Gender (Ages 10–24)

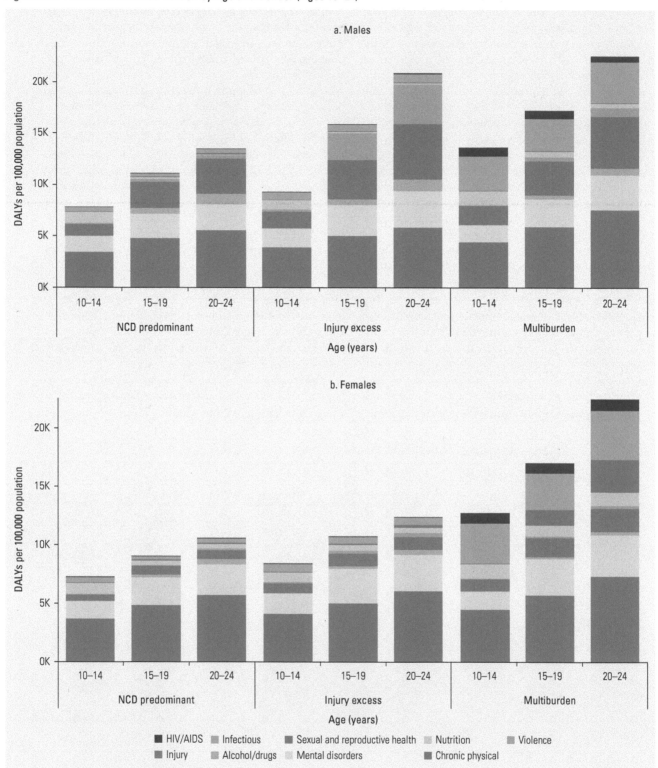

Source: Reprinted from *The Lancet* 387 (10036): G. C. Patton, S. M. Sawyer, J. S. Santelli, D. A. Ross, R. Afifi, and others, "Our Future: A Lancet Commission on Adolescent Health and Wellbeing," 2423–78, © 2016, with permission from Elsevier.
Note: HIV/AIDS = human immunodeficiency virus/acquired immune deficiency syndrome; NCD = noncommunicable disease; DALY = disability-adjusted life year.

framework, HIV/AIDS is in its own category because addressing this condition requires distinct health policy and programmatic responses. The burden of suicide is included within mental disorders. A more detailed description of this framework is provided in chapter 5 in this volume (Patton, Azzopardi, and others 2017). Because it is based on DALYs, this framework does not consider behaviors that, while commencing in adolescence, do not influence health until some years later (for example, tobacco use).

Multiburden countries have a high burden of all nine health conditions, including diseases of poverty (HIV/AIDS and other infectious and vaccine-preventable diseases, undernutrition, and poor sexual and reproductive health, including high maternal mortality), injuries and violence, and noncommunicable diseases (NCDs). These countries also have high adolescent fertility. Injury-excess countries have a high burden of unintentional injuries and violence and a high rate of adolescent fertility, together with NCDs. NCD-predominant countries have a high burden of chronic physical, mental (including suicide), and substance use disorders.

Marked variation is also seen within countries, reflecting, among other factors, inequities in the social determinants of health and access to preventive interventions, education, and health services.

The extent of variation in the profile of adolescent health and health risks between countries (Gore and others 2011; Mokdad and others 2016; Patton and others 2009; Patton, Sawyer, and others 2016) reinforces the opportunities and scope for preventive actions and indicates priority targets. For example, in multiburden countries, health actions need to target the diseases of poverty, while avoiding further rises in injuries, violence, and NCDs. In these countries, addressing the unmet need for contraception should be a priority. Injury-excess countries need to prioritize actions that address their high rates of injury and violence as well as high birth rates among adolescents. NCD-predominant countries need to prioritize actions that address the impact of chronic mental health conditions, substance use disorders, and chronic physical conditions, including obesity.

It is important to understand how the burden of disease increases with age and varies by gender across the life course and during adolescence (figure 21.2), as this has implications for health platforms. For example, boys and girls are more vulnerable road users than adults due to their pattern of road use as pedestrians, cyclists, and motorcyclists (Peden and others 2004). Boys are more likely to die from unintentional injury and violence than girls, much of it related to road traffic accidents (Patton, Sawyer, and others 2016). Thus, in injury-excess countries, the platform of structural actions provides the bedrock for improved road safety (improved roads, traffic control, car safety, drunk-driving legislation, reductions in the speed limit) that will disproportionately benefit adolescents (WHO 2013). Another example is mental health. Across the life course, adolescence is the time of greatest incidence of mental disorders, especially in girls (Kessler and others 2005). Social marginalization, poor school connectedness in early secondary school, and school-based bullying and victimization increase the likelihood of common mental disorders such as depression and anxiety (Bond and others 2007). These conditions also confer risks for health problems such as substance use (Bond and others 2007) and wider developmental outcomes such as early school leaving (Stein and Kean 2000). Not only are preventive actions required to address upstream social determinants, but these interventions also have multiplier effects due to their influence on more than one outcome (Catalano and others 2012).

SIGNIFICANCE OF CHANGING PATTERNS OF HEALTH FOR DELIVERY PLATFORMS

A country's pattern of disease burden has implications for the priority given to different health actions and use of health platforms.

Multiburden Countries

In multiburden countries, the priority is to reduce the excess burden from infectious disease, undernutrition, and sexual and reproductive health, including HIV/AIDS. Health services need to have the human capacity and resources to treat acute and chronic infectious diseases in adolescents. They also have to manage adolescent pregnancies and respond to high unmet needs regarding contraception for adolescent girls, both married and unmarried.

Efforts to promote continued education, especially for girls, are important, as longer participation in schooling reduces the burden of infectious diseases in adolescents (Ngimuh and others 2016) and the risk for too early pregnancy in the context of marriage. To this end, the excess burden from infectious diseases requires structural actions to guarantee fresh water and sanitation, including clean toilets, at schools. Actions are also needed to guarantee the physical and emotional safety of students while at school and en route. Schools provide opportunities to deliver important preventive actions regarding sexual and reproductive health, such as comprehensive sexuality education, and better growth through improved nutrition from school meals. Greater participation in secondary education also expands the opportunities to deliver health services directly through schools, including clinical interventions such as vaccination, antiworming, and iron and folate supplementation.

Beyond schools, social media and community platforms can also be used to promote knowledge of and access to preventive resources for sexual and reproductive health (modern contraception), infectious diseases (insecticide treated bednets), HIV/AIDS (circumcision), and healthy growth and nutrition (nutritional supplements). Opportunities exist to use media and social marketing to explicitly target adolescents in health interventions that increase health literacy, which contributes to adolescent health.

Cash transfers to promote vaccination, school attendance, and HIV/AIDS-free status are also possible. Chapter 18 in this volume (Reavley and others 2017) provides evidence underpinning the strength of evidence for actions in this area.

Given the many barriers that adolescents face accessing health services, multiburden countries need to focus on guaranteeing universal health coverage. Countries that currently provide free health care to children under five should consider extending it to adolescents.

Injury-Excess Countries

In injury-excess countries, health services need to develop accessible trauma services in addition to primary care. Actions across the structural platform need to include legislation regarding driving under the influence of alcohol, graduated driver's licenses, and mandatory use of motorbike helmets. Schools, communities, media, and social marketing can support these actions by delivering messages that seek to change social norms, as have been progressively implemented in many HICs (Sauber-Schatz and others 2016).

To address high adolescent birth rates, schools should provide comprehensive sexuality education to all adolescents and, ideally, link education to the provision of contraception. Health services need to be able to make contraception legally available to adolescents. In some countries, this will require legislation. Other structural actions relate to laws enabling clinicians to provide legal abortions and cash transfers promoting school attendance and discouraging pregnancy in childhood. Once again, aligning actions across sectors is important; schools, media, and social

marketing platforms can each be used to change social norms regarding too-early pregnancy and the role of contraception.

NCD-Predominant Countries

In NCD-predominant countries, health services need to prioritize interventions for chronic physical conditions, mental disorders, and substance abuse disorders. Enabling clinicians, including nurses, to identify and manage common mental disorders requires shifting the focus of medical education and reorienting health services toward NCDs. Most health services require greater clinical capacity to respond to mental health conditions. In addition to human capacity, opportunities exist for mobile health, with m-health applications offering opportunities for well-being (for example, mindfulness apps) and treatment (for example, cognitive behavioral therapy apps, and crisis-support telephone and text services).

Schools in NCD-predominant countries can promote physical activity. Schools, communities, and social media can also help to change social norms regarding tobacco, alcohol, and other drug use, body image, and the stigma of mental disorders.

Most NCD-predominant countries have implemented laws that have greatly reduced adolescents' access to tobacco. Less progress has been made in introducing legislation to reduce adolescents' access to alcohol. As with structural actions to curb substance use among adolescents, there is precedence to use taxation of food and beverages with added salt, sugar, or fats, given early evidence of effect (Colchero and others 2016).

PLATFORMS TO DELIVER ACTIONS FOR HEALTH

The health care system is the sum of the people, institutions, and resources that maintain and improve the health of the people they serve (WHO 2007). Health services are just one of the platforms that can deliver actions and interventions for adolescent health. Indeed, major actions for adolescent health occur outside health services, suggesting that an integrated system of delivery platforms would improve the response to conspicuous and emerging health needs and efforts to prevent other health issues from developing.

The *Lancet* Commission on Adolescent Health and Wellbeing (Patton, Sawyer, and others 2016) described the opportunities for health actions delivered across six platforms: health services, schools, communities, m-health, media and social marketing, and structural actions. These platforms are not mutually exclusive. For example, direct clinical care is delivered mostly by traditional health services such as community clinics and hospitals. However, direct clinical care can also be delivered via school-based clinics and mobile clinics that visit schools and workplaces. M-health approaches can also deliver direct clinical care, as an adjunct to clinical care, and for a wide variety of educational and health-promoting activities.

These platforms are interdependent. For example, the ability of clinicians to prescribe contraception to unmarried girls depends on a nation's legal framework, religious dictates, and community expectations. And, as described in chapter 18 in this volume (Reavley and others 2017), health benefits occur in the context of multicomponent actions. Thus, for any single area of health need, aligning actions across different platforms will bring added benefits.

Health Services

Health services manage adolescents' conspicuous health needs, identify and respond to emerging health issues (for example, contraception for new-onset sexual activity or interventions to address suicidal ideation), and deliver preventive interventions that reduce the likelihood of the onset of a particular health risk (for example, obesity). This requires access to primary care, specialist, and hospital services. Until recently, there has been little focus on health services for adolescents or what is needed to guarantee universal health coverage for this age group. Such a focus is predicated on a robust knowledge of adolescent development, as this influences how adolescents engage with health services and the particular barriers they experience.

Barriers to access reside within the health care system, within health care providers, within families and communities, and within adolescents themselves. The major health system barriers—lack of geographically accessible services and lack of clinicians—are not unique to adolescent health care. In contrast, the direct and indirect costs of health care are significant barriers for adolescents who, for developmental reasons, do not place the same value on current or future health as older adults. Most adolescents rely on family for transportation and payment of health care, making free health care particularly valuable for them.

Regardless of country grouping, health services and clinicians need to have the same competencies (attitudes, knowledge, skills) if they are to work effectively with adolescents (WHO 2015a), summarized in figure 21.3. Adolescents in high-, middle-, and low-income countries alike value patient- and family-centered care with an emphasis on respect, quality communication including confidentiality, appropriate provision of information, involvement in decisions about their care, and coordination of care (Ambresin and others 2013). Routine psychosocial assessment, such as the HEADSS (home, education, activities/employment, drugs, suicidality, sex) approach (Goldenring and Rosen 2004), has been shown to improve the identification of emerging risks (Sanci and others 2000; Sanci and others 2015) and to provide a context for anticipatory guidance and preventive interventions. Adolescents desire privacy and confidentiality regarding their health care. They are quick to feel embarrassment and shame and are often afraid of being judged, all of which are barriers to seeking health care. Health care for adolescents often takes place in the context of families, including parents or extended family members, other caregivers and guardians, or partners. A unique feature for adolescents is concern that their parents and families will be informed about sensitive issues such as sexual behaviors, substance use, and mental disorders (Ford and others 1997). Not only do health care providers need to be nonjudgmental, willing to maintain confidentiality, and able to engage with adolescents and young adults, but they also need to do this while remaining appropriately engaged with families. Health care providers need to understand the legal and ethical challenges of providing health care to legal minors while delivering health care that is consistent with the United Nations Convention on the Rights of the Child, which requires young people to become increasingly involved in their health care as they mature (United Nations General Assembly 1989).

More than a decade ago, the World Health Organization developed a framework for delivering quality primary health care to adolescents. The framework emphasized the importance of adolescent- or youth-friendly health care that has equity of access; is effective, accessible, and acceptable to young people; and is appropriate to their needs (WHO 2002). The principles of what is increasingly referred to as adolescent-responsive health care apply to all levels (clinic, hospital) and all types (mental health) of health services (Sawyer, Proimos, and Towns 2010). More recently, the World Health Organization developed policy guidelines for delivering quality health care to adolescents from the perspective of both individual providers (WHO 2015a) and health services (WHO 2015b). Governments in LMICs are using these guidelines to improve the quality of health care they

Figure 21.3 Domains That Require Special Attention in Health Consultations with Adolescents

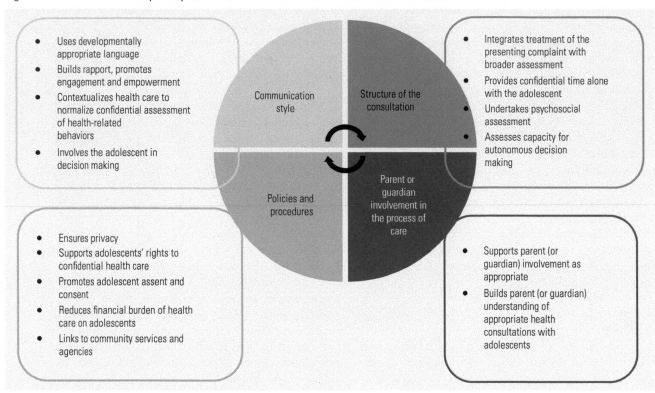

- Uses developmentally appropriate language
- Builds rapport, promotes engagement and empowerment
- Contextualizes health care to normalize confidential assessment of health-related behaviors
- Involves the adolescent in decision making

Communication style

Structure of the consultation

- Integrates treatment of the presenting complaint with broader assessment
- Provides confidential time alone with the adolescent
- Undertakes psychosocial assessment
- Assesses capacity for autonomous decision making

Policies and procedures

Parent or guardian involvement in the process of care

- Ensures privacy
- Supports adolescents' rights to confidential health care
- Promotes adolescent assent and consent
- Reduces financial burden of health care on adolescents
- Links to community services and agencies

- Supports parent (or guardian) involvement as appropriate
- Builds parent (or guardian) understanding of appropriate health consultations with adolescents

Source: © Springer. Used with the permission of Springer. Further permission required for reuse.

provide to adolescents, with some evidence of benefit (Chandra-Mouli, Chatterjee, and Bose 2016).

In HICs, there has been a move toward large primary care clinics that include doctors, nurses, and allied health staff. In LMICs, there is growing interest in using non-physician clinicians to supplement health personnel (Mullen and Frehywot 2007). This model is suitable for providing a range of resources, including nurses who may have fewer communication barriers with adolescents than doctors (AlBuhairan and Olsson 2014).

Historically, specialist pediatric services ceased around the time of puberty, resulting in adolescents from the age of 12–13 years being managed by adult providers in adult settings. Extending specialist pediatric services to a higher upper age is more consistent with adolescent development. In many HICs, the practice of pediatrics now extends up to age 19 years. This practice is starting in LMICs. For example, the Indian Academy of Pediatrics raised the upper age of pediatrics to 19 in 1999. However, adolescents requiring inpatient care in Saudia Arabia continue to be nursed with adults from the age of 14 years (AlBuhairan and Olsson 2014).

Specialist mental health services are usually separate from specialist pediatric and other health services, although hospital services are inconsistently colocated. The age criteria for adolescent mental health services also vary by country.

Specialist adolescent medicine first emerged in the United States more than 50 years ago. An increasing number of countries now support specialist training (Argentina, Canada), while other countries have embedded adolescent health competencies within generalist pediatric, family medicine, and obstetric and gynecology specialties. Specialist pediatric services should be linked with adult services to prevent adolescents from dropping out of health care at key transitions, such as when specialist services end. In HICs, the risk of dropping out of care or poor engagement with adult services is best appreciated for chronic physical health conditions. In LMICs, the issue has arisen especially in the context of HIV/AIDS (Lee and others 2015).

Table 21.1 summarizes the effective and promising actions that can be delivered by health services, categorized by health group. Interventions were deemed to be effective when at least 50 percent of review studies reported positive outcomes. Interventions with some positive evidence not reaching this threshold were deemed as promising and in need of further research.

Table 21.1 Effective and Promising Health Service Actions and Adolescent Health

Health condition	Action
Sexual and reproductive health, including HIV/AIDS	• Condoms and affordable modern contraception, including long-acting reversible contraception • Early diagnosis and treatment of HIV/AIDS and sexually transmitted infections • Male circumcision • Antenatal, delivery, and postnatal care • *Transition to adult care for HIV/AIDS*
Undernutrition	• Screening and micronutrient supplementation
Vaccine-preventable and infectious diseases	• Early identification and treatment • Adolescent vaccinations (human papillomavirus, childhood catch-up) • *Deworming* • *Bednet distribution* • *Seasonal malaria chemoprevention*
Injury and violence	• Trauma care, including first responders (ambulances)
Tobacco, alcohol, and illicit drugs	• *Risk screening* • *Motivational interviewing to promote cessation*
Mental disorders, including suicide	• Management of condition • Practitioner training in recognizing and treating depression • *Routine assessment of mental health, including suicide risk*
Chronic physical disorders	• Management of condition • *Promotion of self-management* • *Promotion of transition to adult health care*
Obesity	• Management of comorbidities

Note: HIV/AIDS = human immunodeficiency virus/acquired immune deficiency syndrome. Actions in italics are promising but lack a strong evidence base in adolescents and young adults.

Training to improve clinician competency is needed in all areas. It is especially important for recognizing and treating depression.

Schools

Schools offer three distinct benefits for adolescent health (chapter 20 in this volume, Bundy, Schultz, and others 2017). First, participation in education is beneficial for an individual's current and future health and well-being. Second, schools provide a setting for delivering preventive actions. Third, schools provide a setting for managing emerging and conspicuous health problems.

Education is a powerful determinant of adolescent health and human capital as well as a driver of socioeconomic progress (Cutler and Lleras-Muney 2012; Plaut and others 2017, chapter 22 in this volume). The Millennium Development Goals have focused attention on universal primary education, and primary school enrollment has expanded rapidly in LMICs (IHME 2015); between 2000 and 2012, the number of out-of-school children of primary school age fell 42 percent (UNESCO 2015). In 2015, at least lower-secondary education (8–10 years of education) was the norm in 34 percent of countries for young men and in 18 percent of countries for young women. Upper-secondary or beyond (10+ years of education) was the norm in 44 percent of countries for young men and 56 percent of countries for young women (IHME 2015).

Participation in secondary education has significant potential to improve adolescent health, yet the health benefits of secondary education for adolescents have been poorly studied in LMICs. In HICs, there may be a threshold effect of upper-secondary education for self-reported health, mental health, and alcohol use, with little additional benefit from tertiary education (Miyamoto and Chevalier 2010). In countries with high participation in secondary education, using schools to promote health explicitly can bring benefits above and beyond the health benefits of educational participation alone.

The benefits of expanding secondary education for health and well-being accrue through various mechanisms, including healthier behaviors, greater cognitive capacity, and longer productive lives (NRC and IOM 2005). While most attention has focused on direct health actions that can be delivered through schools, such as comprehensive sexuality education or school-based health services, indirect actions are just as, if not more, powerful (figure 21.4).

Greater participation in secondary education is associated with reductions in all-cause injury and mortality for ages 15–19, adolescent fertility, and maternal mortality (Patton, Sawyer, and others 2016). The quality of the school environment, or school ethos, also has a profound influence on health (Villa-Torres and Svanemyr 2015). A school's ethos reflects many factors, including the school's management and organization, social and physical environment (including physical and emotional safety, clean toilets, and adequate sanitation), quality of teaching, perceived fairness of discipline, availability of pastoral care, access to health services, whole-of-school health promotion, and access to extracurricular activities, such as sports, art, and music.

As summarized in table 21.2, the most effective actions delivered through schools are multicomponent interventions that involve whole-school activities, changes in the school's policies, curriculum, and social and physical environment, together with family and community engagement (Bonell and others 2013; Fletcher, Bonell, and Hargreaves 2008). These types of actions show consistently positive outcomes for

Figure 21.4 Indirect and Direct Actions for Health That Can Be Delivered in Schools

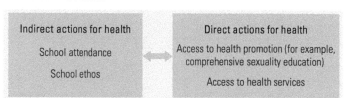

Table 21.2 Effective and Promising School-Based Actions and Adolescent Health

Health condition	Action
Sexual and reproductive health, including HIV/AIDS	• Quality secondary education
	• Comprehensive sexuality education
	• Safe schools with clean toilets and facilities for menstrual care
	• School-based health services with condoms and modern contraceptives
	• *Peer-led interventions*
Undernutrition	• Micronutrient supplements
	• Healthy school meals
Vaccine-preventable and infectious diseases	• Human papillomavirus vaccination
	• *Deworming*
Injury and violence	• Multicomponent interventions targeting violent behavior and substance use
Tobacco, alcohol, and illicit drugs	• Alcohol-free policies
	• Smoke-free policies
	• Multicomponent
Mental disorders, including suicide	• *Educational interventions*
	• *Gatekeeper training*
	• *School-based mental health services*
Chronic physical disorders	• *School-based health services*
Obesity	• *Multicomponent interventions involving education about healthy diet and increasing opportunities for physical education*

Note: HIV/AIDS = human immunodeficiency virus/acquired immune deficiency syndrome. Actions in italics are promising but lack a strong evidence base in adolescents and young adults.

adolescent sexual health, violence, and tobacco smoking and may also be beneficial for other health risks (Shackleton and others 2016).

Providing comprehensive sexuality education through schools, especially when coupled with the provision of contraception and condoms, is increasingly efficient as a site of health promotion as more girls participate in secondary education (Blank and others 2010; Blank and others 2012; Chin and others 2012). Comprehensive sexuality education has been shown to be effective in LMICs as well as HICs. Abstinence-only education has not been found to prevent HIV/AIDS, other STIs, or adolescent pregnancy (Chin and others 2012; DiCenso and others 2002).

Most interventions to increase access to and retention in education have targeted younger adolescents, largely in primary schools. Scholarships, school fee reductions, cash transfers conditional on remaining in school, efforts to reduce grade repetition, school proximity, and mother tongue education are cost-effective actions (Glewwe and Kremer 2006; UNESCO 2015). In some circumstances, providing free school uniforms, abolishing school fees, and offering deworming programs are among the most cost-effective interventions (chapter 29 in this volume, Ahuja and others 2017), while in others providing school meals for students and financial support for parent-teacher associations is less cost-effective (chapter 12 in this volume, Drake and others 2017; chapter 22 in this volume, Plaut and others 2017). Building schools close to students has high up-front costs, but is considered cost-effective, as one school can serve children for many years (UNESCO 2015). Addressing gender disparities in access and targeting more resources to the poorest regions and to disadvantaged students (notably children affected by armed conflict, children whose home language is not used at school, and children with disabilities) are critical to closing equity gaps (UNESCO and UNICEF 2015). Also needed are informal and flexible approaches to reaching children outside of mainstream education, such as child laborers and married adolescents who have left school (Yasunaga 2014).

Many forces operate to exclude or divert adolescents from secondary education. Prominent among these are the costs of education and the opportunity costs to families of the loss of adolescent labor, especially in rural areas. In many LMICs, poor adolescents are less likely to attend secondary school (UNESCO 2015). Early marriage accounts for higher dropout rates among girls in many LMICs (chapter 28 in this volume, Verguet and others 2017). Hence actions to promote continued education in secondary education need to be supported by legislation that prevents child marriage and actions to engage communities and enable them to appreciate the benefits of schooling, especially for girls.

Community

Young people are deeply embedded in their communities and are affected by the behavior, norms, and values of adults, as well as other adolescents. Communities can influence adolescent health in various ways. They can do so directly, by reducing access to harmful substances, preventing violence, or providing safe environments, including transportation to and from school. They can also do so indirectly by encouraging healthy behaviors through community attitudes and norms. Communities provide formal and informal opportunities for young people to engage, participate, and learn, which are beneficial for adolescent health and well-being. Beyond these roles, communities are also places to deliver preventive actions and treatment services.

Community-based youth-focused activities (sports, mentorship, leadership activities) can have multiple benefits. Positive youth development programs seek to promote self-confidence and empowerment, social and emotional skills, and problem solving. Using a variety of strategies (theater, music, and the arts; sports and outdoor education; leadership training and mentorship), these programs also provide opportunities to address and challenge harmful attitudes toward gender, violence, mental health, and disability. Some of these benefits can accrue through informal community programs. For example, the promotion of sports for girls can improve physical fitness, challenge harmful gender norms, and empower girls (Shaw and others 2014). However, it can be challenging to promote access for the most disadvantaged adolescents who have the most to gain from these programs.

Health services can also be delivered in community settings, distinct from primary care clinics. Community-based health care workers are likely to be most effective in places with low levels of trained health workers and few formal health clinics. Unlike the large workforce trained to offer community-based maternal and child health services, in most countries, no equivalent workforce is trained to address adolescents' particular health needs. Adolescents, especially girls who are not in school, can access community-based sexual and reproductive health education. While this will be of benefit, the extent to which community-based sexuality education meets their needs and how well it compares to school-based comprehensive sexuality education is not known. Poor quality is a likely challenge in both contexts. Ethiopia (Health Extension Worker Program),

India (Accredited Social Health Activist Program), and Pakistan (Lady Health Worker Program) have established community-based health worker programs in an effort to overcome critical deficiencies in human resources; if targeted to adolescents and supported by training, these programs could offer important benefits to adolescents, especially girls (Bhutta and others 2010; Liu and others 2011).

In socially and geographically disadvantaged areas, mobile clinics that visit different communities may also provide health services to adolescents. Mobile clinics that are located close to secondary schools, staffed by clinicians who have been trained to work with adolescents, and adequately resourced (especially with contraception) could provide services efficiently to smaller populations. The relative anonymity of mobile health workers may be advantageous for adolescents from small communities who are particularly concerned about confidentiality.

Few programs have been well evaluated or taken to scale. The best examples of community platforms have generally incorporated elements that build on available community structures, use good information on health needs and risks, adopt a multicomponent strategy, and monitor progress (table 21.3). For example, the Communities That Care framework, which has been piloted in several U.S. sites, has been found to have clear benefits for health outcomes such as substance use and violence and to be cost-effective (Catalano and others 2012).

Community-based interactions have particular opportunities to benefit adolescents who are out of school or from marginalized groups. This platform is particularly relevant in LMIC areas with the lowest

Table 21.3 Effective and Promising Community Actions and Adolescent Health

Health condition	Action
Sexual and reproductive health, including HIV/AIDS	• Cash transfer programs, with payments tied to staying in school • *Positive youth development* • *Peer education*
Undernutrition	• Micronutrient supplements (particularly in pregnancy) • Protein-energy supplementation • Deworming • *Cash transfer programs* • *Nutrition education*
Vaccine-preventable and infectious diseases	• *Deworming* • *Bednet distribution*
Injury and violence	• *Promotion of parental skills and parent-child communication* • *Positive youth development* • *Promotion of gender equality* • *Economic empowerment* • *Group training for awareness, knowledge, and skills* • *Police enforcement of traffic injury control*
Tobacco, alcohol, and illicit drugs	• *Promotion of parent-child communication and parenting skills* • *Needle-syringe exchange access* • *Mentoring* • *Interventions to promote parental skills and parent-child communication*
Mental disorders, including suicide	• *Gatekeeper training*
Chronic physical disorders	• *Peer support initiatives*
Obesity	• *Opportunities for maintaining physical activity in daily life*

Note: HIV/AIDS = human immunodeficiency virus/acquired immune deficiency syndrome. Actions in italics are promising but lack a strong evidence base in adolescents and young adults.

enrollment in secondary education. However, these areas also have the least access to community programs. The more that adolescents participate in quality upper-secondary education, the less need there is for parallel community-based interactions.

Mobile Health

Young people are the earliest adopters of information and communication technologies such as mobile phones, the Internet, instant messaging, and social networking. Rapid uptake of these technologies, even in the most remote communities, means that online interventions have the potential to be a powerful platform for adolescent health. These technologies offer a strategy for delivering health care, preventive interventions, and education and health information. Digital media have the potential to reach diverse groups, including geographically and socially marginalized adolescents, while low costs offer the potential to sustain interventions over long periods (Puccio and others 2006).

Using m-health approaches, adolescents can directly engage with clinicians from a distance (for example, by telehealth). Other direct clinical approaches include cognitive behavior therapy or texting with trained counselors (for example, Crisis Text Line) and online prescription and payment of medication. During consultations, clinicians can access online diagrams, videos, or other materials that are likely to educate adolescents more powerfully than traditional means. In time, virtual reality games are likely to be used to deliver health education and promote adolescent health literacy. As adjuncts to clinical care, clinicians can recommend mindfulness or adherence apps for adolescents to use following consultations. M-health approaches can promote efficiency during consultations by facilitating clinically required information before the consultation (for example, online psychosocial assessment). After consultations, m-health can provide opportunities to improve quality or evaluate services, such as using text feedback to assess patient-reported experiences of care or patient-reported outcomes, and to monitor outbreaks of disease (for example, UNICEF's U-Report).

The same benefits pertain to health services themselves, especially in remote regions, where m-health is used to report the quality of medical investigations (for example, medical imaging, electrocardiograms). Benefits are similarly available for training remotely based professionals, where interactive Webinars and more extensive online courses (for example, massive open online courses) are now common aspects of professional development in many parts of the world.

These new tools provide a platform for delivering health services to all populations. Adolescents may be more comfortable accessing m-health services than older adults, especially if confidentiality can be assured. For example, mobile apps could be used to offer treatment for conditions such as mental disorders, where stigma functions as a barrier to accessing treatment. Such interventions would offer particular benefits for adolescents living in countries without an effective mental health workforce. However, adolescents will need adult supervision of their engagement with m-health services, at least initially.

Ready access to free, health-related information and interactive games is a particular feature of new media (for example, PlayForward). While relevant for all adolescent health issues, the benefits are likely to be greater for more sensitive and stigmatized topics that might not otherwise be raised with peers, family, or community-based professionals, such as sexuality, abuse, interpersonal violence, and mental health. Web access is likely to be most important for adolescents whose cultures or religions are most controlling of their access to information, including comprehensive sexuality education (Latifnejad Roudsari and others 2013). Some websites in the United States focus sensitively on adolescent sexual and reproductive health (sexetc.org, bedsider.org). As with all health actions, engaging young people in the development of m-health resources would help to ensure that this approach meets their needs.

At this stage, notwithstanding the enthusiasm for m-health actions, current evidence of effectiveness is very limited regarding the longer-term benefits for health. This means that only promising, rather than effective, interventions are shown in table 21.4.

Table 21.4 Promising Mobile Health Actions and Adolescent Health

Health condition	Action
Sexual and reproductive health, including HIV/AIDS	• *Targeting of knowledge, attitudes, and risk behaviors*
Tobacco, alcohol, and illicit drugs	• *Targeting of knowledge, attitudes, and risk behaviors*
	• *Text messaging to encourage quitting*
Obesity	• *Interactive and personalized feedback*

Note: HIV/AIDS = human immunodeficiency virus/acquired immune deficiency syndrome. Actions in italics are promising but lack a strong evidence base in adolescents and young adults.

Once evidence has been gained, a particular challenge will be finding ways to bring effective interventions to the attention of young people and those who work with them, including families, teachers, and health professionals.

Reflecting their neurodevelopment and life experiences, younger adolescents are less adept at judging the reliability and accuracy of online information, which may render them vulnerable to extreme views (Coiro and others 2015).

The reach of platforms for m-health has greatly expanded (ITU 2015). For example, in Bangladesh, more than 70 percent of women of reproductive age have access to a mobile phone within the household (Labrique and others 2012). So, while access to the Internet is still challenging in many parts of the world, it is changing rapidly, even in remote parts of Sub-Saharan Africa:

- By the end of 2015, there were more than 7 billion mobile cellular subscriptions, corresponding to a penetration rate of 97 percent, up from 738 million in 2000.
- Between 2000 and 2015, global Internet penetration grew sevenfold from 6.5 to 43.0 percent.
- Mobile broadband penetration reached 47 percent in 2015, a twelvefold increase since 2007.
- The proportion of houses with Internet access at home increased from 18 percent in 2005 to 46 percent in 2015.

However, there is still global inequality of access:

- Two-thirds of people from LMICs remained offline in 2015.
- Only 9.5 percent of people in the poorest countries currently use the Internet.

Media and Social Marketing

Media and social marketing have the potential to target the health-related attitudes and values of adolescents as well as those of their families and the broader community. While previously considered distinct, the line between mass media and social marketing is increasingly blurred. Both can be used to shape community and adolescent attitudes, which is one component of setting expectations that support the implementation of other actions, whatever the platform.

Media include traditional approaches (radio, television, newspapers) as well as social and mass media. Social media and marketing have greater capacity than traditional media to target actions according to adolescents' interests. Actions range from the provision of health information, including embedding health messages within traditional media, as well as more focused strategies targeting behavior change. Partnerships with civil society and media professionals are powerful in exploiting the potential of these platforms. Here again, partnerships with young people themselves are an important aspect of meaningful and influential social marketing that targets young people. One example is Youth for Road Safety (YOURS), a global youth-led organization and a member of the UN Road Safety Collaboration. Beyond social media, YOURS uses youth ambassadors to empower young people to develop evidence-based road safety actions that make sense to them. Schools and communities could facilitate access to this platform, creating opportunities to leverage and integrate resources for wider learning.

The strongest evidence of effect pertains to advertising restrictions and multimedia campaigns to reduce tobacco use (table 21.5). These efforts are most effective when linked with structural interventions (taxation and legislation to reduce access). As with m-health, there is remarkably little evidence of health benefits for specific

Table 21.5 Effective and Promising Media and Social Marketing Actions and Adolescent Health

Health condition	Action
Sexual and reproductive health, including HIV/AIDS	• *Promotion of community support for sexual and reproductive health and HIV/AIDS health access for adolescents*
Injury and violence	• Promotion of knowledge of the effects of violence and available services • Promotion of knowledge of risks
Tobacco, alcohol, and illicit drugs	• Advertising restrictions • Campaigns to build community awareness
Mental disorders, including suicide	• *Promotion of adolescent mental health literacy*
Obesity	• *Promotion of physical activity*

Note: HIV/AIDS = human immunodeficiency virus/acquired immune deficiency syndrome. Actions in italics are promising but lack a strong evidence base in adolescents and young adults.

social media interventions. However, the benefits of using social media to change attitudes and behaviors related to the purchase of commercial products suggests that, in time, these approaches will be able to change health-related behaviors, especially in the young.

Structural Actions

Legislation, taxation, and implementation of policies are essential structural actions to improve adolescent health. Indeed, for many health risks, such as tobacco and alcohol, road traffic injuries, violence, unsafe work, and obesity, structural actions are the most effective interventions for adolescent health (table 21.6). In addition to protecting adolescents from hazards, laws are equally important in guaranteeing that adolescents have access to resources for health, such as effective contraception. Other laws function to address social determinants, such as age of marriage, legal driving age, legal working age, and protection from hazards. International agreements are also important for tackling transnational influences such as

Internet advertising and Internet gambling (Patton, Sawyer, and others 2016; Sawyer and others 2012).

Knowledge of adolescent neurodevelopment provides a framework for thinking about how adolescents require both protective and empowering structural actions. Most laws have developed historically without attention to adolescent development. More rational legal frameworks would take greater account of adolescents' evolving cognitive and emotional capacities. With access to knowledge, adolescents demonstrate similar or even greater cognitive capacity than adults to make good judgments in calm and emotionally neutral situations. However, emotions are more likely to drive their decision making in emotionally charged situations of stress or excitement, especially with peers. In addition to protecting adolescents from harm, legal frameworks should ensure age-appropriate autonomy, freedoms, and rights (United Nations General Assembly 1989). Most adolescents are capable of voting at age 16, and doing so both empowers adolescents and promotes civic engagement. This is an example where there are few risks but many

Table 21.6 Effective and Promising Structural Actions and Adolescent Health

Health condition	Action
Sexual and reproductive health, including HIV/AIDS	• *Legislation making 18 years the minimum age of marriage*
	• *Legislation legalizing the provision of contraception to minors*
	• *Legislation legalizing abortion*
Undernutrition	• Fortification of foods with nutrients such as iron and folate
Injury and violence	• Gun control legislation
	• Legislation legalizing homosexuality and using legislation to protect women from violence and sexual coercion
	• Youth justice reform to promote second chances and diversions from custody
	• Legislation making 16 the minimum age for criminal responsibility
	• Graduated drivers' licensing
	• Mandatory wearing of motorcycle helmets
	• Multicomponent traffic injury control
Tobacco, alcohol, and illicit drugs	• Restrictions on alcohol sales to minors
	• Taxes on alcohol
	• Drunk-driving legislation
	• Restrictions on illicit drugs
	• Interventions in licensed premises
Mental disorders, including suicide	• Restricted access (gun control, safe containers)
Obesity	• Tax on foods high in sugar, salt, and fat
	• *Front-of-package nutrition labels*
	• *Restrictions on fast-food advertising*

Note: HIV/AIDS = human immunodeficiency virus/acquired immune deficiency syndrome. Actions in italics are promising but lack a strong evidence base in adolescents and young adults.

benefits from a law that enables younger participation of adolescents. Yet adolescents need laws, policy safeguards, and support for decisions made in contexts where heightened emotion affects the choices they might make (Patton, Sawyer, and others 2016). The notion of graduated laws and policies is one approach to balancing protection with empowerment. For example, graduated driving licenses support young people to acquire appropriate driving skills and experience before they can obtain a full license (Lyon, Pan, and Li 2012).

Structural actions depend on sound governance, implementation capacity, and good information systems to monitor implementation and health outcomes. Thus, legal reforms are unlikely to be successful without addressing the values, knowledge, attitudes, and behavior of the judiciary and police responsible for their implementation. They are more likely to succeed when broader community engagement and education lead to wider support. In fragile states, structural actions are difficult, as the governmental systems for implementation are generally weak. In many other countries, information systems to support structural actions are also weak. Yet, structural actions are the bedrock of any country's capacity to improve adolescent health.

CONCLUSIONS

As children mature through adolescence, the platforms available to deliver health actions need to expand from a sole reliance on families to the inclusion of schools, communities, media, health services, and wider structural actions that shape behaviors through legislative and financial means. Actions are needed that match conspicuous health needs, address emerging health issues, and are oriented toward prevention. Beyond health services, other platforms are critically important in shaping adolescent health. The most effective actions for adolescents are multisectoral and span different platforms. Alignment across sectors provides potent opportunities for amplification of effect. Thus, the relatively modest effect of school-based sexuality education programs on reducing pregnancy is enhanced when aligned with school-based health services that provide ready access to contraception. Without alignment across platforms, certain actions cannot be implemented. For example, health services cannot confidentially provide contraception to adolescents if this contravenes national or customary laws. Given the extent to which these platforms span different government ministries, funding, and programming silos, the development of national adolescent health policies would help to advance the delivery of multisectoral actions.

There are obvious priorities to address in all countries if health actions are to match needs. First, as adolescents have significant need for, but poor access to, health services, efforts to orient the health service platform toward adolescents are urgently required. Such efforts include improving the competencies of the health workforce and considering different financing models. Innovative approaches need to include schools and community-based health care, social media, and m-health actions.

Second, the health benefits from participation in secondary education are clear, especially for girls. Education is one of the smartest investments for adolescent health. Schools also provide a scalable platform for evidence-based actions, including comprehensive sexuality education, condoms and contraception, meals and nutritional supplements, and routine immunization.

Third, as the major determinants of adolescent health, growth, and development lie beyond the health and education sectors, actions for health must also include legislative and financial reforms to limit adolescents' access to hazardous commodities and environments and to promote their access to multisectoral resources for health. Attention needs to be paid to the family and community sectors (cash transfers to reduce poverty and keep adolescent girls in school).

Notwithstanding these clear directions, the evidence base for adolescent health actions is relatively weak, with the predominant evidence from HICs and the focus on sexual and reproductive health. The lack of evidence from LMICs is a particular challenge in planning and selecting interventions for adolescents; more research on the health of adolescents in LMICs is clearly needed, especially regarding efforts to adapt effective interventions from HICs to LMICs. The lack of benefit-cost ratios limits the capacity of governments to be as confident as they would like in taking programs to scale. Better understanding of the costs of implementation and the benefits of interventions is expected to provide more compelling evidence for actions that support adolescent health. However, there are high priority actions to be implemented in every country.

Beyond financial resources, the extent to which these platforms can deliver necessary actions for adolescent health is more often the sum of a country's political and community support and technical capacity, including a trained workforce. Effective interventions will only achieve health outcomes if widely implemented. For this, attention needs to be paid to local communities and cultures, which will entail the involvement of all stakeholders. As much as possible, it will mean using existing system capacities, but additional investments will, without doubt, also be required. Ongoing monitoring and evaluation of interventions in different contexts are critical to building the evidence base (Patton and others 2016).

Regardless of the balance of platforms and actions, ensuring that new investments include strategies to reorient existing workforces (including the education, health, and community workforce) to the health and developmental needs of adolescents is a priority, as is ensuring that mechanisms are put in place to engage adolescents meaningfully so that they can positively influence the systems in which they live and learn and from which they obtain health care.

NOTE

World Bank Income Classifications as of July 2014 are as follows, based on estimates of gross national income (GNI) per capita for 2013:

- Low-income countries (LICs) = US$1,045 or less
- Middle income countries (MICs) are subdivided:
  a) lower-middle-income = US$1,046 to US$4,125
  b) upper-middle-income (UMICs) = US$4,126 to US$12,745
- High-income countries (HICs) = US$12,746 or more.

REFERENCES

Ahuja, A., S. Baird, J. Hamory Hicks, M. Kremer, and E. Miguel. 2017. "Economics of Mass Deworming Programs." In *Disease Control Priorities* (third edition): Volume 8, *Child and Adolescent Health and Development*, edited by D. A. P. Bundy, N. de Silva, S. Horton, D. T. Jamison, and G. C. Patton. Washington, DC: World Bank.

AlBuhairan, F. S., and T. M. Olsson. 2014. "Advancing Adolescent Health and Health Services in Saudi Arabia: Exploring Health-Care Providers' Training, Interest, and Perceptions of the Health-Care Needs of Young People." *Advances in Medical Education and Practice* 5 (September 4): 281–87.

Ambresin, A. E., K. Bennett, G. C. Patton, L. A. Sanci, and S. M. Sawyer. 2013. "Assessment of Youth-Friendly Health Care: A Systematic Review of Indicators Drawn from Young People's Perspectives." *Journal of Adolescent Health* 52 (6): 670–81.

Baltag, V., and S. M. Sawyer. 2016. "Quality Healthcare for Adolescents." In *International Handbook on Adolescent Health and Development: The Public Health Response.* Cham, Switzerland: Springer International Publishing.

Bhutta, Z. A., Z. S. Lassi, G. Pariyo, and L. Huicho. 2010. *Global Experience of Community Health Workers for Delivery of Health-Related Millennium Development Goals: A Systematic Review, Country Case Studies, and Recommendations for Integration into National Health Systems.* Geneva: WHO, Global Health Workforce Alliance.

Blank, L., S. K. Baxter, N. Payne, L. R. Guillaume, and H. Pilgrim. 2010. "Systematic Review and Narrative Synthesis of the Effectiveness of Contraceptive Service Interventions for Young People, Delivered in Educational Settings." *Journal of Pediatric and Adolescent Gynecology* 23 (6): 341–51.

Blank, L., S. K. Baxter, N. Payne, L. R. Guillaume, and H. Squires. 2012. "Systematic Review and Narrative Synthesis of the Effectiveness of Contraceptive Service Interventions for Young People, Delivered in Health Care Settings." *Health Education Research* 27 (6): 1102–19.

Bond, L., H. Butler, L. Thomas, J. Carlin, S. Glover, and others. 2007. "Social and School Connectedness in Early Secondary School as Predictors of Late Teenage Substance Use, Mental Health, and Academic Outcomes." *Journal of Adolescent Health* 40 (4): e9–e18.

Bonell, C., W. Parry, H. Wells, F. Jamal, A. Fletcher, and others. 2013. "The Effects of the School Environment on Student Health: A Systematic Review of Multi-Level Studies." *Health and Place* 21 (May): 180–91.

Bundy, D.A.P., N. de Silva, S. Horton, G. C. Patton, L. Schultz, and D. T. Jamison. 2017. "Child and Adolescent Health and Development: Realizing Neglected Potential." In *Disease Control Priorities* (third edition): Volume 8, *Child and Adolescent Health and Development*, edited by D. A. P. Bundy, N. de Silva, S. Horton, D. T. Jamison, and G. C. Patton. Washington, DC: World Bank.

Bundy, D. A. P., L. Schultz, B. Sarr, L. Banham, P. Colenso, and L. Drake. 2017. "The School as a Platform for Addressing Health in Middle Childhood and Adolescence." In *Disease Control Priorities* (third edition): Volume 8, *Child and Adolescent Health and Development*, edited by D. A. P. Bundy, N. de Silva, S. Horton, D. T. Jamison, and G. C. Patton. Washington, DC: World Bank.

Catalano, R. F., A. A. Fagan, L. E. Gavin, M. T. Greenberg, C. E. Irwin Jr., and others. 2012. "Worldwide Application of Prevention Science in Adolescent Health." *The Lancet* 379 (9826): 1653–64.

Chandra-Mouli, V., S. Chatterjee, and K. Bose. 2016. "Do Efforts to Standardize, Assess, and Improve the Quality of Health Service Provision to Adolescents by Government-Run Health Services in Low and Middle Income Countries, Lead to Improvements in Service-Quality and Service-Utilization by Adolescents?" *Reproductive Health* 13 (February 6): 10. doi:10.1186/s12978-015-0111-y.

Chin, H. B., T. A. Sipe, R. Elder, S. L. Mercer, S. K. Chattopadhyay, and others. 2012. "The Effectiveness of Group-Based Comprehensive Risk-Reduction and Abstinence Education Interventions to Prevent or Reduce the Risk of Adolescent Pregnancy, Human Immunodeficiency Virus, and Sexually Transmitted Infections: Two Systematic Reviews for the Guide to Community Preventive Services." *American Journal of Preventive Medicine* 42 (3): 272–94.

Coiro, J., C. Coscarelli, C. Maykel, and F. Forzani. 2015. "Investigating Criteria That Seventh Graders Use to Evaluate the Quality of Online Information." *Journal of Adolescent and Adult Literacy* 59 (3): 287–97.

Colchero, M. A., B. M. Popkin, J. A. Rivera, and S. W. Ng. 2016. "Beverage Purchases from Stores in Mexico under the Excise Tax on Sugar Sweetened Beverages: Observational Study." *BMJ* 352 (January 6): hh704.

Crone, E. A., and R. E. Dahl. 2012. "Understanding Adolescence as a Period of Social-Affective Engagement and Goal Flexibility." *Nature Reviews Neuroscience* 13 (9): 636–50.

Cutler, D. M., and A. Lleras-Muney. 2012. "Education and Health: Insights from International Comparisons." NBER Working Paper 17738, National Bureau of Economic Research, Cambridge, MA.

DiCenso, A., G. Guyatt, A. Willan, and L. Griffith. 2002. "Interventions to Reduce Unintended Pregnancies among Adolescents: Systematic Review of Randomised Controlled Trials." *BMJ* 324 (7351): 1426.

Drake, L., M. Fernandes, E. Aurino, J. Kiamba, B. Giyosa, and others. 2017. "School Feeding Programs in Middle Childhood and Adolescence." In *Disease Control Priorities* (third edition): Volume 8, *Child and Adolescent Health and Development*, edited by D. A. P. Bundy, N. de Silva, S. Horton, D. T. Jamison, and G. C. Patton. Washington, DC: World Bank.

Fletcher, A., C. Bonell, and J. Hargreaves. 2008. "School Effects on Young People's Drug Use: A Systematic Review of Intervention and Observational Studies." *Journal of Adolescent Health* 42 (3): 209–20.

Ford, C. A., S. G. Millstein, B. L. Halpern-Felsher, and C. E. Irwin Jr. 1997. "Influence of Physician Confidentiality Assurances on Adolescents' Willingness to Disclose Information and Seek Future Health Care." *JAMA* 278 (12): 1029–34.

Glewwe, P., and M. Kremer. 2006. "Schools, Teachers, and Education Outcomes in Developing Countries." In *Handbook of the Economics of Education*, edited by E. Hanushek and F. Welch, 945–1017. Oxford, U. K.: Elsevier.

Goldenring, J. M., and D. S. Rosen. 2004. "Getting into Adolescent Heads: An Essential Update." *Contemporary Pediatrics* 21 (January 1): 64–90.

Gore, F., P. Bloem, G. C. Patton, B. J. Ferguson, V. Joseph, and others. 2011. "A Systematic Analysis of the Global Disease Burden for 10–24 Year Olds." *The Lancet* 377 (9783): 2093–102.

IHME (Institute for Health Metrics and Evaluation). 2015. "Global Educational Attainment 1970–2015." IHME, Seattle.

ITU (International Telecommunication Union). 2015. "ICT Facts and Figures." ITU, Geneva.

Jha, P., and R. Peto. 2014. "Global Effects of Smoking, of Quitting, and of Taxing Tobacco." *New England Journal of Medicine* 370 (January 2): 60–68.

Kessler, R. C., P. Berglund, O. Demler, R. Jin, and K. R. Merikangas. 2005. "Lifetime Prevalence and Age-of-Onset Distributions of DSM-IV Disorders in the National Comorbidity Survey Replication." *Archives of General Psychiatry* 62 (6): 593–602.

Labrique, A. B., S. S. Sikder, S. Mehara, L. Wu, R. Huq, and others. 2012. "Mobile Phone Ownership and Widespread mHealth Use in 168,231 Women of Reproductive Age in Rural Bangladesh." *Journal of Mobile Technology in Medicine* 1 (Suppl 4): 26.

Latifnejad Roudsari, R., M. Javadnoori, M. Hasanpour, S. Hazavehei, and A. Taghipour. 2013. "Socio-Cultural Challenges to Sexual Health Education for Female Adolescents in Iran." *Iranian Journal of Reproductive Medicine* 11 (2): 101–10.

Lee, L., A. L. Agwu, B. Castelnouvo, M. Trent, and A. D. Kambugu. 2015. "Improved Retention in Care for Ugandan Youth Living with HIV Utilizing a Youth-Targeted Clinic at Entry to Adult Care: Outcomes and Implications for a Transition Model." *Journal of Adolescent Health* 56 (2): S50.

Levine, R., C. Lloyd, M. Greene, and C. Grown. 2008. *Girls Count: A Global Investment and Action Agenda; a Girls Count Report on Adolescent Girls.* Washington, DC: Center for Global Development.

Liu, A., S. Sullivan, M. Khan, S. Sachs, and P. Singh. 2011. "Community Health Workers in Global Health: Scale and Scalability." *Mount Sinai Journal of Medicine* 78 (3): 419–35.

Lyon, J. D., R. Pan, and J. Li. 2012. "National Evaluation of the Effect of Graduated Driver Licensing Laws on Teenager Fatality and Injury Crashes." *Journal of Safety Research* 43 (1): 29–37.

Manganello, J. A., R. F. DeVellis, T. C. Davis, and C. Schottler-Thal. 2015. "Development of the Health Literacy Assessment Scale for Adolescents (HAS-A)." *Journal of Communication in Healthcare: Strategies, Media, and Engagement in Global Health* 8 (3): 172–84.

Miyamoto, K., and A. Chevalier. 2010. "Education and Health." In *Improving Health and Social Cohesion through Education*, 111–79. Paris: OECD Publishing.

Mokdad, A., M. H. Forouzanfar, F. Daoud, A. A. Mokdad, C. El Bcheraoui, and others. 2016. "Global Burden of Diseases, Injuries, and Risk Factors for Young People's Health during 1990–2013: A Systematic Analysis for the Global Burden of Disease Study 2013." *The Lancet* 387 (10036): 2383–401. http://dx.doi.org/10.1016/S0140 -6736(16)00648-6.

Mullen, F., and S. Frehywot. 2007. "Non-Physician Clinicians in 47 Sub-Saharan African Countries." *The Lancet* 370 (9605): 2158–63.

Ngimuh, L., B. E. Fokam, J. K. Anchang-Kimbi, and W. Samuel. 2016. "Factors Associated to the Use of Insecticide Treated Nets and Intermittent Preventive Treatment for Malaria Control during Pregnancy in Cameroon." *Archives of Public Health* 74 (February 1): 5. doi:10.1186/s13690-016-0116-1.

NRC (National Research Council) and IOM (Institute of Medicine). 2005. "Growing Up Global: The Changing Transitions to Adulthood in Developing Countries." In *Panel on Transitions to Adulthood in Developing Countries*, edited by C. B. Lloyd. Washington, DC: National Academies Press.

Patton, G. C., P. Azzopardi, E. Kennedy, C. Coffey, and A. Mokdad. 2017. "Global Measures of Health Risks and Disease Burden in Adolescents." In *Disease Control Priorities* (third edition): Volume 8, *Child and Adolescent Health and Development*, edited by D. A. P. Bundy, N. de Silva, S. Horton, D. T. Jamison, and G. C. Patton. Washington, DC: World Bank.

Patton G. C., C. Coffey, S. M. Sawyer, R. M. Viner, D. Haller, and others. 2009. "Global Patterns of Mortality in Young People: A Systematic Analysis of Population Health Data." *The Lancet* 374 (9693): 881–92.

Patton, G. C., S. M. Sawyer, J. S. Santelli, D. A. Ross, R. Afifi, and others. 2016. "Our Future: A Lancet Commission on Adolescent Health and Wellbeing." *The Lancet* 387 (10036): 2423–78.

Peden, M., R. Scurfield, D. Sleet, D. Mohan, A. A. Hyder, and others. 2004. *World Report on Road Traffic Injury Prevention.* Geneva: WHO.

Plaut, D., T. Hill, M. Thomas, J. Worthington, M. Fernandes, and B. Burnett. 2017. "Getting to Education Outcomes: Reviewing Evidence from Health and Education Interventions." In *Disease Control Priorities* (third edition): Volume 8, *Child and Adolescent Health and Development*, edited by D. A. P. Bundy, N. de Silva, S. Horton, D. T. Jamison, and G. C. Patton. Washington, DC: World Bank.

Puccio, J. A., M. Belzer, J. Olson, M. Martinez, C. Salata, and others. 2006. "The Use of Cell Phone Reminder Calls for Assisting HIV-Infected Adolescents and Young Adults to Adhere to Highly Active Anti-Retroviral Therapy: A Pilot Study." *AIDS Patient Care and STDs* 20 (6): 438–44.

Reavley, N., G. C. Patton, S. M. Sawyer, E. Kennedy, and P. Azzopardi. 2017. "Health and Disease in Adolescence." In *Disease Control Priorities* (third edition): Volume 8, *Child and Adolescent Health and Development*, edited by D. A. P. Bundy, N. de Silva, S. Horton, D. T. Jamison, and G. C. Patton. Washington, DC: World Bank.

Sanci, L. A., P. Chondros, S. M. Sawyer, J. Pirkis, E. Ozer, and others. 2015. "Responding to Young People's Health Risks in Primary Care: A Cluster Randomised Trial of Training Clinicians in Screening and Motivational Interviewing." *PLOS One*, September 30.

Sanci, L. A., C. M. M. Coffey, F. C. M. Veit, M. Carr-Gregg, G. C. Patton, and others. 2000. "Evaluation of the Effectiveness of an Educational Intervention for General Practitioners in Adolescent Health Care: Randomised Controlled Trial." *BMJ* 320 (7229): 224–30.

Sauber-Schatz, E. K., D. J. Ederer, A. M. Dellinger, and G. T. Baldwin. 2016. "Vital Signs: Motor Vehicle Injury Prevention—United States and 19 Comparison Countries." *Morbidity and Mortality Weekly Report* 65 (July 8): 26. http://www.cdc.gov/mmwr.

Sawyer, S. M., R. A. Afifi, L. H. Bearinger, S. J. Blakemore, S. J. Ezay, and others. 2012. "Adolescence: A Foundation for Future Health." *The Lancet* 379 (9826): 1630–40.

Sawyer, S. M., J. Proimos, and S. J. Towns. 2010. "Adolescent Friendly Health Services: What Have Children's Hospitals Got to Do with It?" *Journal of Paediatrics and Child Health* 46 (5): 214–16.

Shackleton, N., F. Jamal, R. M. Viner, K. Dickson, G. C. Patton, and others. 2016. "School-Based Interventions Going beyond Health Education to Promote Adolescent Health: Systematic Review of Reviews." *Journal of Adolescent Health* 58 (4): 382–96.

Shaw, A., B. Brady, B. McGrath, M. A. Brennan, and P. Dolan. 2014. "Understanding Youth Civic Engagement: Debates, Discourses, and Lessons from Practice." *Community Development* 45 (4): 300–16.

Stein, M. B., and Y. M. Kean. 2000. "Disability and Quality of Life in Social Phobia: Epidemiological Findings." *American Journal of Psychology* 157 (10): 1606–13.

UNESCO (United Nations Educational, Scientific and Cultural Organization). 2015. *Education for All 2000–2015: Achievements and Challenges.* Paris: UNESCO.

UNESCO Institute for Statistics and UNICEF (United Nations Children's Fund). 2015. *Fixing the Broken Promise of Education for All: Findings from the Global Initiative on Out-of-School Children.* Montreal: UNESCO Institute for Statistics.

UNICEF. 2011. *The State of the World's Children 2011: Adolescence, an Age of Opportunity.* New York: UNICEF.

United Nations General Assembly. 1989. "Convention on the Rights of the Child." United Nations Treaty Series 1577, United Nations General Assembly, New York.

Verguet, S., A. K. Nandi, V. Filippi, and D. A. P. Bundy. 2017. "Postponing Adolescent Parity in Developing Countries through Education: An Extended Cost-Effective Analysis." In *Disease Control Priorities* (third edition): Volume 8, *Child and Adolescent Health and Development*, edited by D. A. P. Bundy, N. de Silva, S. Horton, D. T. Jamison, and G. C. Patton. Washington, DC: World Bank.

Villa-Torres, L., and J. Svanemyr. 2015. "Ensuring Youth's Right to Participation and Promotion of Youth Leadership in the Development of Sexual and Reproductive Health Policies and Programs." *Journal of Adolescent Health* 56 (1): S51–57.

WHO (World Health Organization). 2002. *Adolescent-Friendly Health Services: An Agenda for Change.* Geneva: WHO.

———. 2007. *Everybody's Business: Strengthening Health Systems to Improve Health Outcomes; WHO's Framework for Action.* Geneva: WHO.

———. 2013. *Global Status Report on Road Safety 2013: Supporting a Decade of Action.* Geneva: WHO.

———. 2014. "Second Chance for the Second Decade." WHO, Geneva.

———. 2015a. "Core Competencies in Adolescent Health and Development for Primary Care Providers." WHO, Geneva.

———. 2015b. "Global Standards for Quality Health-Care Services for Adolescents." WHO, Geneva.

Woog, V., S. Singh, A. Browne, and J. Philbin. 2015. *Adolescent Women's Need for and Use of Sexual and Reproductive Health Services in Developing Countries.* New York: Guttmacher Institute.

World Bank. 2007. *World Development Report 2007: Development and the Next Generation.* Washington, DC: World Bank.

Yasunaga, M. 2014. "Non-Formal Education as a Means to Meet Learning Needs of Out-of-School Children and Adolescents." UNESCO Insitute of Statistics, Montreal.

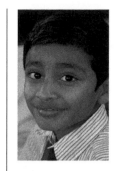

Chapter **22**

Getting to Education Outcomes: Reviewing Evidence from Health and Education Interventions

Daniel Plaut, Milan Thomas, Tara Hill, Jordan Worthington,
Meena Fernandes, and Nicholas Burnett

INTRODUCTION

Over the past several decades, efforts to fight infectious diseases and malnutrition have increased alongside attempts to enroll children in basic education, demonstrating a global commitment to equity and quality in child health and education. Health and education interventions can be complementary, as discussed in chapter 30 of this volume (Pradhan and others 2017). Improvements in access to quality education have contributed to preventing disease—for example, an encouraging drop in infant mortality rates is attributed not only to health services but also to worldwide improvements in education. Work commissioned by the International Commission on Financing Global Education Opportunity found that about 7.3 million lives were saved between 2010 and 2015 in low- and middle-income countries (LMICs) because of increases in educational attainment since 1990 (Pradhan and others 2017). Poor health is linked to poor student outcomes. Disease and malnutrition reduce children's capacity to attend school and their ability to learn, particularly in poor communities lacking quality education services (Jukes, Drake, and Bundy 2008).

Indeed, some development strategies have explicitly pursued cross-sector synergies. For example, the 2015 Incheon Declaration states that quality education instills skills, values, and attitudes that lead to healthy lives. Explicit recognition of the role of health in promoting education is less common. As a complement to the global state of education, as detailed in chapter 4 of this volume (Wu 2017), this chapter outlines the theoretical role of health interventions in increasing education access and quality. It then surveys evidence from LMICs on the extent to which common education interventions and school-based health interventions improve education outcomes. It considers the potential of primary and secondary schools to serve as platforms for health interventions, focusing on interventions targeting middle childhood through adolescence, understood to be the range comprising ages 5–19 years. This focus precludes a discussion of the high returns to investment in early childhood, but the studies included are particularly relevant to policy makers in countries where participation rates in early childhood education are still very low. Definitions of age groupings and age-specific terminology used in this volume can be found in chapter 1 (Bundy, de Silva, and others 2017).

EDUCATION: PROGRESS AND GAPS

Enormous progress has been made in global education in the past few decades, especially with respect to achieving universal primary education and reducing gender

Corresponding author: Daniel Plaut, Results for Development, Washington, DC, United States; dplaut@r4d.org.

disparity (UNESCO 2015). However, several of the Millennium Development Goals (MDGs) for education were not met by 2015. This brief summary of the state of global education provides the background for the ensuing discussion of school-based education and health interventions.

Since the 1990 Jomtien Conference on Education for All, international support for education has focused on improving access and quality (UNESCO 2013). Partly reflecting the MDG focus on primary enrollment and gender parity in primary and secondary school, access has taken overwhelming priority. Quality, initially interpreted mainly as educational inputs (teachers, textbooks), has, since the mid-2000s, come to be interpreted as not just inputs but also as outcomes—that is, learning. Indeed, the Sustainable Development Goals emphasize both access and learning at all levels of education.

Access to primary education has expanded significantly with widespread enrollment efforts. Nearly 60 million additional children enrolled in school between 1999 and 2013 (ISS 2014). Equally impressive has been the progress made in primary school gender parity, illustrated by a female-to-male pupil ratio of 0.94 in low-income countries in 2011 (World Bank 2013). Although this progress is unprecedented, major gaps persist in access to education worldwide. Growth in enrollment has slowed significantly since 2008, and more than 59 million children were still not enrolled in primary school in 2013 (ISS 2014). This figure not only has significant moral implications, but also costs LMIC economies up to 10 percent of gross domestic product (Thomas and Burnett 2013). At the secondary school level, growth in enrollment began from a relatively low base. Secondary enrollment stood at only 65 percent in 2012 (World Bank 2013), and only 63 percent of countries achieved gender parity in secondary education enrollment (UNESCO 2015).

Gaps in global education are even larger when it comes to learning outcomes. About 250 million of the world's 650 million primary schoolchildren are not acquiring basic skills in literacy and mathematics (UNESCO 2014). The Global Partnership for Education's LMIC partners face a learning crisis, with only 44 percent of their 180 million children reaching grade 4 and learning the basic literacy and numeracy skills appropriate for that grade (Global Partnership for Education 2013). Citizen-led assessments of learning in East Africa and India show similarly daunting numbers. In East Africa, Uwezo (2013) found that less than a third of standard three children in 2013 were passing their grade 2 tests on basic numeracy (29 percent) and literacy (25 percent). In India, only 48 percent of grade 5 children are able to read at a grade 2 level (ASER Centre 2014). Major quality-related challenges in education clearly persist in LMICs.

CONCEPTUAL FRAMEWORK

To understand how health interventions might be critical to achieving global education goals, it is important to understand how they fit conceptually alongside education interventions. As illustrated in figure 22.1, health interventions should play a key role in improving education outcomes along with education interventions that seek to improve access to education and student learning. For the purposes of this chapter, health interventions are narrowly defined as programs designed to enhance the physical well-being of students. They can improve education outcomes by preventing and treating health deficiencies that might otherwise deter children from attending school. By enabling children to attend school more often and in better health, these interventions affect access to education and the ability to learn.

Health interventions may also affect education outcomes by improving children's cognitive skills. As demonstrated by Jukes, Drake, and Bundy (2008), malnutrition and infectious disease are linked to poor cognitive skills among school-age children (children ages 5 to 14 years). Conversely, interventions addressing health conditions, particularly malnutrition and malaria, may improve indicators of cognitive skills (Conn 2014).

Although the conceptual link between health interventions and improved education outcomes is clear, there is little consensus regarding the extent of their impact or how it compares with the impact of education interventions. To fill this gap, several meta-analyses have evaluated interventions in LMICs (Banerjee and others 2013; Conn 2014; Evans and Popova 2015; Krishnaratne, White, and Carpenter 2013; McEwan 2015; Petrosino and others 2012). This chapter draws largely from studies that satisfy the inclusion criteria of those meta-analyses to understand the impacts of selected health interventions on education outcomes. As the following sections show, evidence of the impact of these health interventions on increasing access to education (including increasing attendance) is mixed, but generally positive. Their impact on learning is less clear.

SURVEY OF EDUCATION INTERVENTIONS

To address education challenges, governments and non-governmental organizations have implemented a range of education interventions to improve access and learning. This section provides an overview of common education interventions and evidence on their impact.

Figure 22.1 Example of a Conceptual Framework for the Impact of Health and Education Interventions on Education Outcomes

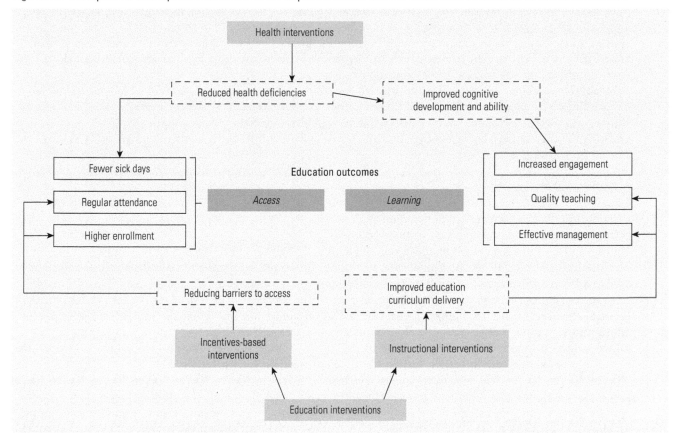

McEwan (2015) distinguishes between incentives-based and instruction-based education interventions:

- *Incentives-based interventions* improve learning by changing incentives for teachers, parents, students, and administrators. Interventions include reducing tuition costs (for example, scholarships, subsidies), introducing performance-based pay for teachers, changing school management structures, and providing families with information about the importance of education.
- *Instruction-based interventions* expand access and improve learning by providing materials and services to schools. They include building physical infrastructure, providing textbooks and technology, and training teachers.

The impact of these interventions is measured by a variety of indicators. Enrollment, attendance, progression, and dropout rates are used to indicate access. Literacy and numeracy test scores are typically used to indicate learning. Evidence about the impact of these interventions is discussed next.

Incentives-Based Interventions

Cost-Reduction Interventions

Among the principal demand-side barriers to education for the poor are household costs: tuition and related expenses, such as textbooks, uniforms, transportation costs, and the opportunity cost of forgone labor by parents and children. Cost-based interventions reduce the price of education for students and households, stimulating demand for education services. The abolition of primary school fees in many countries since the early 2000s has contributed to a rise in enrollment, but rarely to an increase in learning outcomes (UNESCO 2014). Abolishing school fees does not always translate into higher public school enrollment, particularly in countries where households shoulder the burden of costs other than tuition (Foko, Tiyab, and Husson 2012). Furthermore, as demonstrated by Bold and others (2011), free primary education can exacerbate concerns about the low quality of education provided by public schools in LMICs.

Conditional cash transfers (CCTs) are promising cost-reduction interventions for increasing enrollment and attendance rates (chapter 23 in this volume, de Walque and others 2017). Cash transfers are direct and regular cash payments that supplement the income of poor and vulnerable households (Arnold, Conway, and Greenslade 2011). In education, CCTs have been applied to bolster school enrollment, with payments contingent on children's school attendance. CCTs provide incentives for attendance, make education more accessible to the poor, and offset the opportunity costs of enrolling children in school. Although Krishnaratne, White, and Carpenter (2013) claim that CCTs have had a significant impact on access (figure 22.2), their impact on learning is less clear.

School-Based Management

School-based management (SBM) refers to interventions that improve the management and supervision of schools through authority and accountability at the school level (McEwan 2015). SBM is premised on the notion that local communities and parents are most motivated to ensure quality school performance (Banerjee and others 2010). SBM interventions can support existing education management structures, such as the Pratham Initiative in India, which sought to bring about renewed engagement among village education committees (Banerjee and others 2010), as well as new management structures, such as in Pakistan where new committees were established under a community support process (Kim, Alderman, and Orazem 1999).

One category of SBM interventions is the allocation of funds for school improvement through school management committees. For example, the Quality Schools Program in Mexico allowed parents and teachers to develop school improvement plans and provided cash grants over five years to implement them (Skoufias and Shapiro 2006). SBM interventions can also provide community members with the authority to monitor teacher performance and hire and fire teachers (Duflo, Dupas, and Kremer 2009; Kim, Alderman, and Orazem 1999).

Although SBM interventions have demonstrated a positive impact on learning outcomes, McEwan (2015) found the average effects of management and supervision interventions to be small and not robust. According to that review, interventions in The Gambia, Indonesia, and Madagascar showed few effects of SBM and supervision reforms (Blimpo and Evans 2011; Glewwe and Maïga 2011; Pradhan and others 2011). Thus, while the limited evidence base suggests that SBM could positively improve learning outcomes, not enough is known about the mechanisms through which this process occurs (Krishnaratne, White, and Carpenter 2013).

Information-Based Interventions

Information asymmetries can affect access to and quality of education (box 22.1). Providing information about the education system has been shown to have an impact on indicators of both access and quality (Murnane and Ganimian 2014).

Several interventions have sought to increase the perceived value parents and students assign to education, often by providing information on the economic benefits of staying in school. Two studies suggest that providing information on the returns to education can change perceptions, exerting a positive impact on school access and learning outcomes at relatively low cost.

Jensen (2010) targeted grade 8 students in the Dominican Republic with information about the economic returns of continuing to secondary education. Results showed that participating students perceived significantly higher returns to education when they were interviewed several months later. Moreover, dropout rates fell 3.9 percentage points, or 7 percent, the following year; four years later the average years of education was 0.20 year higher. These results were concentrated among students from households above the median income level, and there was little or no effect on schooling for the poorest students. Given that both socioeconomic groups increased their perception of returns to schooling, financial constraints may have prevented the poorest households from continuing their education (Banerjee and others 2013).

Nguyen (2008) similarly found that providing students and parents in Madagascar with statistics about increased earnings from higher levels of education boosted average school attendance by 3.5 percentage points. The information also had a positive effect on language and math test scores, raising scores by 0.20 standard deviation after three months, but only for students who had underestimated the returns to education at baseline.

Figure 22.2 Impact of Conditional Cash Transfers on Improving Access to Education

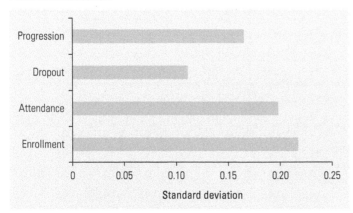

Note: Figure reflects a weighted sum of Cohen's *d* (differences in mean between control and treatment groups, normalized by the study's standard deviation) from the individual studies. The weighted sum is calculated using random effects estimation.

Information Interventions Regarding Learning Outcomes

Several studies have explored the ability of targeted information campaigns about poor learning outcomes to bring about improvements in education quality and school accountability. According to Bruns, Filmer, and Patrinos (2011), providing information on students' educational attainment may have a positive impact on learning outcomes by empowering parents to choose higher-performing schools, encouraging parents and students to monitor school resource allocations and learning outcomes, and pressuring governments and education providers to improve learning outcomes.

Many interventions providing information on children's educational attainment have improved learning outcomes. The Learning and Education Achievement in Pakistan Schools Project provided two report cards to parents in randomly selected villages on the basis of results from learning assessments in English, mathematics, and Urdu (Andrabi, Das, and Khwaja 2015). The first report card included each child's individual test scores and

ranking compared with other students; the second included each school's average score and ranking against other schools. This intervention reduced schools' ability to operate in the context of information asymmetries and applied competitive pressure on schools to improve their quality or reduce their price. Andrabi, Das, and Khwaja (2015) concluded that the intervention improved learning outcomes by 0.10 standard deviation and reduced private school fees 21 percent.

Banerjee and others (2006) analyzed three types of information interventions to encourage local participation in improving education outcomes. While the first two were passive, the third involved a targeted intervention to facilitate community action for improving learning. The targeted intervention was found to have the largest impact on parental engagement. Results suggest that the provision of information alone may be insufficient to affect learning outcomes and that additional interventions are likely needed to generate and sustain impact on students' learning.

Instructional Interventions

Infrastructure

Proximity of schools has been shown to increase participation dramatically, especially for children who live in remote regions or who face cultural barriers to enrollment and participation. A randomized study by Burde and Linden (2009) assessing the impact of the Partnership for Advancing Community-Based Education in Afghanistan demonstrated the importance of school proximity in providing incentives for school participation. They found that enrollment rates were greater than 70 percent in areas where schools were within a mile of home. Enrollment declined significantly as distance from school increased, reaching about 30 percent for children living more than two miles away. These results illustrate the importance of local infrastructure and have significant implications for understanding gender disparity in education. Enrollment of girls in rural Afghanistan proved to be particularly sensitive to school proximity, improving

21 percent with the provision of nearby community-based schools. Overall, community-based schools in rural Afghanistan increased formal school enrollment 47 percent and raised test scores by 0.59 standard deviation.

Kazianga, de Walque, and Alderman (2009) found similar results in their evaluation of the Burkinabé Response to Improve Girls' Chances to Succeed Program in Burkina Faso, which placed well-equipped schools in 132 villages where the potential for primary-school-age girls to attend school was particularly high. The initiative led to a significant improvement in enrollment (19 percent), with the enrollment of girls increasing more than that of boys. Improvement was also seen in test scores, which rose by 0.41 standard deviation (figure 22.3). The study found that "girl-friendly" amenities, including separate latrines for boys and girls, contributed to the improvement in enrollment, demonstrating the potential role of specialized infrastructure in targeting previously neglected populations.

Figure 22.3 Impact of Infrastructure Interventions on Access and Learning

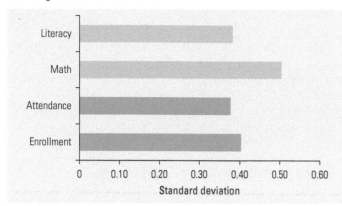

Source: Krishnaratne, White, and Carpenter 2013.
Note: Figure reflects a weighted sum of Cohen's *d* (differences in mean between control and treatment groups, normalized by the study's standard deviation) from the individual studies. The weighted sum is calculated using random effects estimation.

Box 22.2

Impact of Pedagogical Interventions on Learning Outcomes

In a meta-analysis of interventions seeking to improve learning outcomes, Conn (2014) found that the types of learning interventions with the most impact are "those that alter instructional techniques." Two pedagogical interventions have proved effective:

- Adaptive instruction that caters to children's particular learning levels
- Teacher coaching that provides long-term teacher mentoring or coaching, rather than one-off in-service training events.

These sorts of interventions have the largest significant impact on learning outcomes, but differences in categorization illustrate some of the limitations of meta-analysis in providing conclusive and comparable findings regarding intervention types and their impact (Evans and Popova 2015).

Teacher Resources

Because teaching quality is a key determinant of education outcomes, interventions have sought to improve the quality of teaching through various means. These measures include the provision of extra teachers (García-Huidobro 2000), financial rewards for improved student performance (Muralidharan and Sundararaman 2008), and additional and improved

teaching resources and support materials (Lai, Zhang, Qu, and others 2012). Such interventions improve learning outcomes by improving the quality of teaching, reducing class sizes, providing incentives to teachers to do their jobs, and equipping teachers with the necessary resources to teach effectively (box 22.2). Although generally targeted to improving learning outcomes, these interventions can also improve attendance and enrollment because parents are more likely to send their children to school if they trust that teachers are present and believe that children are learning (Krishnaratne, White, and Carpenter 2013).

In general, interventions providing additional teaching resources demonstrate a significant impact on the full range of access and learning education outcomes (Krishnaratne, White, and Carpenter 2013). Although promising, such interventions need to be designed carefully to avoid distorting incentives. For example, while providing financial incentives to teachers on the basis of student performance (test scores) may push teachers to raise the quality of their instruction, it may also adversely provide teachers with incentives to maintain artificially high average exam scores by pressuring poorly performing students to drop out or repeat grades (Glewwe, Ilias, and Kremer 2003).

Materials and Technology

A key category of instructional interventions to improve education outcomes is the provision of additional materials and technology for both students and teachers. Such interventions can include textbooks (Glewwe, Kremer, and Moulin 2009), writing materials and chalkboards (Krishnaratne, White, and Carpenter 2013), flipcharts (Glewwe and others 2004), lesson plans or curriculum guides (Banerjee and others 2007), as well as technology or computer-based learning in the classroom (Barrera-Osorio and Linden 2009; Cristia and others 2012; Lai, Zhang, Hu, and others 2012; Lai, Zhang, Qu, and others 2012). Overall, such interventions have had some positive impact on math test scores, but no effect on attendance, enrollment, or progression (Krishnaratne, White, and Carpenter 2013).

The context and manner in which materials are provided are important in determining impact. Although the provision of materials alone is often ineffective (Glewwe and others 2004; Glewwe, Kremer, and Moulin 2009; Kremer, Moulin, and Namanyu 2003), combining materials with training and a well-defined teaching model augments the efficacy of materials (Friedman, Gerard, and Ralaingita 2010; Lucas and others 2014). According to McEwan (2015), computers and instructional technology interventions have shown the largest effect on learning outcomes.

Summary of the Impacts of Selected Education Interventions

The education interventions described in this section are some of the more promising approaches currently in practice. Each type of intervention has merits, and meta-analyses have explored their impacts relative to each other, with mixed results. Table 22.1 summarizes the education interventions with randomized controlled trials (RCTs) that have shown statistically significant effects on education outcomes in one meta-analysis by Krishnaratne, White, and Carpenter (2013).

Incentives-based interventions such as CCTs and school fees have demonstrated a greater impact on improving access to education (increasing enrollment, attendance, and progression and decreasing dropout), while instruction-based interventions have proved to be more effective at improving learning. The provision of infrastructure and teacher resources shows promise across both access and learning indicators, with pedagogical interventions demonstrating the largest and most significant effect on improving learning outcomes. Instruction-based interventions clearly are promising for improving learning outcomes.

Although these findings reveal several interventions with large and significant effects, Conn (2014) and Evans and Popova (2015) caution against drawing inferences about many of those interventions because of the small number of studies. Findings of the impact of CCTs on access and the impact of teacher resources and materials on learning are based on more studies, so their effect sizes are particularly meaningful (box 22.3).

THE CASE FOR HEALTH INTERVENTIONS

While education interventions are crucial for improving access and learning, health interventions can also play an important role. The role of health in education is particularly important in LMICs, which are burdened with a disproportionate share of morbidity and mortality caused by widespread malnutrition, parasites, and other infectious diseases. Many children in South Asia and Sub-Saharan Africa are unable to access school because of acute and chronic illnesses. For example, a national survey in the Democratic Republic of Congo (ISSP 2012) showed that health issues kept 7 percent of the country's 4 million out-of-school children from enrolling.

Table 22.1 Impact of Incentives-Based and Instructional Education Interventions on Access and Learning

Type of education intervention	Access to Schooling				Learning Outcomes		
	Enrollment	Attendance	Dropout	Progression	Math	Language	Global
Incentives-based interventions							
Cost-reduction interventions							
CCTs	0.22* (16)	0.20* (8)	0.11* (4)	0.17* (4)	−0.02 (2)	−0.03 (1)	0.05 (3)
School fees	0.02 (2)	0.63* (1)	—		0.13* (1)	—	—
Provision of infrastructure	0.40* (4)	0.38* (3)	0.42 (2)	0.20 (1)	0.51* (2)	0.38* (2)	—
Information-based interventions	0.03 (2)	−0.10 (3)	−0.01 (2)	—	0.40 (2)	0.05* (2)	0.03 (2)
Instructional interventions							
Teacher resources	0.23* (2)	0.09* (4)	0.09* (3)	—	0.29* (5)	0.28* (5)	−0.02 (3)
Materials	—	0.05 (8)	0.22 (2)	0.00 (1)	0.16* (10)	0.20 (9)	0.11 (2)
School-based management	0.08 (3)	−0.02 (3)	0.02 (3)	0.06* (3)	0.23* (3)	0.12 (2)	0.20* (1)

Source: Krishnaratne, White, and Carpenter 2013.
Note: Numbers in parentheses indicate the number of studies; — = not available; CCTs = conditional cash transfers. Table reflects a weighted sum of Cohen's *d* (differences in mean between control and treatment groups, normalized by the study's standard deviation) from the individual studies. The weighted sum is calculated using random effects estimation.
*$p < 0.05$.

International Commission on Financing Global Education Opportunity

In 2016, the International Commission on Financing Global Education Opportunity was set up to reinvigorate the case for investing in education. Chaired by Gordon Brown, former prime minister of the United Kingdom, the commission released its report entitled, "The Learning Generation: Investing in Education for a Changing World," at the United Nations in September 2016. The report provides a series of 12 recommendations to ensure all children are learning (International Commission on Financing Global Education Opportunity 2016). A key set of recommendations focuses on promoting inclusion, within which the commission emphasizes the importance of countries investing beyond education to address other barriers that prevent learning. The report draws attention to the fact that up to 500 million school days are lost because of ill health each year

in low-income countries, often from preventable conditions, and recommends that decision makers invest in joint education-health initiatives. Early childhood development and services for adolescent girls are recommended in particular as investments that can deliver strong complementary health and education benefits. Chapter 30 of this volume (Pradhan and others 2017) was prepared as a background paper for the Brown Commission. The chapter estimates the effects of education on under-five mortality, adult mortality, and fertility. In addition, it calculates the economic returns to education resulting from declines in under-five mortality and adult mortality, while also taking into account the effects of education investments on income. Estimates of the internal rate of return to education are about 50 percent higher if the impact of mortality is included in the analysis.

Poor health is a major barrier to educational achievement (Glewwe and Miguel 2008). Addressing chronic health conditions is essential for increasing school enrollment, while preventing and treating acute illness are critical for reducing absenteeism. Even if they are healthy enough to attend school, children in poor health are less able to learn. For example, children with insufficient calories and micronutrients may lack the energy to focus in class, limiting their ability to learn (Gomes-Neto and others 1997).

Health interventions could improve cognitive development and education outcomes by ensuring that enrolled children are present, ready, and able to learn (Bundy, Schultz, and others 2017). Even where the conditions of access and instruction are ideal, cognitive function may constrain learning and achievement. For example, Holding and Snow (2001) examined the lasting, adverse impact of malaria infection on cognition and behavior, and Black (2003) reviewed the effects of micronutrient deficiencies on children's cognitive functioning.

Given the physiological importance of children's health status in determining their readiness to learn, a growing literature has emerged on the impact of health interventions on cognitive skills. However, identifying a relationship between cognition and learning is

complicated by the myriad assessments measuring the two main dimensions of cognitive skills: (1) general intelligence and reasoning and (2) memory and attention. Tests of cognitive skills vary by study, and the choice of tests is determined by budgetary considerations, adaptability to local contexts, and ease of implementation. A related complication is that cognitive skills and learning are cumulative processes, and detectable improvements may require more time to manifest than is typical for health trials.

Effectiveness of health interventions depends on context, specifically disease burden and the education system. For example, the effectiveness of deworming may be greater if delivered regularly to high-risk areas or if delivered at the beginning rather than the end of the school term. The provision of school feeding to children with untreated helminth infection may not lead to improved attendance or learning. The relationship between anemia and cognition is well established, but the condition may be due to nutritional deficiencies, helminth infection, HIV/AIDS, or a combination of factors (Stephenson, Latham, and Kurz 1985). Integrated health interventions are likely to be more effective and cost-effective.

Taking into account these caveats on heterogeneity and the difficulty of measuring the effects of health interventions, this section reviews recent evidence on the effectiveness of deworming, malaria control, school feeding, and nutrition in promoting education outcomes. These health interventions were chosen because they address some of the most prevalent threats to child health in LMICs and because schools have been used as a delivery platform to support their scalability and enhance their cost-effectiveness, as discussed in chapters 20 (Bundy, Schultz, and others 2017) and 25 (Fernandes and Aurino 2017) in this volume.

Deworming Treatment

More than 600 million school-age children are in need of treatment for intestinal worm infection (WHO 2016). Infected children suffer from listlessness, diarrhea, abdominal pain, wasting, stunting, anemia, cognitive impairment, lower productivity, and lower earning capacity (Guyatt 2000).

School-age children are more likely than adults to spread worm infection because they are frequently in contact with other students, less likely to use latrines, and more likely to have poor hygienic practices. School-based interventions have tremendous potential for positive externalities—if a critical mass of students is dewormed in a school, students who do not receive deworming treatment are less likely to be infected by their classmates (Anderson and May 1991). School-based deworming programs distribute oral deworming medicine every 6–12 months to prevent infection. They sometimes also include teacher training on preventive behaviors.

Many studies indicate that deworming has strong impacts on enrollment and attendance, as reviewed by Petrosino and others (2012) and discussed in chapters 13 (Bundy, Appleby, and others 2017) and 29 (Ahuja and others 2017) in this volume. A study of hookworm eradication in the American South found that mass deworming increased enrollment, attention, and literacy (Bleakley 2007). Miguel and Kremer (2004) found that low-cost, single-dose therapies reduced hookworm, roundworm, and schistosomiasis infections by 99 percent and improved school participation by 7 percentage points in a large study (30,000 schoolchildren) in Kenya. These estimates mask heterogeneity given that children who are worse off have the most to gain. Simeon and others (1995) discerned no average impact, but did find significant impacts on attendance for the subset of children who had heavy *Trichuris* infection or were stunted.

Alderman and others (2006) found no impact of albendazole on test scores, while Grigorenko and others (2006) found that praziquantel improved scores on some cognitive tests. Meta-analyses of quasi-experimental results show no clear impact of deworming on learning (Evans and Popova 2015; McEwan 2015). Over the long term, persistent infections are associated with impaired cognitive development and lower educational achievement (Mendez and Adair 1999), and worm infections are estimated to lead to an intelligence quotient (IQ) loss of 3.75 points per child infected, on average, and 200 million years of lost schooling (Jukes, Drake, and Bundy 2008). Ozier (2014) found that, because of externalities, a mass school-based deworming program in Kenya was associated with improved cognitive performance for nontreated infants 10 years after the program. However, just as for learning, conclusive evidence from recent empirical studies with quasi-experimental design is lacking for cognition (Taylor-Robinson and others 2015). The mixed evidence on learning and cognitive impact may be in part due to measurement issues, as discussed in chapter 13 in this volume (Bundy, Appleby, and others 2017).

Malaria Control

More than 500 million school-age children worldwide are at risk of malaria infection, which can be prevented through a variety of interventions, including insecticide-treated bednets and prophylactic antimalarial drugs, as discussed in chapter 14 in this volume (Brooker and others 2017). Although malaria is most severe and common in early childhood, it has serious consequences during the school-age years, accounting for up to 20 percent of mortality in schoolchildren in malaria-ridden countries (World Bank 2015). A range of malaria prevention strategies is typically delivered through schools or communities.

The effect of malaria reduction on educational attainment is indeterminate because of the prevalence of child labor in most malaria-ridden countries (Bleakley 2007). Reducing malaria increases the benefits of education because healthy children are more able to capitalize on opportunities generated by schooling. Conversely, reducing malaria increases the opportunity costs of education because healthy children are more able to supplement household income. The effect on educational attainment of reducing malaria thus requires empirical investigation.

Studies of school-based delivery provide strong evidence that malaria prevention improves attendance and cognition among children in endemic areas. Repeated provision can ensure better results, especially for the most vulnerable. Studies demonstrate that malaria is a significant contributor to absenteeism, accounting for 13 percent to 50 percent of medical absences from school (Nankabirwa and others 2014). In Kenya alone, an estimated 4 million to 10 million school days were lost because of malaria in 2000 (Brooker and others 2000).

School health education programs that promote antimalarial practices were found to reduce absenteeism 25 percent among Kenyan schoolchildren (Ogutu and others 1992). Malaria prevention combined with chloroquine prophylaxis in Sri Lanka was linked to a 62 percent reduction in school absenteeism and a 26 percent increase in mathematics and language test scores (Fernando and others 2006).

Some debate surrounds the impact of malaria on school performance. Bangirana and others (2011) found a minimal impact of malaria on test scores in Uganda, but suggested that the effect of malaria on cognition in schoolchildren may develop too gradually to be observed during the short periods common in controlled studies. Similarly, Clarke and others (2008) found that intermittent preventive treatment of schoolchildren in Kenya had no effect on achievement, but did positively affect performance on attention and memory tests.

Indeed, such results do not preclude an impact of malaria prevention on students' cognitive skills. A strong body of evidence demonstrates that cerebral and uncomplicated malaria can impair cognitive function (Fernando, Rodrigo, and Rajapakse 2010; Kihara, Carter, and Newton 2006; Thuilliez and others 2010), while a consistent association has not been found for asymptomatic parasitemia (Halliday and others 2012). These studies suggest that school-based malaria programs offering diagnostic services, treatment, and prevention may improve education outcomes by promoting readiness to learn.

School Feeding

More than 165 million children worldwide face chronic malnutrition (UNICEF 2013), which can be alleviated to some degree by school feeding—the regular provision of food to children attending schools, discussed in chapter 12 in this volume (Drake and others 2017). Although malaria and deworming treatments are typically limited to low-income countries, school feeding is implemented in almost every country in the world (WFP 2013). The recognition of its potential impacts on education outcomes is also widespread. School feeding programs can help get children into school and keep them there. They can contribute to learning once children are in school, given the well-established link between nutrition and cognition (Adelman, Gilligan, and Lehrer 2008). In LMICs, school feeding programs have traditionally focused on boosting enrollment and attendance, although the emphasis is shifting to assessing their impact on academic achievement, as has been done in high-income countries.

School feeding could affect education outcomes through several channels. First, school feeding can provide incentives for enrollment by lowering the opportunity cost of attendance. On average, school feeding represents an income transfer of US$60 per child per year, as discussed in chapter 12 in this volume (Drake and others 2017). Second, school feeding alleviates hunger, which improves attention span and increases a student's capacity for performance. Third, school feeding provides the nutritional inputs to boost cognitive development, especially in early childhood (Martorell 1996), which could improve performance. Finally, nutrition promotes health by improving resistance to disease, which enables children to stay healthy and maintain better attendance (Buttenheim and others 2011). Thus, school feeding could, in theory, affect education access, cognition, and learning outcomes.

Although the impact of improved nutrition is undisputed, its logistical implementation through school feeding has an ambiguous impact on education outcomes. Several issues associated with the implementation of school feeding could counteract the positive influence of improved nutrition. School feeding could provide food that is insufficiently nutritious. School feeding could also reduce teaching time or overcrowd schools if enrollment increases rapidly, both of which could cause a drop in education quality (Conn 2014). Furthermore, in resource-constrained settings, there could be a substitution effect whereby children who receive school feeding are given less to eat at home, negating any possible gains. In addition, by increasing attendance, school feeding programs could induce a reduction in child labor, which reduces household income and the availability of food at home (Adelman, Gilligan, and Lehrer 2008). It is thus critical to look to the evidence to judge whether the merits of school feeding hold up empirically.

Several reviews have highlighted the positive effects of school feeding on enrollment, attendance, and retention (Jomaa, McDonnell, and Probart 2011). However, the impact of school feeding on cognition and learning is more nuanced and dependent on the quality of schooling. Studies suggest that school feeding can influence the two domains of cognition by reducing micronutrient deficiencies, although the impacts are less than for micronutrient supplementation (Conn 2014). Breakfast programs may be especially important for cognitive function, especially in contexts where breakfast is rarely consumed at home, as discussed in chapter 12 in this volume (Drake and others 2017). Learning effects are stronger for arithmetic tests than for reading, writing, and spelling (Jomaa, McDonnell, and Probart 2011).

Nutrition

Nutrition interventions are also commonly distributed through schools, separately or in conjunction with school meals. These interventions include the provision of supplement tablets as well as micronutrient powders, which can be sprinkled on meals to enhance their nutrient content. By tackling micronutrient deficiencies associated with health status and cognition, nutrition interventions can promote learning and academic achievement.

Nutrition interventions may seek to address one or more micronutrient deficiencies, with one of the most common being iron deficiency. In a review of the literature, Best and others (2011) found positive effects of supplementation of multiple micronutrients on micronutrient and anemia status as compared with supplementation of a single micronutrient. Impact can also depend on the dose, initial micronutrient status, and interactions with other micronutrient supplements. For instance, the inclusion of iron-fortified flour enhanced the iron status of Kenyan schoolchildren (Andang'o and others 2007). However, in Vietnam, iron supplementation alone did not affect anemia status, although the provision of multiple-fortified biscuits did, suggesting that the presence of other nutrients may affect iron absorption and anemia status (Hieu and others 2012). In a review of the literature, Conn (2014) found that nutrition interventions had significant impacts on cognitive function, but not academic achievement, suggesting the need for complementary education interventions.

Summary of the Impacts of Selected Health Interventions

Table 22.2, which is based on a meta-analysis by Krishnaratne, White, and Carpenter (2013), combines effect sizes from disparate, context-specific studies to arrive at a general conclusion. It is based on just one meta-analysis of school-based health interventions, so it should only be taken as suggestive, rather than the final word on these interventions. Similarly, online annexes 22A and 22B combine both health and education intervention effect sizes from Krishnaratne, White, and Carpenter (2013) to illustrate their effect sizes relative to each other. Both demonstrate that, in some cases, health interventions can have as large an effect size on access and learning outcomes as education interventions.

While the size of some of the effects are large and appear to be statistically significant, making these inferences about statistical significance at the 95 percent confidence level hinges on assuming that normal approximation is valid for a very small number of studies. No result for an individual intervention is based on more than four studies. Tipton (2015) highlights the danger of making inferences from small samples. Evans and Popova (2015) considered the results from Krishnaratne, White, and Carpenter (2013) and five other meta-analyses and concluded that they largely agree that school-based health interventions have a significant impact on access indicators (consistent with results in the table), but are not effective in improving test scores.

However, these findings cannot necessarily be taken as evidence that improvements in health are not essential

Table 22.2 Impact of Health Interventions on Access and Learning

Type of health intervention	Access to schooling				Learning outcomes		
	Enrollment	Attendance	Dropout	Progression	Math	Language	Global
School feeding	0.24* (4)	0.26* (4)	—	0.69* (1)	0.40 (1)	0.19 (2)	0.02 (1)
Nutrition	0.04* (1)	0.27* (2)	0.33 (1)	—	0.65* (2)	0.66* (2)	—
Malaria prevention	—	0.59* (1)	0.24* (1)	0.38* (1)	0.62* (1)	0.56* (1)	—
Deworming	0.29 (1)	0.09 (1)	—	—	0.04 (1)	0.02 (1)	−0.03 (1)

Source: Based on data from Krishnaratne, White, and Carpenter 2013.

Note: Numbers in parentheses indicate the number of studies; — = not available. Table reflects a weighted sum of Cohen's *d* (differences in mean between control and treatment groups, normalized by the study's standard deviation) from the individual studies. The weighted sum is calculated using random effects estimation.

*p < 0.05.

for improving learning outcomes. Analyzing impact evaluations from Sub-Saharan Africa, Conn (2014) found that, although deworming had no discernible impact on test scores, it did significantly improve cognitive skills (as measured by tests like Raven's Progressive Matrices). This result suggests that the improvements in health yielded by health interventions may be necessary, but not sufficient, for promoting learning.

Although most experimental studies focus on measuring changes in access and achievement indicators, RCT studies that measure cognitive function also show encouraging results. High-quality evidence is available for nutritional supplements and malaria prevention interventions in particular. For example, Sungthong and others (2004) found that Thai primary schoolchildren receiving iron supplements performed moderately better than the control group on a standardized test of cognitive function (TONI II), while Clarke and others (2008) showed that Kenya schoolchildren treated with a preventive malaria program performed significantly better on attention tests than untreated students. Both studies were placebo controlled and double blind. More should be done to rigorously assess the impact of these and other interventions in other contexts and to link them to learning.

In summary, evidence on the impacts of health interventions is inconclusive, particularly for learning outcomes. More research using cluster-randomized approaches, larger sample sizes, and longer timeframes is needed to assess the impacts of health interventions on learning outcomes.

Evidence on the importance of health in determining readiness to learn and the lack of clear evidence on the impact of health interventions on learning outcomes do not necessarily contradict each other. Rather, other necessary conditions (such as adequate educational resources) may be lacking in the settings where these studies took place, preventing health interventions from improving education outcomes. Cunha and Heckman (2007) discussed a theoretical model involving such

---

Box 22.4

Assessing Cost and Cost-Effectiveness

On the basis of a systematic review of studies by the *Disease Control Priorities* (third edition) Economics Team (which calculated costs per student per year in 2012 U.S. dollars), deworming treatment costs, on average, US$0.93. Programs for malaria control cost US$3.67, and programs for school feeding cost US$75.90, on average. Although these studies cover interventions that varied considerably in scope, the averages provide a sense of the resources required to fund such programs. Although the review did not include studies on nutritional supplements, such interventions have been recognized elsewhere as generally cost-effective (Dhaliwal and others 2012), and on the basis of an observational study of Filipino schoolchildren, Glewwe, Jacoby, and King (2001) suggest that in developing countries, a dollar invested in an early childhood nutrition program returns at least three dollars worth of gains in academic achievement. Chapters 12 (Drake and others 2017), 20 (Bundy, Schultz, and others 2017), 24 (Horton and Black 2017), 26 (Horton and others 2017), and 14 (Brooker and others 2017) in this volume provide more details on the costs of these health interventions.

The comparative cost-effectiveness of interventions for education outcomes has been analyzed. Jensen (2010) found that information-based interventions, which cost as little as US$0.08 per student (Nguyen 2008), may be a highly cost-effective way to promote school access for marginal students. These findings are in sharp contrast to conditional cash transfers like Mexico's Progresa, which costs US$500 per person. Dhaliwal and others (2012) cite examples suggesting that information-based interventions, deworming, and nutritional supplements are highly cost-effective. Kremer, Brannen, and Glennerster (2013) note that pedagogical interventions matching teaching to students' learning levels and providing information might be the most cost-effective interventions for learning. McEwan (2015) found that computer-assisted teaching and textbook distribution are among the least cost-effective learning interventions. Further research and cost-effectiveness analysis of both education and health interventions are needed.

dynamic complementarities in inputs to education. Moreover, conclusions drawn from meta-analyses can be incomplete or misleading because of heterogeneous effects (the impact of interventions could vary by beneficiary gender or socioeconomic status), temporal effects (the size of impacts at the endline of a study does not necessarily indicate lasting effects), and differences in age at exposure (the impacts are age dependent for some health interventions, such as the wealth of evidence on the heightened importance of adequate nutrition in a child's first 1,000 days).

Reviewing the cost and cost-effectiveness of school-based interventions falls outside the remit of this chapter. Furthermore, the vast majority of cost-effectiveness studies measure cost over a single outcome (disability-adjusted life years averted), not taking into account the multisectoral benefits of an intervention. However, because cost-effectiveness has central implications for the feasibility of interventions in resource-constrained settings, box 22.4 briefly notes some cost evidence specific to school-based delivery.

CONCLUSIONS: THE EMERGING NEXUS OF HEALTH AND EDUCATION

Our understanding of the interaction between children's health status and education outcomes has progressed considerably. Indeed, a wealth of evidence on a range of health interventions has been generated from nonexperimental studies and RCTs during the past two decades, including for some health interventions not discussed in this chapter (such as HIV/AIDS prevention and treatment, provision of eyeglasses, disability access, and sanitation).

Overall, the data suggest that health interventions can have a significant impact on education outcomes. Health interventions have been widely shown to improve indicators of access, such as attendance and enrollment. The impact of these interventions on learning and cognitive skills is mixed and uncertain. Despite years of opportunity for definitive research the very plausible hypothesis that sick, malnourished, and hungry children learn less in school remains to be adequately tested. The limited research on interventions to address these problems has so far been inconclusive. This point is but one example of an important theme of this volume as a whole: research on child health and nutrition has been dominated by studies of children younger than age five years, leaving an important gap concerning school-age children.

As discussed in the previous section, the lack of consensus on some interventions is likely due in part to methodological challenges. Furthermore, the lack of universal conclusions about the effects of both health and education interventions is not surprising, given how education and health outcomes are interdependent. In some contexts, education interventions may fail to improve education outcomes because poor health is the binding constraint on educational achievement. In others, health interventions may fail to improve education outcomes because school infrastructure is so poor that improving children's individual abilities to excel in school does not improve actual outcomes. Health interventions alone do not guarantee improved learning outcomes and vice versa; quality education and health services must be provided contemporaneously to maximize the impact of each.

For this reason, focusing on integrated implementation is important. Studies such as Banerjee and others (2006) and Piper and Korda (2010) have shown that incentives-based interventions can have a greater impact when implemented alongside instruction-based interventions. Scant evidence on integrated health and education interventions is available for LMICs. An intervention in Jamaica that combined early stimulation with nutritional supplements for stunted children illustrates the potential impact of integrated interventions: more than two decades after its implementation, the impact on IQ and learning outcomes was still significant (Grantham-McGregor and others 2014). Although the timing of this intervention, which targeted children younger than age four years, was likely a factor in its impact, this promising intervention provides an example of how a more holistic approach to interventions seeking to improve education outcomes by improving cognitive skills could provide significant long-term gains.

However, in more developed settings, even the distinction between health and education outcomes has started to blur as policy makers measure development using more comprehensive measures of well-being. This is evident in theoretical frameworks in which education is recognized as a causal factor for health (Braveman and Gottlieb 2014), as well as in practice. In the United States, programs such as Fast Track and Communities That Care provide comprehensive services for children and their families. The Centers for Disease Control initiative Healthy People 2020 uses high school graduation as a leading indicator of social determinants of health. This merging of education and health in policy and practice may provide guidance for designing programs that integrate education with critical interventions for malnutrition and diseases that are no longer pervasive in high-income countries.

Many chapters in this volume make the economic and social case for investing in health. This chapter has shown that these cases become even stronger when policy makers bear in mind the importance of health interventions for promoting education.

ANNEXES

The annexes to this chapter are as follows. They are available at http://www.dcp-3.org/CAHD.

- Annex 22A. Impact of Interventions on Education Outcomes
- Annex 22B. Median Significant Effect Sizes on Education Outcomes

NOTE

World Bank Income Classifications as of July 2014 are as follows, based on estimates of gross national income (GNI) per capita for 2013:

- Low-income countries (LICs) = US$1,045 or less
- Middle-income countries (MICs) are subdivided:
  a) lower-middle-income = US$1,046 to US$4,125
  b) upper-middle-income (UMICs) = US$4,126 to US$12,745
- High-income countries (HICs) = US$12,746 or more.

REFERENCES

Adelman, S., D. Gilligan, and K. Lehrer. 2008. *How Effective Are Food for Education Programs? A Critical Assessment of the Evidence from Developing Countries*. IFPRI Food Policy Review 9. Washington, DC: International Food Policy Research Institute.

Alderman, H., J. Kunde-Lule, I. Sebuliba, D. A. P. Bundy, and A. Hall. 2006. "Effect on Weight Gain of Routinely Giving Albendazole to Preschool Children during Child Health Days in Uganda: Cluster Randomised Controlled Trial." *BMJ Clinical Research Education* 333 (7559): 122.

Ahuja, A., S. Baird, J. Hamory Hicks, M. Kremer, and E. Miguel. 2017. "Economics of Mass Deworming Programs." In *Disease Control Priorities* (third edition): Volume 8, *Child and Adolescent Health and Development*, edited by D. A. P. Bundy, N. de Silva, S. Horton, D. T. Jamison, and G. C. Patton. Washington, DC: World Bank.

Andang'o, P., S. Osendarp, R. Ayah, C. West, D. Mwaniki, and others. 2007. "Efficacy of Iron-Fortified Whole Maize Flour on Iron Status of Schoolchildren in Kenya: A Randomized Controlled Trial." *The Lancet* 369 (9575): 1799–806.

Anderson, R. M., and R. M. May. 1991. *Infectious Diseases of Humans: Dynamics and Control*. Oxford, U.K.: Oxford University Press.

Andrabi, T., J. Das, and A. Khwaja. 2015. "Report Cards: The Impact of Providing School and Child Test Scores on Educational Markets." Policy Research Working Paper 7226, World Bank, Washington, DC.

Arnold, C., T. Conway, and M. Greenslade. 2011. *Cash Transfers: Literature Review*. London: Department for International Development.

ASER Centre. 2014. "ASER 2014: Main Findings." ASER Centre, New Delhi.

Banerjee, A., R. Banerji, E. Duflo, R. Glennerster, and S. Khemani. 2006. "Can Information Campaigns Spark Local Participation and Improve Outcomes?" Policy Research Working Paper 3967, World Bank, Washington, DC.

Banerjee, A., R. Banerji, R. Glennerster, and S. Khemani. 2010. "Pitfalls of Participatory Programs: Evidence from a Randomized Evaluation of Education in India." *American Economic Journal: Economic Policy* 2 (1): 1–30.

Banerjee, A., S. Cole, E. Duflo, and L. Linden. 2007. "Remedying Education: Evidence from Two Randomized Experiments in India." *Quarterly Journal of Economics* 122 (3): 1235–64.

Banerjee, A., P. Glewwe, S. Powers, and M. Wasserman. 2013. "Expanding Access and Increasing Student Learning in Post-Primary Education in Developing Countries: A Review of the Evidence." Post-Primary Education Initiative Review Paper, Abdul Latif Jameel Poverty Action Lab, Massachusetts Institute of Technology, Cambridge, MA.

Bangirana, P., S. Musisi, M. J. Boivin, A. Ehnvall, C. C. John, and others. 2011. "Malaria with Neurological Involvement in Ugandan Children: Effect on Cognitive Skills, Academic Achievement, and Behaviour." *Malaria Journal* 10 (1): 334.

Barrera-Osorio, F., and L. Linden. 2009. "The Use and Misuse of Computers in Education: Evidence from a Randomized Experiment in Colombia." Policy Research Working Paper, Impact Evaluation Series 4836, World Bank, Washington, DC.

Best, C., N. Neufingerl, J. Del Rosso, C. Transler, T. van den Briel, and others. 2011. "Can Multi-Nutrient Food Fortification Improve the Micronutrient Status, Growth, Health, and Cognition of Schoolchildren? A Systematic Review." *Nutrition Reviews* 69 (4): 186–204.

Black, M. M. 2003. "Micronutrient Deficiencies and Cognitive Functioning." *Journal of Nutrition* 133 (11): S3927–31.

Bleakley, H. 2007. "Disease and Development: Evidence from Hookworm Eradication in the American South." *Quarterly Journal of Economics* 122 (1): 73–117.

Blimpo, M. P., and D. K. Evans. 2011. "School-Based Management and Educational Outcomes: Lessons from a Randomized Field Experiment." Unpublished, World Bank, Washington, DC.

Bold, T., M. Kimenyi, G. Mwabu, and J. Sandefur. 2011. "Why Did Abolishing Fees Not Increase Public School Enrollment in Kenya?" CGD Working Paper 271, Center for Global Development, Washington, DC.

Braveman, P., and L. Gottlieb. 2014. "The Social Determinants of Health: It's Time to Consider the Causes of the Causes." *Public Health Reports* 129 (Suppl 2): 19–31.

Brooker, S. J., S. Clarke, D. Fernando, C. W. Gitonga, J. Nankabirwa, and others. 2017. "Malaria in Middle Childhood and Adolescence." In *Disease Control Priorities* (third edition): Volume 8, *Child and Adolescent Health and Development*, edited by D. A. P. Bundy, N. de Silva, S. Horton, D. T. Jamison, and G. C. Patton. Washington, DC: World Bank.

Brooker, S. J., H. Guyatt, J. Omumbo, R. Shretta, L. Drake, and others. 2000. "Situation Analysis of Malaria in School-Aged Children in Kenya: What Can Be Done?" *Parasitology Today* 16 (5): 183–86.

Bruns, B., D. Filmer, and H. Patrinos. 2011. *Making Schools Work: New Evidence on Accountability Reform.* Human Development Perspectives. Washington, DC: World Bank.

Bundy, D. A. P., L. Appleby, M. Bradley, K. Croke, T. D. Hollingsworth, and others. 2017. "Mass Deworming Programs in Middle Childhood and Adolescence." In *Disease Control Priorities* (third edition): Volume 8, *Child and Adolescent Health and Development*, edited by D. A. P. Bundy, N. de Silva, S. Horton, D. T. Jamison, and G. C. Patton. Washington, DC: World Bank.

Bundy, D. A. P., N. de Silva, S. Horton, G. C. Patton, L. Schultz, and D. T. Jamison. 2017. "Child and Adolescent Health and Development: Realizing Neglected Potential." In *Disease Control Priorities* (third edition): Volume 8, *Child and Adolescent Health and Development*, edited by D. A. P. Bundy, N. de Silva, S. Horton, D. T. Jamison, and G. C. Patton. Washington, DC: World Bank.

Bundy, D. A. P., L. Schultz, B. Sarr, L. Banham, P. Colenso, and others. 2017. "The School as a Platform for Addressing Health in Middle Childhood and Adolescence." In *Disease Control Priorities* (third edition): Volume 8, *Child and Adolescent Health and Development*, edited by D. A. P. Bundy, N. de Silva, S. Horton, D. T. Jamison, and G. C. Patton. Washington, DC: World Bank.

Bundy, D. A. P., S. Shaeffer, M. C. H. Jukes, K. Beegle, A. Gillespie, and others. 2006. "School-Based Health and Nutrition Programs." In *Disease Control Priorities in Developing Countries* (second edition), edited by D. T. Jamison, J. G. Breman, A. R. Measham, G. Alleyne, M. Claeson, D. B. Evans, P. Jha, A. Mills, and P. Musgrove. Washington, DC: World Bank and Oxford University Press.

Burde, D., and L. Linden. 2009. "The Effect of Proximity on School Enrollment: Evidence from a Randomized Controlled Trial in Afghanistan." Working paper, Steinhardt School, New York University, New York; Columbia University, New York.

Buttenheim, A. M., H. Alderman, J. Friedman, and J. Arnold. 2011. "Impact Evaluation of School Feeding Programs in Lao PDR." Policy Research Working Paper 5518, World Bank, Washington, DC.

Clarke, S., M. C. H. Jukes, J. K. Njagi, L. Khasakala, B. Cundill, and others. 2008. "Effect of Intermittent Preventative Treatment of Malaria on Health and Education in Schoolchildren: A Cluster-Randomized, Double-Blind, Placebo-Controlled Trial." *The Lancet* 372 (9633): 127–38.

Conn, K. 2014. "Identifying Effective Education Interventions in Sub-Saharan Africa." PhD dissertation, Columbia University, New York.

Cristia, J. P., P. Ibarraran, S. Cueto, A. Santiago, and E. Severin. 2012. "Technology and Child Development: Evidence from the One Laptop per Child Program." Working Paper 304, Inter-American Development Bank, Washington, DC.

Cunha, F., and J. Heckman. 2007. "The Technology of Skill Formation." Working Paper 12840, National Bureau of Economic Research, Cambridge, MA.

de Walque, D., L. Fernald, P. Gertler, and M. Hibrobo. 2017. "Cash Transfers and Child and Adolescent Development." In *Disease Control Priorities* (third edition): Volume 8, *Child and Adolescent Health and Development*, edited by D. A. P. Bundy, N. de Silva, S. Horton, D. T. Jamison, and G. C. Patton. Washington, DC: World Bank.

Dhaliwal, I., E. Duflo, R. Glennerster, and C. Tulloch. 2012. "Comparative Cost-Effectiveness Analysis to Inform Policy in Developing Countries." Abdul Latif Jameel Poverty Action Lab, Massachusetts Institute of Technology, Cambridge, MA.

Drake, L., M. Fernandes, E. Aurino, J. Kiamba, B. Giyose, and others. 2017. "School Feeding Programs in Middle Childhood and Adolescence." In *Disease Control Priorities* (third edition): Volume 8, *Child and Adolescent Health and Development*, edited by D. A. P. Bundy, N. de Silva, S. Horton, D. T. Jamison, and G. C. Patton. Washington, DC: World Bank.

Duflo, E., P. Dupas, and M. Kremer. 2009. "Additional Resources versus Organizational Changes in Education: Experimental Evidence from Kenya." Unpublished, Abdul Latif Jameel Poverty Action Lab, Massachusetts Institute of Technology, Cambridge, MA.

Evans, D., and A. Popova. 2015. "What Really Works to Improve Learning in Developing Countries?" Policy Research Working Paper 7203, World Bank, Washington, DC.

Fernandes, M. and E. Aurino. 2017. "Identifying an Essential Package for School-Age Child Health: Economic Analysis." In *Disease Control Priorities* (third edition): Volume 8, *Child and Adolescent Health and Development*, edited by D. A. P. Bundy, N. de Silva, S. Horton, D. T. Jamison, and G. C. Patton. Washington, DC: World Bank.

Fernando, D., R. De Silva, K. Carter, N. Mendis, and R. Wickremasinghe. 2006. "A Randomized, Double-Blind, Placebo-Controlled, Clinical Trial of the Impact of Malaria Prevention on the Educational Attainment of School Children." *American Journal of Tropical Medicine* 74 (3): 386–93.

Fernando, D., C. Rodrigo, and S. Rajapakse. 2010. "The Hidden Burden of Malaria: Cognitive Impairment Following Infection." *Malarial Journal* 9 (1): 366.

Foko, B., B. K. Tiyab, and G. Husson. 2012. *Household Education Spending: An Analytical and Comparative Perspective for 15 African Countries.* Dakar: Pole de Dakar, UNESCO-BREDA.

Friedman, W., F. Gerard, and W. Ralaingita. 2010. *International Independent Evaluation of the Effectiveness of Institut pour l'Education Populaire's "Read-Learn-Lead" (RLL) Program in Mali: Mid-Term Report.* Research Triangle Park, NC: RTI International.

García-Huidobro, J. E. 2000. "Educational Politics and Equality in Chile." In *Unequal Schools, Unequal Chances: The Challenges to Equal Opportunity in the Americas*, edited by F. Reimers. Cambridge, MA: Harvard University Press.

Glewwe, P., N. Ilias, and M. Kremer. 2003. "Teacher Incentives." Working Paper 9671, National Bureau of Economic Research, Cambridge, MA.

Glewwe, P., H. Jacoby, and E. King. 2001. "Early Childhood Nutrition and Academic Achievement." *Journal of Public Economics* 81 (3): 345–68.

Glewwe, P., M. Kremer, and S. Moulin. 2009. "Many Children Left Behind? Textbooks and Test Scores in Kenya." *American Economic Journal: Applied Economics* 1 (1): 112–35.

Glewwe, P., M. Kremer, S. Moulin, and E. Zitzewitz. 2004. "Retrospective vs. Prospective Analyses of School Inputs: The Case of Flipcharts in Kenya." *Journal of Development Economics* 74 (1): 251–68.

Glewwe, P., and E. Maïga. 2011. "The Impacts of School Management Reforms in Madagascar: Do the Impacts Vary by Teacher Type?" Department of Applied Economics, University of Minnesota, St. Paul.

Glewwe, P., and E. A. Miguel. 2008. "The Impact of Child Health and Nutrition on Education in Less Developed Countries." In *Handbook of Development Economics*, Vol. 4, edited by T. P. Schultz and J. Strauss. Amsterdam: North-Holland.

Global Partnership for Education. 2013. *Results for Learning Report 2013: Facing the Challenges of Data, Financing, and Fragility*. Washington, DC: Global Partnership for Education.

Gomes-Neto, J. B., E. A. Hanushek, R. H. Leite, and R. C. Frota-Bezzera. 1997. "Health and Schooling: Evidence and Policy Implications for Developing Countries." *Economics of Education Review* 16 (3): 271–82.

Grantham-McGregor, S. M., L. C. H. Fernald, R. M. C. Kagawa, and S. Walker. 2014. "Effects of Integrated Child Development and Nutrition Interventions on Child Development and Nutritional Status." *Annals of the New York Academy of Sciences* 1308 (January): 11–32.

Grigorenko, E. L., R. J. Sternberg, M. C. H. Jukes, K. Alcock, J. Lambo, and others. 2006. "Effects of Antiparasitic Treatment on Dynamically and Statically Tested Cognitive Skills over Time." *Journal of Applied Developmental Psychology* 27 (6): 499–526.

Guyatt, H. 2000. "Do Intestinal Nematodes Affect Productivity in Adulthood?" *Parasitology Today* 16 (4): 153–56.

Halliday, K. E., P. Karanja, E. L. Turner, G. Okello, K. Njagi, and others. 2012. "*Plasmodium falciparum*, Anaemia, and Cognitive and Educational Performance among School Children in an Area of Moderate Malaria Transmission: Baseline Results of a Cluster Randomized Trial on the Coast of Kenya." *Tropical Medicine and International Health* 17 (5): 532–49.

Hieu, N., F. Sandalinas, A. de Sesmaisons, A. Laillou, N. P. Tam, and others. 2012. "Multi-Micronutrient-Fortified Biscuits Decreased the Prevalence of Anaemia and Improved Iron Status, Whereas Weekly Iron Supplementation Only Improved Iron Status in Vietnamese School Children." *British Journal of Nutrition* 108 (8): 1419–27.

Holding, P. A., and R. W. Snow. 2001. "Impact of *Plasmodium falciparum* Malaria on Performance and Learning: Review of the Evidence." *American Journal of Tropical Medicine* 64 (Supp 1–2): 68–75.

Horton, S., and M. M. Black. 2017. "Identifying an Essential Package for Early Childhood Development: Economic Analysis." In *Disease Control Priorities* (third edition): Volume 8, *Child and Adolescent Health and Development*, edited by D. A. P. Bundy, N. de Silva, S. Horton, D. T. Jamison, and G. C. Patton. Washington, DC: World Bank.

Horton, S., E. De la Cruz Toledo, J. Mahon, J. Santelli, and J. Waldfogel. 2017. "Identifying an Essential Package for Adolescent Health: Economic Analysis." In *Disease Control Priorities* (third edition): Volume 8, *Child and Adolescent Health and Development*, edited by D. A. P. Bundy, N. de Silva, S. Horton, D. T. Jamison, and G. C. Patton. Washington, DC: World Bank.

International Commission on Financing Global Education Opportunity. 2016. *The Learning Generation: Investing in Education for a Changing World*. New York: International Commission on Financing Global Education Opportunity

ISS (Institute for Statistics). 2014. *Data Centre*. Paris: UNESCO. http://data.uis.unesco.org/.

ISSP (Institut Supérieur des Sciences de la Population). 2012. "Enquête nationale sur la situation des enfants et adolescents en dehors de l'école." UNICEF, Paris.

Jensen, R. 2010. "The (Perceived) Returns to Education and the Demand for Schooling." *Quarterly Journal of Economics* 125 (2): 515–48.

Jomaa, L., E. McDonnell, and C. Probart. 2011. "School Feeding Programs in Developing Countries: Impacts on Children's Health and Educational Outcomes." *Nutrition Reviews* 69 (2): 83–98.

Jukes, M. C. H., L. J. Drake, and D. A. P. Bundy. 2008. *School Health, Nutrition, and Education for All: Levelling the Playing Field*. Cambridge, MA: CABI Publishing.

Kazianga, H., D. de Walque, and H. Alderman. 2009. "Educational and Health Impacts of Two School Feeding Schemes: Evidence from a Randomized Trial in Rural Burkina Faso." World Bank, Washington, DC.

Kihara, M., J. Carter, and C. Newton. 2006. "The Effect of *Plasmodium falciparum* on Cognition: A Systematic Review." *Tropical Medicine and International Health* 11 (4): 386–97.

Kim, J., H. Alderman, and P. F. Orazem. 1999. "Can Private School Subsidies Increase Enrollment for the Poor? The Quetta Urban Fellowship Program." *World Bank Economic Review* 13 (3): 443–65.

Kremer, M., C. Brannen, and R. Glennerster. 2013. "The Challenge of Education and Learning in the Developing World." *Science* 340 (6130): 297–300.

Kremer, M., S. Moulin, and R. Namanyu. 2003. "Decentralization: A Cautionary Tale." Poverty Action Lab Paper 10, Abdul Latif Jameel Poverty Action Lab, Massachusetts Institute of Technology, Cambridge, MA.

Krishnaratne, S., H. White, and E. Carpenter. 2013. "Quality Education for All Children? What Works in Education in Developing Countries." Working Paper 20, International Initiative for Impact Evaluation (3ie), London.

Lai, F., L. Zhang, X. Hu, Q. Qu, Y. Shi, and others. 2012. "Computer-Assisted Learning as Extracurricular Tutor? Evidence from a Randomized Experiment in Rural Boarding Schools in Shaanxi." Working Paper 235, Rural

Education Action Project (REAP), Stanford University, Stanford, CA.

Lai, F., L. Zhang, Q. Qu, X. Hu, Y. Shi, and others. 2012. "Does Computer-Assisted Learning Improve Learning Outcomes? Evidence from a Randomized Experiment in Public Schools in Rural Minority Areas in Qinghai." Working Paper 237, Rural Education Action Project (REAP), Stanford University, Stanford, CA.

Lucas, A. M., P. J. McEwan, M. Ngware, and M. Oketch. 2014. "Improving Early-Grade Literacy in East Africa: Experimental Evidence from Kenya and Uganda." *Journal of Policy Analysis and Management* 33 (4): 950–76.

Martorell, R. 1996. "Undernutrition during Pregnancy and Early Childhood and Its Consequences for Behavioral Development." Paper prepared for the conference "Early Child Development: Investing in the Future," World Bank, Washington, DC, April 8–9.

McEwan, P. 2015. "Improving Learning in Primary Schools of Developing Countries: A Meta-Analysis of Randomized Experiments." *Review of Educational Research* 85 (3): 353–94.

Mendez, M., and L. Adair. 1999. "Severity and Timing of Stunting in the First Two Years of Life Affect Performance on Cognitive Tests in Late Childhood." *Journal of Nutrition* 129 (8): 1555–62.

Miguel, E., and M. Kremer. 2004. "Worms: Identifying Impacts on Education and Health in the Presence of Treatment Externalities." *Econometrica* 72 (1): 159–217.

Muralidharan, K., and V. Sundararaman. 2008. *Teacher Performance Pay: Experimental Evidence from India.* Cambridge, MA: Harvard University.

Murnane, R. J., and A. J. Ganimian. 2014. "Improving Educational Outcomes in Developing Countries: Lessons from Rigorous Evaluations." Working Paper 20284, National Bureau of Economic Research, Cambridge, MA.

Nankabirwa, J., S. J. Brooker, S. E. Clarke, D. Fernando, C. W. Gitonga, and others. 2014. "Malaria in School-Age Children in Africa: An Increasingly Important Challenge." *Tropical Medicine and International Health* 19 (11): 1294–309.

Nguyen, T. 2008. "Information, Role Models, and Perceived Returns to Education: Experimental Evidence from Madagascar." Unpublished, Abdul Latif Jameel Poverty Action Lab, Massachusetts Institute of Technology, Cambridge, MA.

Ogutu, R., A. Oloo, W. Ekissa, I. Genga, N. Mulaya, and others. 1992. "The Effect of Participatory School Health Programme on the Control of Malaria." *East African Medical Journal* 69 (6): 298–302.

Ozier, O. 2014. "Exploiting Externalities to Estimate the Long-Term Effects of Early Childhood Deworming." Policy Research Working Paper 7052, World Bank, Washington, DC.

Petrosino, A., C. Morgan, T. Fronius, E. Tanner-Smith, and B. Boruch. 2012. "Interventions in Developing Nations for Improving Primary and Secondary School Enrollment of Children: A Systematic Review." Campbell Collaboration, Oslo.

Piper, B., and M. Korda. 2010. "EGRA Plus: Liberia." Program Evaluation Report, RTI International, Research Triangle Park, NC.

Pradhan, E., E. M. Suzuki, S. Martínez, M. Schäferhoff, and D. T. Jamison. 2017. "The Effects of Education Quantity and Quality on Mortality: Their Magnitude and Their Value." In *Disease Control Priorities* (third edition): Volume 8, *Child and Adolescent Health and Development*, edited by D. A. P. Bundy, N. de Silva, S. Horton, D. T. Jamison, and G. C. Patton. Washington, DC: World Bank.

Pradhan, M., D. Suryadarma, A. Beatty, M. Wong, A. Alishjabana, and others. 2011. "Improving Educational Quality through Enhancing Community Participation: Results from a Randomized Field Experiment in Indonesia." Policy Research Working Paper 5795, World Bank, Washington, DC.

Simeon, D. T., S. M. Grantham-McGregor, J. E. Callender, and M. S. Wong. 1995. "Treatment of *Trichuris trichiura* Infections Improves Growth, Spelling Scores, and School Attendance in Some Children." *Journal of Nutrition* 125 (7): 1875–83.

Skoufias, E., and J. Shapiro. 2006. "Evaluating the Impact of Mexico's Quality Schools Program: The Pitfalls of Using Nonexperimental Data." Policy Research Working Paper 4036, World Bank, Washington, DC.

Stephenson, L. S., M. C. Latham, and K. M. Kurz. 1985. "Relationships of *Schistosoma haematobium*, Hookworm, and Malarial Infections and Metrifonate Treatment to Hemoglobin Level in Kenyan School Children." *American Journal of Tropical Medicine and Hygiene* 34 (3): 519–28.

Sungthong, R., L. Mo-Suwan, V. Chongsuvivatwong, and A. F. Geater. 2004. "Once-Weekly and 5-Days a Week Iron Supplementation Differentially Affect Cognitive Function but Not School Performance in Thai Children." *Journal of Nutrition* 134 (9): 2349–54.

Taylor-Robinson, D. C., N. Maayan, K. Soares-Weiser, S. Donegan, and P. Garner. 2015. "Deworming Drugs for Soil-Transmitted Intestinal Worms in Children: Effects on Nutritional Indicators, Haemoglobin, and School Performance (Review)." *Cochrane Database of Systematic Reviews* 4: CD000371.

Thomas, M., and N. Burnett. 2013. *Exclusion from Education: The Economic Cost of Out of School Children in 20 Countries.* Ar-Rayyan, Qatar: Educate A Child; Washington, DC: Results for Development Institute.

Thuilliez, J., M. S. Sissoko, O. B. Toure, P. Kamate, M. B. Niambele, and others. 2010. "Malaria and Primary Education in Mali: A Longitudinal Study in the Village of Donéguébougou." *Social Science and Medicine* 71 (2): 324–34.

Tipton, E. 2015. "Small Sample Adjustments for Robust Variance Estimation with Meta Regression." *Psychological Methods* 20 (3): 375–93.

UNESCO (United Nations Educational, Scientific and Cultural Organization). 2013. *Education for All Global Monitoring Report: Educating Girls Can Save Millions of Lives.* Paris: UNESCO.

———. 2014. *Education for All Global Monitoring Report 2013/4: Teaching and Learning; Achieving Quality for All.* Paris: UNESCO.

———. 2015. *Education for All Global Monitoring Report 2015: Education for All 2000–2015; Achievement and Challenges.* Paris: UNESCO.

UNICEF (United Nations Children's Fund). 2013. *Improving Child Nutrition: The Achievable Imperative for Global Progress*. New York: UNICEF.

Uwezo. 2013. *Are Our Children Learning? Literacy and Numeracy across East Africa*. Nairobi: Uwezo.

WFP (World Food Programme). 2013. *State of School Feeding Worldwide*. Rome: WFP.

WHO (World Health Organization). 2016. "Soil-Transmitted Helminth Infections: Fact Sheet." WHO, Geneva. http://www.who.int/mediacentre/factsheets/fs366/en/.

World Bank. 2013. "Millennium Development Goals Tables." World Bank, Washington, DC.

———. 2015. "Health, Nutrition, and Population Data and Statistics." World Bank, Washington, DC. http://datatopics.worldbank.org/hnp/.

Wu, K. B. 2017. "Global Variation in Education Outcomes at Ages 5 to 19." In *Disease Control Priorities* (third edition): Volume 8, *Child and Adolescent Health and Development*, edited by D. A. P. Bundy, N. de Silva, S. Horton, D. T. Jamison, and G. C. Patton. Washington, DC: World Bank.

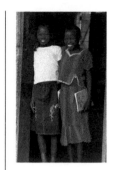

Chapter **23**

Cash Transfers and Child and Adolescent Development

Damien de Walque, Lia Fernald, Paul Gertler, Melissa Hidrobo

INTRODUCTION

Poverty has significant, detrimental, and long-ranging effects on child development (Walker and others 2011). Programs and policies around the world have attempted to address poverty to improve outcomes for children and adolescents, and one popular approach is to use cash transfer (CT) programs (Engle and others 2011). CT programs support vulnerable populations by distributing transfers to low-income households to prevent shocks; protect the chronically poor; promote capabilities and opportunities for vulnerable households; and transform systems of power that exclude certain marginalized groups, such as women or children (Devereux and Sabates-Wheeler 2004). The economic rationale for CT programs is that they can be an equitable and efficient way to address market failures and reach the most vulnerable populations (Fiszbein and others 2009).

When the provision of CTs is tied to mandatory behavioral requirements, they are conditional cash transfer (CCT) programs, which operate by giving cash payments to families only if they comply with a set of requirements (the "conditions" of the cash transfer), usually related to health and education (de Janvry and Sadoulet 2006). For example, many CCT programs distribute benefits conditional on the use of preventive health care services, attendance at health and nutrition education sessions designed to promote positive behavioral changes, or school attendance for school-age children (Barrientos and DeJong 2006; Lagarde, Haines, and Palmer 2007). Definitions of age groupings and age-specific terminology used in this volume can be found in chapter 1 (Bundy and others 2017).

Unconditional cash transfer (UCT) programs are those in which families receive cash benefits because the household falls below a certain income cutoff or lives within a geographically targeted region; however, no conditions are tied to the transfer (Barrientos and DeJong 2006). Given that UCTs do not monitor the behavior of households or require visits to health clinics, these programs are operationally less complex and easier for governments to implement because they do not require a well-functioning health care sector. Thus, administrative costs are often substantially lower for UCTs than for CCTs. School feeding is an example of a noncash transfer and is discussed in chapter 12 of this volume (Drake and others 2017).

Both CCTs and UCTs assume that parents are income constrained, and thus do not have the money to spend to meet the most pressing needs of their families (for example, nutritious food, medical treatment). Providing greater purchasing power allows parents to choose what goods to buy and in what quantity and of what quality. The economic rationale for conditioning transfers on certain behaviors is that individuals or households do not always behave rationally because they have imperfect information, they behave myopically, or there are conflicts of interest between parents and children (Fiszbein and others 2009). In addition, conditioning transfers on human capital creates positive externalities and usually

Corresponding author: Damien de Walque, Development Research Group, World Bank, Washington, DC, United States; ddewalque@worldbank.org.

has more political support. However, many argue that conditioning transfers is paternalistic and costly to monitor and that the neediest households might find it too costly to comply (Grimes and Wängnerud 2010; Handa and Davis 2006; Popay and others 2008; Shibuya 2008).

Mexico's Prospera (previously Progresa and Oportunidades) and Brazil's Bolsa Familia were among the first CCTs to be designed in the late 1990s and have been models for programs throughout Africa, Latin America, and the United States (Aber and Rawlings 2011; Fiszbein and others 2009). By 2011, CT programs covered an estimated 750 million to 1 billion people worldwide; India (48 million households), China (22 million households), Brazil (12 million households), and Mexico (5 million households) were among the countries with the largest programs (DFID 2011). In spite of the common features of many CTs, there is a large degree of heterogeneity across countries and programs with regard to program benefits, conditions, requirements, payments, and targets. For example, in Ecuador and Peru, the transfer is a fixed payment per family per month that does not vary by household size, whereas in Brazil, Malawi, and Mexico the benefits depend on the number, age, and gender of children in the household. In some programs (for example, Prospera in Mexico and Familias en Acción in Colombia), the payment is greater for secondary-school-age children than for primary-school-age children. Similarly, the average transfer amount varies greatly, ranging from 6 percent in Brazil to 22 percent to 29 percent in Mexico and Nicaragua to 200 percent of pretransfer consumption in Malawi (Fiszbein and others 2009; Miller, Tsoka, and Reichert 2010). The size of the transfer reflects the goal of the program, which can be to move households to a minimum level of consumption (Colombia, Jamaica, Mexico) or to base the size of the transfer on the opportunity cost of health care (Honduras) or on the transportation costs to the public health facility (Nepal) (Gaarder, Glassman, and Todd 2010).

This chapter first reviews the evidence from CT programs, both conditional and unconditional, throughout low- and middle-income countries (LMICs), focusing specifically on the direct effects on child and adolescent health and education outcomes. It then discusses the design of CT programs and why and how they could theoretically affect outcomes for young children and adolescents. Although there are other types of social safety net programs, such as voucher schemes, food transfers, and user fee removals, we focus on CTs because many countries are switching to such programs given that they are easier to distribute. In addition, the evidence for many other types of programs is too sparse for them to be included in the analysis.

CT programs are hypothesized to improve child and adolescent outcomes via the family investment model,

according to which families have more money to spend on inputs (Guo and Harris 2000; Yeung, Linver, and Brooks-Gunn 2002) or more time to spend with children (Del Boca, Flinn, and Wiswall 2014), and the family stress model, according to which maternal depression and stress are lower because household resources are higher (Mistry and others 2004).

CCT and UCT programs can vary widely in their objectives, design, and context. While many programs have the broad goals of reducing poverty and improving human capital, some are more focused on decreasing poverty, some on improving education outcomes, some on improving health outcomes, and some on improving nutrition outcomes. Program designs reflect these differences in objectives with differences in conditions, targeting, transfer size, beneficiaries, and complementary components. Consequently, although CCT and UCT programs have the potential to effect multiple outcomes by lessening a household's budget constraints, some programs and contexts may be better suited to improving child and adolescent health and education outcomes. For example, programs in a handful of countries are beginning to experiment with the integration of parenting support or nutritional support—a direct intervention to promote child development—within CT programs (for example, in Colombia, see Attanasio and others 2014; in Mexico, see Fernald and others 2016).

The literature review proceeded as follows. We began by examining the conclusions in the 2011 *Lancet* series on early child development in LMICs (Engle and others 2011; Walker and others 2011) and in five systematic reviews addressing CCTs published since 2011 (Bassani and others 2013; Fernald, Gertler, and Hidrobo 2012; Glassman, Duran, and Koblinsky 2013; Manley, Gitter, and Slavchevska 2013; Ruel, Alderman, and Maternal and Child Nutrition Study Group 2013). We then conducted a literature search to find papers that had been published since those systematic reviews. The search used Google Scholar, JSTOR, and PubMed for peer-reviewed articles and websites of the International Food Policy Research Institute, United Nations Children's Fund, and the World Bank for gray papers. The search was restricted to studies that used experimental or quasi-experimental techniques such as randomization, regression discontinuity, propensity score matching, or difference-in-differences.

We found evidence from studies examining the effects of CTs on birth weight (3 studies); infant mortality (6 studies); height-for-age (or stunting) (23 studies); weight-for-age (or underweight) (12 studies); weight-for-height (or wasting) (10 studies); hemoglobin (or anemia) (10 studies); morbidity (16 studies); cognitive, language, and behavioral development (11 studies); and sexual and reproductive health (9 studies) (table 23.1).

Table 23.1 Summary of Cash Transfer Effects

Indicator	Significant effects of CT on outcome	Significant effects of CT only in subgroups or some measures	No effects or adverse effect of CT
Birth and neonatal outcomes			
Birth weight	Mexico (Barber and Gertler 2010) Uruguay (Amarante and others 2012)	Colombia, urban areas (Attanasio and others 2005)	
Perinatal, neonatal, or infant mortality	Brazil (Shei 2013) Brazil (Rasella and others 2013) India (Lim and others 2010)	Mexico, infant mortality, but not neonatal (Barham 2011)	Indonesia (World Bank 2011) Nepal (Powell-Jackson and others 2009)
Anthropometric measures			
Height, height-for-age, stunting (HAZ)	Mexico (Gertler 2004) Mexico, rural (Neufeld and others 2005) Mexico (Behrman and Hoddinott 2005) Mexico (Fernald, Gertler, and Neufeld 2008) Sri Lanka (Himaz 2008)	Burkina Faso, one-year impact (Akresh, de Walque, and Kazianga 2016) Colombia, children < age 24 months (Attanasio and others 2005) Malawi, children ages 5–18 years (Miller, Tsoka, and Reichert 2010) Mexico, rural, children < age 6 months (Rivera and others 2004) Mexico, urban, children < age 6 months (Leroy and others 2008) Mexico, rural, less-educated mothers (Fernald, Gertler, and Neufeld 2009) Nicaragua, stunting (Maluccio and Flores 2005) Nicaragua, one-year impact (Macours, Schady, and Vakis 2012) South Africa, exposed at age 0–35 months (Agüero, Carter, and Woolard 2009)	Bangladesh (Ahmed and others 2009) Brazil (Morris, Olinto, and others 2004) Ecuador (Paxson and Schady 2010) Ecuador (Fernald and Hidrobo 2011) Indonesia (World Bank 2011) Mexico, urban (Neufeld 2005) Peru (Perova and Vakis 2009) Tanzania (Evans, Holtemeyer, and Kosec 2015) Zambia (Seidenfeld and others 2014)
Weight-for-age, underweight (WAZ)	*Increased weight or decreased underweight:* Nicaragua (Maluccio and Flores 2005) *Decreased weight:* Brazil (Morris, Olinto, and others 2004) Indonesia (World Bank 2011)	Mexico, children < age 6 months (Leroy and others 2008) Mexico, rural, children ages 48–71 months (Neufeld and others 2005) Zambia, WAZ (Seidenfeld and others 2014)	Bangladesh (Ahmed and others 2009) Burkina Faso (Akresh, de Walque, and Kazianga 2016) Malawi (Miller, Tsoka, and Reichert 2010) Nicaragua (Macours, Schady, and Vakis 2012) Peru (Perova and Vakis 2009) Tanzania (Evans, Holtemeyer, and Kosec 2015)
Weight-for-height (wasting, WHZ), BMI	*Decreased BMI or overweight:* Mexico (Fernald, Gertler, and Neufeld 2008)	Mexico, children < age 6 months (Leroy and others 2008) Sri Lanka, children, ages 36–60 months (Himaz 2008) Zambia, WHZ (Seidenfeld and others 2014)	Bangladesh (Ahmed and others 2009) Indonesia (World Bank 2011) Mexico, urban (Neufeld 2005) Mexico (Fernald, Gertler, and Neufeld 2009) Nicaragua (Maluccio and Flores 2005) Tanzania (Evans, Holtemeyer, and Kosec 2015)

table continues next page

Table 23.1 Summary of Cash Transfer Effects *(continued)*

Indicator	Significant effects of CT on outcome	Significant effects of CT only in subgroups or some measures	No effects or adverse effect of CT
Measures of morbidity and anemia			
Illness or sick days	Brazil (Reis 2010)	Mexico, rural areas (Gutiérrez and others 2004)	Ghana (Handa, Park, and others 2014)
	Burkina Faso (Akresh, de Walque, and Kazianga 2016)	Tanzania, two-year evaluation (Evans, Holtemeyer, and Kosec 2015)	Jamaica (Levy and Ohls 2007)
	Malawi (Miller, Tsoka, and Reichert 2010)		Mexico (Fernald, Gertler, and Neufeld 2008)
	Mexico (Gertler 2000)		Peru (Perova and Vakis 2012)
	Mexico (Gertler 2004)		
	Mexico (Gutiérrez and others 2006)		
	Peru (Perova and Vakis 2009)		
Specific illnesses	Uganda (Gilligan and Roy 2014)	Colombia, rural areas, < age 48 months (Attanasio and others 2005)	Brazil (Reis 2010)
			Indonesia (World Bank 2011)
Hemoglobin, anemia	Mexico (Gertler 2004)	Ecuador, poorest quintile, rural (Paxson and Schady 2010)	Mexico (Neufeld and others 2005)
	Uganda (Gilligan and Roy 2014)	Mexico, urban, ages 6–23 months (Neufeld 2005)	Mexico (Fernald, Gertler, and Neufeld 2008)
		Mexico, rural, at one-year, not two-year evaluation (Rivera and others 2004)	Ecuador (Fernald and Hidrobo 2011)
			Nicaragua (Maluccio and Flores 2005)
			Peru (Perova and Vakis 2009)
Developmental outcomes			
Cognition and language	Mexico (Fernald, Gertler, and Neufeld 2008)	Ecuador, poorest quintile of rural population (Paxson and Schady 2010)	Mexico (Fernald, Gertler, and Neufeld 2009)
	Nicaragua (Macours, Schady, and Vakis 2008, 2012)	Ecuador, children of rural mothers with no education (Fernald and Hidrobo 2011)	Peru (Andersen and others 2015)
	Nicaragua (Barham, Macours, and Maluccio 2013)		Zambia (Seidenfeld and others 2014)
	Uganda (Gilligan and Roy 2014)		
Behavior	Mexico (Ozer and others 2009) Mexico (Fernald, Gertler, and Neufeld 2009)		
Indirect effects of cash transfer programs			
Antenatal care	Bangladesh (Nguyen and others 2012)	Mexico, prenatal care quality (Barber and Gertler 2010)	El Salvador (De Brauw and Peterman 2011)
	Honduras (Morris, Flores, and others 2004)	Mexico, urban and rural in 2000 (Hernández Prado and others 2004)	Nepal (Powell-Jackson and others 2009)
	India (Lim and others 2010)	Mexico, certain specifications only (Sosa-Rubí and others 2011)	Peru (Perova and Vakis 2009)
	Indonesia (World Bank 2011)		Zambia (Handa, Peterman, Seidenfeld, and others 2015)
	Uruguay (Amarante and others 2012)		
Presence of skilled birth attendant at birth, in-facility birth	Bangladesh (Nguyen and others 2012)	Indonesia, certain specifications only (World Bank 2011)	Mexico (Urquieta and others 2009)
	El Salvador (De Brauw and Peterman 2011)	Mexico, rural (Hernández Prado and others 2004)	Uruguay (Amarante and others 2012)
	India (Lim and others 2010)	Peru, certain specifications only (Perova and Vakis 2009)	Zambia (Handa, Peterman, Seidenfeld, and others 2015)
	Nepal (Powell-Jackson and others 2009)		
	Nepal (Powell-Jackson and Hanson 2012)		

table continues next page

Table 23.1 Summary of Cash Transfer Effects (continued)

Indicator	Significant effects of CT on outcome	Significant effects of CT only in subgroups or some measures	No effects or adverse effect of CT
Growth monitoring	Colombia (Attanasio and others 2005) Honduras (Morris, Flores, and others 2004) Jamaica (Levy and Ohls 2007) Mexico (Gertler 2000) Mexico (Gutiérrez and others 2004, 2006) Nicaragua (Macours, Schady, and Vakis 2012) Peru (Perova and Vakis 2009) Peru (Perova and Vakis 2012)	Burkina Faso, CCT not UCT (Akresh, de Walque, and Kazianga 2012) Nicaragua, one-year evaluation (Maluccio and Flores 2005) Tanzania, one-year evaluation (Evans, Holtemeyer, and Kosec 2015)	Ecuador (Paxson and Schady 2010) Ecuador (Fernald and Hidrobo 2011) Ghana (Handa, Park, and others 2014)
Child food consumption	Colombia (Attanasio and Mesnard 2006) Nicaragua (Macours, Schady, and Vakis 2008) Uganda (Gilligan and Roy 2014)		Bangladesh (Ahmed and others 2009) Ecuador (Fernald and Hidrobo 2011)
Sexual and reproductive health			
HIV/AIDS	Malawi, UCT and CCT for education (Baird and others 2012) Lesotho, lottery incentives if STI-negative (Björkman Nyqvist and others 2015)		South Africa, CCT for education (Pettifor and others 2015) South Africa (Abdool Karim and others 2015) Malawi, CCT if HIV-negative (Kohler and Thornton 2012)
Sexually transmitted infections	Malawi, UCT and CCT for education (Baird and others 2012) Kenya, education subsidy combined *with* HIV/AIDS education, but not without (Duflo, Dupas, and Kremer 2015) South Africa, CCT for education (Abdool Karim and others 2015) Lesotho, lottery incentives if STI-negative (Björkman Nyqvist and others 2015)	Tanzania, CCT if STI-negative (de Walque and others 2012; de Walque, Dow, and Nathan 2014)	
Sexual behaviors		Malawi, UCT and CCT for education (Baird and others 2012) Kenya, UCT (Handa, Halpern, and others 2014) Kenya, education subsidy combined *with* HIV/AIDS education, but not without (Duflo, Dupas, and Kremer 2015) South Africa, UCT (Cluver and others 2013) South Africa, CCT for education (Pettifor and others 2015) Tanzania, CCT if STI negative (de Walque and others 2012; de Walque, Dow, and Nathan 2014) Lesotho, lottery incentives if STI-negative (Björkman Nyqvist and others 2015)	Malawi, CCT if HIV-negative (Kohler and Thornton 2012)

Note: BMI = body mass index; CT = cash transfer; CCT = conditional cash transfer; HAZ = height-for-age z score; HIV/AIDS = human immunodeficiency virus/acquired immune deficiency syndrome; STI = sexually transmitted infection; UCT = unconditional cash transfer; WAZ = weight-for-age z score; WHZ = weight-for-height.

IMPACT OF CASH TRANSFERS ON HEALTH OUTCOMES

Birth Weight

Low birth weight is a major determinant of health outcomes in childhood and later life. In Latin America, CCTs and UCTs have been found to increase birth weight (Amarante and others 2012; Attanasio and others 2005; Barber and Gertler 2010). In Colombia and Mexico, the effect of CCTs on birth weight was between 0.13 and 0.58 kilograms, although in Colombia, the effect was only significant in urban areas. CTs also decreased the incidence of low birth weight (defined as less than 2,500 grams) by 5 percent in Mexico and 15 percent to 17 percent in Uruguay. Neither the Mexico nor the Uruguay study found any changes in the use of antenatal care associated with participation in the CT programs. However, in Mexico, improvements in birth weight were attributed to improvements in quality of care. In Uruguay, improvements in birth weight were attributed to improvements in mothers' nutrition and a fall in mothers' labor supply and smoking.

Perinatal, Neonatal, or Infant Mortality

Three studies from the review in Fernald, Gertler, and Neufeld (2012) and three more-recent studies investigated the effect of CTs on perinatal mortality (stillbirth after 28 weeks of pregnancy or death of a child within the first week of birth), neonatal mortality (death of a child within the first month of birth), infant mortality (death of a child within the first year of birth), or under-five mortality. Four of the six studies found significant decreases in mortality rates in Brazil, India, and Mexico (Barham 2011; Lim and others 2010; Rasella and others 2013; Shei 2013). More than half of the decline in infant mortality in Mexico resulted from reductions in respiratory and intestinal infections and nutritional deficiencies (Barham 2011). However, studies in Indonesia (World Bank 2011) and Nepal (Powell-Jackson and others 2009) found no significant impact on neonatal or infant mortality.

Self-Reported Child Health: Illness or Morbidity

Of the studies reviewed, 16 investigated the effects of CTs on reported illness or morbidity. Most programs found significant positive effects on measures of illness and morbidity, such as sick days, reported diarrhea, or reported respiratory problems. Studies in Brazil (Reis 2010), Burkina Faso (Akresh, de Walque, and Kazianga 2016), Malawi (Miller, Tsoka, and Reichert 2010), and Tanzania (Evans, Holtemeyer, and Kosec 2015) found

that CTs significantly decreased the number of reported illnesses or sick days. In contrast, program participation had no significant effect on reported illness in Jamaica (Levy and Ohls 2007) and was associated with an increase in reported illness among children ages zero to five years in Ghana (Handa, Park, and others 2014). In Mexico, three evaluations reported a significant decrease in illness rates in the treatment groups (Gertler 2000, 2004; Gutiérrez and others 2006); one evaluation (Gutiérrez and others 2004) found a significant decrease in reported sick days in rural areas, but not urban; and one evaluation (Fernald, Gertler, and Neufeld 2008) found no significant association between the size of the CT received by the family and self-reported sick days of the child. In Peru, results were similarly mixed: a two-year evaluation reported that children in Juntos were less likely to be ill (Perova and Vakis 2009), but a five-year evaluation found no impact on self-reported illness (Perova and Vakis 2012).

Studies in Brazil (Reis 2010), Colombia (Attanasio and others 2005), Indonesia (World Bank 2011), and Uganda (Gilligan and Roy 2014) analyzed the effect of CCTs on specific reported illnesses, such as diarrhea, fever, respiratory conditions, and vomiting. In Uganda (Gilligan and Roy 2014), there was a significant decrease in reported diarrhea rates, while in Colombia, there was a significant decrease in reported diarrhea for rural children, but not for urban children, and there was no impact on respiratory conditions for children in rural or urban areas. In Brazil, although the CT program significantly improved children's morbidity, it had no significant impact on reported vomiting, diarrhea, respiratory conditions, and bed days. Contrary to expectations, in Indonesia, the program significantly increased reports of fever and diarrhea.

Anthropometric Measures

Anthropometric indicators are widely used to assess children's nutritional status. Persistent or severe poor nutrition has direct effects on linear growth and the ability to accumulate muscle mass and fat (Hoddinott and Bassett 2008). Height-for-age z score (HAZ) is a measure of chronic malnutrition, with stunting (HAZ lower than −2 standard deviations) representing an internationally recognized cutoff (WHO 1986). Weight-for-height z score (WHZ) is a measure of acute malnutrition, with wasting (WHZ lower than −2 standard deviations) reflecting a deficit in tissue and fat mass. Weight-for-age z score (WAZ) is a composite indicator of HAZ and WHZ and thus captures both transitory and chronic aspects of malnutrition (Hoddinott and Bassett 2008).

Height-for-Age

The evidence linking CCTs to improvements in child height was mixed, both across and within countries. In Mexico alone, four studies found a significant effect of the program on height (Behrman and Hoddinott 2005; Fernald, Gertler, and Neufeld 2008; Gertler 2004; Neufeld and others 2005), three found significant improvements only for specific subpopulations such as children ages zero to six months (Leroy and others 2008; Rivera and others 2004) or children of mothers with no education (Fernald, Gertler, and Neufeld 2009), and one study found no significant effects in urban areas (Neufeld 2005).

Evaluations of other CCT programs were also inconclusive: in Bangladesh (Ahmed and others 2009), Brazil (Morris, Olinto, and others 2004), Indonesia (World Bank 2011), Peru (Perova and Vakis 2009), and Tanzania (Evans, Holtemeyer, and Kosec 2015), there were no significant effects on children's height. In Nicaragua, a study of the Red de Protección Social Program (Maluccio and Flores 2005) found no impact on HAZ, but a significant decrease in stunting, while a study of the Atención a Crisis Program (Macours, Schady, and Vakis 2012) found a significant improvement in HAZ after adding extended controls, but these impacts had faded two years after the program ended. Similarly, in Burkina Faso, CCTs led to significant improvements in HAZ after one year, but no significant impacts were detected after two years (Akresh, de Walque, and Kazianga 2016). In Colombia, there was a significant improvement in children's HAZ, but only for children younger than age 24 months (Attanasio and others 2005).

The evidence for UCTs was also inconclusive. There was a significant improvement in children's HAZ in Sri Lanka (Himaz 2008), but no effect on young children's HAZ in Ecuador and Zambia (Fernald and Hidrobo 2011; Paxson and Schady 2010; Seidenfeld and others 2014). In South Africa, there was a significant improvement in height for children who had been exposed to the CT program more than 50 percent of the time when they were age 0–35 months (Agüero, Carter, and Woolard 2009). In Malawi, there was a significant improvement in height for children ages 5–18 years, but no significant effect on the prevalence of stunting for children younger than age 5 years, although the sample size for this subpopulation was quite small (Miller, Tsoka, and Reichert 2010).

These mixed findings are consistent with a meta-analysis showing small and nonsignificant impacts of CTs on child HAZ across 17 programs (Manley, Gitter, and Slavchevska 2013). Because of limitations in the study designs, it is not possible to determine whether the lack of significant effects on height in some studies was due to small sample sizes, to children being older and thus less sensitive to nutritional inputs (Victora and others 2010), to a lack of improvement in children's nutritional intake, or to delays and errors in program implementation. Although many studies show improvements in food consumption and health service use, many factors could limit the effectiveness of CTs in improving nutritional status, such as the quality of children's diet and health services, knowledge of adequate feeding practices, and environmental risks such as contaminated water and malaria (Bassett 2008; Manley, Gitter, and Slavchevska 2013).

Weight-for-Height

The evidence of the impact of CTs on WHZ or wasting in general reveals little to no impact. Studies of CTs in Bangladesh (Ahmed and others 2009), Indonesia (World Bank 2011), Nicaragua (Maluccio and Flores 2005), and Tanzania (Evans, Holtemeyer, and Kosec 2015) found no impact on wasting or WHZ. However, a study of a UCT in Zambia (Seidenfeld and others 2014) found an increase in WHZ, but no impact on wasting, and a study of a UCT in Sri Lanka (Himaz 2008) found a significant increase in WHZ, but only among children ages 36–60 months. In Mexico, Neufeld and others (2005) found no effect of the program on WHZ, while Leroy and others (2008) found a significant increase in WHZ, but only for children younger than age 6 months. Also in Mexico, Fernald, Gertler, and Neufeld (2008) found that receiving a greater amount of cash from Oportunidades was associated with lower body mass index– (BMI-) for-age in children ages 3–5 years and a lower prevalence of overweight, but the effect on BMI had disappeared after 10 years (Fernald, Gertler, and Neufeld 2009).

Weight-for-Age

The effects of CCT and UCT programs on WAZ or the prevalence of underweight are mixed, although the majority of studies found no significant effects or only found effects in subgroups. CCT studies in Bangladesh (Ahmed and others 2009), Nicaragua (Macours, Schady, and Vakis 2012), Peru (Perova and Vakis 2009), and Tanzania (Evans, Holtemeyer, and Kosec 2015) found no impact on WAZ or underweight; a different study in Nicaragua (Maluccio and Flores 2005) found a significant reduction in the prevalence of underweight. CCT studies in Brazil (Morris, Olinto, and others 2004) and Indonesia (World Bank 2011) found a decrease in weight. Findings regarding the impacts of UCTs on weight are also inconclusive; a study in Malawi (Miller, Tsoka, and Reichert 2010) found no impact on weight or the prevalence of underweight, and a study in Zambia

(Seidenfeld and others 2014) found an increase in WAZ but no impact on the prevalence of underweight. In Burkina Faso, neither CCTs nor UCTs had an impact on WAZ (Akresh, de Walque, and Kazianga 2016).

In Mexico, results for the effect of Oportunidades on weight outcomes were also mixed. Neufeld and others (2005) found that the prevalence of underweight in rural areas increased in response to the program for children age 48 months and older, but not for younger children and that the program had no significant impact on the prevalence of overweight or on WAZ. A study by Leroy and others (2008), however, found a significant increase in weight for children younger than age six months.

Hemoglobin

Of the nine studies reviewed in Fernald, Gertler, and Hidrobo (2012) and one more-recent study, five found no effects of CT programs on hemoglobin levels or anemia (Fernald, Gertler, and Neufeld 2008; Fernald and Hidrobo 2011; Maluccio and Flores 2005; Neufeld and others 2005; Perova and Vakis 2009). Two studies (one in Ecuador and one in Mexico) found improvements in hemoglobin levels, but only for subgroups (Neufeld 2005; Paxson and Schady 2010). Two studies (one in Mexico and one in Uganda) found that CTs led to significant improvements in hemoglobin or anemia rates (Gertler 2004; Gilligan and Roy 2014); one study (Rivera and others 2004) found significant improvements only in the one-year evaluation, but not in the two-year evaluation, when the late intervention group began receiving the CCT.

Intermediate Pathways

CT programs could affect children's development through several intermediate pathways, such as increased use of health services by pregnant mothers and young children, increased parasite treatments and vitamin supplements, increased food consumption, and improved physical and psychological well-being of mothers. Given space limitations, this chapter provides an overview only of the findings related to the conditions present in many CT programs—health service use for pregnant women and young children and food consumption of individual children.

Health Service Use: Pregnant Women

The programs reviewed varied widely in scope. Programs in Bangladesh, India (Janani Suraksha Yojana Program), and Nepal (Nepal's Safe Delivery Incentive Program) focused on pregnant women with the aim of encouraging antenatal care and professional care at childbirth, while programs in El Salvador, Honduras, Indonesia, Mexico, and Peru were broader in their outreach, but still required pregnant women to seek prenatal care. UCT programs in Uruguay and Zambia had no antenatal care requirements. A systematic review showed that CCTs increased antenatal care, skilled attendance at birth, and births at clinics (Glassman, Duran, and Koblinsky 2013). However, the results were mixed, generally depending on the focus of the program.

There was no significant impact on the number of antenatal visits in El Salvador (De Brauw and Peterman 2011), Nepal (Powell-Jackson and others 2009), or Zambia (Handa, Peterman, Seidenfeld, and others 2015). However, the programs in Bangladesh, Honduras, India, Indonesia, and Uruguay significantly increased either the probability or the number of antenatal visits (Amarante and others 2012; Lim and others 2010; Morris, Flores, and others 2004; Nguyen and others 2012; World Bank 2011), while the CCT in Peru decreased the probability of prenatal visits (Perova and Vakis 2009). In Mexico, prenatal care increased approximately 6 percent in urban areas, but the results for rural areas were mixed and depended on the evaluation method used (Barber and Gertler 2010; Hernández Prado and others 2004; Sosa-Rubí and others 2011). Even though the study by Barber and Gertler (2010) did not find a significant impact on the use of prenatal care, it did find a significant impact on the quality of prenatal care, with beneficiary women receiving, on average, more of the recommended procedures during their prenatal appointments.

The CCT programs in Bangladesh, India, and Nepal had a specific goal of increasing professional care at childbirth, and indeed these programs significantly increased both the probability of having an in-facility birth and the probability of having a skilled birth attendant (Lim and others 2010; Nguyen and others 2012; Powell-Jackson and Hanson 2012; Powell-Jackson and others 2009). CCT programs in El Salvador, Indonesia, and Peru also led to an increase in the probability of having a skilled attendant at birth (De Brauw and Peterman 2011; Perova and Vakis 2012; Triyana 2014; World Bank 2011); however, the impacts in Indonesia and Peru depended on the empirical specification (Perova and Vakis 2009; World Bank 2011). UCT programs in Uruguay and Zambia had no impact on having a skilled attendant present at birth (Amarante and others 2012; Handa, Peterman, Seidenfeld, and others 2015). In Mexico, Hernández Prado and others (2004) found that Oportunidades increased the probability of having a doctor present at birth in rural areas, but decreased the probability in urban areas, while Urquieta and others (2009) found no significant impact on the probability of having a skilled attendant present at birth.

Health Service Use: Young Children

Although a large majority of the studies reviewed found significantly positive effects of CTs on the probability that a child had received growth monitoring or health checkups, the impact depended on whether the transfer was conditional. Of the studies reviewed, 11 (10 from Latin America and the Caribbean and 1 from Africa) examined transfer programs that were conditional on parents taking their children to health visits (Attanasio and others 2005; Evans, Holtemeyer, and Kosec 2015; Gertler 2000; Gutiérrez and others 2004, 2006; Levy and Ohls 2007; Macours, Schady, and Vakis 2012; Maluccio and Flores 2005; Morris, Flores, and others 2004; Perova and Vakis 2009, 2012), 3 examined UCTs either in Ecuador (Fernald and Hidrobo 2011; Paxson and Schady 2010) or in Ghana (Handa, Park, and others 2014), and 1 experimentally varied whether the transfer was conditional on preventive health care of children in Burkina Faso (Akresh, de Walque, and Kazianga 2012). Whereas the studies on conditional programs revealed a significant increase in the percentage of children being taken to health facilities for growth monitoring or preventive care, the studies on UCTs did not find a significant increase.

Food Consumption

Given that CTs increase a household's purchasing power, CT programs could be expected to increase a household's food consumption. Indeed, review studies showed that both UCTs and CCTs had a large positive impact on the quality and quantity of households' food consumption (Fernald, Gertler, and Hidrobo 2012; Hidrobo, Hoddinott, Kumar, and others 2014; Hidrobo, Hoddinott, Peterman, and others 2014). Although households' food consumption improved, these improvements did not necessarily translate into improved nutrition for children. A potential reason for the weak impacts on nutrition may be the intrahousehold allocation of food, such that children did not benefit from the household's increased food consumption, with regard to either quantity or quality. Studies investigating the impacts on food consumption at the level of the individual child found no impacts on children's food consumption in Bangladesh (Ahmed and others 2009) and Ecuador (Fernald and Hidrobo 2011). However, in Colombia (Attanasio and others 2005), Nicaragua (Macours, Schady, and Vakis 2008), and Uganda (Gilligan and Roy 2014), CTs significantly increased the number of days children consumed foods rich in protein and other micronutrients.

Sexual and Reproductive Health

The impact of UCTs on sexual and reproductive health has been assessed, in particular in Sub-Saharan Africa, where the human immunodeficiency virus/acquired immune deficiency syndrome (HIV/AIDS) epidemic makes this issue highly relevant. Baird and others (2012) evaluated an intervention targeting human capital formation as an alternative HIV/AIDS prevention strategy in Malawi. They found that a CT, both conditional and unconditional, of, on average, US$10 per household per month (US$40 every four months) had various impacts on the prevalence of HIV/AIDS and herpes simplex virus-2 (HSV-2) together with pregnancies and sexual relations of girls with men older than age 25 years. They further documented that CTs improved the mental health of the girls, unless the cash was given conditionally to the parents (Baird, de Hoop, and Özler 2013). However, an evaluation of the medium-term impacts of this intervention, two years after it stopped, indicated that most of the impacts were no longer present (Baird and others 2015).

In Kenya, a national CT program for orphans and vulnerable children reduced the risk of sexual debut among young people ages 15–25 years and also reduced the likelihood of pregnancy among women ages 12–24 years by 5 percentage points (Handa, Halpern, and others 2014; Handa, Peterman, Huang, and others 2015). Schooling and peer influences have been found to be the main mediators for the reduction in sexual debut (Brugh and others 2014). Also in Kenya, Duflo, Dupas, and Kremer (2015) found that an education subsidy program had no impact (including in the longer term) on the HSV-2 infection rate. However, an education subsidy combined with HIV/AIDS prevention education focusing on abstinence until marriage resulted in a significant reduction in the HSV-2 infection rate in the intervention compared with the control group.

In a propensity-score-matched case-control study, a child-focused state CT in South Africa was shown to reduce transactional sex and age-disparate sex (Cluver and others 2013). Results from two South African randomized controlled trials suggest that CTs conditional on schooling have mixed results. An individually randomized study of young women conditioned on school attendance with an HIV/AIDS incidence endpoint found no impact on HIV/AIDS incidence, even though the young women who received CTs reported engaging in significantly fewer risk behaviors (Pettifor and others 2015). Another study found that cash incentives conditional on schooling led to a 30 percent reduction in HSV-2 incidence, but could not establish the impact of cash incentives on HIV/AIDS incidence (Abdool Karim and others 2015). Both studies might not have had enough statistical power to detect impacts on HIV/AIDS incidence.

A few randomized field trials have explored the use of financial incentives to encourage safe sexual behavior by making payments contingent on, for example, testing for HIV/AIDS, sexually transmitted infection (STI) status, or school enrollment. These experiments have focused mainly on young adults ages 18–29 years; however, the results are also relevant for adolescents' sexual and reproductive health outcomes. Kohler and Thornton (2012) assessed an experiment in Malawi that offered a single cash reward after one year to individuals who remained HIV-negative. The intervention had no measurable effect on HIV/AIDS status. De Walque and others (2012) and de Walque, Dow, and Nathan (2014) evaluated a conditional cash grant program in Tanzania in which the cash awards of US$10 or US$20 every four months were conditional on receiving negative test results for a set of curable STIs. After one year, the group eligible to receive the US$20 CTs showed a significant reduction in STI prevalence, while the group eligible for the US$10 CT showed no measurable effect. The study was not powered to measure impact on HIV/AIDS incidence.

Björkman Nyqvist and others (2015) assessed the effect on HIV/AIDS incidence of a lottery program in Lesotho with low expected payments but a chance to win a high prize conditional on receiving negative test results for STIs (the expected payment per testing round was about three times lower than in the Tanzania trial discussed above). The intervention resulted in a 21.4 percent reduction in HIV/AIDS incidence over two years. Lottery incentives appear to be particularly effective for individuals willing to take risks. In both the Lesotho and Tanzania studies, the effects were shown to be sustained in one-year postintervention follow-up studies.

IMPACT OF CASH TRANSFERS ON CHILD DEVELOPMENT AND EDUCATION

Early Child Development Outcomes

Evidence from studies examining the effects of CCTs and UCTs on cognitive, language, motor, or socioemotional development was also reviewed (six studies reviewed in Fernald, Gertler, and Hidrobo 2012 and five more-recent studies). The majority of studies from the 2012 review reported small, but significant, positive effects of CCTs on developmental outcomes in children (Fernald, Gertler, and Neufeld 2008, 2009; Fernald and Hidrobo 2011; Macours, Schady, and Vakis 2008; Ozer and others 2009; Paxson and Schady 2010). The studies published since the 2012 review showed mixed results. In Uganda, food and CTs were linked directly to preschool participation, and cash, but not food, was found to increase children's cognitive scores significantly

(Gilligan and Roy 2014). In Zambia, the UCT had no impact on a highly abbreviated language and cognition scale (Seidenfeld and others 2014). Evidence from Peru showed no effects of the Juntos CCT on language outcomes in children (Andersen and others 2015), but two studies in Nicaragua showed benefits to cognitive development from participation in two different CT programs (Barham, Macours, and Maluccio 2013; Macours, Schady, and Vakis 2012).

Two Latin American countries have tried to improve child development outcomes using the existing structure of CCTs to deliver parenting support, including stimulation and nutrition supplementation. In Colombia, the home-visiting program included as part of a CCT had positive effects on child development (Attanasio and others 2014), as did the integration of Mexico's CCT Prospera with Educación Inicial, a large-scale, group-based, parenting-support program (Fernald and others 2016).

Education Outcomes

Beyond health, CT programs can have broad impacts on the overall development of children and adolescents and their households (Handa, Seidenfeld, and others 2014). In their systematic review, Baird and others (2014) used data from 75 reports covering 35 studies to complement the evidence on the effectiveness of CT programs in improving schooling outcomes and to inform the debate surrounding the design of such programs. They found that both CCTs and UCTs improve the odds of being enrolled in and attending school compared with no CT program.

While the positive impact of CTs on human capital accumulation suggests that those improvements would also translate into better labor market outcomes, such as employment and wages, such long-term impacts have not yet been documented, probably because of the length of the study period required to make such assessments. However, CTs have been shown to improve household productivity by being invested in agricultural assets, reducing participation in low-skilled labor, and limiting child labor outside the home (Covarrubias, Davis, and Winters 2012).

COMPARING CASH TRANSFER DESIGNS, INCLUDING COST AND COST-EFFECTIVENESS

Conditional versus Unconditional

An important question is whether and how the conditions attached to CCTs affect the outcomes they seek to improve. CCT programs represent a top-down approach in which individuals or organizations decide what is best for poor children and provide incentives to their parents to achieve these objectives. In contrast, UCT programs assume that, once a budget constraint is relaxed, parents are in a better position to make appropriate decisions regarding their child's human capital. CCT programs are more costly per recipient to administer than UCT programs because of the costs associated with monitoring conditions.

In their systematic review, Baird and others (2014) specifically examined the role of conditions. They found that the effects for enrollment and attendance are always larger for CCTs than for UCTs, but the difference is not statistically significant. When programs are categorized as having no schooling conditions, having some conditions with minimal monitoring and enforcement, and having explicit conditions that are monitored and enforced, a much clearer pattern emerges: programs that are explicitly conditional, monitor compliance, and penalize noncompliance have substantively larger effects (60 percent improvement in odds of enrollment). Unlike enrollment and attendance, the effectiveness of CT programs for improving test scores is small at best.

Few studies have explicitly compared CCTs and UCTs in the same context. One experiment (Baird, McIntosh, and Özler 2011) examined the impact of CCTs and UCTs on adolescent girls' schooling and health outcomes in Malawi, concluding that CCTs outperformed UCTs for schooling outcomes, but UCTs outperformed CCTs for several other outcomes—for example, delaying marriage and childbearing. Benhassine and others (2015) used a randomized experiment in Morocco to estimate the impact of a labeled CT program: a small cash transfer made to fathers of school-age children in poor rural communities, not conditional on school attendance but explicitly labeled as an education support program. They documented large gains in school participation and concluded that adding conditionality and targeting mothers made almost no difference in that context.

A pilot program in rural Burkina Faso incorporated a random experimental design to evaluate the relative effectiveness of four social protection programs targeting poor households: CCTs given to fathers, CCTs given to mothers, UCTs given to fathers, and UCTs given to mothers (Akresh, de Walque, and Kazianga 2016). In the same context, this study also investigated the role of conditionality and the gender of the recipient in a CT program targeting all children—boys and girls up to age 15 years—and the impact of different CT modalities on a broad range of education, health, and household welfare outcomes. The results indicated that CTs improved the education and health of children as well as the socioeconomic conditions of households and adults.

They substantially increased school enrollment, unconditional attendance, and grade progression, but they had a more limited impact on learning outcomes as measured by standardized tests. They also improved the health outcomes of children ages zero to five years, leading to more preventive visits to health clinics, fewer illnesses (both as reported by parents and as measured by a biomarker for inflammation), and better nutritional outcomes (as indicated by anthropometric measurements). However, the conditionality led to differentiated impacts. For school enrollment and several health outcomes, CCTs outperformed UCTs.

The results from Burkina Faso further indicated that CCTs were more effective than UCTs in improving the enrollment of "marginal" children—those who were not enrolled in school or were less likely to go to school, including girls, younger children, and lower-ability children (Akresh, de Walque, and Kazianga 2013). These results shed new light on the role of conditionality in CT programs. In resource-poor settings, both UCTs and CCTs relax the budget constraint and allow households to enroll more children than they would traditionally prioritize for human capital investments. But the conditions attached to CCTs play a critical role in improving the outcomes of children in whom parents are less likely to invest.

Role of the CT Recipient

Another important question is whether the gender of the CT recipient matters. Numerous intrahousehold bargaining research papers indicate that resources under the mother's control have a stronger positive impact on a child's health and schooling than resources controlled by the father (Lundberg, Pollak, and Wales 1997; Schultz 1990; Thomas 1990, 1993). However, almost all current CT programs give resources to the mother, so it is not possible to disentangle how much of any impact is due to the recipient's gender, how much is due to the income effect, and how much is due to the change in relative prices associated with the conditionality. Furthermore, the recipient's gender might affect outcomes differently for conditional as opposed to unconditional CTs. While Benhassine and others (2015) and Haushofer and Shapiro (2016) found no important differences in measured impacts depending on the recipient's gender, Akresh, de Walque, and Kazianga (2016) found more contrasting results when they explicitly investigated the gender of the transfer recipient in Burkina Faso.

While giving cash to mothers seems slightly, but not significantly, better for education outcomes, giving cash to fathers leads to significantly better nutritional outcomes during years when the harvest has been poor.

In the context of a CCT program, another interesting question is the role of parental and child returns to schooling or health decisions regarding school attendance or safe sexual behaviors, especially with adolescents who can more easily make their own decisions. Parents and children may have different views about when it is optimal for a child to invest in human capital. In addition, the actions of children are unlikely to be perfectly observed by their parents, which potentially leads to a moral hazard problem that may prevent investments in schooling or health even when such investments would be optimal from the point of view of the parent-child pair under perfect information (Bursztyn and Coffman 2012).

Bursztyn and Coffman (2012) found that parents attach a value to the monitoring of attendance provided by CCTs in Brazil. However, Baird, McIntosh, and Özler (2011) obtained inconclusive results when comparing the effectiveness of giving one extra dollar to children with the effectiveness of giving one extra dollar to parents in the context of joint transfers to parents and children in Malawi.

CONCLUSIONS

This chapter reviews the evidence from CT programs throughout LMICs and their direct effects on the health and education outcomes of children and adolescents. It also discusses the design of CT programs and why and how they could theoretically affect the outcomes of young children and adolescents. It is very difficult to compare results across countries and contexts, because, as illustrated in table 23.1, UCTs and CCTs have heterogeneous objectives, targeting, conditions applied to the transfer, amount of the transfer, and complementary services. CCT programs also differ because of country-level differences in the supply of health services. For example, even if households comply with the specified conditions, increased use of health services may not result in improved health outcomes if health services have poor infrastructure, high absenteeism, or inadequate supplies. Policy makers should not assume that CT programs will be the most efficient intervention for improving the health outcomes of children and adolescents. The specific context, design, and objectives of each successful experience should be carefully considered before it is replicated and implemented in other settings. Our review shows mostly positive effects of CT programs on some child outcomes, including birth weight; infant mortality; illness or morbidity; and cognitive, language, and behavioral development. Outcomes with large mixed or subgroup effects included HAZ or stunting. Outcomes with large null results included WAZ or

underweight, WHZ or wasting, and hemoglobin or anemia. With regard to indirect effects of CTs, results were strong and significant for participation in prenatal care, presence of a skilled birth attendant, and growth monitoring.

CTs may not show clear and consistent effects on anthropometric results or anemia for several reasons. CT programs try to address many issues at multiple levels (parental, community) that influence child development, but they do not directly work to change the broader factors that have previously been linked with improving nutrition and decreasing stunting and anemia, such as safe water and sanitation, infant and young child feeding practices, and country-level food availability (Smith and Haddad 2014). Similarly, programs promoting child development that have an educational or stimulation component have shown larger cognitive effects than cash-only or nutrition-only programs, both in the United States (Nores and Barnett 2010) and in Latin America (Attanasio and others 2014; Fernald and others 2016). In spite of this evidence, there are clear cost constraints—for example, the estimated annual unit cost of an early child development or child care intervention including nutrition supplementation has been estimated to be three to four times the cost of a conditional CT program (Shekar, Heaver, and Lee 2006).

Strong evidence indicates that CT programs keep adolescent students enrolled in school longer. Some of these programs, but not all, have also been effective in controlling the spread of HIV/AIDS among adolescents, primarily by keeping them in school. Some experiments with direct incentives to stay free of STIs have also been promising. However, further experiments with CCT programs and their implementation on a larger scale are needed before it can be concluded that they offer an efficient, scalable, and sustainable HIV/AIDS-prevention strategy.

In our review, CCTs generally showed greater effects than UCTs, although there were still far fewer UCTs than CCTs, so it is difficult to generalize. Moreover, UCTs are more common in Sub-Saharan Africa, while CCTs are more common in Latin America, so it is difficult to disentangle the conditionalities from regional differences. In a large review of studies examining CCTs versus UCTs, the largest effects on education outcomes were found for programs that were explicitly conditional, had a clear system for monitoring compliance, and had penalties for noncompliance (Baird and others 2014). Thus, CT programs appear to be most effective when the receipt of cash is linked with a specific intervention that can maximize the potential impact of the transfer. However, there may be a limit to the number of conditions that households can handle because of the possibilities for misunderstanding (Gaarder, Glassman, and Todd 2010). Moreover, programs with multiple objectives may find that conditionality leads to greater improvements in some outcomes than in others.

CCTs and UCTs attempt to break the cycle of poverty, but there are still many questions relating to how CCTs and UCTs function, how CCTs and UCTs differ in effectiveness, what can be done to improve the effectiveness of CT programs in general, and whether the CCT model can be used throughout the world. Future research relating to CTs could focus on a wide range of topics: for example, examining the CT "black box" to understand mechanisms and pathways linking program participation to child development outcomes; testing potential additions to CT programs (intensive parenting education, child care availability) that could make the programs more effective, particularly for child development; varying the CT amount or program requirements to understand and identify potential threshold effects; understanding the contextual factors (community or household characteristics) that could maximize the effectiveness of CTs; and modifying existing CT programs to have a greater focus on obesity and chronic disease prevention in countries experiencing the nutrition transition, such as many Latin America countries. With a greater understanding of how and why CTs function, their effectiveness can be improved for children and adolescents throughout the world.

NOTE

World Bank Income Classifications as of July 2014 are as follows, based on estimates of gross national income (GNI) per capita for 2013:

- Low-income countries (LICs) = US$1,045 or less
- Middle-income countries (MICs) are subdivided:
  a) lower-middle-income = US$1,046 to US$4,125
  b) upper-middle-income (UMICs) = US$4,126 to US$12,745
- High-income countries (HICs) = US$12,746 or more.

REFERENCES

Abdool Karim, Q., K. Leask, A. Kharsany, H. Humphries, F. Ntombela, and others. 2015. "Impact of Conditional Cash Incentives on HSV-2 and HIV Prevention in Rural South African High School Students: Results of the CAPRISA 007 Cluster Randomized Controlled Trial." Abstract presented at the 2015 International AIDS Society Conference, Vancouver, Canada, July 18–22.

Aber, L., and L. B. Rawlings. 2011. "North-South Knowledge Sharing on Incentive-Based Conditional Cash Transfer Programs." Social Protection Discussion Paper No. 1101, World Bank, Washington, DC. http://ejournal.narotama .ac.id/files/North-South%20knowledge%20sharing%20 on%20incentive-based%20conditional%20cash%20 transfer%20programs.pdf.

Agüero, J. M., M. R. Carter, and I. Woolard. 2009. "The Impact of Unconditional Cash Transfers on Nutrition: The South African Child Support Grant." Paper prepared for the North American Summer Meetings, Econometric Society, Boston, MA, June 4–7.

Ahmed, A. U., A. R. Quisumbing, M. Nasreen, J. Hoddinott, and E. Bryan. 2009. Comparing Food and Cash Transfers to the Ultra Poor in Bangladesh. Washington, DC: International Food Policy Research Institute.

Akresh, R., D. de Walque, and H. Kazianga. 2012. "Alternative Cash Transfer Delivery Mechanisms: Impacts on Routine Preventative Health Clinic Visits in Burkina Faso." Working Paper 17785, National Bureau of Economic Research, Cambridge, MA.

———. 2013. "Cash Transfers and Child Schooling: Evidence from a Randomized Evaluation of the Role of Conditionality." Policy Research Working Paper 6340, World Bank, Washington, DC.

———. 2016. "Evidence from a Randomized Evaluation of the Household Welfare Impacts of Conditional and Unconditional Cash Transfers Given to Mothers or Fathers." Policy Research Working Paper 7730, World Bank, Washington, DC.

Amarante, V., M. Manacorda, E. Miguel, and A. Vigorito. 2012. "Do Cash Transfers Improve Birth Outcomes? Evidence from Matched Vital Statistics, Program, and Social Security Data." Working Paper 17690, National Bureau of Economic Research, Cambridge, MA.

Andersen, C. T., S. A. Reynolds, J. R. Behrman, B. T. Crookston, K. A. Dearden, and others. 2015. "Participation in the Juntos Conditional Cash Transfer Program in Peru Is Associated with Changes in Child Anthropometric Status but Not Language Development or School Achievement." Journal of Nutrition 145 (10): 2396–405.

Attanasio, O. P., E. Battistin, E. Fitzsimons, A. Mesnard, and M. Vera-Hernández. 2005. "How Effective Are Conditional Cash Transfers? Evidence from Colombia." Briefing Note 54, Institute for Fiscal Studies, London. http://www.ifs.org .uk/bns/bn54.pdf.

Attanasio, O. P., C. Fernandez, E. O. A. Fitzsimons, S. M. Grantham-McGregor, C. Meghir, and others. 2014. "Using the Infrastructure of a Conditional Cash Transfer Program to Deliver a Scalable Integrated Early Child Development Program in Colombia: Cluster Randomized Controlled Trial." BMJ 349 (September 29): g5785.

Attanasio, O. P., and A. Mesnard. 2006. "The Impact of a Conditional Cash Transfer Programme on Consumption in Colombia." Fiscal Studies 27 (4): 421–42.

Baird, S., E. Chirwa, C. McIntosh, and B. Özler. 2015. "What Happens Once the Intervention Ends? The Medium-Term Impacts of a Cash Transfer Programme in Malawi." 3ie Impact Evaluation Report 27.: International Initiative for Impact Evaluation (3ie), New Delhi.

Baird, S., J. de Hoop, and B. Özler. 2013. "Income Shocks and Adolescent Mental Health." *Journal of Human Resources* 48 (2): 370–403.

Baird, S., F. H. G. Ferreira, B. Özler, and M. Woolcock. 2014. "Conditional, Unconditional, and Everything in Between: A Systematic Review of the Effects of Cash Transfer Programmes on Schooling Outcomes." *Journal of Development Effectiveness* 6 (1): 1–43.

Baird, S., R. S. Garfein, C. McIntosh, and B. Özler. 2012. "Effect of a Cash Transfer Programme for Schooling on Prevalence of HIV and Herpes Simplex Type 2 in Malawi: A Cluster Randomized Trial." *The Lancet* 379 (9823): 1320–29.

Baird, S., C. McIntosh, and B. Özler. 2011. "Cash or Condition? Evidence from a Cash Transfer Experiment." *Quarterly Journal of Economics* 126 (4): 1709–53.

Barber, S., and P. J. Gertler. 2010. "Empowering Women: How Mexico's Conditional Cash Transfer Programme Raised Prenatal Care Quality and Birth Weight." *Journal of Development Effectiveness* 2 (1): 51–73.

Barham, T. 2011. "A Healthier Start: The Effect of Conditional Cash Transfers on Neonatal and Infant Mortality in Rural Mexico." *Journal of Development Economics* 94 (1): 74–85.

Barham, T., K. Macours, and J. A. Maluccio. 2013. "Boys' Cognitive Skill Formation and Physical Growth: Long-Term Experimental Evidence on Critical Ages for Early Childhood Interventions." *American Economic Review Papers and Proceedings* 103 (3): 467–71.

Barrientos, A., and J. DeJong. 2006. "Reducing Child Poverty with Cash Transfers: A Sure Thing?" *Development Policy Review* 24 (5): 537–52.

Bassani, D. G., P. Arora, K. Wazny, M. F. Gaffey, L. Lenters, and others. 2013. "Financial Incentives and Coverage of Child Health Interventions: A Systematic Review and Meta-Analysis." *BMC Public Health* 13 (Suppl 3): S30.

Bassett, L. 2008. "Can Conditional Cash Transfer Programs Play a Greater Role in Reducing Child Undernutrition?" Social Protection Discussion Paper 0835, World Bank, Washington, DC.

Behrman, J. R., and J. Hoddinott. 2005. "Program Evaluation with Unobserved Heterogeneity and Selective Implementation: The Mexican Progresa Impact on Child Nutrition." *Oxford Bulletin of Economics and Statistics* 67 (4): 547–69.

Benhassine, N., F. Devoto, E. Duflo, P. Dupas, and V. Pouliquen. 2015. "Turning a Shove into a Nudge? A Labeled Cash Transfer for Education." *American Economic Journal: Economic Policy* 7 (3): 86–125.

Björkman Nyqvist, M., L. Corno, D. de Walque, and J. Svensson. 2015. "Using Lotteries to Incentivize Safer Sexual Behavior: Evidence from a Randomized Controlled Trial on HIV Prevention." Policy Research Working Paper 7215, World Bank, Washington, DC.

Brugh, K., C. T. Halpern, A. Pettifor, H. Thirumurty, and S. Handa. 2014. "Do Schooling and Peer Influences Mediate the Impact of Cash Transfer on Adolescent Sexual Debut in Kenya?" Unpublished, University of North Carolina at Chapel Hill.

Bundy, D. A. P., N. de Silva, S. Horton, G. C. Patton, L. Schultz, and D. T. Jamison. 2017. "Child and Adolescent Health and Development: Realizing Neglected Potential." In *Disease Control Priorities* (third edition): Volume 8, *Child and Adolescent Health and Development*, edited by D. A. P. Bundy, N. de Silva, S. Horton, D. T. Jamison, and G. C. Patton. Washington, DC: World Bank.

Bursztyn, L., and L. C. Coffman. 2012. "The Schooling Decision: Family Preferences, Intergenerational Conflict, and Moral Hazard in the Brazilian Favelas." *Journal of Political Economy* 120 (3): 359–97.

Cluver, L., M. Boyes, M. Orkin, M. Pantelic, M. Thembela, and others. 2013. "Child-Focused State Cash Transfers and Adolescent Risk of HIV Infection in South Africa: A Propensity-Score-Matched Case Control Study." *The Lancet* 1 (6): e362–70.

Covarrubias, K., B. Davis, and P. Winters. 2012. "From Protection to Production; Productive Impacts of the Malawi Social Cash Transfer Scheme." *Journal of Development Effectiveness* 4 (1): 50–77.

De Brauw, A., and A. Peterman. 2011. "Can Conditional Cash Transfers Improve Maternal Health and Birth Outcomes? Evidence from El Salvador's Comunidades Solidarias Rurales Program." IFPRI Discussion Paper 01080, International Food Policy Research Institute, Washington, DC.

de Janvry, A., and E. Sadoulet. 2006. "Making Conditional Cash Transfer Programs More Efficient: Designing for Maximum Effect of the Conditionality." *World Bank Economic Review* 20 (1): 1–29.

de Walque, D., W. H. Dow, and R. Nathan. 2014. "Rewarding Safer Sex: Conditional Cash Transfers for HIV/STI Prevention." Policy Research Working Paper 7099, World Bank, Washington, DC.

de Walque, D., W. H. Dow, R. Nathan, R. Abdul, F. Abilahi, and others. 2012. "Incentivising Safe Sex: A Randomised Trial of Conditional Cash Transfers for HIV and Sexually Transmitted Infection Prevention in Rural Tanzania." *BMJ Open* 2 (February 8): e000747. doi:10.1136/bmjopen-2011-000747.

Del Boca, D., C. Flinn, and M. Wiswall. 2014. "Household Choices and Child Development." *Review of Economic Studies* 81 (1): 137–85.

Devereux, S., and R. Sabates-Wheeler. 2004. "Transformative Social Protection." IDS Working Paper 232, Institute of Development Studies, Brighton, U.K.

DFID (Department for International Development). 2011. "Cash Transfers: Evidence Paper." DFID, London.

Drake, L., M. Fernandes, E. Aurino, J. Kiamba, B. Giyosa, C. Burbano, H. Alderman, L. Mai, A. Mitchell, and A. Gelli. 2017. "School Feeding Programs in Middle Childhood and Adolescence." In *Disease Control Priorities* (third edition): Volume 8, *Child and Adolescent Health and Development*, edited by D. A. P. Bundy, N. de Silva, S. Horton, D. T. Jamison, and G. C. Patton. Washington, DC: World Bank.

Duflo, E., P. Dupas, and M. Kremer. 2015. "Education, HIV, and Early Fertility: Experimental Evidence from Kenya."

American Economic Review 105 (9): 2757–97. http://dx.doi.org/10.1257/aer.20121607.

Engle, P. E., L. C. H. Fernald, J. Alderman, J. Behrman, C. O'Gara, and others. 2011. "Strategies for Reducing Inequalities and Improving Developmental Outcomes for Young Children in Low- and Middle-Income Countries." *The Lancet* 378 (9799): 1339–53.

Evans, D., B. Holtemeyer, and K. Kosec. 2015. "Cash Transfers and Health: Mechanisms and Impacts." World Bank, Washington, DC.

Fernald L. C. H., P. J. Gertler, and M. Hidrobo. 2012. "Conditional Cash Transfer Programs: Effects on Growth, Health, and Development in Young Children." In *The Oxford Handbook of Poverty and Child Development*, edited by R. King and V. Maholmes. New York: Oxford University Press.

Fernald, L. C. H., P. J. Gertler, and L. M. Neufeld. 2008. "The Role of Cash in Conditional Cash Transfer Programmes for Child Health, Growth, and Development: An Analysis of Mexico's Oportunidades." *The Lancet* 371 (9615): 828–37.

———. 2009. "Ten-Year Impact of Oportunidades—Mexico's Conditional Cash Transfer Program—on Child Growth, Cognition, Language, and Behavior." *The Lancet* 374 (9706): 1997–2005.

Fernald, L. C. H., and M. Hidrobo. 2011. "Effect of Ecuador's Cash Transfer Program (Bono de Desarrollo Humano) on Child Development in Infants and Toddlers: A Randomized Effectiveness Trial." *Social Science and Medicine* 72 (9): 1437–46.

Fernald L. C., R. M. Kagawa, R. M. Knauer, L. Schnaas, A. G. Guerra, and L. M. Neufeld. 2016. "Promoting Child Development Through Group-Based Parent Support Within a Cash Transfer Program: Experimental Effects on Children's Outcomes." *Developmental Psychology*. Epub ahead of print October 17. https://www.ncbi.nlm.nih.gov/pubmed/?term=fernald+knauer.

Fiszbein, A., and N. Schady, with F. H. G. Ferreira, M. Grosh, N. Kelleher, and others. 2009. *Conditional Cash Transfers: Reducing Present and Future Poverty*. Washington, DC: World Bank.

Gaarder, M. M., A. Glassman, and J. E. Todd. 2010. "Conditional Cash Transfers and Health: Unpacking the Causal Chain." *Journal of Development Effectiveness* 2 (1): 6–50.

Gertler, P. J. 2000. "Final Report: The Impact of Progresa on Health." International Food Policy Research Institute, Washington, DC.

———. 2004. "Do Conditional Cash Transfers Improve Child Health? Evidence from Progresa's Controlled Randomized Experiment." *American Economic Review* 94 (2): 336–41.

Gilligan, D., and S. Roy. 2014. "Resources, Stimulation, and Cognition: How Transfer Programs and Preschool Shape Cognitive Development in Uganda." International Food Policy Research Institute, Washington, DC.

Glassman, A., D. Duran, and M. Koblinsky. 2013. "Impact of Conditional Cash Transfers on Maternal and Newborn Health." *Journal of Health, Population, and Nutrition* 31 (4, Suppl 2): S48–66.

Grimes, M., and L. Wängnerud. 2010. "Curbing Corruption through Social Welfare Reform? The Effects of Mexico's Conditional Cash Transfer Program on Good Government." *American Review of Public Administration* 40 (6): 671–90.

Guo, G., and K. M. Harris. 2000. "The Mechanisms Mediating the Effects of Poverty on Children's Intellectual Development." *Demography* 37 (4): 431–47.

Gutiérrez, J. P., S. Bautista, P. J. Gertler, M. Hernandez Avila, and S. M. Bertozzi. 2004. "Impacto de Oportunidades en la morbilidad y el estado de salud de la población beneficiana y en la utilización de los servicios de salud: Resultados de corto plazo en zonas urbanas y de mediano plazo en zonas rurales." In *Evaluación externa de impacto del Programa Oportunidades 2004*, edited by B. H. Prado and M. H. Avila. Mexico, DF: Instituto Nacional de Salud Pública.

———. 2006. "Impacto de Oportunidades en el estado de salud, morbilidad y utilización de servicios de salud de la población beneficiaria en zonas urbanas." In *Evaluación externa de impacto del Programa Oportunidades 2006*, edited by M. H. Ávila, B. H. Prado, and J. E. U. Salomón. Mexico, DF: Instituto Nacional de Salud Pública.

Handa, S., and B. Davis. 2006. "The Experience of Conditional Cash Transfers in Latin America and the Caribbean." *Development Policy Review* 24 (5): 513–36.

Handa, S., C. T. Halpern, A. Pettifor, and H. Thirumurthy. 2014. "The Government of Kenya's Cash Transfer Program Reduces the Risk of Sexual Debut among Young People Age 15–25." *PLoS One* 9 (1): e85473.

Handa, S., M. Park, R. Osei Darko, I. Osei-Akoto, B. Davis, and others. 2014. "Livelihood Empowerment against Poverty Program Impact Evaluation." University of North Carolina, Carolina Population Center, Chapel Hill, NC.

Handa, S., A. Peterman, C. Huang, C. T. Halpern, A. Pettifor, and others. 2015. "Impact of the Kenya Cash Transfer for Orphans and Vulnerable Children on Early Pregnancy and Marriage of Adolescent Girls." *Social Science and Medicine* 141 (September): 36–45.

Handa, S., A. Peterman, D. Seidenfeld, and G. Tembo. 2015. "Income Transfers and Maternal Health: Evidence from a National Randomized Social Cash Transfer Program in Zambia." *Health Economics* 25 (2): 225–36.

Handa, S., D. Seidenfeld, B. Davis, G. Tembo, and the Zambia Cash Transfer Evaluation Team. 2014. "Are Cash Transfers a Silver Bullet? Evidence from the Zambian Child Grant." Innocenti Working Paper 2014–08, United Nations Children's Fund Office of Research, Florence.

Haushofer, J., and J. Shapiro. 2016. "The Short-Term Impact of Unconditional Cash Transfers to the Poor: Experimental Evidence from Kenya." *Quarterly Journal of Economics*, July 19. doi: 10.1093/qje/qjw025.

Hernández Prado, B., J. Urquieta Salomon, M. Ramirez Cilalobos, and J. Figueroa. 2004. "Impacto de Oportunidades en la salud reproductiva de la poblacion beneficiaria." In *Evaluacion externa de impacto del Programa Oportunidades 2004*, edited by B. H. Prado and M. H. Avila. Mexico, DF: Instituto Nacional de Salud Pública.

Hidrobo, M., J. Hoddinott, N. Kumar, and M. Olivier. 2014. "Social Protection and Food Security." International Food Policy Research Institute, Washington, DC.

Hidrobo, M., J. Hoddinott, A. Peterman, A. Margolies, and V. Moreira. 2014. "Cash, Food, or Vouchers? Evidence from a Randomized Experiment in Northern Ecuador." *Journal of Development Economics* 107 (March): 144–56.

Himaz, R. 2008. "Welfare Grants and Their Impact on Child Health: The Case of Sri Lanka." *World Development* 36 (10): 1843–57.

Hoddinott, J., and L. Bassett. 2008. "Conditional Cash Transfer Programs and Nutrition in Latin America: Assessment of Impacts and Strategies for Improvement." International Food Policy Research Institute, Washington, DC.

Kohler, H. P., and R. Thornton. 2012. "Conditional Cash Transfers and HIV/AIDS Prevention: Unconditionally Promising?" *World Bank Economic Review* 26 (2): 165–90.

Lagarde, M., A. Haines, and N. Palmer. 2007. "Conditional Cash Transfers for Improving Uptake of Health Interventions in Low- and Middle-Income Countries: A Systematic Review." *JAMA* 298 (16): 1900–10.

Leroy, J. L., A. García-Guerra, R. García, C. Domínguez, J. Rivera, and others. 2008. "The Oportunidades Program Increases the Linear Growth of Children Enrolled at Young Ages in Urban Mexico." *Journal of Nutrition* 138 (4): 793–98.

Levy, D., and J. Ohls. 2007. "Evaluation of Jamaica's PATH Program: Final Report." Mathematica Policy Research, Princeton, NJ.

Lim, S. S., L. Dandona, J. A. Hoisington, S. L. James, M. C. Hogan, and others. 2010. "India's Janani Suraksha Yojana, a Conditional Cash Transfer Programme to Increase Births in Health Facilities: An Impact Evaluation." *The Lancet* 375 (9730): 2009–23.

Lundberg, S., R. Pollak, and T. Wales. 1997. "Do Husbands and Wives Pool Their Resources? Evidence from the United Kingdom Child Benefit." *Journal of Human Resources* 32 (3): 463–80.

Macours, K., N. Schady, and R. Vakis. 2008. "Cash Transfers, Behavioral Changes, and the Cognitive Development of Young Children: Evidence from a Randomized Experiment." World Bank, Washington, DC.

———. 2012. "Cash Transfers, Behavioral Changes, and Cognitive Development in Early Childhood: Evidence from a Randomized Experiment." *American Economic Journal: Applied Economics* 4 (2): 247–73.

Maluccio, J. A., and R. Flores. 2005. "Impact Evaluation of a Conditional Cash Transfer Program: The Nicaraguan Red de Protección Social." Research Report 141, International Food Policy Research Institute, Washington, DC.

Manley, J., S. Gitter, and V. Slavchevska. 2013. "How Effective Are Cash Transfers at Improving Nutritional Status?" *World Development* 48 (August): 133–55.

Miller, C., M. Tsoka, and K. Reichert. 2010. "Cash Transfers and Child Health in Malawi: Early Findings on the Impact of $14 per Month." University of York, York, UK.

Mistry, R. S., J. C. Biesanz, L. C. Taylor, M. Burchinal, and M. J. Cox. 2004. "Family Income and Its Relation to Preschool Children's Adjustment for Families in the NICHD Study of Early Child Care." *Developmental Psychology* 40 (5): 727–45.

Morris, S. S., R. Flores, P. Olinto, and J. M. Medina. 2004. "Monetary Incentives in Primary Health Care and Effects on Use and Coverage of Preventive Health Care Interventions in Rural Honduras: Cluster Randomised Trial." *The Lancet* 364 (9450): 2030–37.

Morris, S. S., P. Olinto, R. Velasquez Flores, E. A. Nilson, and A. C. Figueiró. 2004. "Conditional Cash Transfers Are Associated with a Small Reduction in the Rate of Weight Gain of Preschool Children in Northeast Brazil." *Journal of Nutrition* 134 (9): 2336–41.

Neufeld, L. 2005. "Estudio comparativo sobre el estado nutricional y la adquisición de lenguaje entre ninos de localidades urbana con y sin Oportunidades." In *Evaluación externa de impacto del Programa Oportunidades 2004.* Vol. III: *Salud,* edited by M. Hernandez Avila. Mexico, DF: Instituto Nacional de Salud Pública.

Neufeld, L., D. Sotres Alvarez, P. J. Gertler, L. Tolentino Mayo, J. Jimenez Ruiz, and others. 2005. "Impacto de Oportunidades en el crecimiento y estado nutricional de niños en zonas rurales." In *Evaluación externa de impacto del Programa Oportunidades 2004.* Vol. III: *Alimentación,* 17–52, edited by M. Hernandez Avila. Mexico, DF: Instituto Nacional de Salud Pública.

Nguyen, H. T., L. Hatt, M. Islam, N. L. Sloan, J. Chowdhury, and others. 2012. "Encouraging Maternal Health Service Utilization: An Evaluation of the Bangladesh Voucher Program." *Social Science and Medicine* 74 (7): 989–96.

Nores, M., and W. S. Barnett. 2010. "Benefits of Early Childhood Interventions across the World: (Under) Investing in the Very Young." *Economics of Education Review* 29 (2): 271–82.

Ozer, E. J., L. C. H. Fernald, J. G. Manley, and P. J. Gertler. 2009. "Effects of a Conditional Cash Transfer Program on Children's Behavior Problems." *Pediatrics* 123 (4): e630–377. doi:10.1542/peds.2008-2882.

Paxson, C., and N. Schady. 2010. "Does Money Matter? The Effects of Cash Transfers on Child Development in Rural Ecuador." *Economic Development and Cultural Change* 59 (1): 187–229.

Perova, E., and R. Vakis. 2009. "Welfare Impacts of the 'Juntos' Program in Peru: Evidence from a Non-Experimental Evaluation." World Bank, Washington, DC.

———. 2012. "5 Years in Juntos: New Evidence on the Program's Short and Long-Term Impacts." *Economía* 35 (69): 53–82.

Pettifor, A., C. MacPhail, A. Selin, X. Gomez-Olivé, J. Hughes, and others. 2015. "HPTN 068 Conditional Cash Transfer to Prevent HIV Infection among Young Women in South Africa: Results of a Randomized Controlled Trial." Abstract presented at the 2015 International AIDS Society conference, Vancouver, Canada, July 18–22.

Popay, J., S. Escorel, M. Hernández, H. Johnston, J. Mathieson, and L. Rispel. 2008. "Understanding and Tackling Social Exclusion." Final Report to the WHO

Commission on Social Determinants of Health from the Social Exclusion Knowledge Network. World Health Organization, Geneva.

Powell-Jackson, T., and K. Hanson. 2012. "Financial Incentives for Maternal Health: Impact of a National Programme in Nepal." *Journal of Health Economics* 31 (1): 271–84.

Powell-Jackson, T., B. Neupane, S. N. Tiwari, K. Tumbahangphe, D. Manandhar, and others. 2009. "The Impact of Nepal's National Incentive Programme to Promote Safe Delivery in the District of Makwanpur." In *Innovations in Health System Finance in Developing and Transitional Economies*, edited by D. Chernichovsky and K. Hanson, 221–49. Advances in Health Economics and Health Services Research 21. Bingley, U.K.: Emerald Group Publishing.

Rasella, D., R. Aquino, S. Tiwari, K. Tumbahangphe, D. Manandhar, and others. 2013. "Effect of a Conditional Cash Transfer Programme on Childhood Mortality: A Nationwide Analysis of Brazilian Municipalities." *The Lancet* 382 (9886): 57–64.

Reis, M. 2010. "Cash Transfer Programs and Child Health in Brazil." *Economics Letters* 108 (1): 22–25.

Rivera, J. A., D. Sotres-Alvarez, J. P. Habicht, T. Shamah, and S. Villalpando. 2004. "Impact of the Mexican Program for Education, Health, and Nutrition (Progresa) on Rates of Growth and Anemia in Infants and Young Children: A Randomized Effectiveness Study." *JAMA* 291 (21): 2563–70.

Ruel, M. T., H. Alderman, and Maternal and Child Nutrition Study Group. 2013. "Nutrition-Sensitive Interventions and Programmes: How Can They Help to Accelerate Progress in Improving Maternal and Child Nutrition?" *The Lancet* 382 (9891): 536–51.

Schultz, T. P. 1990. "Testing the Neoclassical Model of Family Labor Supply and Fertility." *Journal of Human Resources* 25 (4): 599–634.

Seidenfeld, D., S. Handa, G. Tembo, S. Michelo, C. H. Scott, and others. 2014. "The Impact of an Unconditional Cash Transfer on Food Security and Nutrition: The Zambia Child Grant Program." Institute of Development Studies, Brighton, U.K.

Shei, A. 2013. "Brazil's Conditional Cash Transfer Program Associated with Declines in Infant Mortality Rates." *Health Affairs (Millwood)* 32 (7): 1274–81.

Shekar, M., R. Heaver, and Y.-K. Lee. 2006. *Repositioning Nutrition as Central to Development: A Strategy for Large-Scale Action*. Washington, DC: World Bank.

Shibuya, K. 2008. "Conditional Cash Transfer: A Magic Bullet for Health?" *The Lancet* 371 (9615): 789–91. doi: 10.1016 /S0140-6736(08)60356-6.

Smith, L., and L. Haddad. 2014. "Reducing Child Undernutrition: Past Drivers and Priorities for the Post-MDG Era." Institute of Development Studies, Brighton, U.K. http://opendocs.ids.ac.uk/opendocs/bitstream/handle /123456789/3816/Wp441R.pdf?sequence=4.

Sosa-Rubí, S. G., D. Walker, E. Serván, and S. Bautista-Arredondo. 2011. "Learning Effect of a Conditional Cash Transfer Programme on Poor Rural Women's Selection of Delivery Care in Mexico." *Health Policy and Planning* 26 (6): 496–507.

Thomas, D. 1990. "Intrahousehold Resource Allocation: An Inferential Approach." *Journal of Human Resources* 25 (4): 635–64.

———. 1993. "The Distribution of Income and Expenditure within the Household." *Annales de Economie et de Statistiques* 29 (January–March): 109–36.

Triyana, M. 2014. "Do Health Care Providers Respond to Demand-Side Incentives? Evidence from Indonesia." Stanford University, Stanford, CA.

Urquieta, J., G. Angeles, T. A. Mroz, H. Lamadrid-Figueroa, and B. Hernández. 2009. "Impact of Oportunidades on Skilled Attendance at Delivery in Rural Areas." *Economic Development and Cultural Change* 57 (3): 539–58.

Victora, C. G., M. de Onis, P. C. Hallal, M. Blössner, and R. Shrimpton. 2010. "Worldwide Timing of Growth Faltering: Revisiting Implications for Interventions." *Pediatrics* 125 (3): e473–80.

Walker, S. P., T. D. Wachs, S. Grantham-McGregor, M. M. Black, C. A. Nelson, and others. 2011. "Inequality Begins in Early Childhood: Risk and Protective Factors for Early Child Development." *The Lancet* 378 (9799): 1325–38.

WHO (World Health Organization). 1986. "Use and Interpretation of Anthropometric Indicators of Nutritional Status." *Bulletin of the World Health Organization* 64 (6): 929.

World Bank. 2011. "Program Keluarga Harapan: Main Findings from the Impact Evaluation of Indonesia's Pilot Household Conditional Cash Transfer Program." World Bank, Jakarta.

Yeung, W. J., M. R. Linver, and J. Brooks-Gunn. 2002. "How Money Matters for Young Children's Development: Parental Investment and Family Processes." *Child Development* 73 (6): 1861–79.

Chapter 24

Identifying an Essential Package for Early Child Development: Economic Analysis

Susan Horton and Maureen M. Black

INTRODUCTION

The eight other volumes in this third edition of *Disease Control Priorities* focus on health; this volume complements their focus by examining the synergies between health and education outcomes. Most of the chapters in this volume focus on children ages five years and older and on adolescents. This chapter deals with children younger than age five years, serving as a counterpart to the detailed analysis of young child health in volume 2 (Black and others 2016).

The importance and effectiveness of interventions to enrich early child development (ECD) are discussed in chapter 19 of this volume (Black, Gove, and Merseth 2017). Surveys of the literature for low- and middle-income countries (LMICs) include Engle and others (2007), Engle and others (2011), and Nores and Barnett (2010).

Recent literature has begun to consider the synergies in delivering interventions focusing on nutrition or health in conjunction with child development. Surveys have examined whether codelivery enhances outcomes, reduces costs, and increases cost-effectiveness or benefit-cost ratios (Batura and others 2014; Grantham-McGregor and others 2014).

This chapter examines the costs and benefit-cost ratios of interventions that incorporate responsive stimulation to achieve better child outcomes. The purpose is to develop and cost an essential package of ECD interventions appropriate across LMICs that will complement health and nutritional interventions.

We use the term *responsive stimulation* when discussing ECD interventions that highlight the importance of positive interactions between children and caregivers. Other terms are used in the literature, including *parenting*, *caregiving*, and *psychosocial stimulation*; these terms imply a unidirectional concept, rather than the bidirectional concept that underlies many theories of child development.

The most appropriate interventions vary according to children's ages. Children younger than age three years spend much of their time with parents, family members, or caregivers. Infants and young children need care and adult attention, and the ratio of children per adult needs to be low, making group settings less feasible and more costly. Between age three years and the age of school entry, children are more likely to be in a group setting outside of the home for at least part of the day; 54 percent of this age group worldwide is enrolled in preschool (UNESCO 2015). This practice is dictated in part by economics—the ratio of children per adult supervisor can be higher—and by children's developmental needs as they begin to interact more with peers.

The main public services with which children younger than age three years interact are those for health, nutrition, and social protection. Young children can benefit from community-based interventions (Singla, Kumbakumba, and Aboud 2015), but these interventions do not generally have national coverage. Delivering interventions for responsive stimulation in coordination

Corresponding author: Susan Horton, University of Waterloo, Ontario, Canada; sehorton@uwaterloo.ca.

with health and nutrition services for these younger children may be an effective approach in this age group.

After age three years, it is more appropriate to integrate health and nutrition interventions into preschools and schools because children have few regularly scheduled health visits unless they are ill. Accordingly, our discussion of the economics of ECD is divided into the two age groups: children younger than age three years and children ages three to five years.

Factors other than age also affect the best way to deliver interventions. The likelihood that children participate in preschool depends on income. Enrollment in preschool is lower in poorer countries and higher in richer ones; within countries, enrollment is higher in families in the highest wealth quintile compared with other quintiles (UNESCO 2015). Enrollment in group settings is likely to be higher in urban areas than in areas of lower population density. This means that program design has potential impacts on equity—urban and rural areas and countries at different income levels may need different services.

This chapter focuses on responsive stimulation interventions delivered through health and nutrition services for young children when they are usually accompanied by family members and preschool experiences for children ages three to five or six years. We do not discuss day care arrangements for younger children at length because they tend to be more informal and not necessarily of high quality, at least for Latin America and the Caribbean (Berlinski and Schady 2015). Because of the degree of dispersion, high required staff-to-child ratios, and problems in monitoring (Leroy, Gadsden, and Guijarro 2012), day care is not an easy modality by which to deliver interventions to improve responsive stimulation. We also do not cover interventions specifically intended to address the mental health of caregivers; mental health is the subject of volume 4 (Patel and others 2015).

We first briefly discuss the methods used for the literature search and the results on costs per child and benefit-cost ratios of interventions. We use this information to develop and cost an essential package and to derive some brief conclusions. Definitions of age-specific groupings and age-specific terminology used in this volume can be found in chapter 1 (Bundy and others 2017).

METHODS

We began with a systematic search of the published literature. The original searches of the literature for this volume undertaken in July 2014 and January 2015 did not yield any cost-effectiveness or benefit-cost studies for preschool children (Horton and Wu 2016), most likely because the search terms were not specific enough.

A second, more specific, search was undertaken in July 2015 with additional search terms (annex 24A) that yielded three relevant articles, two of which contained benefit-cost or unit cost information. Other articles were obtained through consultation with experts, searches of bibliographies of relevant articles, and searches of gray literature.

In all, 11 articles that provide economic estimates were identified. One contained information on benefit-cost ratios only, three on unit cost only, and seven on both. These articles cover a broad range of LMICs, although coverage of Latin America and the Caribbean was the most in-depth (five studies). One study was found for multiple countries in the Middle East, two for Turkey, one for Mozambique, and one for Pakistan, and one covers a broad range of LMICs. Although South-East Asia has large preschool programs and center-based care programs, no articles providing economic estimates were found for that region.

The 11 identified studies of the economics of ECD cover regions similar to those addressed in the larger literature on effectiveness of ECD discussed in chapter 19 in this volume (Black, Gove, and Merseth 2017). A survey and meta-analysis of the effectiveness literature outside Canada and the United States was undertaken by Nores and Barnett (2010). They restricted their coverage to experimental studies and to quasi-experimental studies with stronger designs, identifying 28 studies in 13 countries (4 in Latin America and the Caribbean, 4 in Asia, 3 in Western Europe, and 1 each in Mauritius and Turkey). Four of the programs identified in Nores and Barnett's (2010) survey are also covered in the economic literature—the interventions in Bolivia, Jamaica, Turkey, and Uruguay that are discussed in the next two sections. It is a noticeable omission that no effectiveness and benefit-cost studies are available for Sub-Saharan Africa.

Our survey of cost and benefit-cost is therefore likely to be fairly representative of the larger literature on effectiveness, and there is overlap of actual programs covered. We know quite a lot about the few programs that have been the subject of well-designed research studies. These programs may be more effective than the average, but because they are more intensive, they may cost more. The same would be true for the United States, where the Perry Preschool Project, Head Start, and the Abecedarian Project were intensively studied, with long-term follow-up. Other programs that have not been studied may be less costly, but they may also be less effective and less cost-effective. However, the objective should be to try to replicate good-quality, effective programs.

The literature on both effectiveness and economic aspects also has a regional bias. Studies focus more on middle-income countries; in particular, we know very little about cost and effectiveness in Sub-Saharan Africa, where coverage is lowest and expansion of coverage is most needed.

BENEFIT-COST RATIOS OF EARLY CHILD DEVELOPMENT INTERVENTIONS

Children Younger than Age Three Years

Recent studies have examined the effectiveness of combined health, nutrition, and early childhood interventions in LMICs for children, typically younger than age three years (Grantham-McGregor and others 2014; Nores and Barnett 2010). Table 24.1 presents our benefit-cost findings based on our literature search.

Two randomized controlled trials for Pakistan and the Caribbean had positive economic evaluations. The benefit-cost ratio for an intervention in Antigua, Jamaica, and St. Lucia that developed videos and showed them to parents waiting in health centers, followed by group discussion, was 5.3 (Walker and others 2015). In Pakistan, a randomized controlled trial compared nutrition alone, responsive stimulation alone, and the two combined against a control receiving usual care (Gowani and others 2014). The combined option had the best outcome and cost less than the other two interventions. The lower costs were unrepresentative of an intervention at scale because they were due to two vacant supervisor positions, and the research study may have helped compensate for the absence of usual levels of supervision.

López Boo, Palloni, and Urzua (2014) estimated a benefit-cost ratio of 1.5 for an intervention in Nicaragua that combined responsive stimulation and a nutrition intervention of multiple micronutrient powders for children younger than age three years. However, the entire benefit is based on reduction of anemia, which is likely to be predominantly due to the nutrition intervention; it does not take into account any cognitive benefits

Table 24.1 Benefit-Cost Ratios of Early Child Development Interventions

Study	Country or region	Comments	Benefit-cost ratio (d = discount rate)
Ages zero to two years			
Berlinski and Schady 2015	Latin America	Home visits; modeled costs and returns, using 3 percent discount rate. Outcomes: child cognitive skills; mother's employment.	3.6 (Guatemala) 2.6 (Colombia) 3.5 (Chile)
Walker and others 2015	Jamaica, St. Lucia, Antigua	Details not yet published; summary results cited in Berlinski and Schady 2015.[a]	5.3
Gowani and others 2014	Pakistan	Parenting intervention took advantage of spare capacity (home visits without intervention were "too short"); combined intervention was less costly because two regular supervisory posts vacant; likely not replicable in nonresearch setting.[a]	Not calculated, but combined nutrition and parenting very favorable
López Boo, Palloni, and Urzua 2014	Nicaragua	Benefit-cost ratio is for combined effect of Sprinkles[b] and early child development, but effect calculated on the basis of anemia (likely to be primarily effect of Sprinkles).[a]	1.5
Ages three to five years: Preschool programs			
Behrman, Cheng, and Todd 2004	Bolivia	Range depends on assumptions about gain in earnings from increased educational attainment, and cost of education.[a]	2.28–3.66 (d = 3%) 1.37–2.48 (d = 5%)
Berlinski and Schady 2015	Latin America	Modeled benefits (child cognitive skills hence future earnings, and mother's employment) compared to preschool costs.	5.1 (Guatemala) 3.4 (Colombia) 4.3 (Chile)
Berlinski, Galiani, and Manacorda 2008	Uruguay	Modeled benefits of increased school grade completion, net of cost of preschool and additional school cost.	19.1 (d = 3%) 3.2 (d = 10%)

table continues next page

Table 24.1 Benefit-Cost Ratios of Early Child Development Interventions (continued)

Study	Country or region	Comments	Benefit-cost ratio (d = discount rate)
Engle and others 2011	73 low- and middle-income countries	Modeled change in wages due to increased school attainment, associated with increased preschool participation. Includes additional preschool cost but not school cost.	14.3–17.6 (d = 3%) 6.4–7.8 (d = 6%)
Kaytaz 2004	Turkey	Considers cost of preschool education plus forgone earnings of students staying longer in school. Range depends on assumptions on share continuing to tertiary education.[a]	2.18–3.43 (d = 6%) 1.12–1.69 (d = 10%)

Note: For details of interventions, see table 24.2. Berlinski and Schady (2015) also model the benefit-cost ratio of day care provision to children ages zero to five years as 1.2 (Guatemala), 1.1 (Colombia), and 1.5 (Chile), also using a modeling exercise and discount rate of 3 percent. Psacharopoulos (2015) provides benefit-cost estimates of 3:1 for preschool in the Philippines citing Patrinos (2007), and 77:1 in Kenya, citing Orazem, Glewwe, and Patrinos (2009). Patrinos (2007) cites Glewwe, Jacoby, and King (2001), which is a study of the return to nutrition interventions in preschools in the Philippines; and Orazem, Glewwe, and Patrinos (2009) cite Vermeersch and Kremer (2004), which is a study of the return to school meals in Kenya. We have not included these estimates.
a. Measured outcomes are described in table 24.2.
b. Sprinkles is a brand of multiple micronutrient powders.

resulting from responsive stimulation. Finally, one study for Latin America and the Caribbean models the effect of a home visiting program that educates mothers in child development (Berlinski and Schady 2015); however, this program is not combined with a nutrition or health intervention. Benefit-cost ratios for the three countries ranged from 2.6 to 3.6. There may be other benefit-cost studies of home visiting programs in LMICs that we did not survey given that our search focused on combined programs that included health interventions. More economic studies of combined interventions would be helpful.

Children Ages Three to Five Years

There is a larger literature on preschool programs than on programs for younger children (table 24.1). Benefit-cost ratios of preschool for five countries—Bolivia, Chile, Colombia, Turkey, and Uruguay—generally exceeded 3 (using a discount rate of 3 percent or higher); in Uruguay, the benefit-cost ratio was 19.1, using a discount rate of 3 percent. Benefit-cost ratios for preschool ages remained generally greater than 1 for discount rates up to 10 percent. A cross-country study generated a benefit-cost ratio of 14.3–17.6, but it did not incorporate the requisite additional costs of greater school enrollment (Engle and others 2011).

A nutritional add-on to preschool—a breakfast of porridge—generated an extraordinarily high benefit-cost ratio of 77 in Kenya (Psacharopoulos 2015, citing Orazem, Glewwe, and Patrinos 2009, who in turn use Vermeersch and Kramer 2004). However, the underlying empirical study does not appear to have been published,

and it is not clear that Psacharopoulos (2015) accounted for the cost of the breakfast in the calculations.

The benefit-cost ratios estimated for LMICs are slightly lower than those estimated for well-known preschool studies in the United States, which ranged from 2.7 to 7.2 for three programs (Temple and Reynolds 2007). One difference is that the type of longitudinal studies available in the United States has not been conducted in LMICs; Gertler and others (2014), one of the first, is a 20-year follow-up to a seminal intervention in Jamaica. For LMICs, there are estimates of the benefits in cognitive achievement, school attainment, and wages. There are few data, however, on some of the substantial costs avoided by quality preschool programs in the United States, such as the costs of crime. LMIC estimates probably underestimate the benefits of ECD interventions; Gertler and others (2014) found large effects on wages for Jamaica that were associated with increases in international migration for the treated group.

Comparing across all programs irrespective of child age, the benefit-cost ratio of integrated programs tends to be higher than that of stand-alone programs. This outcome may be due in part to lower marginal costs of the intervention, as well as possible synergies in outcomes. This inference relies on four studies (Gowani and others 2014; López Boo, Palloni, and Urzua 2014; Walker and others 2015; and a subsequent interpretation by Psacharopoulos 2015 of Vermeersch and Kremer 2004). Because two of these are not or not yet published (Walker and others 2015; Vermeersch and Kremer 2004), and the study designs of the other two have unique features, additional studies are needed to confirm this tendency.

UNIT COST OF INTERVENTIONS

Unit cost data are presented in table 24.2. There are some inconsistencies in the data, for example, Araujo, López Boo, and Puyana (2013) reported financial costs that do not take account of volunteers, donations, and parental contributions. Programs for younger children are more heterogeneous in structure. They vary from day care (Araujo, López Boo, and Puyana 2013; Behrman, Cheng, and Todd 2004), to programs to educate mothers of children ages five and six years in groups (Chang and others 2015; Sirali, Bernal, and Naudeau 2015), to home visits (Gowani and others 2014; van Ravens and Aggio 2008). What is covered in the costs for preschool programs is more uniform because the programs are somewhat more standardized, but preschool programs also vary in intensity, for example, hours per week and ratio of children to teachers.

Costs are updated to 2012 U.S. dollars to permit comparisons, and comparing costs as a percentage of per capita gross national income (GNI) is also useful. Berlinski and Schady (2015) and van Ravens and Aggio (2008) model costs, arguing that the salary of an ECD educator has approximately a constant relation to the salary of a primary teacher; that primary teachers' salaries have a predictable relationship to GNI; and that the educator-to-child ratio is fairly predictable, depending on child age (very high for day care, lower for preschool, and lower still for group education programs for parents and caregivers).

Table 24.2 Unit Costs of Early Child Development Interventions

Study	Country or region	Intervention and outcomes measured	Cost in study	Unit	Currency (year)	Annual cost per child in 2012 US$	Annual cost per child as share of GNI (percent)
Ages zero to two years							
Araujo, López Boo, and Puyana 2013	Latin America and the Caribbean	Financial costs for four parenting programs across Latin America and the Caribbean, ranging from US$13 to US$599 per child; median = Mexico and Ecuador. No outcome measured.	188 (median)	Child per year	US$	220	2.2 for median countries
Walker and others 2015	Antigua, Jamaica, and St. Lucia	Parents were shown a video on responsive stimulation at routine health visits, engaged in group discussion, and received small books and puzzles to use at home. Outcome: parenting scale, Griffith Mental Development Scale, Communicative Development Index.	100	Child over 15-month period	2012 US$	100[a]	2.0
Gowani and others 2014	Pakistan	Lady Health Workers (who provide health and nutrition advice in home visits) were trained to also give responsive stimulation; also monthly group meetings held with mothers; 2x2 factorial design. Outcomes: cognition, motor, language scores.	4	Child per month, birth to 24 months	2012 US$	48	3.8
López Boo, Palloni, and Urzua 2014	Nicaragua	PAININ program provided three-hour care per day in centers (with ECD and Sprinkles[b]) in urban areas; home parenting visits twice a week in rural areas by volunteer mothers. Outcomes: anemia, hemoglobin, verbal and numeric memory.	37	Child per year	2012 US$	37	2.1
van Ravens and Aggio 2008	Middle East	Home visiting: develop formula that cost per child is 16/(total fertility rate), as % of per capita GDP; range of costs US$13–US$1,393 for 19 countries. No outcomes.	85 in median country (Jordan)	Child per year	2006 US$	117	2.3

table continues next page

Table 24.2 Unit Costs of Early Child Development Interventions (continued)

Study	Country or region	Intervention and outcomes measured	Cost in study	Unit	Currency (year)	Annual cost per child in 2012 US$	Annual cost per child as share of GNI (percent)
Ages three to five years							
Araujo, López Boo, and Puyana 2013	Latin America and the Caribbean	Financial costs from 28 child care programs, ranging from US$257 to US$3,264 per child; median = Mexico and Ecuador. No outcomes measured.	836 median	Child per year	2010 US$	977	10 for median countries
Behrman, Cheng, and Todd 2004	Bolivia	PIDI: provides day care to children ages 6–72 months in poor, largely urban areas; 40 percent of cost is food. Outcomes: motor, language, psychosocial skills; nutritional status.	43	Child per month	1996 US$	600	26.0
Berlinski, Galiani, and Manacorda 2008	Uruguay	Government-provided preschool for ages four to five years. Outcomes: subsequent school attainment.	1,164.80 (US$129.10)	Child per year	1997 Uruguayan pesos	198	1.4
Kaytaz 2004	Turkey	Preschool. Outcomes: subsequent school attainment.	886,424,000 (US$552)	Child per year	2002 Turkish liras	1,245	11.5
Martinez, Naudeau, and Pereira 2012; Sirali, Bernal, and Naudeau 2015	Mozambique	Preschool for three and a quarter hours per day; cost in pilot phase (Martinez, Naudeau, and Pereira 2012) was only half of cost in scale up (Sirali, Bernal, and Naudeau 2015). Outcomes: subsequent enrollment in primary school; scores on various development tests; spillover to older sibling school enrollment and parents' work time.	25 (pilot); 50 scale up	Child per year	2010[c] US$ 2012[c] US$	50 (at scale-up)	9.4
Sirali, Bernal, and Naudeau 2015	Turkey	MOCEP 25-week training program for mothers and children ages five to six years; lectures and discussions once per week, kits for use at home, home visits by trainers. No outcomes discussed.	40	Participant (25 weeks)	2010 US$	90[a]	0.8
van Ravens and Aggio 2008	Middle East	Preschool: develop formula that cost per child is 12.5 percent of per capita GDP; range of costs US$54–US$3,482 for 19 countries. No outcomes discussed.	239 median country Jordan	Child per year	2006 US$	330	6.5 for median country

Note: ECD = early child development; GDP = gross domestic product; GNI = gross national income; MOCEP = Mother and Child Education Program; PAININ = Comprehensive Childcare Program; PIDI = Programa de Atención Integral a la Niñez Nicaragüense, Proyecto Integral de Desarollo Infantil.
a. Cost is for duration of program per child; duration is not exactly one year.
b. Sprinkles are a brand of multiple micronutrient powders.
c. Original authors do not specify dates; these are estimated by current authors.

Berlinski and Schady (2015) explained that the cost of preschool programs varies systematically with process quality. More intensive supervision adds about 10 percent to the cost of preschool programs, while structural quality—quality of buildings, higher pay for teachers, smaller class sizes—can add up to 300 percent to the basic cost of preschool programs. The data are insufficient to examine the benefit-cost ratio variations of basic, improved process quality, and improved structural quality programs, although Berlinski and Schady (2015) argued that the benefit-cost ratio of enhancing process quality is likely higher than that of enhancing structural quality. This is, however, a contested literature, because trained teachers who can improve process quality may not stay long in low-quality school environments, such as those with dilapidated buildings. Vermeer and others (2016) undertook an international meta-analysis and commented on how different factors affect a measure of program quality that can be measured by observers, and in turn is known to correlate with longer-term outcomes.

Children Younger than Age Three Years

The cost of integrating a component on responsive stimulation with regular visits for nutrition and health is more modest than that of establishing either a day care or a preschool program. Table 24.2 provides unit cost data for five programs for younger children that primarily seek to benefit mothers and children in their homes or in community-based day care with volunteer mothers.

Programs for younger children vary considerably in their format, and annual costs per child range from about 0.8 percent of per capita GNI for financial costs of day care and home visit programs in Latin America and the Caribbean, as well as a mother-child education program in Turkey, to 3.8 percent of per capita GNI for a home visit program in Pakistan. The median share of per capita GNI is 2.2 percent. Programs tend to cost more per child in absolute amount as country income increases because salaries increase, and where the educators are paid rather than serve as volunteers. Home visit programs cost more than programs in which groups of mothers attend centers for parenting education. However, center-based programs may simply transfer the costs of attendance to families rather than trainers, and these programs may reduce participation by those in poorer households or those living in more remote locations.

Children Ages Three to Five Years

Preschool programs are more costly than programs involving educating mothers or caregivers. The annual costs per child range from 1.4 percent of per capita GNI in Uruguay to 26 percent in Bolivia. However, the very lowest and highest costs are probably outliers. The Uruguay program is in an upper-middle-income country and provides a half-day program, which may reduce costs, while the program cost in Bolivia is 16 percent of per capita GNI if cost of food is excluded. The median cost is approximately 10 percent of per capita GNI. This amount is roughly consistent with a formula developed by van Ravens and Aggio (2008), who used salaries and staff-to-child ratios and estimated the cost to be 12.5 percent of gross domestic product (GDP). Preschool programs are consistently more costly than group parenting education because of the higher staff-to-child ratio that is necessary.

Parenting programs are less common in this age group, but one program summarized in the table for children ages three to five years provides group parental education for mothers of older children (Sirali, Bernal, and Naudeau 2015), the Mother and Child Education Program in Turkey. This program has been widely disseminated to other countries.

THE ESSENTIAL PACKAGE AND ITS COST

Assumptions

Parenting programs are more likely to be oriented to children younger than age three years and to entail the participation of mothers. The Mother and Child Education Program delivered to mothers of older children is somewhat unusual in this respect (Sirali, Bernal, and Naudeau 2015). Some parenting programs are delivered to groups of mothers (see table 24.2 for examples for the Caribbean and Turkey); others are delivered primarily through home visits (see table 24.2 for examples from the Middle East and Latin America and the Caribbean); and hybrid programs use both group and home visit components (see table 24.2 for one program in Pakistan). Preschool programs typically focus on ages three to five years, although they may include younger children.

The cost of ECD programs is driven primarily by salary costs. Costs depend on several factors, including the ratio of educators to children, country GNI because salaries tend to increase with country income, and the specific design of individual programs.

Program type has a substantial impact on cost because there are systematic differences in the ratio of staff to children and families. Parenting programs provided to groups can have higher child-to-staff ratios than those involving home visiting; the lowest ratios observed are for preschool programs, where teachers educate children rather than parents. The ratios might be approximately 50 to 1, 25 to 1, and 12 to 1, respectively (estimate based on Araujo, López Boo, and Puyana 2013; Gowani and others 2014; and van Ravens and Aggio 2008). Based on these staffing ratios, we estimate that home visiting programs might cost about twice as much per child as group parenting programs, while preschool programs might cost about four times as much per child as group parenting programs. All three types of programs—parenting programs, home visiting programs, and preschool programs—may vary in effectiveness.

Similarly, we can estimate that the per capita income of lower-middle-income countries is about three times that of low-income countries, and that of upper-middle-income countries is about nine times that of low-income countries, using the World Bank definitions. Table 24.2 includes information from one low-income country, Mozambique.

We developed the following estimates for costs per child per year in 2012 U.S. dollars, based on table 24.2, also using the ratios discussed:

- **Group parenting programs**: US$30–US$35 per child in lower-middle-income countries and US$90–US$100 per child in upper-middle-income countries
- **Home visiting programs**: US$60–US$70 per child in lower-middle-income countries and US$200 per child in upper-middle-income countries
- **Preschool programs**: US$300 per child in lower-middle-income countries and US$600 per child in upper-middle-income countries.

We have no data for low-income countries in Sub-Saharan Africa, other than one preschool program that cost US$50 per child per year for a three hour per day program once the program moved beyond the pilot phase.

These estimates are roughly consistent with the country data (table 24.2) and the staffing ratios presented. Costs for individual countries will vary with per capita GNI and program design. It is always possible to make programs cheaper by, for example, reducing intensity or using volunteers, but doing so can be detrimental to effectiveness. We assume that programs delivered to mothers need to be delivered once per lifetime of children, whereas children may participate in preschool programs for two or three years until they begin formal schooling. The cost of US$30–US$35 for a group parenting program per child born is modest compared with the larger investment in health per child born. Routine immunization alone with six or more vaccines now costs US$46.50 per fully immunized child (Brenzel, Young, and Walker 2015; see Black and others 2016).

Evidence from programs (table 24.1) suggests that the benefit-cost ratio of a well-designed and well-implemented program is in the range of 2–5, using a modest 3 percent to 5 percent social discount rate. Although some benefit-cost estimates are higher than these, they may be from studies that underestimate the full program cost.

Recommendations for an Essential Package

Based on considerations of cost, our subjective assessment of feasibility, and benefit-cost, we recommend the following.

Essential Package
Countries should aim to cover all first-time parents (at a minimum) and all births (preferably) with a group parenting program that is integrated into the provision of health services. This program could be conventional (in person) or could take advantage of innovative methods, such as videos combined with facilitated group discussion. Parenting programs could be integrated into existing home visiting programs that provide health services, in which case the program could be offered instead of or in combination with group delivery. The programs should be provided in one year of the child's first three years, preferably as early as possible to have the greatest impact.

Countries might also choose to implement the program differently in different regions, providing group sessions in more densely populated areas and home visits to more remote households and to poorer households. Costs will increase as the proportion receiving home visits increases, but equity and impact will also increase.

Programs must have a certain intensity to have an impact. In the Caribbean pilot (Walker and others 2015), mothers participated in group discussions five times over approximately 15 months; each session took about 25 minutes of the mother's time (a combination of viewing a video and participating in a group discussion, with one-on-one reinforcement during the visit with the nurse). In Pakistan, mothers received home visits of approximately 30 minutes about once a month, and the pilot program followed children in their first two years of life (Gowani and others 2014). In Latin American programs, parents generally met with community workers for slightly more than an hour a week for 10 months of the year over a two-year period (Araujo, López Boo, and Puyana 2013). A group program in Uganda for both parents that entailed 12 sessions is discussed in chapter 19 in this volume (Black, Gove, and Merseth 2017); the content of the parenting programs is also important. Programs that do not have sufficient quality and intensity will not be effective.

Preschool Programs
Evidence suggests that children are more ready for school cognitively, socially, and emotionally if they have preschool education; this is particularly important for children from more vulnerable households. The estimated cost per child is US$300 per child per year in lower-middle-income countries and US$600 per child per year in upper-middle-income countries. We assume that governments would subsidize or pay the full cost of this education for vulnerable households but require parental contribution or full payment for more affluent households. This approach is more common in upper-middle-income countries.

When estimating preschool costs, van Ravens and Aggio (2008) assume a half-day program and use a ratio of 20 children per teacher. UNICEF (2008) recommends 15 hours per week and a 15:1 maximum ratio, but even many countries in Europe do not achieve this goal, and this objective would certainly imply higher costs than provided here.

CONCLUSIONS

Codelivery of health, nutrition, and responsive stimulation programs can benefit child development and be cost-effective. For children younger than age three years, codelivery is best achieved by integrating responsive stimulation elements into existing health and nutrition programs. For children ages three to five years, codelivery can be achieved by integrating health and nutrition interventions into preschool programs.

For children younger than age three years, group parenting programs cost about US$30–US$35 per year in lower-middle-income countries, and about twice that if home visiting is included. Some home visiting is likely to be required to reach some populations and improve equity. The benefit-cost ratio for existing programs ranges from about 2:1 to about 5:1. Group parenting programs need facilitators but can also incorporate media, such as videos.

Preschool programs cost about US$300 per child in lower-middle-income countries, and the benefit-cost estimates for existing programs similarly range from about 2:1 to 5:1 (higher benefit-cost ratios have been obtained, but typically where costs are underestimated). Countries can usually afford to subsidize preschool for only selected groups, such as poor households and marginalized groups.

Programs for individual children and families need to be complemented by appropriate national policies for child development. National policies include policies proscribing child abuse and facilitating behavior change communication to support positive parenting behaviors.

Evidence on cost and cost-effectiveness is quite modest, and we rely heavily on a relatively few longitudinal studies of high-quality programs. Some researchers have used innovative methods, such as using national data retrospectively (for example, Berlinski, Galiani, and Manacorda 2008) or linking across national datasets. It would also not be too difficult or costly to augment the cost and cost-effectiveness literature by collecting cost data for existing studies of effectiveness.

Evidence on cost and cost-effectiveness is presently insufficient for low-income countries in Sub-Saharan Africa. Although children in this region likely will benefit from ECD programs, well-evaluated pilot programs are required to identify program designs that will work well in this context and that are scalable.

For all of these interventions, program quality is extremely important. Good training and supervision are critical. If ECD is seen as a low-cost add-on to existing health and nutrition programs, and current staff is overburdened by yet more tasks, the outcomes are likely to be of low quality. Well-designed and well-supervised interventions can affordably improve the likelihood that vulnerable children will be better able to reach their full potential.

ANNEX

The annex to this chapter is as follows. It is available at http://www.dcp-3.org/CAHD.

• Annex 24A. Literature Search Terms and Methods

ACKNOWLEDGMENT

The authors would like to thank Vittoria Lutje for running the systematic searches, Florencia López Boo for providing helpful references, and Daphne Wu for providing excellent research assistance.

NOTE

World Bank Income Classifications as of July 2014 are as follows, based on estimates of gross national income (GNI) per capita for 2013:

• Low-income countries (LICs) = US$1,045 or less
• Middle-income countries (MICs) are subdivided:
    a) lower-middle-income = US$1,046 to US$4,125
    b) upper-middle-income (UMICs) = US$4,126 to US$12,745
• High-income countries (HICs) = US$12,746 or more.

REFERENCES

Araujo, M. C., F. López Boo, and J. M. Puyana. 2013. *Overview of Early Childhood Development Services in Latin America and the Caribbean.* Washington, DC: Inter-American Development Bank.

Batura, N., Z. Hill, H. Haghparast-Bidgoli, R. Lingham, T. Colbourn, and others. 2014. "Highlighting the Evidence Gap: How Cost-Effective Are Interventions to Improve Early Childhood Nutrition and Development?" *Health Policy and Planning* 30 (6): 813–21. doi:10.1093/healpol/czu055.

Behrman, J., Y. Cheng, and P. Todd. 2004. "Evaluating Preschool Programs Where Length of Exposure to the Program Varies: A Nonparametric Approach." *Review of Economics and Statistics* 86: 108–32.

Berlinski, S., S. Galiani, and M. Manacorda. 2008. "Giving Children a Better Start: Preschool Attendance and School-Age Profiles." *Journal of Public Economics* 92 (5–6): 1416–40.

Berlinski, S., and N. Schady, eds. 2015. *The Early Years: Child Well-Being and the Role of Public Policy*. New York: Palgrave Macmillan.

Black, M. M., A. Gove, and K. A. Merseth. 2017. "Platforms to Reach Children in Early Childhood." In *Disease Control Priorities* (third edition): Volume 8, *Child and Adolescent Health and Development*, edited by D. A. P. Bundy, N. de Silva, S. Horton, D. T. Jamison, and G. C. Patton. Washington, DC: World Bank.

Black, R., N. Walker, R. Laxminaryan, and M. Temmerman. 2016. "Reproductive, Maternal, Newborn, and Child Health: Key Messages of this Volume." In *Disease Control Priorities* (third edition): Volume 2, *Reproductive, Maternal, Newborn, and Child Health*, edited by R. Black, R. Laxminarayan, M. Temmerman, and N. Walker. Washington, DC: World Bank.

Brenzel, L., D. Young, and D. G. Walker. 2015. "Costs and Financing of Routine Immunization: Approach and Findings of a Multi-Country Study (EPIC)." *Vaccine* 335 (Suppl 1): A13–20.

Bundy, D. A. P., N. de Silva, S. Horton, G. C. Patton, L. Schultz, and D. T. Jamison. 2017. "Child and Adolescent Health and Development: Realizing Neglected Potential." In *Disease Control Priorities* (third edition): Volume 8, *Child and Adolescent Health and Development*, edited by D. A. P. Bundy, N. de Silva, S. Horton, D. T. Jamison, and G. C. Patton. Washington, DC: World Bank.

Chang, S. M., S. M. Grantham-McGregor, C. A. Powell, M. Vera-Hernández, F. López-Boo, and others. 2015. "Integrating a Parenting Intervention with Routine Primary Health Care: A Cluster-Randomized Trial." *Pediatrics* 136: 272–80.

Engle, P., M. Black, J. R. Behrman, M. Cabral de Mello, P. J. Gertler, and others. 2007. "Strategies to Avoid the Loss of Development Potential in More than 200 Million Children in the Developing World." *The Lancet* 369 (9557): 229–42.

Engle, P., L. C. H. Fernald, H. Alderman, J. Behrman, C. O'Gara, and others. 2011. "Strategies for Reducing Inequalities and Improving Developmental Outcomes for Young Children in Low-Income and Middle-Income Countries." *The Lancet* 378 (9799): 1339–53.

Gertler, P., J. Heckman, R. Pinto, A. Zanolini, C. Vermeersch, and others. 2014. "Labor Market Returns to Early Childhood Stimulation Intervention in Jamaica." *Science* 344 (6187): 998–1001.

Glewwe, P., H. G. Jacoby, and E. M. King. 2001. "Early Childhood Nutrition and Academic Achievement: A Longitudinal Analysis." *Journal of Public Economics* 81: 345–68.

Gowani, S., A. K. Yousafzai, R. Armstrong, and Z. A. Bhutta. 2014. "Cost-Effectiveness of Responsive Stimulation and Nutrition Intervention on Early Child Development Outcomes in Pakistan." *Annals of the New York Academy of Sciences* 1308: 149–61.

Grantham-McGregor, S. M., L. C. H. Fernald, R. M. C. Kagawa, and S. Walker. 2014. "Effects of Integrated Child Development and Nutrition Interventions on Child Development and Nutritional Status." *Annals of the New York Academy of Sciences* 1308: 11–32.

Horton, S., and D. C. N. Wu. 2016. "Methodology and Results of Systematic Search, Cost and Cost-Effectiveness Analysis, for *Child and Adolescent Health and Development*." Working Paper, DCP3, Seattle, WA. http://www.dcp-3.org/resources /working-papers.

Kaytaz, M. 2004. "A Cost-Benefit Analysis of Preschool Education in Turkey." ACEV (Mother Child Education Foundation). http://siteresources.worldbank.org/INTTURKEY/Resources /361616-1142415001082/Preschool_by_Kaytaz.pdf.

Leroy, J. L., P. Gadsden, and M. Guijarro. 2012. "The Impact of Daycare Programmes on Child Health, Nutrition and Development in Developing Countries: A Systematic Review." *Journal of Development Effectiveness* 4 (3): 472–96.

López Boo, F. L., G. Palloni, and S. Urzua. 2014. "Cost-Benefit Analysis of a Micronutrient and Early Childhood Stimulation Program in Nicaragua." *Annals of the New York Academy of Sciences* 1308: 139–48.

Martinez, S., S. Naudeau, and V. Pereira. 2012. "The Promise of Preschool in Africa: A Randomized Impact Evaluation of Early Childhood Development in Rural Mozambique." World Bank and Save the Children, Washington, DC. http:// siteresources.worldbank.org/INTAFRICA/Resources/The _Promise_of_Preschool_in_Africa_ECD_REPORT.pdf.

Nores, M., and W. S. Barnett. 2010. "Benefits of Early Childhood Interventions across the World: (Under) Investing in the Very Young." *Economics of Education Review* 29 (2): 271–82.

Orazem, P., P. Glewwe, and H. Patrinos. 2009. "The Benefits and Costs of Alternative Strategies to Improve Educational Outcomes." In *Global Crises, Global Solutions*, edited by B. Lomborg. Cambridge, U.K.: Cambridge University Press.

Patel, V., D. Chisholm, T. Dua, R. Laxminarayan, and M. E. Medina-Mora, eds. 2015. *Disease Control Priorities* (third edition): Volume 4, *Mental, Neurological, and Substance Use Disorders*. Washington, DC: World Bank.

Patrinos, H. A. 2007 "The Living Conditions of Children." Policy Research Working Paper 4251, World Bank, Washington, DC.

Psacharopoulos, G. 2015. "Education Assessment Paper: Benefits and Costs of the Education Targets for the Post-2015 Development Agenda." Copenhagen Consensus Centre. http://www.copenhagenconsensus.com/publication/post -2015-consensus-education-assessment-psacharopoulos.

Singla, D. R., E. Kumbakumba, and F. E. Aboud. 2015. "Effects of an Integrated Intervention on Child Development and Maternal Depressive Symptoms in Rural Uganda: A Cluster-Randomized Trial." *The Lancet Global Health* 3 (8): e458–69.

Sirali, Y., R. Bernal, and S. Naudeau. 2015. "Early Childhood Development: What Does It Cost to Provide It at Scale?" Brookings Education + Development Blogs. http://www .brookings.edu/blogs/education-plus-development /posts/2015/01/20-scaling-early-childhood-development -sirali-bernal-naudeau.

Temple, J. A., and A. J. Reynolds. 2007. "Benefits and Costs of Investments in Preschool Education: Evidence from the Child: Parent Centres and Related Programs." *Economics of Education Review* 26: 126–44.

UNESCO (United Nations Educational, Scientific and Cultural Organization). 2015. *EFA Global Monitoring Report 2015: Achievements and Challenges*. Paris: UNESCO.

UNICEF (United Nations Children's Fund). 2008. "The Child Care Transition." UNICEF Innocenti Centre Report Card 8. https://www.unicef-irc.org/publications/pdf/rc8_eng.pdf.

van Ravens, J., and C. Aggio. 2008. "Expanding Early Childhood Care and Education: How Much Does It Cost?" Working Paper 46, Bernard van Leer Foundation, The Hague.

Vermeer, H. J., M. H. van Uzendoorn, R. A. Cárcamo, and L. J. Harrison. 2016. "Quality of Child Care Using the Environment Rating Scales: A Meta-Analysis of International Studies." *International Journal of Early Childhood* 48 (1): 33–60.

Vermeersch, C., and M. Kremer. 2004. "School Meals, Education Achievement and School Competition: Evidence from a Randomized Evaluation." Policy Research Working Paper 3523, World Bank, Washington, DC. http://elibrary.worldbank.org/doi/pdf/10.1596/1813-9450-3523.

Walker, S. P., C. Powell, S. M. Chang, H. Baker-Henningham, S. Grantham-McGregor, and others. 2015. "Delivering Parenting Interventions through Health Services in the Caribbean: Impact, Acceptability and Costs." Working Paper IDB-WB-642, Inter-American Development Bank, Washington, DC.

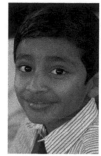

Chapter 25

Identifying an Essential Package for School-Age Child Health: Economic Analysis

Meena Fernandes and Elisabetta Aurino

INTRODUCTION

This chapter presents the investment case for providing an integrated package of essential health services for children attending primary schools in low- and middle-income countries (LMICs). In doing so, it builds on chapter 20 in this volume (Bundy, Schultz, and others 2017), which presents a range of relevant health services for the school-age population and the economic rationale for administering them through educational systems. This chapter identifies a package of essential health services that low- and middle-income countries (LMICs) can aspire to implement through the primary and secondary school platforms. In addition, the chapter considers the design of such programs, including targeting strategies. Upper-middle-income countries and high-income countries (HICs) typically aim to implement such interventions on a larger scale and to include and promote additional health services relevant to their populations. Studies have documented the contribution of school health interventions to a range of child health and educational outcomes, particularly in the United States (Durlak and others 2011; Murray and others 2007; Shackleton and others 2016). Health services selected for the essential package are those that have demonstrated benefits and relevance for children in LMICs. The estimated costs of implementation are drawn from the academic literature. The concept of a package of essential school health interventions and its justification through a cost-benefit perspective was pioneered by Jamison and Leslie (1990).

As chapter 20 notes, health services for school-age children can promote educational outcomes, including access, attendance, and academic achievement, by mitigating earlier nutrition and health deprivations and by addressing current infections and nutritional deficiencies (Bundy, Schultz, and others 2017). This age group is particularly at risk for parasitic helminth infections (Jukes, Drake, and Bundy 2008), and malaria has become prevalent in school-age populations as control for younger children delays the acquisition of immunity from early childhood to school age (Brooker and others 2017). Furthermore, school health services are commonly viewed as a means for building and reinforcing healthy habits to lower the risk of noncommunicable disease later in life (Bundy 2011).

This chapter focuses on packages and programs to reach school-age children, while the previous chapter, chapter 24 (Horton and Black 2017), focuses on early childhood interventions, and the next chapter, chapter 26 (Horton and others 2017), focuses on adolescent interventions. These packages are all part of the same continuum of care from age 5 years to early adulthood, as discussed in chapter 1 (Bundy, de Silva, and others 2017). A particular emphasis of the economic rationale for targeting school-age children is to promote their health and education while they are in the process of learning; many of the interventions that are part of the package have been shown to yield substantial benefits in educational outcomes (Bundy 2011; Jukes, Drake, and Bundy 2008). They might be viewed as health interventions that leverage the investment in education.

Corresponding author: Meena Fernandes, Partnership for Child Development, Imperial College, London, United Kingdom; meenaf@gmail.com.

Schools are an effective platform through which to deliver the essential package of health and nutrition services (Bundy, Schultz, and others 2017). Primary enrollment and attendance rates increased substantially during the Millennium Development Goals era, making schools a delivery platform with the potential to reach large numbers of children equitably. Furthermore, unlike health centers, almost every community has a primary school, and teachers can be trained to deliver simple health interventions, resulting in the potential for high returns for relatively low costs by using the existing infrastructure.

This chapter identifies a core set of interventions for children ages 5–14 years that can be delivered effectively through schools. It then simulates the returns to health and education and benchmarks them against the costs of the intervention, drawing on published estimates. The investment returns illustrate the scale of returns provided by school-based health interventions, highlighting the value of integrated health services and the parameters driving costs, benefits, and value for money (the ratio of benefits to costs). Countries seeking to introduce such a package need to undertake context-specific analyses of critical needs to ensure that the package responds to the specific local needs.

CONDITIONS AND POSSIBLE INTERVENTIONS

Possible interventions for the essential package were considered from the perspective of four domains of child development. Three of which (physical, nutrition, and psychosocial) pertain primarily to health, and one (cognition) primarily to education. Table 25.1 presents an overview of low-cost interventions in each domain and the possible delivery platforms identified in the literature.

Although interventions promoting psychosocial health may be beneficial for primary-school-age children, most studies focus on secondary school and adolescents. Interventions delivered through population-based mechanisms, such as the media, are likely targeted to decision makers and to adolescents rather than children. For some conditions, such as oral health, identification and prevention may be through one platform (schools or communities), and remedial treatment may be through another (primary health centers).

Most of the interventions have potential impacts on education as a consequence of improvements in health, although the specific pathways vary. Providing meals in schools may help mitigate the energy intake gap for children experiencing low to moderate undernutrition, thereby promoting overall health status and school participation. The regular provision of iron-folate pills or meals fortified with micronutrient powders may reduce the prevalence of anemia and so improve cognitive ability, thereby improving school attendance and learning. Correcting refractive error may have a direct impact on future economic productivity by improving learning and academic achievement.

The benefits of interventions such as oral hygiene and vaccines are related primarily to health. Although most vaccines are delivered in early childhood, primary schools can be optimal delivery platforms for primary doses of the human papillomavirus (HPV) vaccine and booster doses of tetanus vaccine (LaMontagne and

Table 25.1 Platforms for Delivering School-Based Health Interventions

Domain		Platform		
	Population level	Community	School	Primary health center
Physical health	Education	Refractive error	**Deworming; insecticide-treated bednets; malaria chemoprevention; tetanus toxoid and HPV vaccination; oral health prevention;** sex education messages; **refractive error**	**Deworming; insecticide-treated bednets; tetanus toxoid and HPV vaccination; oral health and dentistry**
Nutrition	Nutrition education messages	**Micronutrient supplementation; multifortified foods**	**Micronutrient supplementation; multifortified foods; school feeding;** nutrition education messages	**Micronutrient supplementation**
Psychosocial	Mental health messages	n.a.	Mental health education and counseling	Mental health counseling
Cognition	Conditional cash transfers	School promotion	**Vision screening**	**Vision screening**

Note: HPV = human papillomavirus; n.a. = not applicable. Interventions in bold are covered in this chapter.

others 2017), while health centers can target out-of-school children and marginalized girls. In a global survey, 95 of 174 countries used schools to deliver some vaccines, but the prevalence was much lower among LMICs than HICs, 28 percent and 64 percent, respectively (Vandelaer and Olaniran 2015). Effective immunization from tetanus requires several doses in infancy through early childhood, with boosters in middle childhood (around ages 4–7 years) and adolescence (ages 12–15 years). The World Health Organization (WHO) recommends delivering tetanus-diphtheria toxoid combination immunizations rather than a single antigen tetanus toxoid (WHO 2006). At least 80 countries include the tetanus toxoid and booster immunizations in school-based programs, making it the vaccine most commonly delivered through schools (Vandelaer and Olaniran 2015) and part of the essential package.

An estimated 80 percent of the global burden of cervical cancer is concentrated in LMICs, underscoring the relevance of the HPV vaccine as a preventive measure. The essential package promotes the administration of two doses of the HPV vaccine to girls in a given grade in primary school, with the selected grade containing the largest share of the target age group.

The package includes hygiene education, but not the water and sanitation components of WASH. This decision reflects the high cost of intervention, especially the construction of water supply infrastructure and school facility infrastructure and maintenance (Snilstveit and others 2015)-the costs of which would exceed the costs of all other candidate interventions for the essential package.

Table 25.2 estimates the burden of conditions treatable by interventions in the essential package in LMICs, underscoring the potential global impact of school-based health services.

ESTIMATING THE COSTS

Table 25.3 summarizes the evidence on the costs and outcomes of interventions in the essential package. The estimates typically focus on average annual costs incurred in delivering the intervention; they exclude

Table 25.2 Burden of Conditions Affecting the Health and Development of School-Age Children

Domain and condition or infection	Estimated school-age population at risk	Possible interventions
Physical health		
Schistosoma and STHs, including hookworm, roundworm, whipworm	Schistosomiasis: 207 million cases globally STHs: 870 million cases in 2014[a]	Deworming treatment
Malaria	568 million at risk globally; more than 200 million cases of *Plasmodium falciparum* in ages 5–14 years in 2010 in Sub-Saharan Africa alone	ITNs, intermittent preventive screening and administration of malaria chemoprevention, indoor residual spraying
Tetanus	All school-age children	Tetanus toxoid vaccine
HPV	All girls ages 9–14 years	HPV vaccine
Tooth decay	40 percent to 90 percent of children age 12 years in LMICs[b]	Provision of toothbrushes, promotion of oral care, dental screening and referrals
Nutrition		
Micronutrient deficiencies	Anemia: 304.6 million[c]	Micronutrient powders, food fortification, micronutrient-rich foods
Underweight	Girls: 16 percent; boys: 25 percent[d]	School feeding
Cognition		
Uncorrected refractive error	13 million[e]	Vision screening and provision of inexpensive eyeglasses

Note: HPV = human papillomavirus; ITNs = insecticide-treated bednets; LMICs = low- and middle-income countries; STHs = soil-transmitted helminths.
a. Fenwick 2012.
b. Bagramian, Garcia-Godoy, and Volpe 2009.
c. McLean and others 2009.
d. Manyanga and others 2014. Seven African countries (Benin, Djibouti, the Arab Republic of Egypt, Ghana, Malawi, Mauritania, and Morocco) reported prevalence for students ages 11–17 years.
e. Resnikoff and others 2008.

Table 25.3 Costs of Potential Interventions

Costs per year (2012 US$ unless otherwise noted)

Domain	Intervention	Cost per child	Cost per case averted	Cost per death averted	Cost per DALY averted
Nutrition	School meals[a]	41 (2008)	100 kilocalorie gain: 10.22	—	n.a.
	Micronutrient powder supplementation[b]	2.92 (2014)	Anemia: 8.59	—	n.a.
Infectious disease	Deworming: Mass drug administration[c]	0.35	Helminth infection: 0.93–5.28	n.a.	3.36–6.92
	Malaria: Intermittent parasite clearance[d]	1.88–4.03 (2009) (White and others 2011)	Infection: 5.36–9 (Horton and Wu 2015); 1.45–33 (2009) (White and others 2011); anemia: 29.84–50 (Horton and Wu 2015)	110–4,961 (2009)	24 (2009)
	Malaria: Insecticide treated bednets[d]	0.40	Infection: 10–48	950–2,500 (2009)	20–48 (2009)
Vision screening	Refractive error screening and provision of corrective glasses[e]	Ready-made glasses: 2–3; Screening kit: 9 each	Poor vision: 0.71–1.07	—	84
Oral health	Toothbrush provision and education[f]	0.60	Caries reduction: 40 percent, 1.25 per child	—	n.a.
Vaccines	Tetanus toxoid vaccine[g]	0.40 (2003)	—	117 (2003)	3.61 (2003)
	HPV bivalent vaccine[h]	Vaccine cost: 0.55–2.00 per dose for Gavi-eligible countries; Delivery: 4.88–6.73 per fully vaccinated girl (2009)		2,161–2,608	QALY gained for reduced cervical cancer risk: 4,500–8,890 (2011 international $)

Note: — = not available; n.a. = not applicable; DALY = disability-adjusted life year; HPV = human papillomavirus; LMICs = low- and middle-income countries; QALY = quality-adjusted life year.

a. Standardized cost of school meals in LMICs in 2008 US$ (Kristjanssen and others 2015). Cost is standardized to 401 kilocalories. School meals should contribute at least 30 percent to international recommendations, or 555 kilocalories.

b. Cost estimate from Stopford and others, forthcoming. Cost per case averted was calculated assuming that micronutrient powders reduce anemia by 34 percent, based on a review of the evidence (Salam and others 2013).

c. Cost per case averted from Horton and Wu 2015.

d. Cost per death and DALY averted from Horton and Wu 2015; White and others 2011.

e. Cost per DALY for ages 5–10 years from Baltussen, Naus, and Limburg 2009. Cost per case averted assumes that eyeglasses have a useful lifespan of four years, one teacher has one kit for 165 schoolchildren, and compliance is 70 percent, similar to Baltussen, Naus, and Limburg 2009.

f. Monse and others 2013.

g. Griffiths and others 2004.

h. Change in recommendation from a three-dose to a two-dose schedule is likely to improve cost-effectiveness. Gavi eligibility is based on average gross national income. At least 54 LMICs qualify for support (http://www.gavi.org/support/apply/countries-eligible-for-support/). Estimate of cost per death averted from Levin and others 2015.

teacher training, policy development, and monitoring and evaluation. The estimates are drawn from existing studies; therefore the components of each cost estimate are not presented or standardized.

Training Costs

Regular training and refresher courses are needed for teachers delivering the interventions. Training could cover all interventions in the essential package and be integrated with other teacher training courses. Refresher courses are particularly critical in contexts with high teacher turnover. Appropriate monitoring and evaluation are also strongly recommended to ensure appropriate implementation.

Nutrition Costs

School meals can contribute to the recommended energy intake for undernourished children (Drake and others 2017). The three possible modalities include meals, biscuits or snacks, and take-home rations. Almost every country in the world offers school feeding in some form, and meals are the most common modality. The essential package includes the provision of meals or alternatively of snacks in contexts where meals are not possible. Snacks such as packaged biscuits or milk may be more appropriate in emergency contexts or where schools do not have the infrastructure to prepare or serve meals. The inclusion of micronutrients may increase costs, but also benefits. Various studies assess the value of iron-folate pills for girls, especially those entering adolescence. The intervention in the essential package focuses on addressing micronutrient deficiencies.

Infectious Disease Treatment Costs

The cost-effectiveness estimates for infectious diseases—in particular, malaria and helminth infection—may vary with the transmission setting and level of treatment coverage. Deworming treatment is included in the essential package, given the prevalence of soil-transmitted helminths (STHs) and *Schistosoma* infection in this age group (Bundy, Appleby, and others 2017). The pills are free to public health systems because they are donated by the global pharmaceutical industry via the WHO, and costs are related primarily to delivery. In some contexts, one oral treatment provided to each child annually is sufficient; in contexts with higher prevalence, two treatments may be needed. The cost of delivering schistosomiasis treatment in addition to STH treatment is marginal and assumed to be absorbed almost fully in the modeling of costs. The alternative of screening for worm infections, for example by using the Kato-Katz test, and treating only those who are infected is significantly more expensive and is not included in the package (Speich and others 2010).

For malaria, three school-based interventions were considered for inclusion in the essential package. The alternative of intermittent preventive treatment (Stuckey and others 2014)—that is, the distribution of antimalarials to all children at specific times, for example, when malaria is seasonally epidemic—was also ruled out because there is no affordable treatment available that is recommended by the WHO for this use in school-age children.

The evidence clearly demonstrates the cost-effectiveness of ITNs to lower the risk of malaria (Lim and others 2011), as well as the low usage rate among school-age children (Noor and others 2009). The essential package includes malaria education in schools for endemic countries because it is deemed to be the most effective way to promote use of ITNs (Nankabirwa, Wandera, and others 2014).

Vision and the Correction of Refractive Error

Refractive error can be detected through basic screening and can be corrected by the provision of inexpensive corrective lenses (Graham and others 2017). Schools are important in this context as a focus for identifying children with poor vision: children are typically unaware of their impairment and health systems in LMICs rarely have community outreach. The prevalence of refractive error is low, and the costs of corrective lenses can be spread across the target population, reducing the cost per child and increasing the affordability of the intervention. Studies suggest that uncorrected refractive error affects 2.34 per 1,000 people in Africa and 6.59 per 1,000 people in South-East Asia (Baltussen, Naus, and Limburg 2009); however, the proportion in Africa will likely rise as more children have access to schools and books. Studies suggest that the corrective lenses affordable in LMICs are likely to be ready-made.

Oral Health Costs

Two options for oral health are dental services and prevention through skills-based oral health education (Benzian and others 2017). In LMICs, oral health services are typically provided in clinics and hospitals, and are limited by the availability of qualified personnel; the ratio of dentists to population is roughly 1 to 2,000 in HICs, compared with 1 to 150,000 in Sub-Saharan Africa. Oral disease is an expensive condition to treat and is poorly integrated in primary health systems in LMICs (Kandelman and others 2012).

Dental screening at schools and referrals to mobile health teams with dental expertise may be possible in some settings but was not considered affordable and generalizable to be included in the essential package. In contrast, oral health promotion through schools is low cost and has the potential to shape long-term oral hygiene behaviors and is included. Oral health promotion can take place through information provided in health education classes regarding the benefits of using a toothbrush and fluorination; it may involve daily group brushing with fluoride toothpaste at school. The essential package proposes the inclusion of the Fit for School integrated oral health intervention, which has been tested in Cambodia, Indonesia, the Lao People's Democratic Republic, and the Philippines. The program, which cost US$0.60 per child per year for supplies in the Philippines, reduced school absences as well as caries by one-third after one year (Monse and others 2013).

Vaccine Costs

Evidence on the costs of administering the tetanus toxoid vaccine in schools is lacking for LMICs, hence the estimates are based on studies of the cost of antenatal vaccination in primary health clinics. The share of children reached through schools is likely to be higher, depending on attendance rates. School-based delivery is unlikely to have significant economies of scale compared with interventions such as school feeding that reach all children on a daily basis. The tetanus toxoid booster vaccine is typically administered once a year to all children at the beginning and end of primary school, in accordance with the national immunization schedule.

Vaccination to prevent HPV includes two doses administered to girls between ages 9 and 13 years. The costing exercise reflects the administration of two doses to girls in one grade in primary school. The cost of the vaccine is highly dependent on the price of the vaccine itself, which may be subsidized through GAVI, the Vaccine Alliance. On average, the cost of administering HPV immunizations in LMICS is greater than for other routine immunizations, which range from US$0.75 to US$1.40 per dose. However, the cost has dropped in recent years, enabling HPV vaccination to be delivered in low-resource settings. Some studies have found that delivering HPV vaccines through schools costs more than delivering them through health facilities and integrated school-health centers (Hutubessy and others 2012; Levin and others 2014), but coverage may also be higher. School-based delivery is likely to reach a larger share of the population, including children from disadvantaged households.

ESTIMATING THE BENEFITS

Each intervention in the essential package is justified by its low costs of delivery and high ratio of benefits to costs, making it a sound and affordable investment for LMIC governments. Improved education and health outcomes translate into improved productivity and higher national gross domestic product (GDP). To permit comparisons with costs, these benefits must be quantified in financial terms.

This section summarizes the economic benefits of each intervention and the pathways through which they are achieved, based on the literature. Estimates for the benefits of school feeding are based on evidence on specific pathways leading to health and educational outcomes.

Nutrition and Food

School feeding has at least three objectives: social protection, education, and health (Drake and others 2017). School meals transfer a significant amount of noncash income to households, which can cushion shocks such as high food prices. School meals can draw children to school, support learning, and support physical growth by reducing energy deficits. Meals enhanced with micronutrients can also support child nutrition and enhance cognition. Iron-deficiency anemia is one of the top five causes of years lost to disability, contributing nearly 50 percent of the total for ages 10–19 years (Murray and others 2013). While these multiple benefits support the case for school feeding, they are difficult to quantify and aggregate (see chapter 12 in this volume, Drake and others 2017 for more discussion on school feeding).

A recent systematic review (Snilstveit and others 2015) synthesizes the findings from 16 studies (15 unique programs) published in 21 papers, of the effects of school feeding (where feeding occurs in school, that is, does not include take-home rations). The review examines three access outcomes (enrollment, drop-out, and attendance), as well as four measures of schooling outcomes (cognitive scores, math scores, language arts scores, and composite achievement scores). A meta-analysis indicated that although in many cases the point estimate of the effect of school feeding was in the expected direction (improving enrollment, reducing drop-out, and improving scores), none of the effects was statistically significant, other than an increase in attendance.

We use the effect on enrollment (a 9 percent increase, equivalent to 8 extra days in school [Snilstveit and others 2015]), the cost per school meal of $41 per child (table 25.4), and mean per capita GDP in 2015 of $620 in low-income countries and $2035 in lower-middle income countries in 2015 (World Bank 2016a). We assume that the average child eating school meals for one year is 10 years old, enters the labor force at age 15, and continues working until age 55. Annual wage income per person of working age was therefore about $574 in low-income countries and about $1,489 in lower-middle-income countries in 2015 (based on the proportion of the population of working age, 15–64 years, being 54 percent in low-income countries and 64 percent in lower-middle-income countries [World Bank 2016b], and labor income being approximately half of GDP). The returns to an extra year of education are 12 percent per annum in Sub-Saharan Africa (Montenegro and Patrinos 2014;

Figure 25.1 Estimated Cumulative Per-Child Benefits from Receipt of One Year of School Feeding in LICs and lower-middle-income countries

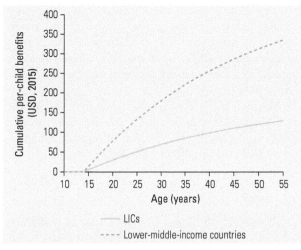

Note: LICs = low-income countries.

Pradhan and others 2017, chapter 30, estimate somewhat lower but still substantial returns to education across low- and middle-income countries).

With these assumptions, we can calculate that eight days of increased attendance increases future wages by 1.08 percent (12 percent multiplied by 0.09). A stream of future wages of $W per year (starting 5 years in the future and continuing for 40 years) is worth about 20W currently, when discounted at 3 percent. Figure 25.1 presents the estimated trajectory of benefits that accrue due to the delivery of school feeding for one year based on the calculation described.

Combining these assumptions implies that the benefit-cost of school meals is around 3 in low-income countries and exceeds 7 for lower-middle income countries. With more optimistic assumptions (for example, that there are additional benefits from improved cognitive scores), the benefit-cost ratio would be even higher.

Infectious Disease

Children infected with intestinal worms are often too sick or tired to attend school or to concentrate in school when they do attend. Persistent worm infections are associated with impaired cognitive development and lower educational achievement (Mendez and Adair 1999; Simeon, Grantham-McGregor, and Wong 1995). A study from Kenya found that after a deworming program, enrollment increased 7 percent and school absenteeism decreased 25 percent (Miguel and Kremer 2004). However, these effects mask heterogeneity; children who are worse off to begin with are likely to gain more. Simeon, Grantham-McGregor, and Wong (1995) found significant impacts on

attendance for children who had heavy *Trichuris* infection or were stunted. Two studies have calculated the economic and social returns to deworming in the United States and Kenya, respectively, through long-term follow-ups (Baird and others 2015; Bleakley 2007). In the United States, hookworm eradication led to gains in income and returns to schooling. In Kenya, deworming increased labor and educational outcomes among men and women, respectively. The authors estimated a conservative internal rate of return to deworming of 32 percent.

Schools can provide significant economies of scale for deworming treatment. The cost for delivery through schools was US$0.03 (Tanzania) and US$0.04 (Ghana) per child per year, compared with delivery through mobile health teams coordinated by primary health centers of US$0.21 in Tanzania and US$0.51 in Montserrat (Guyatt 2003). See also chapters 13 (Bundy, Appleby, and others 2017) and 29 (Ahuja and others 2017) in this volume for discussion of these issues.

Malaria places a significant burden on health care systems and productivity in endemic countries. In Sub-Saharan Africa, malaria is responsible for at least 15 percent of disability-adjusted life years (DALYs) (WHO 2001). Furthermore, mortality from malaria is concentrated among the poor. An estimated 60 percent of malaria-related deaths occur in the poorest 20 percent of the global population, a higher share than other common infectious diseases and conditions. Various studies have estimated the impact of malaria with regard to nutritional, cognitive and educational impairments among school-age children, such as anemia, diminished cognitive function and motor and language skills, and school absenteeism (Boivin and others 2007; Clarke and others 2004; John and others 2008; Nankabirwa, Brooker, and others 2014; Nankabirwa, Wandera, and others 2014). Malaria is associated with GDP losses of 1 percent to 20 percent, averaging 10 percent in Sub-Saharan Africa (Gallup and Sachs 2001). The regional loss in economic output is about US$12 billion a year (WHO 2001).

Several strategies are in place to control and eradicate malaria. Ultimately, effectiveness varies with the intensity of transmission and other factors contributing to anemia, such as undernutrition and helminth infection. Global policy efforts have focused on pregnant women and children younger than age five years because of strong evidence on the effectiveness of interventions such as ITNs (White and others 2011). Recent efforts have shifted to providing ITNs to everyone, not only the most vulnerable. Less attention has been given to school-age children, although the prevalence of malaria in the school-age population is often high and can explain approximately one-half of mortality occurring in this age group (Nankabirwa, Brooker, and others 2014).

For the school-age population, strategies to control and eradicate malaria can provide benefits, such as averted cases of malaria and anemia; reduced absenteeism; enhanced attention span and cognitive function; and lowered risk of cerebral malaria, which may alter speech, language, and motor skills.

ITNs are a cost-effective intervention for reducing malaria and anemia among asymptomatic cases (White and others 2011). School-age children are the least likely to use ITNs, although studies generally find positive evidence that they face a lower risk when they do (chapter 14 in this volume, Brooker and others 2017). Based on data from 18 Sub-Saharan African countries, about 40 percent of school-age children are not protected (Noor and others 2009).

As demonstrated in studies from Ghana, Kenya, Lao PDR, and Thailand, skills-based health education in schools can increase knowledge about malaria and the correct use of ITNs and decrease parasite prevalence (Ayi and others 2010; Nonaka and others 2008; Okabayashi and others 2006; Onyango-Ouma, Aagaard-Hansen, and Jensen 2005). In Ghana, school-based education regarding ITN use was associated with a decline in malaria prevalence to 10 percent from 30 percent over the course of one year (Ayi and others 2010). Averting even a single episode of malaria may bring substantial benefits, such as increased participation in higher education and improved cognitive development over the life of the child.

Vision and the Correction of Refractive Error

The benefits of correcting poor vision are related primarily to education pathways and gains in labor market outcomes. An estimated 153 million people globally suffer from poor vision, including 13 million school-age children (Resnikoff and others 2008; Smith and others 2009). Economic losses due to impaired vision exceed an estimated US$200 billion a year globally (Fricke and others 2012). Although little is known about the prevalence of uncorrected refractive error among school-age children, an estimated 9 percent of children in Ethiopia (Yared and others 2012) and 13 percent in China (Glewwe, Park, and Zhao 2012) have undiagnosed or untreated vision problems. In Brazil, poor vision resulted in a 10 percentage point higher probability of dropping out and an 18 percentage point higher probability of repeating a grade (Gomes-Neto and others 1997). In China, poor vision decreased students' academic performance, as measured by test scores, by 0.2–0.3 standard deviations, equivalent to a loss of 0.3 years of schooling (Glewwe, Park, and Zhao 2012).

Providing eye care screening and free glasses in schools can overcome the barriers of cost and lack of skilled eye care personnel (Limburg, Kansara, and d'Souza 1999; Sharma and others 2008; Wedner and others 2000). Training teachers to assess whether children should be examined and potentially receive glasses has been tested in various contexts; in a rural region in Cambodia, fewer than 100 teachers in less than four weeks screened 13,175 students and referred 44 to a team of refractionists to be assessed for eyeglasses (Keeffe 2012).

The essential package recommends periodic screening of children in a specific grade for refractive error and provision of glasses, with the aim of screening all children at risk over time (Baltussen and Smith 2012).

Oral Health

The burden of poor oral health and hygiene is concentrated in upper-middle-income countries and HICs, although the share of the population that is untreated is highest in LMICs. Tooth decay can affect psychosocial well-being and lead to school absenteeism (Kakoei and others 2013; Krisdapong and others 2013; Naidoo, Chikte, and Sheiham 2001). Prevention of cavities may also reduce undernutrition because of the pain associated with severe tooth decay (Benzian and others 2011). The risk of poor oral health is expected to rise as diets in LMICs shift to greater consumption of processed foods and sugars (Viswanath and others 2014). Between 1990 and 2012, the average increase in DALYs due to dental caries was between 42 percent and 78 percent in most countries in Sub-Saharan Africa (Dye and others 2013; Kassebaum and others 2015). Building healthy habits in childhood may provide benefits over the life course. Group activities in school may be an effective means for establishing these norms (Claessen and others 2008).

Vaccines

Although the HPV vaccine is substantially more expensive than the tetanus toxoid vaccine, both are cost-effective. At the global level, cervical cancer caused 6.9 million DALYs in 2013, with more than 80 percent of cases occurring in LMICs (Fitzmaurice and others 2015). Country- and region-specific studies have been conducted on the benefits of HPV vaccination, with a focus on health benefits. The overwhelming majority of these studies indicate that HPV vaccination of preadolescent girls (usually ages 8–14 years, depending on the specific country) has the potential to substantially reduce the morbidity and mortality associated with cervical cancer. Assuming coverage of 70 percent, effective over a lifetime, HPV vaccination could avert more than 670,000 cervical cancer cases in Sub-Saharan Africa over five consecutive birth cohorts of girls vaccinated as young adolescents (Kim and others 2013).

The HPV vaccination is now part of the recommended national schedule in more than 60 countries or territories, but only 8 of these are LMICs (WHO and UNICEF 2013). However, more than 25 LMICs, about one-third in Africa, have piloted the vaccine in one or more urban and rural districts. Recommendations to replace the three-dose schedule with a two-dose schedule, with a minimum interval of six months between doses, would increase the benefits in relation to the costs (WHO 2014). More information on the HPV vaccine can be found in volume 3, chapter 4 (Denny and others 2015).

Delivery of the tetanus toxoid vaccine lowers the risk of contracting tetanus, both for recipients and for their children who have not yet been vaccinated, providing an intergenerational benefit. In Africa, tetanus has caused 3 million DALYs (Ehreth 2003). For the essential package, countries need to administer the tetanus toxoid vaccine to children in the grade that captures the largest proportion of children ages 4–7 or 12–15 years.

COMPARING COSTS AND BENEFITS OF THE ESSENTIAL PACKAGE

Figure 25.2 provides an illustrative mapping of the benefits and costs for all of the interventions in the essential package. Some interventions should be delivered to all children, while others should be targeted geographically or by age to limit overall costs.

Table 25.4 presents the essential package of school health interventions for LMICs, based on costs and benefits. Differences between LICs and lower-middle-income countries are due to differences in resources. Upper-middle-income countries can augment the essential package with additional interventions or expand coverage of targeted interventions to a wider age group or to more schools. All countries may tailor the package to the context and add additional components.

The essential package addresses a variety of health risks facing school-age children. Some are tackled directly; others seek to change behaviors associated with poor health outcomes, including the use of ITNs and promotion of oral health. The frequency of delivery is also noteworthy. Some interventions are delivered just once over the course of primary school (HPV vaccination), while others recur daily (school feeding) or annually (deworming and vision screening). All costs are standardized to one calendar year.

In total, the essential package costs an estimated US$10.30 per child per year in LICs. The average cost per

child of each intervention draws on the cost per treated child in table 25.3. For targeted interventions, the cost per treated child exceeds the average cost per child. Some efficiencies can be expected. In this exercise, a 20 percent reduction in costs for the integrated delivery of malaria and oral health education was assumed (figure 25.3).

The delivery of some interventions is recommended for all children (oral hygiene). For other interventions, screening of all children and treatment for an identified subset of children is recommended (eyeglass screening). For some interventions, the economic returns are greater when targeted to a subset of the population, such as school feeding for food-insecure areas or for children at risk of dropping out.

These estimates exclude start-up costs, which could include the costs of establishing policies or guidelines or undertaking mapping exercises. For example, a national mapping exercise of helminth worms would indicate where deworming treatment is needed, and mapping of poverty and food security would support

Figure 25.2 Indicative Mapping of Benefits and Costs of Essential Package Interventions

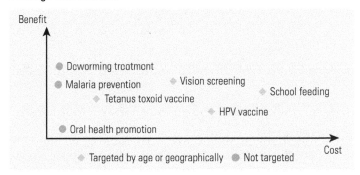

Note: HPV = human papillomavirus.

Figure 25.3 Cost Shares of the Essential Package, by Country Income Level
U.S. dollars

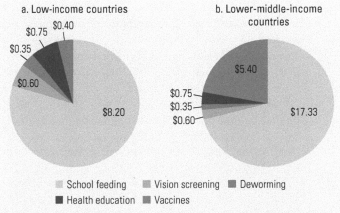

Table 25.4 Costs of the Essential Package of Health Interventions for School-Age Children

Domain	Intervention	Target	Average annual cost per child (US$)	Intervention	Target	Average annual cost per child (US$)
	Low-Income Countries			**Lower-Middle-Income Countries**		
School feeding	Daily snacks or meals with micronutrient fortification	All children in at least 20% of schools in regions with the highest levels of poverty and food insecurity	8.20	Daily meals with micronutrient fortification	All children in at least 40% of schools in regions with the highest level of poverty and food insecurity	16.40
Deworming	Deworming treatment	All children attending schools in areas endemic for STHs and schistosomiasis[a]	0.35	Deworming treatment	All children attending schools in areas endemic for STHs and schistosomiasis[a]	0.35
Vision screening	Screening and provision of ready-made glasses	All children in a select grade	0.60	Screening and provision of custom or ready-made glasses	All children in a select grade	0.60
Oral health and malaria	Health education about prevention of tooth decay and usage of ITNs	All children for oral health promotion and all children attending schools in endemic areas for malaria[a]	0.75	Health education about prevention of tooth decay and usage of ITNs	All children for oral health promotion and all children attending schools in endemic areas for malaria[a]	0.75
Vaccines	Tetanus toxoid vaccine	Children in a select grade in all schools	0.40	Tetanus toxoid vaccine	Children in a select grade in all schools	0.40
	HPV vaccine			HPV vaccine	Girls from a select grade in all schools (two doses)	5

Note: HPV = human papillomavirus; ITNs = insecticide-treated bednets; STHs = soil transmitted helminths.
a. Assuming 50 percent of child population at risk.

the targeting of school feeding to the most disadvantaged households. Costs of the total package are aggregated by size of population in low-income and lower-middle income countries in chapter 1 (Bundy, de Silva, and others 2017).

CONCLUSIONS

Several low-cost health interventions to support the development of children can be delivered through schools. The health and education benefits for each intervention are significant, but there is comparatively less evidence on the combined benefits of providing several interventions jointly. The provision of a set of integrated basic interventions may create cost efficiencies and increase the benefit-cost ratio. For example, health education classes can include material on both oral hygiene and malaria prevention.

This chapter defines an affordable package of school-based health interventions for LMICs and estimates the costs and potential benefits. The interventions can improve the quality and the quantity of schooling, generating a high benefit-cost ratio. The returns to education are highest in LICs, but this finding is due, in part, to higher per capita income in lower-middle-income countries. More research is needed on how to support countries in financing the essential package as well as evaluating the benefits over the life course.

Interventions for school-age children can have significant impacts on schooling, earnings, health status, and productivity in LMICs. The estimated benefit-cost ratios for such interventions consistently exceed one, suggesting that the discounted value of gains exceeds the costs. These results support the case for placing school health high on the policy agenda and for promoting coherence with early childhood health intervention programs to maximize benefit gains. Causal estimates of the impacts of interventions stem mostly from small-scale local interventions and are likely to be sensitive to population heterogeneity (social, economic, and cultural differences), differences in program implementation (administrative capacity and trust), and differences in the wider political economy of reform. As a result, available impact estimates may have limited external validity. In addition, benefit-cost ratios based on these impact estimates are sensitive to the choice of rates of return and discount rates applied in evaluating future impacts against costs.

If benefit-cost ratios associated with interventions for the school-age child are so attractive, why have governments not implemented them at scale? Benefits may not scale up, despite scale economies, and the benefit-cost ratio for nationwide implementation may be lower. Moreover, governments may not be sufficiently aware of the benefits of the interventions; indeed, the documents guiding national and international policy tend to evaluate immediate reductions in clinical morbidity and mortality and to give low priority to the long-term socioeconomic benefits. Furthermore, the health and development of school-age children has historically been given low priority in health system planning, so even where governments recognize the net benefits of interventions for the school-age child, they may face budgetary constraints and conflicting priorities, especially given the strong vested interests in existing programs for other age groups.

NOTE

World Bank Income Classifications as of July 2014 are as follows, based on estimates of gross national income (GNI) per capita for 2013:

- Low-income countries (LICs) = US$1,045 or less
- Middle-income countries (MICs) are subdivided:
  a) lower-middle-income = US$1,046 to US$4,125
  b) upper-middle-income (UMICs) = US$4,126 to US$12,745
- High-income countries (HICs) = US$12,746 or more.

REFERENCES

Ahuja, A. S. Baird, J. Hamory Hicks, M. Kremer, and E. Miguel. 2017. "Economics of Mass Deworming Programs." In *Disease Control Priorities* (third edition): Volume 8, *Child and Adolescent Health and Development*, edited by D. A. P. Bundy, N. de Silva, S. Horton, D. T. Jamison, and G. C. Patton. Washington, DC: World Bank.

Ayi, I., D. Nonaka, J. K. Adjovu, S. Hanafusa, M. Jimba, and others. 2010. "School-Based Participatory Health Education for Malaria Control in Ghana: Engaging Children as Health Messengers." *Malaria Journal* 9: 98.

Bagramian, R. A., F. Garcia-Godoy, and A. R. Volpe. 2009. "The Global Increase in Dental Caries: A Pending Public Health Crisis." *American Journal of Dentistry* 22 (1): 3–8.

Baird, S., J. H. Hicks, M. Kremer, and E. Miguel. 2015. "Worms at Work: Long-Run Impacts of a Child Health Investment." Working Paper 21428, National Bureau of Economic Research, Cambridge, MA.

Baltussen, R., J. Naus, and H. Limburg. 2009. "Cost-Effectiveness of Screening and Correcting Refractive Errors in School Children in Africa, Asia, America and Europe." *Health Policy* 89 (2): 201–15.

Baltussen, R., and A. Smith. 2012. "Cost Effectiveness of Strategies to Combat Vision and Hearing Loss in sub-Saharan Africa and South East Asia: Mathematical Modelling Study." *BMJ* 344: e615. doi:10.1136/bmj.e615.

Benzian, H., M. Hobdell, C. Holmgren, R. Yee, B. Monse, and others. 2011. "Political Priority of Global Oral Health: An Analysis of Reasons for International Neglect." *International Dental Journal* 61 (3): 124–30.

Benzian, H., B. Varenne, N. Stauf, R. Garg, and B. Monse. 2017. "Promoting Oral Health through Programs in Middle Childhood and Adolescence." In *Disease Control Priorities* (third edition): Volume 8, *Child and Adolescent Health and Development*, edited by D. A. P. Bundy, N. de Silva, S. Horton, D. T. Jamison, and G. C. Patton. Washington, DC: World Bank.

Bleakley, H. 2007. "Disease and Development: Evidence from Hookworm Eradication in the American South." *Quarterly Journal of Economics* 122 (1): 73–116.

Boivin, M. J., P. Bangirana, J. Byarugaba, R. O. Opoka, R. Idro, and others. 2007. "Cognitive Impairment after Cerebral Malaria in Children: A Prospective Study." *Pediatrics* 119 (2): 360–66.

Brooker, S. J., S. Clarke, D. Fernando, C. W. Gitonga, J. Nankabirwa, and others. 2017. "Malaria in Middle Childhood and Adolescence." In *Disease Control Priorities* (third edition): Volume 8, *Child and Adolescent Health and Development*, edited by D. A. P. Bundy, N. de Silva, S. Horton, D. T. Jamison, and G. C. Patton. Washington, DC: World Bank.

Bundy, D. A. P. 2011. *Rethinking School Health. A Key Component of Education for All*. Directions in Development. Washington, DC: World Bank.

Bundy, D. A. P., L. Appleby, M. Bradley, K. Croke, T. D. Hollingsworth, R. Pullan, H. Turner, and N. de Silva. 2017. "Mass Deworming Programs in Middle Childhood and Adolescence." In *Disease Control Priorities* (third edition): Volume 8, *Child and Adolescent Health and Development*, edited by Bundy, D. A. P., N. de Silva, S. Horton, D. T. Jamison, and G. C. Patton. Washington, DC: World Bank.

Bundy, D. A. P., N. de Silva, S. Horton, G. C. Patton, L. Schultz, and D. T. Jamison. 2017. "Child and Adolescent Health and Development: Realizing Neglected Potential." In *Disease Control Priorities* (third edition): Volume 8, *Child and Adolescent Health and Development*, edited by Bundy, D. A. P., N. de Silva, S. Horton, D. T. Jamison, and G. C. Patton. Washington, DC: World Bank.

Bundy, D. A. P., L. Schultz, B. Sarr, L. Banham, P. Colenso, and others. 2017. "The School as a Platform for Addressing Health in Middle Childhood and Adolescence." In *Disease Control Priorities* (third edition): Volume 8, *Child and Adolescent Health and Development*, edited by D. A. P. Bundy, N. de Silva,

S. Horton, D. T. Jamison, and G. C. Patton. Washington, DC: World Bank.

Claessen, J.-P., S. Bates, K. Sherlock, F. Seepsarsand, and R. Wright. 2008. "Design Interventions to Improve Tooth Brushing." *International Dental Journal* 58 (Suppl 5): 307–20.

Clarke, S. E., S. Brooker, J. K. Njagi, E. Njau, B. Estambale, and others. 2004. "Malaria Morbidity among School Children Living in Two Areas of Contrasting Transmission in Western Kenya." *American Journal of Tropical Medicine and Hygiene* 71 (6): 732–38.

Denny, L., R. Herrero, C. Levin, and J. J. Kim. 2015. "Cervical Cancer." In *Disease Control Priorities* (third edition): Volume 3, *Cancer*, edited by H. Gelbrand, P. Jha, R. Sankaranarayanan, and S. Horton. Washington, DC: World Bank.

Drake, L., M. Fernandes, E. Aurino, J. Kiamba, B. Giyose, and others. 2017. "School Feeding Programs in Middle Childhood and Adolescence." In *Disease Control Priorities* (third edition): Volume 8, *Child and Adolescent Health and Development*, edited by D. A. P. Bundy, N. de Silva, S. Horton, D. T. Jamison, and G. C. Patton. Washington, DC: World Bank.

Durlak, J. A., R. P. Weissberg, A. B. Dymnicki, R. D. Talor, and K. B. Schellinger. 2011. "The Impact of Enhancing Students' Social and Emotional Learning: A Meta-Analysis of School-Based Universal Interventions." *Child Development* 82 (1): 405–32.

Dye, C., T. Mertens, G. Hirnschall, W. Mpanju-Shumbusho, R. D. Newman, and others. 2013. "WHO and the Future of Disease Control Programmes." *The Lancet* 381 (9864): 413–18.

Ehreth, J. 2003. "The Global Value of Vaccination." *Vaccine* 21 (7): 596–600.

Fenwick, A. 2012. "The Global Burden of Neglected Tropical Diseases." *Public Health* 126 (3): 233–36.

Fitzmaurice, C., D. Dicker, A. Pain, H. Hamavid, M. Moradi-Lakeh, and others. 2015. "The Global Burden of Cancer 2013." *JAMA Oncology* 1 (4): 505–27.

Fricke, T. R., B. A. Holden, D. A. Wilson, G. Schlenther, K. S. Naidoo, and others. 2012. "Global Cost of Correcting Vision Impairment from Uncorrected Refractive Error." *Bulletin of the World Health Organization* 90 (10): 728–38.

Gallup, J. L., and J. D. Sachs. 2001. "The Economic Burden of Malaria." *American Journal of Tropical Medicine and Hygiene* 64 (1): 85–96.

Glewwe, P., A. Park, and M. Zhao. 2012. "Visualizing Development: Eyeglasses and Academic Performance in Rural Primary Schools in China." Working paper 12-2, Center for International Food and Agricultural Policy, University of Minnesota.

Gomes-Neto, J. B., E. A. Hanushek, R. H. Leite, and R. C. Frota-Bezzera. 1997. "Health and Schooling: Evidence and Policy Implications for Developing Countries." *Economics of Education Review* 16 (3): 271–82.

Graham, N., L. Schultz, S. Mitra, and D. Mont. 2017. "Disability in Middle Childhood and Adolescence." In *Disease Control Priorities* (third edition): Volume 8, *Child and Adolescent Health and Development*, edited by Bundy, D. A. P., N. de Silva, S. Horton, D. T. Jamison, and G. C. Patton. Washington, DC: World Bank.

Griffiths, U. K., L. J. Wolfson, A. Quddus, M. Younus, and R. A. Hafiz. 2004. "Incremental Cost-Effectiveness of Supplementary Immunization Activities to Prevent Neonatal Tetanus in Pakistan." *Bulletin of the World Health Organization* 82 (9): 643–51.

Guyatt, H. 2003. "The Cost of Delivering and Sustaining a Control Programme for Schistosomiasis and Soil-Transmitted Helminthiasis." *Acta Tropica* 86 (2–3): 267–74.

Horton, S., and M. Black. 2017. "Identifying an Essential Package for Early Childhood Development: Economic Analysis." In *Disease Control Priorities* (third edition): Volume 8, *Child and Adolescent Health and Development*, edited by D. A. P. Bundy, N. de Silva, S. Horton, D. T. Jamison, and G. C. Patton. Washington, DC: World Bank.

Horton, S., De la Cruz Toledo, J. Mahon, J. Santelli, and J. Waldfogel. 2017. "Identifying an Essential Package for Adolescent Health: Economic Analysis." In *Disease Control Priorities* (third edition): Volume 8, *Child and Adolescent Health and Development*, edited by D. A. P. Bundy, N. de Silva, S. Horton, D. T. Jamison, and G. C. Patton. Washington, DC: World Bank.

Horton, S., and R. H. Steckel. 2013. "Malnutrition: Global Economic Losses Attributable to Malnutrition 1900–2000 and Projections to 2050." In *How Much Have Global Problems Cost the Earth? A Scorecard from 1900 to 2050*, edited by B. Lomborg and B. R. Lomborg, 247–72. Cambridge, U.K.: Cambridge University Press.

Horton, S., and D. Wu. 2015. "Methodology and Results for Systematic Search, Cost, and Cost-Effectiveness Analysis." Working Paper for Child and Adolescent Health and Development, *DCP3*, Seattle, Washington.

Hutubessy, R., A. Levin, S. Wang, W. Morgan, M. Ally, and others. 2012. "Costing Nationwide HPV Vaccine Delivery in Low- and Middle-Income Countries Using the WHO Cervical Cancer Prevention and Control Costing Tool: A Case Study of the United Republic of Tanzania." *BMC Medicine* 10 (1): 136.

Jamison, D. T., and J. Leslie. 1990. "Health and Nutrition Considerations in Education Planning. 2. The Cost and Effectiveness of School-Based Interventions." *Food and Nutrition Bulletin* 12 (3): 204–14.

John, C. C., P. Bangirana, J. Byarungaba, R. O. Opoka, R. Idro, and others. 2008. "Cerebral Malaria in Children Is Associated with Long-Term Cognitive Impairment." *Pediatrics* 122 (1): 92–99.

Jukes, M. C. H., L. J. Drake, and D. A. P. Bundy. 2008. *School Health, Nutrition, and Education for All: Levelling the Playing Field*. Cambridge, MA: CABI Publishing.

Kakoei, S., M. Parirokh, N. Nakhaee, F. Jamshidshirazi, M. Rad, and others. 2013. "Prevalence of Toothache and Associated Factors: A Population-Based Study in Southeast Iran." *Iran Endodontic Journal* 8 (3): 123–28.

Kandelman, D., S. Arpin, R. J. Baez, P. C. Baehni, and P. E. Petersen. 2012. "Oral Health Care Systems in Developing and Developed Countries." *Periodontology 2000* 60 (1): 98–109.

Kassebaum, N. J., E. Bernabe, M. Dahiya, B. Bhandari, C. J. Murray, and others. 2015. "Global Burden of Untreated Caries: A Systematic Review and Metaregression." *Journal of Dental Research* 94 (October): 1355–61.

Keeffe, J. 2012. "The Need for Correction of Refractive Error in Children: Cambodia." Centre for Eye Research Australia and WHO Collaborating Centre for Prevention on Blindness.

Kim, J. J., M. Sharma, M. O'Shea, S. Sweet, M. Diaz, and others. 2013. "Model-Based Impact and Cost-Effectiveness of Cervical Cancer Prevention in the Middle East and Northern Africa." *Vaccine* 31 (Suppl 6): G65–77.

Krisdapong, S., P. Prasertsom, K. Rattanarangsima, and A. Sheiham. 2013. "School Absence Due to Toothache Associated with Sociodemographic Factors, Dental Caries Status, and Oral Health-Related Quality of Life in 12- and 15-Year-Old Thai Children." *Journal of Public Health Dentistry* 73 (4): 321–28.

Kristjanssen, E., A. Gelli, V. Welch, T. Greenhalgh, S. Liberato, and others. 2015. "Costs, and Cost-Outcome of School Feeding Programmes and Feeding Programmes for Young Children. Evidence and Recommendations." *International Journal of Education Development* 48 (May): 79–83. doi:10.1016/j.ijedu-dev.2015.11.011.

LaMontagne, D. S., T. Cernuschi, A. Yabuku, P. Bloem, D. Watson-Jones, and J. Kim. 2017. "School-Based Delivery of Vaccines to 5 to 19 Year Olds." In *Disease Control Priorities* (third edition): Volume 8, *Child and Adolescent Health and Development*, edited by D. A. P. Bundy, N. de Silva, S. Horton, D. T. Jamison, and G. C. Patton. Washington, DC: World Bank.

Levin, A., S. A. Wang, C. Levin, V. Tsu, and R. Hutubessy. 2014. "Costs of Introducing and Delivering HPV Vaccines in Low- and Lower-Middle-Income Countries: Inputs for Gavi Policy on Introduction Grant Support to Countries." *PLoS One* 9 (6): e101114.

Levin, C. E., M. Sharma, Z. Olson, S. Verguet, J. F. Shi, and others. 2015. "An Extended Cost-Effectiveness Analysis of Publicly Financed HPV Vaccination to Prevent Cervical Cancer in China." *Vaccine* 33 (24): 2830–41.

Lim, S. S., N. Fullman, A. Stokes, N. Ravishankar, F. Masiye, and others. 2011. "Net Benefits: A Multicountry Analysis of Observational Data Examining Associations between Insecticide-Treated Mosquito Nets and Health Outcomes." *PLoS Medicine* 8: e1001091.

Limburg, H., H. T. Kansara, and S. d'Souza. 1999. "Results of School Eye Screening of 5.4 Million Children in India: A Five-Year Follow-Up Study." *Acta Ophthalmologica Scandinavica* 77 (3): 310–14.

Manyanga, T., H. El-Sayed, D. T. Doku, and J. R. Randall. 2014. "The Prevalence of Underweight, Overweight, Obesity, and Associated Risk Factors among School-Going Adolescents in Seven African Countries." *BMC Public Health* 14 (1): 1.

McLean, E., M. Cogswell, I. Egli, D. Wojdyla, and B. De Benoist. 2009. "Worldwide Prevalence of Anaemia, WHO Vitamin and Mineral Nutrition Information System, 1993–2005." *Public Health Nutrition* 12 (4): 444–54.

Mendez, M., and L. Adair. 1999. "Severity and Timing of Stunting in the First Two Years of Life Affect Performance on Cognitive Tests in Late Childhood." *Journal of Nutrition* 129 (8): 1555–62.

Miguel, E., and M. Kremer. 2004. "Worms: Identifying Impacts on Education and Health in the Presence of Treatment Externalities." *Econometrica* 72 (1): 159–217.

Monse, B., H. Benzian, E. Naliponguit, V. J. Belizario, A. Schratz, and others. 2013. "The Fit for School Health Outcome Study: A Longitudinal Survey to Assess Health Impacts of an Integrated School Health Programme in the Philippines." *BMC Public Health* 13: 256.

Montenegro, C. E., and H. A. Patrinos. 2014. "Comparable Estimates of Returns to Schooling around the World." Policy Research Working Paper 7020, World Bank, Washington, DC.

Murray, N. G., B. J. Low, C. Hollis, A. W. Cross, and S. M. Davis. 2007. "Coordinated School Health Programs and Academic Achievement: A Systematic Review of the literature." *Journal of School Health* 77: 589–600.

Murray, C. J., T. Vos, R. Lozano, M. Naghavi, A. D. Flaxman, and others. 2013. "Disability-Adjusted Life Years (DALYs) for 291 Diseases and Injuries in 21 Regions, 1990–2010: A Systematic Analysis for the Global Burden of Disease Study 2010." *The Lancet* 380 (9859): 2197–223.

Naidoo, S., U. M. Chikte, and A. Sheiham. 2001. "Prevalence and Impact of Dental Pain in 8–10-Year-Olds in the Western Cape." *Journal of the South African Dental Association* 56 (11): 521–23.

Nankabirwa, J. I., S. J. Brooker, S. J. Clarke, D. Fernando, C. W. Gitonga, and others. 2014. "Malaria in School-Age Children in Africa: An Increasingly Important Challenge." *Tropical Medicine and International Health* 19 (11): 1294–309.

Nankabirwa, J. I., B. Wandera, P. Amuge, N. Kiwanuka, G. Dorsey, and others. 2014. "Impact of Intermittent Preventive Treatment with Dihydroartemisinin-Piperaquine on Malaria in Ugandan Schoolchildren: A Randomized, Placebo-Controlled Trial." *Clinical Infectious Diseases* 58 (10): 1404–12.

Nonaka, D., J. Kobayashi, M. Jimba, B. Vilaysouk, K. Tsukamoto, and others. 2008. "Malaria Education from School to Community in Oudomxay Province, Lao PDR." *Parasitology International* 57 (1): 76–82.

Noor, A. M., V. C. Kirui, S. J. Brooker, and R. W. Snow. 2009. "The Use of Insecticide Treated Nets by Age: Implications for Universal Coverage in Africa." *BMC Public Health* 9: 369.

Okabayashi, H., P. Thongthien, P. Singhasvanon, J. Waikagul, S. Looareesuwan, and others. 2006. "Keys to Success for a School-Based Malaria Control Program in Primary Schools in Thailand." *Parasitology International* 55 (2): 121–26.

Onyango-Ouma, W., J. Aagaard-Hansen, and B. B. Jensen. 2005. "The Potential of Schoolchildren as Health Change Agents in Rural Western Kenya." *Social Science and Medicine* 61 (8): 1711–22.

Pradhan, E., E. M. Suzuki, S. Martínez, M. Schäferhoff, and D. T. Jamison. 2017. "The Effects of Education Quantity and Quality on Child and Adult Mortality: Their Magnitude and Their Value." In *Disease Control Priorities* (third edition): Volume 8, *Child and Adolescent Health and Development*, edited by Bundy, D. A. P., N. de Silva, S. Horton, D. T. Jamison, and G. C. Patton. Washington, DC: World Bank.

Resnikoff, S., D. Pascolini, S. P. Mariotti, and G. P. Pokharel. 2008. "Global Magnitude of Visual Impairment Caused by Uncorrected Refractive Errors in 2004." *Bulletin of the World Health Organization* 86 (1): 63–70.

Salam, R. A., C. MacPhail, J. K. Das, and Z. A. Bhutta. 2013. "Effectiveness of Micronutrient Powders (MNP) in Women and Children." *BMC Public Health* 13 (Suppl 3): S22.

Shackleton, N., F. Jamal, R. M. Viner, K. Dickson, G. Patton, and C. Bonell. 2016. "School-Based Interventions to Promote Adolescent Health: Systematic Review of Reviews." *Journal of Adolescent Health* 58 (4): 382–96.

Sharma, A., L. Li, Y. Song, K. Choi, D. S. Lam, and others. 2008. "Strategies to Improve the Accuracy of Vision Measurement by Teachers in Rural Chinese Secondary Schoolchildren: Xichang Pediatric Refractive Error Study (X-PRES) Report No. 6." *Archives of Ophthalmology* 126 (10): 1434–40.

Simeon, D. T., S. M. Grantham-McGregor, and M. S. Wong. 1995. "*Trichuris trichiura* Infection and Cognition in Children: Results of a Randomized Clinical Trial." *Parasitology* 110 (04): 457–64.

Smith, T. S. T., K. D. Frick, B. A. Holden, T. R. Fricke, and K. S. Naidoo. 2009. "Potential Lost Productivity Resulting from the Global Burden of Uncorrected Refractive Error." *Bulletin of the World Health Organization* 87 (6): 431–37.

Snilstveit, B., J. Stevenson, D. Phillips, M. Vojtkova, E. Gallagher, and others. 2015. *Interventions for Improving Learning Outcomes and Access to Education in Low- and Middle-Income Countries: A Systematic Review, 3ie Final Review.* London: International Initiative for Impact Evaluation (3ie).

Speich, B., S. Knopp, K. A. Mohammed, I. S. Khamis, L. Rinaldi, and others. 2010. "Comparative Cost Assessment of the Kato-Katz and FLOTAC Techniques for Soil-Transmitted Helminth Diagnosis in Epidemiological Surveys." *Parasites and Vectors* 3 (71): 1–11.

Stopford, I., E. Aurino, F. Amese, S. Hamdani, and M. Fernandes. Forthcoming. "A Cost Analysis of the Inclusion of Micronutrient Powders in the Ghana School Feeding Programme."

Stuckey, E. M., J. Stevenson, K. Galactionova, A. Y. Baidjoe, T. Bousema, and others. 2014. "Modeling the Cost Effectiveness of Malaria Control Interventions in the Highlands of Western Kenya." *PloS One* 9 (10): e107700.

Vandelaer, J., and M. Olaniran. 2015. "Using a Schools-Based Approach to Deliver Immunization: Global Update." *Vaccine* 33 (5): 719–25.

Viswanath, D., V. L. Jayasimha, M. L. V. Prabhuji, and V. Vasudevan. 2014. "A Critical Appraisal of Diet and Nutrition on Oral Health in Children: A Review." *International Journal of Health Sciences and Research* 4 (1): 165–73.

Wedner, S. H., D. A. Ross, R. Balira, L. Kaji, and A. Foster. 2000. "Prevalence of Eye Diseases in Primary School Children in a Rural Area of Tanzania." *British Journal of Ophthalmology* 84 (11): 1291–97.

WFP (World Food Programme). 2012. *The State of School Feeding.* Rome: WFP.

White, M., L. Conteh, R. Cibulskis, and A. C. Ghana. 2011. "Costs and Cost-Effectiveness of Malaria Control Interventions: A Systematic Review." *Malaria Journal* 10: 337.

WHO (World Health Organization). 2001. "Malaria at a Glance." WHO, Geneva. http://www.who.int/management /Malaria_at_a_glance%20WB.pdf.

———. 2006. "Tetanus Vaccines: WHO Position Paper." *Weekly Epidemiological Record* 20 (81): 197–208.

———. 2014. "Human Papillomavirus Vaccines: WHO Position Paper." *Weekly Epidemiological Record* 43 (89): 465–92.

WHO and UNICEF (United Nations Children's Fund). 2013. *Immunization, Vaccines, and Biologics: WHO/UNICEF Joint Reporting Process.* Geneva: WHO.

World Bank. 2016a. World Development Indicators: Size of the Economy, 2015. http://wdi.worlbank.org/table/1.1 Accessed November 7 2016.

———. 2016b. World Development Indicators: Population dynamics, 2015. http://wdi.worlbank.org/table/2.1 Accessed November 7 2016.

Yared, A. W., W. T. Belaynew, S. Destaye, T. Ayanaw, and E. Zelalem. 2012. "Prevalence of Refractive Errors among School Children in Gondar Town, Northwest Ethiopia." *Middle East African Journal of Ophthalmology* 19 (4): 372.

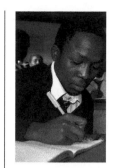

Chapter 26

Identifying an Essential Package for Adolescent Health: Economic Analysis

Susan Horton, Elia De la Cruz Toledo, Jacqueline Mahon, John Santelli, and Jane Waldfogel

INTRODUCTION

Adolescents form a large proportion of the population in many low- and middle-income countries (LMICs)—more than 20 percent in the countries with the fastest-growing populations (WHO 2014). The adolescent period, defined as ages 10 through 19 years, is key to future health because it is during these years that health decisions and habits are formed that have long-term impacts. Adolescents who are enabled to make healthy eating and exercise choices, to adopt healthy sexual behaviors, and to avoid addictive substances and excessive risks have the best opportunities for health in later life. Equally important, some mental health issues are manifested in late adolescence, and early detection is important.

Despite the pivotal nature of this age, adolescents until recently have been relatively neglected in international donor strategies for maternal, newborn, and child health. Specific areas where funding is lacking include preventing unsafe abortion and coerced sex, and providing antenatal, childbirth, and postnatal care (iERG 2013). Many adolescents are entitled to appropriate health care under the Convention on the Rights of the Child, but those ages 18 and 19 years are not specifically included.

Recent reports and studies seek to bring greater attention to adolescent health needs (Gorna and others 2015; Laski and others 2015; Patton and others 2016; UNICEF 2011, 2012; WHO 2014). Groups such as the International Health Partnership (http://www.internationalhealthpartnership.net) have begun to modify the well-known term *RMNCH*

(Reproductive, Maternal, Newborn, and Child Health) to *RMNCAH* to include adolescents. The Every Woman Every Child (2015) strategy is titled "The Global Strategy for Women's, Children's and Adolescents' Health 2016–2030" and signals a positive change. It highlights research indicating that the health of women, children, and adolescents is central to the Sustainable Development Goals for 2030. The term *youth* is mentioned 10 times in the Outcome Declaration of the Sustainable Development Agenda (UN 2015), and the term *adolescent* is mentioned once in reference to adolescent girls.

This chapter provides an overview of methods and examines the economic case for investment in adolescent health by surveying what is known on cost, cost-effectiveness, and cost-benefit ratios of interventions. We then use these economic data to examine the cost of an essential package of health and behavioral interventions that all countries need to provide. The essential package draws on packages developed elsewhere (Every Woman Every Child 2015; Patton and others 2016; WHO 2013). Useful information also comes from costing studies of related packages (Deogan, Ferguson, and Stenberg 2012; Temin and Levine 2009). Countries can modify this package depending on their specific needs and resource availability. Finally, we estimate what such a package might cost in 2012 U.S. dollars and provide brief conclusions. Definitions of age groupings and age-specific terminology used in this volume can be found in chapter 1 (Bundy, de Silva, and others 2017).

Corresponding author: Susan Horton, University of Waterloo, Ontario, Canada; sehorton@uwaterloo.ca.

METHODS

Our focus is on the costs and cost-effectiveness of certain areas of health of particular concern in adolescence. Topics we do not address are discussed in other volumes in this series:

- Human papillomavirus (HPV) (volume 3, Gelband and others 2015; volume 6, Holmes and others 2017)
- Reproductive health more generally (volume 2, Black and others 2016)
- Interventions in nonhealth areas, such as education and child marriage, that have strong impacts on health
- Conditional cash transfers (chapter 23 in this volume, de Walque and others 2017)
- Cost-effectiveness results from the second edition of *Disease Control Priorities* (*DCP2*), which included substantial modeling of interventions for smoking (Jha and others 2006), alcohol (Rehm and others 2006), obesity (Willett and others 2006), injury (Norton and others 2006), and mental health (Hyman and others 2006); these are all health issues for which adolescence is a particularly vulnerable age. *DCP2* included a chapter on adolescent health (Lule and others 2006) that reviewed the economic literature before 2000.

- Interventions covered in the chapter on school-age children (chapter 25 in this volume, Fernandes and Aurino 2017) are more appropriate with younger age groups, although some overlap occurs between school age and adolescence. Table 26.1 shows how the discussion is divided between this chapter and the preceding chapter on school-age children.

We searched the literature on the economics of interventions that were aimed specifically at adolescents or that would primarily benefit adolescents. The main areas where we anticipated finding studies included nutrition, sexual and reproductive health, mental health, alcohol, injury, and smoking and other addictive substances.

There are relatively few cost and cost-effectiveness studies on these topics in the peer-reviewed literature in English for LMICs. We drew first on systematic reviews of cost and cost-effectiveness for high-income countries (HICs), which were identified using a search in PubMed (see details in annex 26A). We identified seven such systematic reviews published since 2000.

We then undertook a systematic review of the literature in English for LMICs (see annex 26A for details) to identify individual studies since 2000. We augmented this review with an expert search and identified seven studies.

Table 26.1 Platforms for Delivering Different Interventions for Adolescents, Compared with School-Age Children

Health area	Population level	Community	School	Primary health center
Physical health	Healthy lifestyle messages: tobacco, alcohol, injury Sexual health messages	*Deworming* *Malaria prevention and treatment* *Tetanus toxoid and HPV vaccination* *Oral health promotion* Adolescent-friendly health services	*Deworming* *Malaria prevention and treatment* *Tetanus toxoid and HPV vaccination* *Oral health promotion* Sexual health education Healthy lifestyle education Adolescent-friendly health services	*Deworming* *Malaria prevention and treatment* *Tetanus toxoid and HPV vaccination* *Oral health promotion and treatment* Adolescent-friendly health services
Nutrition	Nutrition education messages	*Micronutrient supplementation* *Multifortified foods*	*Micronutrient supplementation* *Multifortified foods* *School feeding* Nutrition education	
Mental health	Mental health messages		Mental health education and counseling	Mental health treatment
Cognitive development		School promotion	*Vision screening*	*Vision screening*

Note: HPV = human papillomavirus. Blue colored interventions are covered in chapter 25 in this volume, Fernandes and Aurino 2017, on school-age children.

Costs and cost-effectiveness are expressed in the original currency units; for LMICs they are also converted to 2012 U.S. dollars, first by adjusting using the consumer price index in the currency of the studied country, and then using the 2012 market exchange rate to the U.S. dollar. The WHO (2001) benchmark for cost-effectiveness is the point at which an intervention's cost per disability-adjusted life year (DALY) averted is less than three times a country's per capita gross national income (GNI), and an intervention is very cost-effective if the cost per DALY averted is less than per capita GNI.

We did not convert the cost-effectiveness numbers for HICs. The benchmark for acceptability for public financing would be about US$50,000 per quality-adjusted life year (QALY) saved in the United States or £30,000 per QALY saved in the United Kingdom; we simply specify in the text whether the interventions are or are not cost-effective. All figures refer to 2012 U.S. dollars, unless otherwise noted.

Cost and cost-effectiveness studies do not cover all the areas of interest for adolescent health interventions. It is particularly difficult to find costs and cost-effectiveness of interventions at the national level (for example, for policy change or mass media campaigns), given that there is no easy way to identify the effectiveness of interventions in the absence of a control group. Clearly, however, interventions at the national level can be important. We also did not find studies of the cost and cost-effectiveness of social media, which may be an effective way to reach adolescents. These interventions are relatively new, and the literature may not yet have caught up.

UNIT COST, COST-EFFECTIVENESS, AND BENEFIT-COST RATIOS OF INTERVENTIONS

Given the relative neglect of adolescent health in LMICs, the paucity of economic analysis is not surprising. Even evidence of effectiveness of interventions is scanty. More pilot programs using innovative methods are needed, and existing successful pilot interventions need to be brought to scale.

Adolescents are also a diverse group, and interventions that succeed in some contexts may not do so in others. Some adolescents are in school, but others are not, and there are generally fewer cost-effective ways to reach those not in school. Some adolescents are married and face very different health challenges from those who are not. Adolescents living in rural areas face different circumstances than those in cities; there are also big differences across world regions, for example, in the experience of violence by adolescents.

Table 26.1 categorizes interventions by the type of delivery platform, as well as the broad program outcome; the four groupings are physical health, nutrition, mental health, and cognitive development. Many programs delivered in person need to be supplemented by national-level policy changes as well as by supportive messages in the media. Most programming for adolescents will be delivered either in the community or in school (for those in school).

Neuroscience has given us new insights into the difficulties in effecting behavior change in adolescents. In this age range, the brain develops in ways that stimulate innovation and risk-taking. Peer influence becomes increasingly important, and input from parents and adults less salient (see discussion in chapter 6 in this volume, Bundy and Horton 2017, and chapter 10 in this volume, Grigorenko 2017). Risk-taking may have evolutionary benefits, in that this is the period in which adolescents have traditionally been expected to leave the parental home and set up a new, independent household. Risk-taking also has a downside, in that executive control functions are still developing and can be overridden in the heat of the moment, particularly in the company of peers. Steinberg (2007) suggests that interventions limiting the scope of potential damage may work better than education alone. For example, graduated driving licenses may more successfully reduce automobile injuries than educational programs about safe driving behavior. At the same time, adolescence is such a crucial time for establishing habits and behaviors with lifelong consequences that it would seem impossible not to include educational interventions.

Two methodological issues affect the economic evaluation of school-based interventions. First, the same intervention can vary substantially in quality depending on the context in which it is implemented, and hence also in effectiveness. Second, very few school-based programs track outcomes longitudinally. This shortcoming is particularly an issue for the myriad studies of obesity; short-term weight gain outcomes may be a very poor guide to long-term outcomes. Lack of longitudinal studies may be less of an issue in the areas of smoking and early pregnancy. In both cases, avoiding the risky behavior for three or four years may suffice to avoid the undesired outcomes. Adolescents who reach early adulthood without becoming smokers are substantially less likely to become lifelong smokers. Similarly, postponing first pregnancy until the end of the teenage years can have a significant effect on schooling attainment for young women as well as health benefits for both the young women and their babies.

Findings for High-Income Countries

Our literature search identified six systematic reviews for HICs (Guo and others 2010; Korber 2014; Romeo, Byford, and Knapp 2005; Shepherd and others 2010; Vos and others 2010; Wu and others 2011). We also draw on nonsystematic reviews by De la Cruz and others (2015) and McDaid and others (2014). Given the amount that is spent on, for example, educational programs, it is surprising that the cost-effectiveness literature is relatively spotty.

Obesity

For HICs, we identified two systematic reviews of cost-effectiveness of physical activity as a way to address obesity (see table 26.2) (Korber 2014; Wu and others 2011); McDaid and others (2014) also reference studies on obesity. These three reviews identify some interventions that are cost-effective and others that are not. In some cases, interventions that are cost-effective are costly and may not be affordable (Wu and others 2011). De la Cruz and others (2015) surveyed individual studies

Table 26.2 Summary of Reviews of Cost-Benefit and Cost-Effectiveness of Interventions for Adolescent Health, High-Income Countries

Study	Scope of review or study	Study findings
Guo and others 2010	Study of school-based **health care** in four school districts in the United States	• School-based health care could have saved Medicare US$35 per student per year; cost of intervention US$180 per student per year for children and adolescents ages 5–14 years. • School-based care also narrowed gap between disadvantaged groups (African American) and other students.
Korber 2014	Systematic review of 13 economic evaluations of interventions to promote **physical activity**	5 studies of United States, 4 Australia, 2 Germany, 1 United Kingdom, 1 New Zealand • Cost per DALY averted for Australia ranged from $A 20,227 to $A 760,000 per DALY (Walking School Bus). • Cost per QALY saved for United States ranged from US$900 to US$4,305. • Cost per QALY saved for United Kingdom was £94–£103.
McDaid and others 2014	**Alcohol**: Review of 2 studies	• Education sessions with 11–12-year-olds and parents (one study) have a benefit-cost ratio of 9:1; various interventions (other study) have benefit-cost ratios ranging from 5:1 to 100:1 in United States.
McDaid and others 2014	**Smoking**: Review of 7 studies, largely school based (2 include mass media as well)	• The Netherlands: Cost US$25,174 per QALY saved • Germany: 3.6:1 benefit-cost ratio • United States: (4 studies) US$5,860–US$405,277 per QALY saved; US$7,333–US$24,271 per QALY saved; highly cost-effective; and cost-effective or cost saving, respectively • Canada: Results similar to United States
McDaid and others 2014	**Sexual health**: 1 study	• Net savings for a program to prevent early pregnancy among adolescents in low-income areas in United States is US$11,262 per participant.
McDaid and others 2014	**Mental well-being**: 5 studies	• US$3,500 per DALY for program to screen Australian teenagers with depressive symptoms and treat with psychiatrist • US$9,725 per DALY for program in United States to offer 15 sessions of CBT to at-risk teens ages 13–18 years with one parent with depressive disorder • Three interventions to promote well-being in schools in United States had benefits of 28:1, 5:1–10:1, and 25:1 for reduced drug dependency, smoking, and delinquency, respectively.
McDaid and others 2014	**Obesity prevention**: 3 studies	• Various programs in Australia were cost saving over lifetime; others (Walking School Bus, gastric banding, and drug therapy) were not. • Program in United States to reduce TV watching, improve physical activity, and improve diet effective in girls at cost of US$5,076 per QALY saved. • Study in United Kingdom found lifestyle interventions effective at cost of US$20,589 per QALY saved.

table continues next page

Table 26.2 Summary of Reviews of Cost-Benefit and Cost-Effectiveness of Interventions for Adolescent Health, High-Income Countries (continued)

Study	Scope of review or study	Study findings
Romeo, Byford, and Knapp 2005	Systematic review of **mental health interventions** for children and adolescents	21 studies: 10 United States, 4 United Kingdom, 3 Canada, 1 Australia, 1 Sweden, 1 Norway, and 1 the Netherlands • Programs heterogeneous in design and in outcome measures, not readily converted to a common health outcome metric.
Shepherd and others 2010	Systematic review of school-based interventions for prevention of transmission of **sexually transmitted infections**; modeled for economic cost-effectiveness	• Examined 15 RCTs: 13 for United States, 2 for United Kingdom • Review found significant changes in knowledge and in some measures of self-efficacy but few significant differences in behavior (only short follow-up). • Estimated cost of teacher-led programs at £4.30/pupil; peer-led £15/pupil; incremental cost-effectiveness ratio £20,223 per QALY saved for teacher led; £80,782 per QALY saved for peer led
Vos and others 2010	Modeling of cost-effectiveness of broad range of interventions for Australia (costs in $A); **drugs and mental well-being**	• School-based program for illicit drug education cost $A 59,000 per DALY averted. • Screen and treat with a psychologist in school for child and adolescent depression cost $A 5,400 per DALY averted. • Screen and treat with bibliotherapy in school for child and adolescent depression cost $A 180 per DALY averted, but evidence of effectiveness limited.
Wu and others 2011	Systematic review and cost-effectiveness of programs to promote **physical activity**	91 studies (141 interventions) of which 48 RCTs; predominantly for United States, almost all for HICs. Of these, the cost per MET per person per year varied considerably: • Point-of-decision prompts had the lowest cost per MET but very small effect on overall physical activity levels. • School and community-based programs had middle cost per MET and middle effect on physical activity levels. • Individually adapted behavior change and social support programs had highest cost per MET but highest effect on physical activity levels.

Source: Horton 2015.

Note: Costs are in year of original study. CBT = cognitive behavioral therapy; DALY = disability-adjusted life year; HICs = high-income countries; MET = Metabolic Equivalent of Task; QALY = quality-adjusted life year; RCTs = randomized controlled trials.

for HICs and identified two studies for obesity: Haynes and others (2010) suggesting that reducing consumption of carbonated drinks can be very cost-effective; and Carter and others (2009), indicating that physical activity promotion is cost-effective, although barely.

Smoking, Alcohol Use, and Illicit Drug Use

No systematic reviews were identified for smoking, alcohol use, or illicit drug use. Individual studies may not include keywords related to adolescence, although it is well understood that adolescence is a key period for experimentation with (and in some cases becoming addicted to) these substances. For the United States, there are examples of cost-effective, as well as cost-ineffective, smoking prevention interventions for adolescents (surveyed in McDaid and others 2014). De la Cruz and others (2015) highlight one study for smoking, in which increased cigarette taxation combined with

subsidies for quitting aids has attractive cost-effectiveness ratios in the Netherlands (Over and others 2014). Vos and others (2010) survey examples of programs to prevent or reduce use of illicit substances, some of which are cost-effective.

Reproductive and Sexual Health

Two systematic reviews (Guo and others 2010; Shepherd and others 2010) cover school-based health care, which often has a focus on sexual and reproductive health, and at times, on mental health. Some school-based programs are cost-effective in preventing sexually transmitted infections (Shepherd and others 2010). Some school-based interventions on reproductive health are even cost saving (Guo and others 2010), as was one program aimed at preventing early pregnancy among adolescents living in a low-income area (McDaid and others 2014).

Mental Health

School-based programs can also be effective for mental health (Romeo, Byford, and Knapp 2005), although cost may make them difficult to afford. De la Cruz and others (2015) identify a study combining cognitive behavioral therapy with a change in medication that improves mental health, but this intervention is not quite cost-effective (Lynch and others 2011).

Overall Findings

In each of the reviewed health areas in HICs, it is possible to find some interventions for adolescents that are cost-effective, using the country's own threshold, and others that are not. Lack of cost-effectiveness has several causes, among them, poor implementation, poor monitoring, and poor design. Monitoring behavior change interventions is more challenging than, for example, monitoring vaccinations. Poor design may arise when modeling or communicating behavior changes in ways that do not appeal to adolescents. Some interventions may be effective but relatively high cost, so that even if they are cost-effective, they are not affordable.

The lessons from HICs are that schools are an appropriate venue for interventions since adolescence is a key age at which interventions should occur; however, it is crucial to have programs that are well conceptualized, well targeted, and well implemented. Programs need to be evidence based. In the United States, the Department of Health and Human Services (2014) funds evaluations for pilot programs and lists the types of evidence required for a program to be eligible for evaluation. As outlined in the methodology section, implications have to be drawn cautiously. The context of HICs differs from that of LMICs; and even in HICs, the number of studies with long-term follow-up is limited.

Findings for Low- and Middle-Income Countries

We identified seven studies in LMICs, most of a single country, but one has results for six middle-income countries (MICs). Two are of obesity; four are of sexual and reproductive health; and one is of smoking prevention (table 26.3). Most of the studies were conducted in MICs.

Obesity

For MICs, school-based interventions to reduce obesity are affordable at less than US$1 or US$1.50 per person in the overall population; however, they are not cost-effective, according to Cecchini and others' (2010) comprehensive modeling study of interventions in MICs. In comparison, restrictions on the advertising of food to children cost about one-tenth as much per person in the

population; although only marginally cost-effective over a 20-year horizon, these restrictions become cost saving or cost-effective or very cost-effective in all the countries over a 50-year horizon. Cecchini and others (2010) also model five other interventions aimed at adults that are not discussed here.

A large trial of school-based interventions in China (Meng and others 2013) finds that nutritional or physical activity interventions alone are not effective, but a combined program is effective, albeit not significantly so. This observation that comprehensive interventions are required is consistent with the general literature on obesity prevention that is not restricted to children and adolescents or to LMICs. Meng and others (2013) do not calculate cost-effectiveness per DALY or QALY. Accordingly, it is not possible to infer whether the intervention is cost-effective; however, it is not inexpensive at US$4.41 per participant over two years, and at US$31.10 if teachers' time is included. In comparison, per capita annual health expenditure from the public budget in 2013 was, on average, US$15.36 for low-income countries, US$30.67 for lower-middle-income countries, and US$260.96 for upper-middle-income countries (World Bank 2016).

Smoking

Findings from a study of a school-based intervention for smoking in India (Brown and others 2012) are similar. Although the program is cost-effective per QALY saved, the cost of US$45.81 per student is not inexpensive; removing the cost of teachers' time reduces the cost of this particular intervention by only 5 percent. This was a large-scale pilot; it is possible that costs could be reduced by embedding the training involved into the regular teacher training curriculum rather than delivering it via special workshops that require travel and per diem expenses.

Reproductive and Sexual Health

Of the four studies of interventions for sexual and reproductive health, only one (Duflo and others 2006) provides cost-effectiveness estimates. Their findings suggest that providing adolescent girls with information they can use to make more informed decisions (advising them of the age profile of human immunodeficiency virus/acquired immune deficiency syndrome [HIV/AIDS] status in men) is the most cost-effective at US$253 per DALY averted. More general educational interventions regarding HIV/AIDS, and subsidies designed to help girls stay in school also fall into the very cost-effective zone for Kenya at less than one times per capita GNI (WHO 2001). Unit costs are modest; Duflo and others (2006) do not present unit costs for the curriculum-based

Table 26.3 Cost And Cost-Effectiveness of Interventions Relevant for Adolescent Health in Low- and Middle-Income Countries, from Systematic Review

Study	Country/region	Intervention/condition	Cost per unit as presented in article	Unit	Currency (year)	Cost per unit in 2012 US$
Obesity						
Cecchini and others 2010	Brazil, China, India, Mexico, Russian Federation, South Africa	Modeling effects of two interventions aimed at obesity at school age, and five others aimed at adults:				
		• School-based interventions	0.82 (Brazil)	Per head of population	2005 US$	1.44
			0.53 (China)			0.86
			0.73 (India)			1.09
			1.22 (Mexico)			1.35
			0.51 (Russian Federation)			0.87
			0.99 (South Africa)			1.19
		• Food advertising regulations for children	0.04 (Brazil)	Per head of population	2005 US$	0.07
			0 (China)			0
			0 (India)			0
			0.09 (Mexico)			0.10
			0.13 (Russian Federation)			0.22
			0.08 (South Africa)			0.10
		• School-based interventions (20-year horizon)	> 1 million (except Russian Federation)	Per DALY averted	2005 US$	> 1 million in all countries
			830,177 (Russian Federation)			
		• Food advertising regulations for children (20-year horizon)	CS (Brazil)	Per DALY averted	2005 US$	CS
			556 (China)			902
			3,186 (India)			4,753
			11,151 (Mexico)			12,340
			5,718 (Russian Federation)			9,725
			13,241 (South Africa)			15,892

table continues next page

Table 26.3 Cost And Cost-Effectiveness of Interventions Relevant for Adolescent Health in Low- and Middle-Income Countries, from Systematic Review (continued)

Study	Country/region	Intervention/condition	Cost per unit as presented in article	Unit	Currency (year)	Cost per unit in 2012 US$
		• School-based interventions (50-year horizon)	93,350 (Brazil)	Per DALY averted	2005 US$	174,918
			35,174 (China)			57,031
			59,665 (India)			89,009
			235,957 (Mexico)			261,123
			261,114 (Russian Federation)			444,098
			153,233 (South Africa)			183,911
		• Food advertising regulations for children (50-year horizon)	CS (Brazil)	Per DALY averted	2005 US$	CS
			CS (China)			CS
			752 (India)			1,122
			658 (Mexico)			728
			4,823 (Russian Federation)			8,209
			3,352 (South Africa)			4,023
Meng and others 2013	China	Combined nutrition and physical education intervention in schools (also reports nutrition alone, physical education alone; no significant effect)	26.80	Per student	US$ (year not given; likely 2009–10)	31.10
			3.80 excluding cost of time of teachers			4.41 excluding cost of time of teachers
			1,308.90	Per case of overweight or obesity averted	US$ (year not given; likely 2009–10)	1,519
Sexual and reproductive health						
Duflo and others 2006	Kenya	• Education of school students on HIV/AIDS (cost $9 per student in a specific grade in 2003, estimated by authors of this chapter)	575	Per pregnancy averted (proxy for unprotected sex)	US$ (year not given; likely 2003)	1,600
		• Informing girls in school of age profile of HIV in men	91	Per pregnancy averted	US$ (year not given; likely 2003)	253
		• Free school uniforms once in each of two years for grade 6 students (uniform cost $6 in 2003)	749 (full cost)	Per pregnancy averted	US$ (year not given; likely 2003)	2,084

table continues next page

Table 26.3 Cost And Cost-Effectiveness of Interventions Relevant for Adolescent Health in Low- and Middle-Income Countries, from Systematic Review (continued)

Study	Country/region	Intervention/condition	Cost per unit as presented in article	Unit	Currency (year)	Cost per unit in 2012 US$
Kempers, Ketting, and Lesco 2014	Moldova	Adolescent-friendly sexual and reproductive health services	2.55	Per person in population covered	2011 US$	2.59
			12.10	Per user		12.58
Kivela, Ketting, and Baltussen 2013	Nigeria	School-based intervention for sexuality education (costs for pilot programs also for India, Indonesia, and Kenya)	7 (Nigeria)	Per student	2009 US$	9.40
Terris-Prestholt and others 2006	Tanzania	An adolescent sexual health program, with school-based education component plus condom distribution	13.46	Per student	2001 US$	17.92
			1.54	Per condom distributed		2.05
Smoking						
Brown and others 2012	India	School-based education intervention against smoking (MYTRI)	31.73 per student for 2-year program	Per student	2006 US$	45.81
			2,492	Per QALY	2006 US$	3,598
			(2,769 if students' time included)			(3,998 if students' time included)

Note: CS = cost saving; HIV/AIDS = human immunodeficiency virus/acquired immune deficiency syndrome; MYTRI = Mobilizing Youth for Tobacco-Related Initiatives in India.

interventions, but calculations using their data suggest these cost approximately US$25 per student in one grade. Duflo and others (2006) present figures for a subsidy to keep students in school of 2012 US$16.69 per student (cost of a uniform) per year, and US$33.38 for the intervention that provided uniforms in two different years.

Two other studies provide costs per student for educational interventions on sexual and reproductive health. Kivela, Ketting, and Baltussen (2013) examine costs in four LMICs; for a program at scale in Nigeria; and pilot programs in India, Indonesia, and Kenya. The two extracurricular programs in Indonesia and Kenya cost significantly more than the intracurricular ones. Costs were US$85 and US$205 per student, respectively, compared with US$9.40 in Nigeria, and US$16.30 in India. The budgetary outlays were a quarter or less of the total cost for the three countries with intracurricular programs because governments are already paying teachers' salaries. International standards recommend that there should be 12–20 lessons of 45–60 minutes each, spread over more than one year, for such interventions to be effective.

Kivela, Ketting, and Baltussen (2013) point out some of the issues of including sexuality education in the curriculum. Their study notes that opposition to the programs in India and Nigeria caused implementation delays of several years, with attendant increased costs.

A study for Tanzania (Terris-Prestholt and others 2006) estimated that an adolescent sexual health intervention cost US$17.92 for the school-based education component. Other components included adolescent-friendly health services, peer distribution of condoms, and community mobilization efforts; the educational component accounted for 70 percent of the costs. Information about the net budgetary cost was not presented, including how much of the educational program cost was allotted to teacher's salaries when presenting the program, as opposed to the additional costs for teacher training.

The last study of sexual and reproductive health (Kempers, Ketting, and Lesco 2014) presents the cost of an adolescent-friendly sexual and reproductive health service in Moldova. Four well-performing centers were picked for study out of 38. The centers provide services for sexually transmitted infection, early pregnancy and contraception, and HIV/AIDS. Costs were US$6.14 per visit; assuming each participant required on average two visits, the cost was US$12.58 per user per year. Slightly less than 20 percent of the covered youth population used the services, such that the cost per young person in the population covered was US$2.59.

Although the youth-friendly health services in Moldova were potentially cost saving for potential numbers of sexually transmitted infections averted, unwanted pregnancies averted, and cases of HIV/AIDS averted, funding the services was difficult. A little more than 50 percent of the cost came from the National Health Insurance Company; services also relied on contributions from donors, nongovernmental organizations, and local authorities, as well as substantial amounts of volunteer time.

Implications for Program Development

This review of evidence from HICs and LMICs provides some guidance for the economics of an essential package of interventions. At the same time, we must recognize that evidence on what works is still being amassed.

First, data are simply insufficient in a number of areas, including national media campaigns, national policy making, and social media, which are likely all important ways to support any intervention delivered to individual adolescents. The modeling results on restrictions on food advertising to young people (Cecchini and others 2010) are promising, but the estimated effectiveness of advertising interventions relies on very limited evidence.

Second, programs delivered through schools are a mainstay (Bundy, Schultz, and others 2017). Their unit costs are not inexpensive, but school-based programs may be less costly than community-based ones. Costs of educational programs in schools can be reduced by providing intracurricular programs at scale and incorporating training into the teacher education curriculum. Teacher involvement in educational interventions is crucial, and effective training can reduce costs and improve affordability in the long term. At the same time, neuroscience suggests that education programs alone are insufficient in areas in which adolescents make "hot" decisions. Education may need to be complemented with risk reduction efforts based on behavioral theory and skill development. The likelihood of success for simply preventing an undesirable outcome for a few years may be higher than that for establishing lifelong healthy habits.

One limitation of the evidence is that education programs are very heterogeneous. Program design, context, and intensity of effort in implementation all matter. Another limitation is that the duration of follow-up studies of school-based interventions is usually short. Thus, evidence on long-term impact is lacking. This differs from the literature on early childhood development and preschool interventions, where there are a modest number of high-quality research studies with long-term follow-up, both for HICs and LMICs (see chapter 19 in this volume, Black and others 2017, and chapter 24 in this volume, Horton and Black 2017).

Finally, youth-friendly health services may be important and cost-effective, but they are time intensive to deliver, and issues of affordability in LMICs may arise.

COSTING AN ESSENTIAL PACKAGE

Promoting adolescent health requires a broad range of actions across several sectors. Education is key and affects skills and employment opportunities; for girls, education helps delay marriage and early childbearing. Policies and laws that allow flexibility in adolescents' access to health services without necessarily requiring parental authorization are vital, as are policies and laws controlling their exposure to unhealthy products and activities (Laski and others 2015). Empowerment and involvement of adolescents in decision making concerning their well-being is essential. Although ministries of health will be involved in promoting adolescent health in all of these areas, they will not necessarily lead the efforts.

The focus of this chapter is on the more narrowly defined interventions to promote adolescent health in which ministries of health have the primary responsibility. The adolescent package costed here draws on several other sources. The WHO (2013) provides policy advice on programs for preconception care, which overlaps substantially with the initiatives discussed in the previous section. Patton and others (2016) include recommendations for adolescent health as well as other supportive nonhealth services. The Global Strategy for Women's, Children's and Adolescents' Health (Every Woman Every Child 2015) includes recommendations in five priority areas for adolescent health interventions (Laski and others 2015).

Two other studies provide cost estimates. The Centre for Global Development's *Start with a Girl* discusses an agenda for adolescent girl health that was also costed (Temin and Levine 2009). Deogan, Ferguson, and Stenberg (2012) provide estimates for a package of adolescent-friendly health services, as well as the cost of providing this package in 74 LMICs. These services are one component of a desirable package for promoting adolescent health.

The WHO's (2013) guidelines on preconception care recommend interventions in 13 areas. These areas are primarily directed at women but apply to older adolescent girls, given the younger age at first birth in many LMICs. The areas comprise the following:

- Nutritional conditions
- Vaccine-preventable diseases
- Genetic conditions
- Environmental health
- Infertility and subfertility

- Female genital mutilation
- Too early, unwanted, and rapid-succession pregnancies
- Sexually transmitted infections
- HIV/AIDS
- Interpersonal violence
- Mental health
- Psychoactive substance use
- Tobacco use.

Nutritional conditions and vaccine-preventable diseases are discussed in the package for school-age children (Fernandes and Aurino 2017); others are consistent with topics discussed in this chapter.

Priority actions for adolescent health in the Global Strategy for Women's, Children's and Adolescents' Health are summarized by Laski and others (2015) as follows:

- Health education, including comprehensive sexuality education
- Access to and use of integrated health services
- Immunization
- Nutrition, including healthy eating and exercise, and supplementation of key micronutrients
- Psychosocial support for detection and management of mental health problems.

Start with a Girl is an ambitious agenda with eight components recommended for adolescent girls in LMICs (Temin and Levine 2009). The total package is US$359.31 per girl per year. (We have not updated their cost estimates to 2012 since doing so is not straightforward for a multicountry estimate). The eight components specific to girls, with associated costs per girl per year, are youth-friendly health services (US$8.50), iron supplements (US$2.00), HPV vaccination (US$17.50), reducing harmful traditional practices (US$80.85), male engagement (US$113.85), obesity reduction (US$0.11), edutainment programs (US$0.57), safe spaces (US$130.51), and comprehensive sexuality education (US$6.02). The edutainment intervention, which combines computer games with educational elements, is directed at issues of sexual and reproductive health, gender-based violence, and other health challenges facing girls. The ninth component is male engagement for young men ages 15–24 years living on less than US$2 per day (US$113.25). Smoking reduction is not costed because it is expected that revenue from higher taxation would more than cover interventions. This package is somewhat different from what is costed in this chapter. It is, on the one hand, much more comprehensive; on the other hand, it does not consider the health of male adolescents.

Deogan, Ferguson, and Stenberg (2012) have undertaken a comprehensive costing of adolescent-friendly health services for 74 countries. The package includes contraception; maternity care; management of sexually transmitted infections; HIV/AIDS testing and counseling, harm reduction, and care and treatment; safe abortion services; and care of injuries due to intimate partner violence and sexual violence. It also includes costs of activities to improve quality of care and increase uptake of services by adolescents. Once full coverage is achieved, the cost is estimated to be US$4.70 per adolescent, or US$0.82 averaged over the whole population. There is some degree of overlap between costs for adolescent-friendly health services; estimates of expanding contraceptive services are discussed in volume 9, chapter 3 (Watkins and others 2018). The overall cost of US$4.3 billion in aggregate covers 74 countries. We have not converted these figures to 2012 U.S. dollars because their projections are in current U.S. dollars for 2011–15 and the conversion would not be straightforward.

The essential package costed in this chapter draws on the economic assessment of existing interventions and the key interventions outlined in recent strategy documents where ministries of health have a leading or major role. The package that we cost includes the following components:

- Adolescent-friendly health services
- School-based educational programming covering such topics as sexual and reproductive health, mental health, smoking, alcohol, and illicit drugs
- National media and policy efforts to support a healthy lifestyle program to complement school-based programming

These interventions correlate fairly well with the burden of disease in adolescence: the top five causes of death are road injury, HIV/AIDS, suicide, lower respiratory infections, and interpersonal violence; and the top five causes of years lived with disability are depression, road injuries, anemia, HIV, and suicide (WHO 2014). Because road traffic injuries are an important topic in volume 7 of this series (Mock and others 2017), they are not discussed in the present chapter.

We use Deogan, Ferguson, and Stenberg's (2012) estimates for adolescent-friendly health services. We use Ebbeler's (2009) estimates for the national media cost for a sexuality education campaign of US$0.58 per girl or boy reached, and we assume that double this amount could incorporate a more comprehensive campaign against various harms. Ebbeler's (2009) estimates provide the detailed assumptions underpinning the costing in Temin and Levine's (2009) *Start with a Girl*.

Finally, we use estimates from the previous section for the costs of school-based education programs. Three programs (table 26.3) cost US$9, US$18, and US$25, approximately. The Indian antismoking program (Brown and others 2012), at almost US$46, relies heavily on per diem and travel costs as a start-up, and it is unrepresentative of what a mature program might cost. We include a cost of US$18 per adolescent per year and assume that adolescents would participate in such a program each year for three years (ages 14–16 years). Of this cost, 25 percent represents additional budget costs to the government of developing the program, training the trainers, and refreshing the curriculum periodically; the balance is the cost of teachers' time. We specifically exclude obesity from the educational package. The evidence base is weak, and current programs are not unequivocally effective. This is an area where more pilot programs and evaluations are required.

The cost of the recommended package is as follows:

- US$4.70 per adolescent ages 10–19 years for adolescent-friendly health services
- US$1.16 per adolescent ages 10–19 years for national media campaigns and national policy efforts
- US$9.00 per adolescent ages 14–16 years for the net budget cost of a school-based education program, excluding cost of teachers' time; this amount is equivalent to US$3.00 per adolescent ages 10–19 years.

The total package, therefore, costs roughly US$8.90 per year for each adolescent ages 10–19 years.

Deogan, Ferguson, and Stenberg's (2012) estimate for adolescent-friendly health services is carefully constructed using detailed data; the other two items are simply rough estimates and require further refinement. Costs of the total package are aggregated by size of population in low-income and lower-middle income countries in chapter 1 (Bundy, de Silva, and others 2017).

CONCLUSIONS

Adolescent health, overlooked for years, is now achieving much-needed prominence in the international health agenda. Adolescence is a key point in the life course, a point at which important health behaviors are established that determine the path of chronic disease at older ages. It is a key time at which to invest in and benefit the health of the working-age population, older adults, and through new mothers and their babies, the next generation. The relative neglect of adolescents in research and programming means that knowledge of how to design cost-effective programs is inadequate relative to needs. This is an area in which there may be a payoff to trying innovative approaches and in which pilot programs require rigorous evaluation.

Economic evaluations for HICs suggest that a number of health interventions for adolescents can be cost-effective or very cost-effective, including screening and treating for selected mental health conditions as well as school-based programs on education regarding smoking, alcohol, and sexual health. Whether interventions aimed at obesity are cost-effective is uncertain because data on long-term outcomes are lacking.

For LMICs, we were able to find only two cost-effectiveness studies using QALYs or DALYs as outcomes. One concluded that restrictions on advertising of unhealthy foods was cost-effective (or even cost saving) in preventing obesity across a range of countries, while school-based interventions were not. The other study concluded that a school-based antismoking pilot program in India was cost-effective, although not very cost-effective; it is likely that if it became part of the routine curriculum it could become less costly and therefore likely more cost-effective.

An essential package for adolescent health should include at least three elements: national-level policy combined with communication of social norms, accessible and respectful services, and targeted education. National and subnational governments need to create an appropriate environment through legislation and through social marketing of key messages. Access to services that recognize adolescents' desires for confidentiality and treat them respectfully will facilitate uptake. Education in health and wellness will provide this group with the means to be active participants in their own health and improve outcomes. This education can be provided in schools as well as in other venues where it is cost-effective to reach those who are no longer in school. These elements need to be complemented with broader social policy and initiatives outside the health area that affect adolescent well-being.

The essential package in this chapter costs approximately US$8.90 per adolescent in lower-middle-income countries (in 2012 U.S. dollars). The costs will be somewhat higher in upper-middle-income countries. Compared with per capita annual public health expenditure of US$31 in lower-middle-income countries in 2013 (World Bank 2016), this amount is not unreasonable. Low- and lower-middle-income countries, in particular, face pressing unmet needs for treatment of existing illnesses. The economic evidence summarized in this chapter can help make the case for the substantial returns on preventive investments in adolescent health.

The future research needs are large, given the paucity of existing evidence. Cost-effectiveness studies should be undertaken for promising pilot programs before they are scaled up. It is not too difficult to collect cost information retrospectively to calculate cost-effectiveness or the benefit-cost ratio if a program proves to be effective. Another priority is for longitudinal studies, particularly for the rapidly growing problem of obesity, but there is considerable uncertainty about whether school-based programs have any lasting effect. A third knowledge gap is how to reach adolescents who are not in school. It is possible that social media and mass media can be used innovatively to reach this group, and perhaps the health sector can learn how to design appealing health messages from advertisers of commercial products.

ANNEX

This annex to this chapter is as follows. It is available at http://www.dcp-3.org/CAHD.

- Annex 26A. Methodology and Results of Systematic Search, Cost-Effectiveness Analysis

NOTE

World Bank Income Classifications as of July 2014 are as follows, based on estimates of gross national income (GNI) per capita for 2013:

- Low-income countries (LICs) = US$1,045 or less
- Middle-income countries (MICs) are subdivided:
  a) lower-middle-income = US$1,046 to US$4,125
  b) upper-middle-income (UMICs) = US$4,126 to US$12,745
- High-income countries (HICs) = US$12,746 or more.

REFERENCES

Black, R., R. Laxminarayan, M. Temmerman, and N. Walker. 2016. *Reproductive, Maternal, Newborn and Child Health.* Volume 2 in *Disease Control Priorities* (third edition), edited by D. T. Jamison, H. Gelband, S. Horton, P. Jha, R. Laxminarayan, and R. Nugent. Washington, DC: World Bank.

Black, M., A. Grove, and K. Merseth. 2017. "Platforms to Reach Children in Early Childhood." In *Disease Control Priorities* (third edition): Volume 8, *Child and Adolescent Health and Development*, edited by D. A. P. Bundy, N. de Silva, S. Horton, D. T. Jamison, and G. C. Patton. Washington, DC: World Bank.

Brown, H. S., M. Stigler, C. Perry, P. Dhavan, M. Arora, and others. 2012. "The Cost-Effectiveness of a School-Based Smoking Prevention Program in India." *Health Promotion International* 28 (2): 178–86.

Bundy, D. A. P., N. de Silva, S. Horton, G. C. Patton, L. Schultz, and D. T. Jamison. 2017. "Child and Adolescent Health and Development: Realizing Neglected Potential." In *Disease*

Control Priorities (third edition): Volume 8, *Child and Adolescent Health and Development*, edited by Bundy, D. A. P., N. de Silva, S. Horton, D. T. Jamison, and G. C. Patton. Washington, DC: World Bank.

Bundy, D. A. P., and S. Horton. 2017. "Impact of Interventions on Health and Development during Childhood and Adolescence: a Conceptual Framework." In *Disease Control Priorities* (third edition): Volume 8, *Child and Adolescent Health and Development*, edited by D. A. P. Bundy, N. de Silva, S. Horton, D. T. Jamison, and G. C. Patton. Washington, DC: World Bank.

Bundy, D. A. P., L. Schultz, B. Sarr, L. Banham, P. Colenso, and L. Drake. 2017. "The School as a Platform for Addressing Health in Middle Childhood and Adolescence." In *Disease Control Priorities* (third edition): Volume 8, *Child and Adolescent Health and Development*, edited by D. A. P. Bundy, N. de Silva, S. Horton, D. T. Jamison, and G. C. Patton. Washington, DC: World Bank.

Carter, R., M. Moodie, A. Markwick, A. Magnus, T. Vos, and others. 2009. "Assessing Cost-Effectiveness in Obesity (ACE-Obesity): An Overview of the ACE Approach, Economic Methods and Cost Results." *BMC Public Health* 9: 11.

Cecchini, M., F. Sassi, J. A. Lauer, Y. Y. Lee, V. Guajardo-Barron, and D. Chisholm. 2010. "Tackling of Unhealthy Diets, Physical Inactivity, and Obesity: Health Effects and Cost-Effectiveness." *The Lancet* 376 (9754): 1775–84.

De la Cruz, T. E., J. Mahon, J. Santelli, and J. Waldfogel. 2015. "Economic perspectives on Adolescent Health: A Review of Research on the Cost-Effectiveness of Interventions to Improve Adolescent Health." Unpublished, Columbia University, New York.

Deogan, C., J. Ferguson, and K. Stenberg. 2012. "Resource Needs for Adolescent-Friendly Health Services: Estimates for 74 Low- and Middle-Income Countries." *PLoS One* 7: e51420.

Department of Health and Human Services, United States. 2014. "HSS Office of Adolescent Health's Teen Pregnancy Program: Investing in Evidence-Based and Innovative Programs to Prevent Teen Pregnancy and Promote Adolescent Health." Department of Health and Human Services, Washington, DC. http://www.hhs.gov/ash/oah /oah-initatives/teen_pregnancy/about/Assets/tpp-overview -brochure.pdf.

de Walque, D., L. Fernald, P. Gertler, and M. Hidrobo. 2017. "Cash Transfers and Child and Adolescent Development." In *Disease Control Priorities* (third edition): Volume 8, *Child and Adolescent Health and Development*, edited by D. A. P. Bundy, N. de Silva, S. Horton, D. T. Jamison, and G. C. Patton. Washington, DC: World Bank.

Duflo, E., M. Kremer, P. Dupas, and S. Sinei. 2006. "Education and HIV/AIDS Prevention: Evidence from a Randomized Evaluation in Western Kenya." Research Paper, Brookings Institution, Washington, DC. http://www.brookings.edu /research/papers/2006/02/development-kremer.

Ebbeler, J. 2009. *Financial Requirements for Global Investments in Priority Health Interventions for Adolescent Girls*. New York: Centre for Global Development. http://www.cgdev .org/doc/GHA/Start_with_a_Girl-Annex2.pdf.

Every Woman Every Child. 2015. *The Global Strategy for Women's, Children's and Adolescents' Health 2016–2030: Survive, Thrive, Transform*. Geneva: WHO. http://www .who.int/life-course/partners/global-strategy/.

Fernandes, M., and E. Aurino. 2017. "Identifying the Essential Package for School-Age Child Health: Economic Analysis." In *Disease Control Priorities* (third edition): Volume 8, *Child and Adolescent Health and Development*, edited by D. A. P. Bundy, N. de Silva, S. Horton, D. T. Jamison, and G. C. Patton. Washington, DC: World Bank.

Gelband, H., P. Jha, R. Sankaranarayanan, and S. Horton, editors. 2015. *Disease Control Priorities* (third edition): Volume 3, *Cancer*, edited by H. Gelband, P. Jha, R. Sankaranarayanan, and S. Horton. Washington, DC: World Bank.

Gorna, R., N. Klingen, K. Senga, A. Soucat, and K. Takemi. 2015. "Women's, Children's, and Adolescents' Health Needs Universal Health Coverage." *The Lancet* 386 (1011): 2371–72.

Grigorenko, E. 2017. "Brain Development: The Effect of Interventions on Children and Adolescents." In *Disease Control Priorities* (third edition): Volume 8, *Child and Adolescent Health and Development*, edited by D. A. P. Bundy, N. de Silva, S. Horton, D. T. Jamison, and G. C. Patton. Washington, DC: World Bank.

Guo, J. J., T. J. Wade, W. Pan, and K. N. Keller. 2010. "School-Based Health Centers: Cost-Benefit Analysis and Impact on Health Care Disparities." *American Journal of Public Health* 100 (9): 1617–23.

Haynes, S. M., G. F. Lyons, E. L. McCombie, M. S. McQuigg, S. Mongia, and others. 2010. "Long-Term Cost-Effectiveness of Weight Management in Primary Care." *International Journal of Clinical Practice* 64 (6): 775–83.

Holmes, K., S. Bertozzi, B. Bloom, and P. Jha, editors. 2017. *Disease Control Priorities* (third edition): Volume 6, *Major Infectious Diseases*, edited by D. T. Jamison, H. Gelband, S. Horton, P. Jha, R. Laxminarayan, and R. Nugent. Washington, DC: World Bank.

Horton, S., and M. Black. 2017. "Identifying an Essential Package for Early Childhood Development: Economic Analysis." In *Disease Control Priorities* (third edition): Volume 8, *Child and Adolescent Health and Development*, edited by D. A. P. Bundy, N. de Silva, S. Horton, D. T. Jamison, and G. C. Patton. Washington, DC: World Bank.

Horton, S. 2015. *Investment Case for Child and Adolescent Health, and Health System Strengthening*. Draft prepared for UNICEF. Waterloo, ON, Canada: University of Waterloo.

Hyman, S., D. Chisholm, R. Kessler, V. Patel, and H. Whiteford. 2006. "Mental Disorders." In *Disease Control Priorities in Developing Countries* (second edition), edited by D. T. Jamison, J. G. Breman, A. R. Measham, G. Alleyne, M. Claeson, and D. B. Evans, P. Jha, A. Mills, and P. Musgrove. Washington, DC: World Bank and Oxford University Press.

iERG (Independent Expert Review Group). 2013. *Every Woman, Every Child: Strengthening Equity and Dignity through Health*. Geneva: World Health Organization.

Jha, P., F. J. Chaloupka, J. Moore, V. Gajalakshmi, P. C. Gupta, and others. 2006. "Tobacco Addiction." In *Disease Control Priorities in Developing Countries* (second edition), edited by D. T. Jamison, J. G. Breman, A. R. Measham, G. Alleyne, M. Claeson, and D. B. Evans, P. Jha, A. Mills, and P. Musgrove. Washington, DC: World Bank and Oxford University Press.

Kempers, J., E. Ketting, and G. Lesco. 2014. "Cost Analysis and Exploratory Cost-Effectiveness of Youth-Friendly Sexual and Reproductive Health Services in the Republic of Moldova." *BMC Health Services Research* 14: 316–24.

Kivela, J., E. Ketting, and R. Baltussen. 2013. "Cost Analysis of School-Based Sexuality Education Program in Six Countries." *Cost Effectiveness and Resource Allocation* 11: 17–23.

Korber, K. 2014. "Potential Transferability of Economic Evaluations of Programs Encouraging Physical Activity in Children and Adolescents across Different Countries: A Systematic Review of the Literature." *International Journal of Environmental Research and Public Health* 11 (10): 10606–621.

Laski, L., Z. Matthews, S. Neal, G. Adeyemo, G. C. Patton, and others 2015. "Realising the Health and Wellbeing of Adolescents." *BMJ* 351: h4119.

Lule, E., J. E. Rosen, S. Singh, J. C. Knowles, and J. R. Behrman. 2006. "Adolescent Health Programs." In *Disease Control Priorities in Developing Countries* (second edition), edited by D. T. Jamison, J. G. Breman, A. R. Measham, G. Alleyne, M. Claeson, and D. B. Evans, P. Jha, A. Mills, and P. Musgrove. Washington, DC: World Bank and Oxford University Press.

Lynch, F. L., J. F. Dickerson, G. Clarke, B. Vitiello, G. Porta, and others. 2011. "Incremental Cost-Effectiveness of Combined Therapy vs. Medication Only for Youth with Selective Serotonin Reuptake Inhibitor-Resistant Depression: Treatment of SSRI-Resistant Depression in Adolescents Trial Findings." *Archives of General Psychiatry* 68 (3): 253–26.

McDaid, D., A. L. Park, C. Currie, and C. Zanotti. 2014. "Investing in the Wellbeing of Young People: Making the Economic Case." In *Wellbeing: A Complete Reference Guide Vol. 5: The Economics of Wellbeing*, edited by D. MacDaid and C. Copper, 181–214. Oxford, U.K.: Wiley-Blackwell.

Meng, L., H. Xu, A. Liu, J. van Raaij, W. Bemelmans, and others. 2013. "The Costs and Cost-Effectiveness of a School-Based Comprehensive Intervention Study on Obesity in China." *PLoS One* 8 (10): e7771.

Mock, C. N., O. Kobusingye, R. Nugent, and K. Smith, editors. 2017. *Injury Prevention and Environmental Health.* Volume 7, *Disease Control Priorities* (third edition), edited by D. T. Jamison, H. Gelband, S. Horton, P. Jha, R. Laxminarayan, and R. Nugent. Washington, DC: World Bank.

Norton, R., A. A. Hyder, D. Bishai, and M. Peden. 2006. "Unintentional Injuries." In *Disease Control Priorities in Developing Countries* (second edition), edited by D. T. Jamison, J. G. Breman, A. R. Measham, G. Alleyne, M. Claeson, and D. B. Evans, P. Jha, A. Mills, and P. Musgrove. Washington, DC: World Bank and Oxford University Press.

Over, E. A., T. L. Feenstra, R. T. Hoogenveen, M. Droomers, E. Usters, and others. 2014. "Tobacco Control Policies Specified According to Socioeconomic Status: Health Disparities and Cost-Effectiveness." *Nicotine and Tobacco Research* 16 (6): 725–32.

Patton, G. C., S. M. Sawyer, J. Santelli, D. A. Ross, R. Afifi, and others. 2016. "Our Future: A Lancet Commission on Adolescent Health and Wellbeing." *The Lancet* 387 (10036): 2423–78.

Rehm, J., D. Chisholm, R. Room, and A. D. Lopez. 2006. "Alcohol." In *Disease Control Priorities in Developing Countries* (second edition), edited by D. T. Jamison, J. G. Breman, A. R. Measham, G. Alleyne, M. Claeson, and D. B. Evans, P. Jha, A. Mills, and P. Musgrove. Washington, DC: World Bank and Oxford University Press.

Romeo, R., S. Byford, and M. Knapp. 2005. "Annotation: Economic Evaluations of Child and Adolescent Mental Health Interventions: A Systematic Review." *Journal of Child Psychology* 46 (9): 919–30.

Shepherd, J., J. Kavanagh, J. Picot, K. Cooper, A. Harden, and others. 2010. "The Effectiveness and Cost-Effectiveness of Behavioural Interventions for the Prevention of Sexually Transmitted Infections in Young People Aged 13–19: A Systematic Review and Economic Evaluation." *Health Technology Assessments* 14 (7). doi:103310/hta 14070.

Steinberg, L. 2007. "Risk Taking in Adolescence: New perspectives from Brain and Behavioral Science." *Current Direction in Psychological Science* 16 (2): 55–59.

Temin, M., and R. Levine. 2009. *Start with a Girl: A New Agenda for Global Health.* Washington, DC: Center for Global Development.

Terris-Prestholt, F., L. Kumaranayake, A. I. Obasi, B. Cleophas-Mazige, M. Makokha, and others. 2006. "From Trial Intervention to Scale-Up: Costs of an Adolescent Sexual Health Program in Mwanza, Tanzania." *Sexually Transmitted Infections* 33 (S10): S133–39.

UN (United Nations). 2015. "Tranforming Our World: The 2030 Agenda for Sustainable Development." A/RES/70/1. UN General Assembly, New York. http://sustainabledevelopment .un.org/content/documents/21252030%20Agenda%20 for%20Sustainable%20Development%20web.pdf.

UNICEF (United Nations Children's Fund). 2011. *The State of the World's Children 2011: Adolescence: An Age of Opportunity.* New York: UNICEF.

———. 2012. *Progress for Children: A Report Card on Adolescents.* Number 10. New York: UNICEF.

Vos, T., T. Carter, J. Barendregt, C. Mihalopoulos, L. Veerman, and others. 2010. *Assessing Cost-Effectiveness in Prevention (ACE-Prevention): Final Report.* Melbourne: University of Queensland, Brisbane, and Deakin University.

Watkins, D. A., Dean T. Jamison, A. Mills, R. Atun, K. Danforth, and others. 2018. "Universal Health Coverage and Essential Packages of Care." In *Disease Control Priorities* (third edition): Volume 9, *Disease Control Priorities: Improving Health and Reducing Poverty*, edited by D. T. Jamison, R. Nugent, H. Gelband, S. Horton, P. Jha, R. Laxminarayan, and C. N. Mock. Washington, DC: World Bank.

WHO (World Health Organization). 2001. *Macroeconomics and Health: Investing in Health for Economic Development.* Geneva: WHO.

———. 2013. *Preconception Care: Maximizing the Gains for Maternal and Child Health.* WHO Policy Brief. Geneva: WHO. http://www.who.int/maternal_child_adoles cent/documents/concensus_preconception_care/en/.

———. 2014. *Health for the World's Adolescents: A Second Chance in the Second Decade.* Geneva: WHO. http://www.who.int /adolescent/second-decade/section1.

Willett, W. C., J. P. Koplan, R. Nugent, C. Dusenbury, P. Puska, and others. 2006. "Prevention of Chronic Disease by Means of Diet and Lifestyle Change." In *Disease Control Priorities in Developing Countries* (second edition), edited by D. T. Jamison, J. G. Breman, A. R. Measham, G. Alleyne, M. Claeson, and D. B. Evans, P. Jha, A. Mills, and P. Musgrove. Washington, DC: World Bank and Oxford University Press.

World Bank. 2016. *World Development Indicators.* Washington, DC: World Bank. http://data.worldbank.org.

Wu, S., D. Cohen, Y. Shi, M. Peason, and R. Sturm. 2011. "Economic Analysis of Physical Activity Interventions." *American Journal of Preventive Medicine* 40 (2): 149–58.

Chapter 27

The Human Capital and Productivity Benefits of Early Childhood Nutritional Interventions

Arindam Nandi, Jere R. Behrman, Sonia Bhalotra,
Anil B. Deolalikar, and Ramanan Laxminarayan

INTRODUCTION

By 2012, child mortality had fallen to almost half its level in 1990.[1] The next major challenge is to improve early-life conditions to harness developmental potential. An estimated 200 million children under age five years in low- and middle-income countries (LMICs) are unlikely to reach their developmental potential because of inadequate health, nutritional, and other investments in early life (Grantham-McGregor and others 2007).[2] This inability to achieve full potential implies substantial losses of welfare and future economic productivity for these children and for their societies (Akresh and others 2012; Behrman, Alderman, and Hoddinott 2004; Bhalotra and Venkataramani 2011; Bhutta and others 2008; Currie and Vogl 2013; Hoddinott and others 2008; Horton, Alderman, and Rivera 2009) and increases the risk of adult morbidities and lower life expectancy (Bhalotra, Karlsson, and Nilsson 2015; Hjort, Solvesten, and Wust 2014). This chapter supplements previous work focusing on estimates of economic benefits from early-life nutritional interventions in LMICs.[3]

Figure 27.1 shows the pathways through which early-life interventions can affect later-life economic outcomes. Prenatal and early childhood interventions affect outcomes at every stage of the lifecycle. These impacts accumulate, making it important to study long-term dynamic effects of interventions. Familial and public investments enter during all lifecycle stages, often induced by the initial intervention. Later investments may in principle complement or substitute for those early in the lifecycle, but some evidence suggests they may be reinforcing (Almond and Mazumder 2013; Bhalotra and Venkataramani 2011, 2013), consistent with recent models that describe human capital production as involving dynamic complementarities across types of investment (for example, health and schooling) and across ages, such that investments early in life increase rates of return to investments later in life (Cunha and Heckman 2007; see also Alderman and others 2017, chapter 7 in this volume).

In the first section, we provide a selected review of evidence of long-term human capital and economic benefits from early-life interventions and then some illustrative calculations of benefit-cost ratios for these interventions. We focus on interventions affecting maternal and early childhood health, including micronutrient supplementation and breastfeeding, and maternal survival. We then present evidence of effects of early interventions on low birth weight (LBW), stunting, and cognitive development in the second section. The third section discusses issues in the estimation of benefit-cost ratios of early-life interventions and presents simulations, illustrating sensitivity of estimates to alternative parameters. The fourth section

Corresponding author: Arindam Nandi, Tata Centre for Development, University of Chicago, Chicago, Illinois, United States; anandi@uchicago.edu.

Figure 27.1 Lifecycle Approach to Early Childhood Interventions

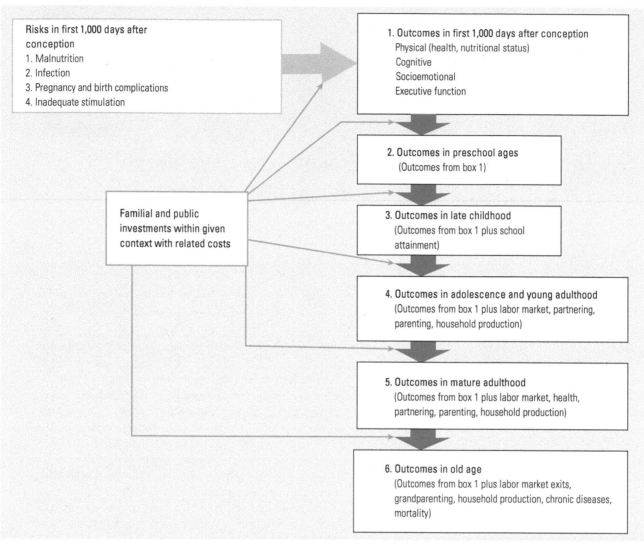

Source: Adapted from Hoddinott, Alderman, and others 2013.

discusses issues of designing policy based on the growing body of estimates from randomized trials in LMICs. Definitions of age groupings and age-specific terminology used in this volume can be found in chapter 1 (Bundy and others 2017).

MATERNAL AND CHILDHOOD INTERVENTIONS

Since Barker's (1990) pioneering "fetal origins" hypothesis linking the prenatal environment to indicators of adult health, including diabetes and heart disease risk, the importance of in utero influences on physical and cognitive development during the first thousand days after conception (figure 27.1, top right box) has gained increasing recognition. Maternal stress and nutritional deprivation tend to stimulate permanent changes in tissue structure and function that help the fetus survive but that are associated with abnormal structure, function, and disease in adult life. Almond and Currie (2011, 167) summarize the implications of the fetal origins hypothesis: "One can best help children (throughout their life course) by helping their mothers. That is, we need to focus on pregnant women or perhaps women of child-bearing age if the key period turns out to be so early in pregnancy that many women are unaware of the pregnancy. Such preemptive targeting would constitute a radical departure from current policies that steer nearly all healthcare resources to the sick."

Maternal health could improve later-life child outcomes through at least two avenues. First, improved maternal health can lead to better delivery outcomes, such as avoidance of premature birth and reduced likelihood of LBW, which are associated with negative economic consequences in later life (Alderman and Behrman 2006).[4] Bhalotra and Rawlings (2011) show that, by numerous indicators, poor maternal health is significantly associated with risks of LBW, infant mortality, and growth faltering. A one standard deviation decrease in a mother's height is associated with increased LBW risks of 7.4 percent of the sample mean rate and with increased neonatal mortality risk of 9.3 percent of the sample rate. A one standard deviation decrease in body mass index is associated with higher LBW risks by 10.8 percent of the mean and with higher neonatal mortality risks by 13.1 percent of the mean. LBW and neonatal mortality risks are lower by 5.7 percent and 16.9 percent of their mean rates, respectively, among nonanemic mothers relative to anemic mothers. These tendencies are widespread. Many current interventions focus on improving mothers' health during pregnancy and tend to influence mothers' body mass index and anemia status. However, the estimated associations of maternal height with birth and early childhood outcomes underscore that mothers' health *stocks* when they give birth, in the accumulation of which nutritional investments in mothers' childhoods count, are also important for reproductive and next-generation outcomes. In addition to maternal health indicators, evidence suggests that maternal behaviors, such as smoking and drinking during pregnancy, compromise fetal development (Almond and Currie 2011; Currie and Vogl 2013; Gilman, Gardener, and Buka 2008; Nilsson 2008; Stratton, Howe, and Battaglia 1996; Victora and others 2008; Weitzman, Gortmaker, and Sobol 1992).

Second, maternal health can affect later-life economic outcomes conditional on birth outcomes. For instance, breastfeeding and stimulation are associated with children's cognitive and socioemotional skills, and maternal mental health tends to influence breastfeeding, stimulation, and mother-child bonding (Attanasio and others 2014; Bennett and others 2014; Krutikova and others 2015; Maselko and others 2015; Rahman and others 2008; Rees and Sabia 2009).

The limiting case of poor maternal health, of course, is maternal death. Deaths of mothers who contribute to household resources reduce such resources and thereby investments in children. Fathers' deaths tend to reduce household resources more, but mothers' deaths may reduce the share of resources going to children more. However, because mothers tend to spend more time with young children, mothers' deaths are likely to have larger impacts on children's skill development. Mothers' deaths may have gender-specific impacts on children if daughters substitute for mothers in home production. Higher maternal mortality risks also may lower human capital investments in girls relative to boys because they shorten expected horizons over which returns to investments in girls flow. Male mortality risks, higher on average than female mortality risks, for the same reason lower the incentives for human capital investments in boys.

The rest of this section reviews some empirical evidence on impacts of maternal and reproductive health interventions on later-life outcomes of children.

Prenatal Interventions

Field, Robles, and Torero (2009) evaluate the effects of iodine supplementation during pregnancy in Tanzania. Iodine deficiency is widespread in many developing countries. Compelling evidence indicates that iodine matters most during fetal brain development, and iodine deficiencies have adverse effects on children's cognitive abilities. In the early 1970s, 40 percent of the Tanzanian population lived in iodine-deficient areas and 25 percent had iodine-deficiency disorders. Tanzania subsequently launched a large and intensive early iodine supplementation program, which ultimately reached nearly a quarter of the population for an average of four years. Field, Robles, and Torero (2009) assess whether children who benefited from supplements in utero exhibited higher grade progression rates 10–15 years later. They also compare those exposed to the sporadic iodization efforts with unexposed siblings, thereby controlling for selective uptake by families.

They find large and robust impacts. Children protected from iodine deficiency during their first trimester in utero attain an average of 0.3 schooling grades more than siblings and older and younger children in their district who were not protected, confirming that first trimesters are critical for cognitive development. The effects are substantially larger for girls, indicating potentially important roles of micronutrient deficiencies in explaining gender differences in schooling attainment.

To verify their findings, Field, Robles, and Torero (2009) present cross-country regressions of school participation on baseline iodine-deficiency disorders and fractions of populations consuming adequately iodized salt. The results show a negative correlation between baseline iodine-deficiency disorders and female secondary schooling and a positive correlation between early salt iodization and female primary schooling attainment. Given the low cost of iodine supplementation and the persistence of iodine deficiency in poor countries,

Field, Robles, and Torero (2009) conclude that prenatal supplementation offers an efficient, cost-effective means of improving human capital. Studies of introduction of iodized salt in Sweden and the United States similarly show that it raised schooling attainment (especially for women) and cognitive performance, respectively (Feyrer, Politi, and Weil 2013; Politi 2011).

Recent studies estimate substantial economic benefits of micronutrient supplementation. Five of the top 10 most cost-effective solutions for addressing the world's 10 biggest challenges, according to the Copenhagen Consensus Expert Panel (2008), were micronutrient-related early childhood interventions (table 27.1). The 2012 Copenhagen Consensus Expert Panel also ranked micronutrient supplementation and fortification as the top priority, but the micronutrient-related interventions were combined as "Bundled Interventions to Reduce Undernutrition in PreSchoolers" (Lomborg 2014). Updating the estimates in

Table 27.1 Top Priorities for Addressing the World's 10 Biggest Challenges, Ranked by the Expert Panel of the Copenhagen Consensus, 2008

	Solution	Challenge
1	Micronutrient supplements for children (vitamin A and zinc)	Malnutrition
2	The Doha Development Agenda	Trade
3	Micronutrient fortification (iron and salt iodization)	Malnutrition
4	Expanded immunization coverage for children	Diseases
5	Biofortification	Malnutrition
6	Deworming and other nutrition programs at school	Malnutrition and education
7	Lowering the price of schooling	Education
8	Increase and improve girls' schooling	Women
9	Community-based nutrition promotion	Malnutrition
10	Provide support for women's reproductive role	Women
11	Heart attack acute management	Diseases
12	Malaria prevention and treatment	Diseases
13	Tuberculosis case finding and treatment	Diseases
14	R&D in low-carbon energy technologies	Global warming
15	Bio-sand filters for household water treatment	Water
16	Rural water supply	Water
17	Conditional cash transfers	Education
18	Peacekeeping in postconflict situations	Conflicts
19	HIV combination prevention	Diseases
20	Total sanitation campaign	Water
21	Improving surgical capacity at district hospital level	Diseases
22	Microfinance	Women
23	Improved stove intervention	Air pollution
24	Large, multipurpose dam in Africa	Water
25	Inspection and maintenance of diesel vehicles	Air pollution
26	Low sulfur diesel for urban road vehicles	Air pollution
27	Diesel vehicle particulate control technology	Air pollution
28	Tobacco tax	Diseases
29	R&D and mitigation	Global warming
30	Mitigation only	Global warming

Source: Copenhagen Consensus Expert Panel 2008.
Note: HIV = human immunodeficiency virus; R&D = research and development.

Behrman, Alderman, and Hoddinott (2004) and Horton, Alderman, and Rivera (2009), Hoddinott, Rosegrant, and Torero (2013) report benefit-cost ratios (BCRs) for iodized salt (BCR=81), iron supplements for mothers and children ages 6–24 months (BCR=24), vitamin A supplementation (BCR=13), and zinc supplements for children (BCR=3). The evidence thus suggests that micronutrient supplementation and fortification have very high economic returns relative to costs.

Horton and Ross (2003, 51) review evidence for causal relationships between iron deficiency and a variety of "functional consequences with economic implications (motor and mental impairment in children and low work productivity in adults)." Using plausible impact estimates, they simulate annual physical and cognitive productivity losses due to iron deficiency for 10 developing countries and obtain a median value of 4 percent of GDP, with a range of 2.4 percent (Arab Republic of Egypt) to 7.9 percent (Bangladesh).

A few studies have examined the association between interventions that address acute undernutrition and future health, educational, and economic outcomes. A study by the Institute of Nutrition of Central America and Panama (INCAP) provided a protein-rich nutritional supplement to 2,392 children under age seven years starting in 1969. The intervention was later found to be associated with higher schooling grades of women, improved cognitive outcomes of men and women, and higher male wages (Hoddinott, Behrman, and others 2013; Maluccio and others 2006, 2009). The Andhra Pradesh Children and Parents Study is a similar trial of nutritional supplementation provided to pregnant women and young children in 29 villages of southern India from 1987 through 1990. Adolescent children born during the trial period in intervention areas were taller and had better cardiovascular health and educational outcomes (Kinra and others 2008; Nandi and others 2016).

Canning and others (2011) analyze effects of antenatal maternal vaccination against tetanus, which is expected to prevent children from acquiring tetanus at birth through blood infection and to thereby reduce infant mortality. They follow up a randomized controlled trial of maternal tetanus toxoid immunization conducted in 1974 in Bangladesh, looking at schooling outcomes for children born in 1975–79. They find, in cases in which parents had no schooling, that tetanus toxoid vaccination of mothers reduced the probability of no schooling for children by 4.5 percent and increased the probability of children completing one to seven grades of schooling by 1.5 percent and of children completing eight or more schooling grades by 3 percent. On average, schooling attainment increases by about 0.25 grades. They do not correct for the fact that about one-fourth of children had died by the year of follow up, arguing that the relevant parameter for policy purposes is the impact of maternal tetanus on child education conditional on survival. Driessen and others (2011) show that an intensive measles vaccination program in Bangladesh was associated with an increase in the probability that a boy has enrolled in school of 9.5 percentage points, while having no effect on girls' enrollment.

Breastfeeding Interventions

Numerous studies indicate positive short- and long-term associations of breastfeeding of newborn babies, in particular exclusive breastfeeding, with desirable outcomes (Horta and Victora 2013; Ip and others 2007; Kramer and Kakuma 2012; Victora 2000). The relationship is especially pronounced in LMICs. Anderson, Johnstone, and Remley (1999); Horta and Victora (2013); and Victora and others (2015) conclude that breastfeeding may significantly improve children's cognitive performance and reduce future risk factors and cardiovascular disease incidence.

There is a growing literature on breastfeeding promotion across the world. Renfrew and others (2009) provide a systematic review of nine types of breastfeeding promotion interventions in 48 studies, 65 percent of which are randomized controlled trials: increased mother and baby contact (kangaroo mother care [KMC], advocated by the World Health Organization [2003] and Conde-Agudelo, Diaz-Rossello, and Belizan [2003]), variation in feeding methods (cup feeding, gavage feeding, bottle feeding), methods of expressing breastmilk (use of pumps), increasing breastmilk production (use of galactagogues and relaxation techniques), supporting optimal nutritional intake from breastmilk, breastfeeding education and peer support, training of health care staff, early hospital discharge with home support, and better organization of care. They conclude that KMC and breastfeeding education and peer support are the two most effective methods of increasing breastfeeding uptake and adherence rates. Home-based education and peer support for breastfeeding for mothers of LBW babies is estimated to more than double breastfeeding rates up to 24 weeks and increase exclusive breastfeeding rates by even more in low-income settings. Support programs that are jointly based at home and in facilities also have similar effectiveness in increasing breastfeeding rates up to 12 weeks. Renfrew and others (2009) report evidence that short periods of KMC skin-to-skin contact significantly increase the duration of any breastfeeding at up to one month after hospital discharge in developed country settings and that daily contact between mothers and babies, which results in increased breastfeeding rates, is estimated to improve child health outcomes at two months and six months across the world.

Jolly and others (2012) conduct a systematic review and meta-regression analysis of peer-support breastfeeding programs. They find that peer support reduces risks of no breastfeeding by 30 percent in LMICs and 7 percent in high-income countries. Peer support also reduces risks of nonexclusive breastfeeding by 37 percent in developing countries.

Some methodological concerns about the causal relationship between breastfeeding and future outcomes need to be mentioned. Most available studies generally are associative and do not control for selection into breastfeeding on the basis of child characteristics such as innate health or expected survival chances or family characteristics such as socioeconomic status (Colen and Ramey 2014; Drane and Logemann 2000; Jain, Concato, and Leventhal 2002).

Some studies attempt to mitigate such biases. Doyle and Denny (2010) compare ordinary least squares and instrumental variables estimates and conclude that there is no significant selection into breastfeeding in their sample of British children. In view of evidence in other studies that less-educated women are less likely to breastfeed, this finding suggests context specificity in selection. Using sibling comparisons, Der, Batty, and Deary (2006) argue that cross-sectional relationships between breastfeeding and child cognitive outcomes are overestimates of causal effects and that family background explains most of the positive associations. Colen and Ramey (2014) find that perceived positive effects of breastfeeding on a series of child health, cognitive, and behavioral outcomes in the United States are completely nullified in sibling comparisons. However, Rees and Sabia (2009), using sibling fixed effects estimators, find positive breastfeeding effects on children's high school test scores and college attendance, and Rothstein (2013) and Belfield and Kelly (2012) use propensity score matching and find positive effects of breastfeeding on young American children's health and cognitive outcomes. Borra, Iacovou, and Sevilla (2012) also use propensity score matching and find that breastfeeding for four weeks improves cognitive test scores among British children. Kramer and others (2008), based on a large randomized controlled trial, find that longer and exclusive breastfeeding improves Belarussian children's IQs. Using hospital-level variation in coverage of the Baby-Friendly Hospital Initiative, a breastfeeding support program initiated in 1991 and led by the World Health Organization and the United Nations Children's Fund, Del Bono and Rabe (2012) find significantly positive impacts of breastfeeding on children's cognitive and emotional development but not on any indicators of their physical health. In addition, they find that breastfeeding has significantly positive effects on mothers' mental health. Using variation in breastfeeding generated by whether births occur on weekends when hospital staffing is more limited or on weekdays, Fitzsimons and Vera-Hernandez (2014) estimate large impacts of breastfeeding on cognitive development but no effects on noncognitive development or health in a sample of less-educated mothers in the United Kingdom.

Maternal Survival

Mothers' deaths can profoundly affect their children's emotional and educational well-being, thereby affecting their future schooling attainment and labor productivity. Ainsworth and Semali (2000) analyze effects that maternal deaths (from AIDS) have on Tanzanian children's schooling. They find that female adult deaths—irrespective of whether they were parents—are associated with delayed school enrollment among children ages 7–11 years and early dropout among children ages 15–19 years. In contrast, prime-age male deaths do not have significant effects on children's school enrollment. This finding is consistent with teenage children substituting for adult women's time in home-production activities. Impacts of adult deaths on child schooling are largest among poor households.

Ainsworth and Semali (2000) also find that children ages zero to five years who lost their mothers are much more likely to be stunted than children who lost their fathers or children with both parents living. The children whose nutritional status is most affected by mothers' deaths are those whose mothers had no schooling (and who were therefore likely to be from poor households). Similarly, Case and Ardington (2006), using longitudinal data from KwaZulu-Natal, South Africa, find that maternal orphans are significantly less likely to be enrolled in school and complete significantly fewer schooling grades than children whose mothers are alive, but no significant effects are observed for paternal orphans.

Using a large Indonesian panel dataset, Gertler, Levine, and Ames (2004) observe that recent parental death lowered children's school enrollment, with the largest effects for youth at transitions between primary and junior secondary and between junior secondary and secondary. Their results suggest that children in bereaved families drop out of school at roughly 50 percent higher rates than their classmates. They find no significant difference between effects on child schooling of maternal versus paternal deaths. The impact on human capital investment in girls of improvements in women's life expectancies from large concentrated reductions in Sri Lankan maternal mortality is analyzed in Jayachandran and Lleras-Muney (2009). They study district-level data for 1946–53, a period in which maternal mortality rates fell by 70 percent. The "treatment" group was individuals who were ages 2–11 years in 1946, just before the maternal mortality decline; the "control" group was individuals ages 18–37 years in 1946 whose schooling preceded the maternal mortality decline. Their results suggest that the maternal mortality rate decline increased female literacy by 2.5 percent, a 1 percentage point increase (relative to changes in male literacy), and raised completed schooling by about 0.2 grades or 4 percent.

ANTHROPOMETRIC AND COGNITIVE OUTCOMES OF EARLY-LIFE INTERVENTIONS

Interventions That Reduce Low Birth Weight

Alderman and Behrman (2006) estimate the economic benefits of reducing LBW in LMICs through seven pathways: reduced infant mortality, reduced neonatal care, reduced costs of infant and child illness, productivity gains from reduced stunting, productivity gains from increased cognitive ability, reductions in prevalence (and thereby costs) of chronic disease, and intergenerational benefits. Based on their review of relevant empirical studies, they estimate that economic benefits from reducing LBW in LMICs are fairly substantial, with a present discounted value of US$510 (using a 5 percent discount rate) for each infant moved from the LBW to the non-LBW category. They decompose the economic benefits of reducing LBW status into the seven individual components and calculate

estimates for different discount rates (table 27.2). Their results suggest that the largest economic gains come from productivity increases due to increased cognitive ability (about 40 percent of the total with a 5 percent discount rate), followed by productivity increases from reduced stunting (17 percent) and reduced infant mortality (16 percent). The present discounted value of moving an infant from LBW to non-LBW status ranges from US$832 with a discount rate of 3 percent to US$257 at a discount rate of 10 percent. The implication of these results is that any intervention that costs less than these amounts per child moved from LBW to non-LBW status is worthwhile to undertake purely on the grounds of saving resources or increasing productivity.

Nutritional Interventions That Reduce Stunting

Stunting reflects cumulative effects of chronic poverty, poor maternal health, inadequate nutrient consumption, and infections, among others (Bhalotra and Rawlings 2011, 2013; Martorell, Khan, and Schroeder 1994; Victora and others 2008). It has been claimed that growth faltering up to age two years is irreversible in its effects on an important set of adult outcomes, including not only stature but also education, health, and productivity (Bhutta and others 2008; Victora and others 2008; Victora and others 2010). Alderman, Hoddinott, and Kinsey (2006); Hoddinott, Alderman, and others (2013); Hoddinott, Behrman, and others (2013); and Hoddinott, Rosegrant, and Torero (2013) discuss the pathways through which stunting generates economic losses—loss

Table 27.2 Estimates of Present Discounted Value of Seven Major Classes of Benefits of Shifting One LBW Infant to Non-LBW Status

US dollars, except as noted

	Annual discount rate					
	1%	2%	3%	5%	10%	20%
1. Reduced infant mortality	97	96	95	93	89	81
2. Reduced neonatal care	42	42	42	42	42	42
3. Reduced costs of infant and child illness	40	40	39	38	36	33
4. Productivity gain from reduced stunting	350	250	180	100	29	4
5. Productivity gain from increased ability	850	600	434	240	70	10
6. Reduction in costs of chronic diseases	240	133	74	23	1.5	0
7. Intergenerational benefits	422	220	122	45	8	1
Sum of PDV of seven benefits	2,041	1,381	986	581	275.5	171
Sum as percentage of that for 5%	351%	238%	170%	100%	47%	30%

Source: Alderman and Behrman 2006.
Note: LBW = low birth weight; PDV = present discounted value.

of physical growth potential (and physical strength that is often needed to be productive in manual occupations), delayed enrollment in school, cognitive impairment, and increased risk of chronic diseases.

Recent studies, however, suggest the following:

- Although early-life nutritional status predicts significantly later child nutritional status, about half the variance in later child nutritional status is not predicted by early-life nutritional status.
- The unpredicted component of later child nutritional status is associated with parental and community characteristics and appears to be malleable and responsive to some possible interventions.
- The unpredicted growth in nutritional status between early and late childhood is significantly associated with late childhood cognitive skills (Crookston and others 2010; Crookston and others 2011; Crookston and others 2013; Prentice and others 2013; Schott and others 2013).

This revisionist literature raises questions about whether the conventional wisdom overemphasizes the first thousand days of life, at least with regard to irreversibility (though whether cost considerations may still imply that early-life interventions have relatively high rates of return remains a question). A bigger threat to conventional wisdom may be studies in process that find no evidence of significant causal impacts on late childhood schooling and cognitive skills if early-life household resources and the endogenous choices that lead to early-life nutritional status are controlled for (Georgiadis 2015).

Building on the work of three studies (Bhutta and others 2008; Hoddinott and others 2011; Horton and others 2010), two studies (Bhutta and others 2013;

Hoddinott, Alderman, and others 2013) calculate average benefit-cost ratios for interventions that reduce stunting in 14 selected LMICs in Asia and Africa (figure 27.2). Among the interventions considered are universal salt iodization, iron fortification of staples, iron–folic acid supplementation, community-based nutrition programs, vitamin A supplementation, deworming, and therapeutic zinc supplementation. Figure 27.2 shows that the median benefit-cost ratio is 18.7 (Kenya), with a range from 3.8 (Democratic Republic of Congo) to 34.1 (India). The benefit-cost ratios for most countries, moreover, appear to be significantly greater than 1.0 under a range of more conservative assumptions than in the base simulations.

Hoddinott, Behrman, and others (2013) use data from a randomized controlled trial in Guatemala to examine adult consequences at ages 25–42 years of growth faltering by age two years. The adults were participants in an INCAP food-supplementation trial in four Guatemalan villages when they were under age seven years in 1969–77. The trial was designed to test effects on physical and cognitive development of a nutritious protein-rich supplement, atole. The study uses instrumental variable methods to correct for estimation bias and control for potentially confounding factors. The authors find that growth failure had large significant effects on numerous adult outcomes, including schooling attainment, family formation, reproduction, cognitive skills, men's wage rates, and poverty avoidance. However, no impact was observed on female wage rates, possibly because most adult women were engaged in low-productivity activities such as agricultural production and processing. Also, no significant associations were observed between growth failure and several measures of adult health, including metabolic syndrome and cardiovascular disease risk factors. This paper suggests that interventions that improve childhood nutrition and promote linear growth from conception to age two years confer lifelong benefits to individuals as well as to their families. Indeed, Behrman and others (2009) provide evidence, using the same data, of intergenerational benefits in that women, but not men, in atole-supplied communities during their childhood, though not just up to age two years, three to four decades later had children with significantly greater birth weights and long-term nutritional status.

Nutritional Interventions That Improve Cognitive Development

Early childhood is critical for cognitive skill formation (Cunha and Heckman 2007; Grantham-McGregor and others 2007; Heckman, Stixrud, and Urzua 2006),

Figure 27.2 Average Benefit-Cost Ratios for Interventions to Reduce Stunting in Selected High-Burden Countries

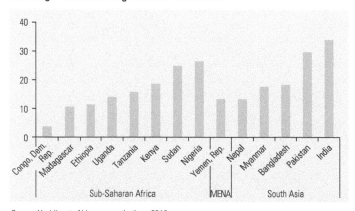

Source: Hoddinott, Alderman, and others 2013.
Note: MENA = Middle East and North Africa.

as illustrated by analysis of how the preschool environment, for example, the U.S. Perry Preschool Program, influences adult test scores and other attainments (Schweinhart and others 2005). In fact, the early childhood health and nutritional environment also influences cognitive performance because nutritional deficiency or infection (which reduces net nutrition by consuming metabolic resources) may impair neurological development (Eppig, Fincher, and Thornhill 2010; Fischer Walker and others 2013). If investments in human capital through childhood and adolescence reinforce cognitive investments in early life, then the longer-term cognitive gains from early-life nutritional interventions may be even larger than might appear from short-term cognitive gains.

Numerous studies using quasi-experimental or experimental design provide evidence of the positive impacts on cognitive function or test scores. Almond, Mazumder, and Van Ewijk (2015) show that Muslim British children who are in utero during Ramadan have lower test scores. Majid (2015) shows that Muslim Indonesian children who are in utero during Ramadan have lower birth weights; study fewer hours during elementary school; do more child labor; score lower on cognitive and math tests; and as adults, work fewer hours and are more likely to be self-employed. Maluccio and others (2009) and Stein and others (2005) show that the INCAP early-life nutritional supplement resulted in higher cognitive attainments. Barham (2012) shows impacts from a health and family planning program in the Matlab area of Bangladesh. Venkataramani (2012) shows impacts from malaria eradication in Mexico. Almond, Edlund, and Palme (2009) identify cognitive deficits associated with exposure to radioactive fallout. Bhalotra and Venkataramani (2013) show that a Mexican clean water reform that led to sharp drops in diarrhea led to better cognitive performance. Bharadwaj, Loken, and Neilson (2013) show that the assignment of neonatal care facilities to babies who fall just below the LBW threshold resulted in their having better test scores relative to babies who fall just above the LBW threshold.

BENEFIT-COST RATIOS

Most studies that evaluate interventions provide estimates of impacts of early-life nutritional interventions on later-life education, health, and earnings. In this section, we construct somewhat generic benefit-cost estimates incorporating both immediate and longer-term impacts and costs of early-life nutritional interventions. However crude, such estimates are useful in assessing the viability of specific investments in maternal and early child health that compete with one another and with other interventions. Estimating benefit-cost ratios is challenging because of the paucity of information on longer-term benefits that can be causally associated with specific interventions and on relevant costs, all of which tend to vary by context. We provide illustrative estimates (table 27.3) based on evidence available from international experience and explore how sensitive our estimates are to key assumptions.

Benefits

We assume that the primary economic benefit for children treated by the intervention arises from increasing lifetime productivity and therefore earnings through increasing schooling, health, or both (Almond 2006; Behrman, Alderman, and Hoddinott 2004; Bhalotra and Venkataramani 2011; Engle and others 2011; Hoddinott, Alderman, and others 2013; Hoddinott, Rosegrant, and Torero 2013). The estimates we use to obtain the benefits depend on (1) the relationship between interventions and human capital (schooling attainment, health) and (2) the relationship between human capital and earnings or productivity. Some recent studies combine (1) and (2) by estimating direct effects of early-life interventions on adult earnings using approaches that also incorporate any externalities and general equilibrium effects (for example, Baird and others 2016; Bhalotra and Venkataramani 2011; Bleakley 2007). The illustrative simulations presented here isolate earnings impacts that flow from schooling increases generated by an early-life health intervention.

For the base case simulations in table 27.3, we use 0.5 additional schooling grades, as estimated in Field, Robles, and Torero (2009). For simulation, as shown in column 2 in table 27.3, we assume that schooling rates of return in labor markets equal schooling rates of return in other activities (for example, household production), as implied by models in which people allocate their time between wage activities and other activities so that at the margin, rates of return are equalized among all activities. This is a more plausible assumption for many developing economies where most of the working population is engaged in small- and medium-scale agricultural and other informal activities with less rigidities in work and pay schedules than those that dominate in, say, Western Europe. We assume workers live through age 64 years (but see later discussion on survival rates). We use as our base estimates for rates of return to schooling attainment in developing countries those summarized by Orazem, Glewwe, and Patrinos (2009): 7.5 percent for rural areas. Given the dominance of rural areas in South Asia and Sub-Saharan Africa, where

Table 27.3 Illustrative Simulations of Benefit-Cost Ratios of Early-Life Nutritional Interventions

Assumptions	Base case	Base case except				Base case with changes in columns (2)–(5)	Higher discount rate	
		Higher intervention impact on schooling	Higher rate of return to schooling attainment	Lower costs	Higher positive externalities		Base case except discount rate = 6%	Case in column (6) except discount rate = 6%
	(1)	(2)	(3)	(4)	(5)	(6)	(7)	(8)
Impact of intervention on schooling attainment (Grades)	0.5	1	0.5	0.5	0.5	1	0.5	1
Rate of return to increased schooling attainment (%)	7.5	7.5	11.5	7.5	7.5	11.5	7.5	11.5
Direct cost of intervention (% of annual basic wage)	4.0	4.0	4.0	2.0	4.0	2.0	4.0	4.0
Direct cost of additional grade of school (% of basic wage)	15.0	15.0	15.0	10.0	15.0	10.0	15.0	10.0
Opportunity cost of additional year of school (% of basic wage)	75.0	75.0	75.0	50.0	75.0	50.0	75.0	50.0
Discount rate (%)	3.0	3.0	3.0	3.0	3.0	3.0	6.0	6.0
Externality as percentage of labor market rate of return	10.0	10.0	10.0	10.0	25.0	25.0	10.0	25.0
Benefit-cost ratio	2.3	2.4	3.5	3.6	2.6	6.9	1.4	4.2
PDV of benefits (US$)	1,000	2,100	1,600	1,000	1,000	3,800	640	2,350
PDV of costs (US$)	450	870	450	300	450	550	440	560
Annual basic wage (US$)	1,000	1,000	1,000	1,000	1,000	1,000	1,000	1,000

Note: PDV = present discounted value.

undernutrition prevalence is highest, we assume 7.5 percent for our base case. We explore the robustness of our results to increasing this rate of return to 11.5 percent in simulation, as shown in column 3 of table 27.3.

Costs

In many relevant interventions, one primary cost is the time cost of program implementers and, for interventions that extend schooling, opportunity costs of time of school-age students and school teachers. We characterize time costs relative to wages of adults with basic schooling levels, which we label "basic wages." We assume a basic wage of US$1,000 per year, roughly the threshold per capita income used by the World Bank to define low-income countries. Changing this basic wage would not change the benefit-cost ratios presented in table 27.3 if beneficiaries and service providers receive comparable wages because it would change benefits and costs in the same proportions. If service providers are

paid more than beneficiaries, the benefit-cost ratios in table 27.3 would be smaller.

We consider three components of resource costs:

- *Direct costs per child of interventions.* The primary emphasis in the literature is on supplier costs of providing interventions, which include time of individuals engaged in the interventions, costs of micronutrients and other materials that may vary with program scale, and fixed costs such as program-related infrastructure. There may also be important private costs, such as the financial and time costs that families (usually mothers) incur to ensure that their children benefit from interventions. In addition, there may be distortion costs of raising funds for public sector expenditures on interventions that have been estimated to be a quarter or more of public expenditures (Harberger 1997). For our basic simulations, we assume that all these costs for interventions for an additional child, such as in Field, Robles, and

Torero (2009), total 4 percent of the basic wage (that is, US$40 if the basic wage is US$1,000). We explore the sensitivity of our estimates to reducing this to 2 percent in simulation (4).

- *Direct costs of one additional year of schooling for one child.* We assume that early-life nutritional interventions raise children's final schooling attainment. The added direct cost of extending schooling again includes time costs of additional teachers, but also variable costs such as books and other materials and fixed costs related to school buildings. Private costs include families' costs for transportation and school materials. There may be distortion costs associated with taxation. For our basic simulations, we assume that all these costs for an additional child per school year total 15 percent of the basic wage, but we explore the sensitivity to a reduction to 10 percent in simulation (4). We assume that these costs are incurred when children are about age 14 years, the margin of completing basic schooling in most low-income countries.

- *Opportunity costs of time of extending schooling for children.* If schooling attainment is extended because of interventions, not only are there additional direct schooling costs, there are also opportunity costs of children being in school instead of engaged in other activities, including work. For our basic simulations, we assume that these costs for an additional child per school year are 75 percent of the basic wage, but we explore the sensitivity of our estimates to 50 percent in simulation (4). Again, we assume that these costs are incurred when children are about age 14 years.

Often relatively little attention is paid to costs, particularly private costs, even though private and public resource costs are as important as impacts in assessing the priority of particular interventions. There is often confusion between budgetary costs of suppliers, such as governmental entities, and real resource costs, private and public. Although policy makers need to be cognizant of budgetary constraints, allocation of public resources should be based on the present discounted value of benefits (perhaps weighted to reflect desired distributional goals, such as poverty alleviation) relative to the present discounted value of real resource costs. Those real resource costs include opportunity costs of alternative uses of public *and* private resources and any distortion costs of raising public funds. Public transfers should not be included in real resource costs although they are part of governmental outlays, a matter that has caused some confusion in assessing, for example, benefit-cost ratios of conditional and unconditional transfer programs.

Other Central Assumptions

Discount Rates

Most benefits of preschool programs accrue, and some costs are incurred, years after the interventions. For instance, if maternal health programs increase the adult productivity of the children of the targeted women attaining higher schooling, these benefits may flow one to six decades after the interventions. To account for this delay, future costs and benefits are discounted to the present. Evaluations of commercial projects often involve discount rates of 10 percent or 12 percent, but discount rates of 3 percent and 6 percent are often used in social sectors (Engle and others 2011). We therefore produce estimates using 3 percent and 6 percent.

Survival Rates

Another reason that timing may be important is that not all children will survive to be productive adults through age 64 years. Therefore, our estimates of future benefits and costs (but primarily benefits given that they may flow for long periods or only be realized many years after interventions) are adjusted for survival probabilities based on World Health Organization Life Tables for Uganda for 2009 (as representative of a Sub-Saharan African country).[5] This adjustment reduces benefits from earnings for intervention-treated children at ages 45–49 years by about 10 percent and at ages 55–59 years by about 15 percent. For countries with longer life expectancies, these adjustments will be smaller, and vice versa.

Externalities

Schooling is perceived to have positive externalities—benefits to others in society beyond the person schooled—by, for example, reducing crime or increasing political participation, though systematic empirical evidence on such externalities remains fairly limited. To illustrate impacts of possible externalities, we assume that social rates of return to schooling increases induced by interventions are 10 percent higher than private rates of return (we also investigate the sensitivity of our estimates to an assumed 25 percent higher rate).

General Equilibrium Effects

If the programs we consider were scaled up, resulting schooling expansions may be substantial, and this outward shift in supply of educated adults may, all else equal, reduce schooling rates of return. This tendency may, however, be limited by outward shifts in demand for more-schooled adults because of productivity increases or, for instance, because more-schooled consumers consume more schooling-intensive goods and services. Because the outcome is ambiguous, we do not directly adjust for it, but it is effectively allowed for when we vary rates of return to schooling.

Benefit-Cost Estimates

Table 27.3 summarizes benefit-cost ratios for interventions such as iodine provision in pregnancy studied in Field, Robles, and Torero (2009) under the assumptions just discussed. Because the ratios attempt to include all benefits and costs, including externalities, these are social benefit-cost ratios. Private benefits are assumed to be smaller because they do not include externalities, but private costs also may be smaller if any of the costs are covered by public subsidies, as is likely. Therefore, private benefit-cost ratios may be larger or smaller than the public benefit-cost ratios in the table.

The first column presents base estimates, with somewhat conservative assumptions regarding key parameters. The base-case social benefit-cost ratio is 2.3, implying that benefits are 130 percent greater than costs. The next four columns vary the assumed parameters underlying the base case by making them less conservative and, as expected, benefit-cost ratios increase. The increase is relatively small, to 2.4, for simulation (2), which allows larger impacts of the intervention on schooling attainment. This is because the increase of 100 percent in impacts of interventions on schooling attainment not only increases benefits due to greater schooling attainment, but also increases costs, raising both direct and opportunity costs of schooling. For the next two cases, the benefit-cost ratios rise to 3.5–3.6, which implies that benefits are more than triple the costs. These two variations highlight different channels through which benefit-cost ratios might be higher: higher program impacts (in the second case perhaps through improved school quality) and reduced costs. The increase in simulation (5), for which assumed positive externalities cause social rates of return to schooling to be 25 percent rather than 10 percent greater than private rates of return, is to 2.6, about the same as for simulation (2). Simulation (6) gives benefit-cost ratios that would be obtained if all of the changes from the base simulation were implemented together and if their impacts were additive. Under this combined set of more optimistic assumptions, the benefit-cost ratio is 6.9, suggesting that early-life nutritional investments are definitely attractive.

The estimates, however, are sensitive to discount rates. The penultimate column makes the base-case assumptions but uses the more conservative assumption of a 6 percent discount rate. The estimated benefit-cost ratio is 1.4, that is, benefits are slightly greater than costs.

The last column makes all the assumptions in column 6 except that the discount rate is assumed to be 6 percent instead of 3 percent. This change reduces the estimated benefit-cost ratio to 4.2. The substantial reduction reflects the importance of the appropriate discount rate. Even with this reduction, the benefit-cost ratio implies that benefits are more than four times as large as costs.

These estimates are based on a number of assumptions and illustrate substantial sensitivity to some assumptions, such as the appropriate discount rate. But all in all, they suggest the possibility of fairly large potential gains in children's lifetime productivity from interventions that improve maternal health, as in Field, Robles, and Torero (2009), with possibly very satisfactory benefit-cost ratios.

We must note that our analysis of iodine supplementation is an illustrative example and we are not advocating it over any other nutritional intervention. There is a large body of knowledge on the benefits of other micronutrient interventions including food fortification. In two clinical trials, Andersson and others (2008) and Haas and others (2014) find that double fortification of salt is associated with higher levels of hemoglobin and other body iron measures among Indian children and women. Horton, Wesley, and Mannar (2011) evaluate the effect of double fortification of salt using iron and iodine on hemoglobin levels in India to find a benefit-cost ratio ranging from 2.4 to 5.0. There are several systematic reviews and meta-analyses of the relationship between fortification and child health outcomes across the world (Aaron, Dror, and Yang 2015; Das and others 2013; De-Regil and others 2011; Ojukwu and others 2009; Pachón and others 2015). Farebrother and others (2015) provide a summary of these systematic reviews.

POLICY DESIGN: MECHANISMS AND SCALE UP

Rapid growth in randomized controlled trials and other systematic studies has expanded the evidence base, documenting the way in which cost-effective local or small-scale childhood interventions have led to improvements in health and educational capital and later-life productivity. However, two major challenges arise in using this evidence as the basis for policy. First, although there are notable exceptions, many trials identify intervention impacts without identifying the mechanisms driving the impact, and, in many cases, multiple mechanisms are plausible (Deaton 2010). This is important because external validity or transferability of interventions may depend upon understanding the mechanisms and relevant contextual dimensions (Cartwright and Hardie 2012).

The second, related, issue is that an intervention that is scaled up may not have the same impact as it does on a small scale, for instance, because of general equilibrium effects, endogenous political reactions, or heterogeneity across beneficiaries and implementers (Allcott and Mullainathan 2012). A vivid illustration is Bold and others (2013), who analyze provision of contract teachers to Kenyan schools. They find that pupils in schools in which a nongovernmental organization managed interventions experienced test score improvements, but there were no test score gains when the same interventions were implemented by the Ministry of Education. Their findings caution against assuming that the evidence gathered from good field trials can be used to guide policy as suggested, for instance, by Banerjee and He (2008).

Probably the most-studied social program with an important health and nutritional component in the developing world is the Mexican Oportunidades (originally PROGRESA) conditional cash transfer program, introduced in 1997 (Behrman 2007, 2010; Levy 2006; Levy and Rodriguez 2004). This program provided transfers conditional on various behaviors, including attending health clinics regularly and, among others, obtaining micronutrients for infants and young children. An important program component was the establishment of an evaluation strategy from the very start, with baseline data and periodic household surveys collected from about 25,000 families (both program eligible and noneligible) with about 125,000 individuals living in 508 small, poor, rural communities (population less than 2,500) to which the initial program was directed, 320 of which were randomly selected to receive the program initially with the remainder enrolled after about 18 months. The initial program results were instrumental in evaluations that resulted not only in program modifications but also in ensuring the political support necessary for scaling up the program to cover about 30 million Mexicans and to continue the program with changes in the government, including the first change in the governing party in more than seven decades.

With respect to impacts of the child nutrition component of the program, Behrman and Hoddinott's (2005) preferred estimates (child fixed effects estimates that control for unobserved heterogeneity correlated with access to the supplement) indicate significantly positive and fairly substantial program effects on children ages 12–36 months. The findings imply an increase of about one-sixth in mean growth per year for these children and a lower probability of stunting. The authors estimate that the long-term consequences of these improvements are nontrivial; the impact working through adult height alone could result in a 2.9 percent increase in lifetime earnings.

CONCLUSIONS

Evidence is accumulating that early-life health and nutritional interventions, including those that act to improve the health and nutritional status of potential mothers and pregnant women and those that directly treat children in early life, have significant impacts on schooling, earnings, and productivity over the lifecycle in LMICs. Our estimates of benefit-cost ratios for such interventions, obtained under a range of plausible parameters, consistently exceed one, suggesting that the present discounted value of gains exceeds costs. These results motivate the case for placing early-life health and nutrition high on the policy agenda. Causal estimates of impacts of early-life nutritional interventions mostly stem from small-scale local interventions; therefore, these estimates are likely to be sensitive to population heterogeneity (social, economic, and cultural differences), differences in program implementation (administrative capacity and trust), and differences in the wider political economy of reform. As a result, available impact estimates may have limited external validity. In addition, estimation of benefit-cost ratios using these impact estimates is, as we have illustrated, sensitive to choices of rates of return and discount rates applied in evaluating estimated future impacts against costs.

If, in fact, benefit-cost ratios associated with early-life health interventions are as attractive as some estimates in the literature and our simulations indicate, then it is natural to ask why governments have not implemented them at scale. Benefits may not scale up, and even if there are scale economies in costs, the benefit-cost ratio for nationwide implementation may be lower. Other possibilities are that governments are not sufficiently aware of the benefits of the studied interventions and, indeed, perusal of documents that guide national and international policy suggests that the tendency is to evaluate immediate reductions in morbidity, growth retardation, or mortality, and that the dynamic socioeconomic benefits of health interventions are often ignored. A third possibility is that even where governments recognize the net benefits of early-life interventions, they face budgetary constraints or conflicting political priorities in policy choices that are difficult to adjust given strong vested interests in existing programs.

ACKNOWLEDGMENTS

The authors thank Grand Challenges Canada Grant 0072-03 for partial support for undertaking this study. The authors alone are responsible for all interpretations.

NOTES

World Bank Income Classifications as of July 2014 are as follows, based on estimates of gross national income (GNI) per capita for 2013:

- Low-income countries (LICs) = US$1,045 or less
- Middle-income countries (MICs) are subdivided:
  a) lower-middle-income = US$1,046 to US$4,125
  b) upper-middle-income (UMICs) = US$4,126 to US$12,745
- High-income countries (HICs) = US$12,746 or more.

1. See the Millennium Development Goals Factsheet No. 290 (http://www.who.int/mediacentre/factsheets/fs290/en/).
2. The estimate of Grantham-McGregor and others (2007) of the number of children at risk of not reaching their development potential relies primarily on the prevalence of stunting.
3. Reviews of the economic benefits of early childhood stimulation and education include Behrman, Fernald, and Engle (2014); Behrman and Urzúa (2013); Engle and others (2007); and Engle and others (2011). Hoddinott, Rosegrant, and Torero (2013) review agricultural interventions and information and communications technology investments that have impacts on child nutrition.
4. The association between LBW and worse health, cognitive, and economic outcomes is, however, not free from criticism. Other indicators of the birth endowment are preterm birth, the Apgar score, and neonatal mortality. See review by Wilcox (2001) who finds that the literature on birth weight and health outcomes often reports a noncausal or biased positive relationship. The author proposes several modifications to the basic birth weight indicator along with alternative measures of fetal growth.
5. Global Health Observatory data repository, Life Tables, Uganda (http://apps.who.int/gho/data/view.main.61730?lang=en; accessed April 28, 2015).

REFERENCES

Aaron, G. J., D. K. Dror, and Z. Yang. 2015. "Multiple-Micronutrient Fortified Non-Dairy Beverage Interventions Reduce the Risk of Anemia and Iron Deficiency in School-Aged Children in Low-Middle Income Countries: A Systematic Review and Meta-Analysis (i–iv)." *Nutrients* 7 (5): 3847–68.

Ainsworth, M., and I. Semali. 2000. "The Impact of Adult Deaths on Children's Health in Northwestern Tanzania." Policy Research Working Paper 2266, World Bank, Washington, DC.

Akresh, R., S. Bhalotra, M. Leone, and U. Osili. 2012. "War and Stature: Growing up during the Nigerian Civil War." *American Economic Review Papers and Proceedings* 102 (3): 273–77.

Alderman, H., J. Behrman, P. Glewwe, L. Fernald, and S. Walker. 2017. "Evidence of Impact of Interventions on Growth and Development during Early and Middle Childhood." In *Disease Control Priorities* (third edition): Volume 8, *Child and Adolescent Health and Development*, edited by D. A. P. Bundy, N. de Silva, S. Horton, D. T. Jamison, and G. C. Patton. Washington, DC: World Bank.

Alderman, H., and J. R. Behrman. 2006. "Reducing the Incidence of Low Birth Weight in Low-Income Countries Has Substantial Economic Benefits." *World Bank Research Observer* 21 (1): 25–48.

Alderman, H., J. Hoddinott, and B. Kinsey. 2006. "Long Term Consequences of Early Childhood Malnutrition." *Oxford Economic Papers* 58 (3): 450–74.

Allcott, H., and S. Mullainathan. 2012. "External Validity and Partner Selection Bias." Working Paper 18373, National Bureau of Economic Research, Cambridge, MA.

Almond, D. 2006. "Is the 1918 Influenza Pandemic Over? Long-Term Effects of in Utero Influenza Exposure in the Post-1940 US Population." *Journal of Political Economy* 114 (4): 672–712.

Almond, D., and J. Currie. 2011. "Killing Me Softly: The Fetal Origins Hypothesis." *Journal of Economic Perspectives* 25 (3): 153–72.

Almond, D., L. Edlund, and M. Palme. 2009. "Chernobyl's Subclinical Legacy: Prenatal Exposure to Radioactive Fallout and School Outcomes in Sweden." *Quarterly Journal of Economics* 124 (4): 1729–72.

Almond, D., and B. Mazumder. 2013. "Fetal Origins and Parental Responses." *Annual Review of Economics* 5 (1): 37–56.

Almond, D., B. Mazumder, and R. Van Ewijk. 2015. "In Utero Ramadan Exposure and Children's Academic Performance." *Economic Journal* 125 (589): 1501–33.

Anderson, J. W., B. M. Johnstone, and D. T. Remley. 1999. "Breast-Feeding and Cognitive Development: A Meta-Analysis." *American Journal of Clinical Nutrition* 70 (4): 525–35.

Andersson, M., P. Thankachan, S. Muthayya, R. B. Goud, A. V. Kurpad, and others. 2008. "Dual Fortification of Salt with Iodine and Iron: A Randomized, Double-Blind, Controlled Trial of Micronized Ferric Pyrophosphate and Encapsulated Ferrous Fumarate in Southern India." *American Journal of Clinical Nutrition* 88 (5): 1378–87.

Attanasio, O., C. P. Fernández, E. O. A. Fitzsimons, S. M. Grantham-McGregor, C. Meghir, and others. 2014. "Using the Infrastructure of a Conditional Cash Transfer Program to Deliver a Scalable Integrated Early Child Development Program in Colombia: Cluster Randomized Controlled Trial." *BMJ* 349: g5785.

Baird, S., J. H. Hicks, M. Kremer, and E. Miguel. 2016. "Worms at Work: Long-Run Impacts of a Child Health Investment." *Quarterly Journal of Economics.* 131 (4): 1637–80. doi:10.1093/qje/qjw022.

Baker, M., and K. Milligan. 2008. "Maternal Employment, Breastfeeding, and Health: Evidence from Maternity Leave Mandates." *Journal of Health Economics* 27 (4): 871–87.

Banerjee, A., and R. He. 2008. "Making Aid Work." In *Reinventing Foreign Aid*, edited by W. Easterly. Cambridge, MA: MIT Press.

Barham, T. 2012. "Enhancing Cognitive Function: Medium-Term Effects of a Health and Family Planning Program in Matlab." *American Economic Journal: Applied Economics* 4 (1): 245–73.

Barker, D. J. 1990. "The Fetal and Infant Origins of Adult Disease." *BMJ* 301 (6761): 1111.

Behrman, J. R. 2007. "Policy-Oriented Research Impact Assessment (PORIA) Case Study on the International Food Policy Research Institute (IFPRI) and the Mexican PROGRESA Anti-Poverty and Human Resource Investment Conditional Cash Transfer Program." Impact Assessment Discussion Paper 27, International Food Policy Research Institute, Washington, DC. http://www.ifpri.org/sites/default/files/publications/ia27.pdf.

———. 2010. "The International Food Policy Research Institute (IFPRI) and the Mexican PROGRESA Anti-Poverty and Human Resource Investment Conditional Cash Transfer Program." *World Development* 38 (10): 1473–85.

Behrman, J. R., H. Alderman, and J. Hoddinott. 2004. "Hunger and Malnutrition." In *Global Crises, Global Solutions*, edited by B. Lomborg, 363–420. Cambridge, U.K.: Cambridge University Press.

Behrman, J. R., M. C. Calderon, S. H. Preston, J. F. Hoddinott, R. Martorell, and others. 2009. "Nutritional Supplementation of Girls Influences the Growth of Their Children: Prospective Study in Guatemala." *American Journal of Clinical Nutrition* 90 (5): 1372–79.

Behrman, J. R., P. L. Engle, and L. Fernald. 2014. "Preschool Programs in Developing Countries." In *Education Policy in Developing Countries*, edited by P. Glewwe, 65–106. Chicago, IL: University of Chicago Press.

Behrman, J. R., and J. F. Hoddinott. 2005. "Program Evaluation with Unobserved Heterogeneity and Selective Implementation: The Mexican Progresa Impact on Child Nutrition." *Oxford Bulletin of Economics and Statistics* 67 (4): 547–69.

Behrman, J. R., and S. Urzúa. 2013. "Economic Perspectives on Some Important Dimensions of Early Childhood Development in Developing Countries." In *Handbook of Early Childhood Development: Translating Research to Global Policy*, edited by P. R. Britto, P. L. Engle, and C. M. Super, 123–41. Oxford, U.K.: Oxford University Press.

Belfield, C. R., and I. R. Kelly. 2012. "The Benefits of Breast Feeding across the Early Years of Childhood." *Journal of Human Capital* 6 (3): 251–77.

Bennett, I., W. Schott, S. Krutikova, and J. R. Behrman. 2014. "Maternal Depression Predicts Poor Concurrent and Subsequent Child Anthropometric, Cognitive and Social Outcomes: Ethiopia, India, Peru and Vietnam." Unpublished, University of Pennsylvania, Philadelphia, PA.

Bhalotra, S., M. Karlsson, and T. Nilsson. 2015. "Infant Health and Longevity: Evidence from a Historical Trial in Sweden." Discussion Paper 8969, Institute for the Study of Labor, Bonn.

Bhalotra, S., and S. Rawlings. 2011. "Intergenerational Persistence in Health in Developing Countries: The Penalty of Gender Inequality?" *Journal of Public Economics* 95 (3–4): 286–99.

———. 2013. "Gradients of the Intergenerational Transmission of Health in Developing Countries." *Review of Economics and Statistics* 95 (2): 660–72.

Bhalotra, S., and A. Venkataramani. 2011. "The Captain of the Men of Death and His Shadow: Long-Run Impacts of Early Life Pneumonia Exposure." Discussion Paper 6041, Institute for the Study of Labor, Bonn.

———. 2013. "Cognitive Development and Infectious Disease: Gender Differences in Investments and Outcomes." Discussion Paper 7833, Institute for the Study of Labor, Bonn.

Bharadwaj, P., K. V. Loken, and C. Neilson. 2013. "Early Life Health Interventions and Academic Achievement." *American Economic Review* 103 (5): 1862–91.

Bhutta, Z. A., T. Ahmed, R. E. Black, S. Cousens, K. Dewey, and others. 2008. "Maternal and Child Undernutrition 3: What Works? Interventions for Maternal and Child Undernutrition and Survival." *The Lancet* 371 (9610): 417–40.

Bhutta, Z. A., J. K. Das, A. Rizvi, M. F. Gaffey, N. Walker, and others. 2013. "Evidence-Based Interventions for Improvement of Maternal and Child Nutrition: What Can Be Done and at What Cost?" *The Lancet* 382 (9890): 452–77.

Bleakley, H. 2007. "Disease and Development: Evidence from Hookworm Eradication in the American South." *Quarterly Journal of Economics* 122 (1): 73–117.

Bold, T., M. Kimenyi, G. Mwabu, A. Ng'ang'a, and J. Sandefur. 2013. "Scaling-up What Works: Experimental Evidence on External Validity in Kenyan Education." Working Paper 321, Centre for Global Development, London.

Borra, C., M. Iacovou, and A. Sevilla. 2012. "The Effect of Breastfeeding on Children's Cognitive and Noncognitive Development." *Labour Economics* 19 (4): 496–515.

Bundy, D. A. P., N. de Silva, S. Horton, G. C. Patton, L. Schultz, and D. T. Jamison. 2017. "Child and Adolescent Health and Development: Realizing Neglected Potential." In *Disease Control Priorities* (third edition): Volume 8, *Child and Adolescent Health and Development*, edited by D. A. P. Bundy, N. de Silva, S. Horton, D. T. Jamison, and G. C. Patton. Washington, DC: World Bank.

Canning, D., A. Razzaque, J. Driessen, D. G. Walker, P. K. Streatfield, and others. 2011. "The Effect of Maternal Tetanus Immunization on Children's Schooling Attainment in Matlab, Bangladesh: Follow-up of a Randomized Trial." *Social Science and Medicine* 72 (9): 1429–36.

Cartwright, N., and J. Hardie. 2012. *Evidence-Based Policy: A Practical Guide to Doing It Better*. Oxford, U.K.: Oxford University Press.

Case, A., and C. Ardington. 2006. "The Impact of Parental Death on School Outcomes: Longitudinal Evidence from South Africa." *Demography* 43 (3): 401–20.

Colen, C. G., and D. M. Ramey. 2014. "Is Breast Truly Best? Estimating the Effects of Breastfeeding on Long-Term Child Health and Wellbeing in the United States Using Sibling Comparisons." *Social Science and Medicine* 109: 55–65.

Conde-Agudelo, A., J. L. Diaz-Rossello, and J. M. Belizan. 2003. "Kangaroo Mother Care to Reduce Morbidity and Mortality in Low Birthweight Infants." *Cochrane Database of Systematic Reviews* 2: CD002771.

Copenhagen Consensus Expert Panel. 2008. *Copenhagen Consensus 2008: Results*. Denmark: Copenhagen Consensus Center.

Crookston, B. T., K. A. Dearden, S. C. Alder, C. A. Porucznik, J. B. Stanford, and others. 2011. "Impact of Early and Concurrent Stunting on Cognition." *Maternal and Child Nutrition* 7 (4): 397–409.

Crookston, B. T., M. E. Penny, S. C. Alder, T. T. Dickerson, R. M. Merrill, and others. 2010. "Children Who Recover from Early Stunting and Children Who Are Not Stunted Demonstrate Similar Levels of Cognition." *Journal of Nutrition* 140 (11): 1996–2001.

Crookston, B. T., W. Schott, S. Cueto, K. A. Dearden, P. Engle, and others. 2013. "Post-Infancy Growth, Schooling, and Cognitive Achievement: Young Lives." *American Journal of Clinical Nutrition* 98 (6): 1555–63.

Cunha, F., and J. Heckman. 2007. "The Technology of Skill Formation." *American Economic Review* 97 (2): 31–47.

———. 2008. "Formulating, Identifying and Estimating the Technology of Cognitive and Noncognitive Skill Formation." *Journal of Human Resources* 43 (4): 738–82.

Currie, J., and T. Vogl. 2013. "Early-Life Health and Adult Circumstance in Developing Countries." *Annual Review of Economics* 5 (1): 1–36.

Das, J. K., R. Kumar, R. A. Salam, and Z. A. Bhutta. 2013. "Systematic Review of Zinc Fortification Trials." *Annals of Nutrition and Metabolism* 62 (Suppl. 1): 44–56.

Deaton, A. 2010. "Instruments, Randomization, and Learning about Development." *Journal of Economic Literature* 48 (2): 424–55.

Del Bono, E., and B. Rabe. 2012. "Breastfeeding and Child Cognitive Outcomes: Evidence from a Hospital-Based Breastfeeding Support Policy." ISER Working Paper Series 2012-29, Institute for Social and Economic Research, University of Essex.

Der, G., G. D. Batty, and I. J. Deary. 2006. "Effect of Breast Feeding on Intelligence in Children: Prospective Study, Sibling Pairs Analysis, and Meta-Analysis." *BMJ* 333 (7575): 945.

De-Regil, L. M., P. S. Suchdev, G. E. Vist, S. Walleser, and J. P. Peña-Rosas. 2011. "Home Fortification of Foods with Multiple Micronutrient Powders for Health and Nutrition in Children under Two Years of Age." *Cochrane Database of Systematic Reviews* Sep 7 (9): CD008959. doi:10.1002/14651858.CD008959.pub2.

Doyle, O., and K. J. Denny. 2010. "The Causal Effect of Breastfeeding on Children's Cognitive Development: A Quasi-Experimental Design." Working Paper 201020, School of Economics, University College Dublin.

Drane, D. L., and J. A. Logemann. 2000. "A Critical Evaluation of the Evidence on the Association between Type of Infant Feeding and Cognitive Development." *Paediatric and Perinatal Epidemiology* 14: 349–56.

Driessen, J., A. Razzaque, D. Walker, and D. Canning. 2011. "The Effect of Childhood Measles Vaccination on School Enrollment in Matlab, Bangladesh." PGDA Working Papers 8111, Program on the Global Demography of Aging, Harvard T. H. Chan School of Public Health, Cambridge, MA.

Engle, P. L., M. M. Black, J. R. Behrman, M. C. de Mello, P. J. Gertler, and others. 2007. "Strategies to Avoid the Loss of Developmental Potential in More Than 200 Million Children in the Developing World." *The Lancet* 369 (9557): 229–42.

Engle, P. L., L. C. H. Fernald, H. Alderman, J. R. Behrman, C. O'Gara, and others. 2011. "Strategies for Reducing Inequalities and Improving Developmental Outcomes for Young Children in Low and Middle Income Countries." *The Lancet* 378 (9799): 1339–53.

Eppig, C., C. L. Fincher, and R. Thornhill. 2010. "Parasite Prevalence and the Worldwide Distribution of Cognitive Ability." *Proceedings of the Royal Society B* 277 (1701): 3801–8.

Farebrother, J., C. E. Naude, L. Nicol, M. Andersson, and M. B. Zimmermann. 2015. "Iodised Salt and Iodine Supplements for Prenatal and Postnatal Growth: A Rapid Scoping of Existing Systematic Reviews." *Nutrition Journal* 14 (1): 1.

Feyrer, J., D. Politi, and D. N. Weil. 2013. "The Cognitive Effects of Micronutrient Deficiency: Evidence from Salt Iodization in the United States." Working Paper 19233, National Bureau of Economic Research, Cambridge, MA.

Field, E., O. Robles, and M. Torero. 2009. "Iodine Deficiency and Schooling Attainment in Tanzania." *American Economic Journal: Applied Economics* 1 (4): 140–69.

Fischer Walker, C. L., I. Rudan, L. Liu, H. Nair, E. Theodoratou, and others. 2013. "Global Burden of Childhood Diarrhoea and Pneumonia." *The Lancet* 381 (9875): 1405–16.

Fitzsimons, E., and M. Vera-Hernandez. 2014. "Food for Thought? Breastfeeding and Child Development." Working Paper 14–04, Institute of Education, London.

Georgiadis, A. 2015. "The Sooner the Better but It's Never Too Late: The Impact of Child Growth at Different Stages of Infancy and Childhood on Cognitive Development." Oxford University, Oxford, U.K.

Gertler, P., D. I. Levine, and M. Ames. 2004. "Schooling and Parental Death." *Review of Economics and Statistics* 86 (1): 211–25.

Gilman, S. E., H. Gardener, and S. L. Buka. 2008. "Maternal Smoking during Pregnancy and Children's Cognitive and Physical Development: A Causal Risk Factor?" *American Journal of Epidemiology* 168 (5): 522–31.

Grantham-McGregor, S., Y. B. Cheung, S. Cueto, P. Glewwe, L. Richter, and others. 2007. "Developmental Potential in the First 5 Years for Children in Developing Countries." *The Lancet* 369 (9555): 60–70.

Haas, J. D., M. Rahn, S. Venkatramanan, G. S. Marquis, M. J. Wenger, and others. 2014. "Double-Fortified Salt Is Efficacious in Improving Indicators of Iron Deficiency in Female Indian Tea Pickers." *Journal of Nutrition* 144 (6): 957–64.

Harberger, Arnold C. 1997. "New Frontiers in Project Evaluation? A Comment on Devarajan, Squire, and Suthiwart-Narueput." *World Bank Research Observer* 12 (1): 73–79.

Heckman, J. J., J. Stixrud, and S. Urzua. 2006. "The Effects of Cognitive and Noncognitive Abilities on Labor Market Outcomes and Social Behavior." *Journal of Labor Economics* 24: 411–82.

Hjort, J., M. Solvesten, and M. Wust. 2014. "Universal Investment in Infants and Long-Run Health: Evidence from

Denmark's 1937 Home Visiting Program." Unpublished, Technical report, SFI, Denmark.

Hoddinott, J., H. Alderman, J. R. Behrman, and L. Haddad. 2013. "The Economic Rationale for Investing in Stunting Reduction." *Maternal and Child Nutrition* 9 (Suppl. 2): 69–82. doi:10.1111/mcn.12080. PMID: 24074319.

Hoddinott, J., J. R. Behrman, J. A. Maluccio, P. Melgar, A. R. Quisumbing, and others. 2013. "Adult Consequences of Growth Failure in Early Childhood." *American Journal of Clinical Nutrition* 98 (5): 1170–78.

Hoddinott, J., J. A. Maluccio, J. R. Behrman, R. Flores, and R. Martorell. 2008. "Effect of a Nutrition Intervention during Early Childhood on Economic Productivity in Guatemalan Adults." *The Lancet* 371 (9610): 411–16.

Hoddinott, J. J., J. Maluccio, J. R. Behrman, P. Martorell, A. R. Melgar, and others. 2011. "The Consequences of Early Childhood Growth Failure over the Life Course." Discussion Paper 1073, International Food Policy Research Institute, Washington, DC.

Hoddinott, J., M. Rosegrant, and M. Torero. 2013. "Investments to Reduce Hunger and Undernutrition." In *Global Problems, Smart Solutions. About Copenhagen Consensus 2012 Conference Results*, edited by B. Lomborg, 332–67. Cambridge, U.K.: Cambridge University Press.

Horta, B. L., and C. G. Victora. 2013. *Long-Term Effects of Breastfeeding: A Systematic Review.* Geneva: World Health Organization.

Horton, S., H. Alderman, and J. A. Rivera. 2009. "Copenhagen Consensus 2009 Challenge Paper: Hunger and Malnutrition." In *Global Crises, Global Solutions*, edited by Bjorn Lomborg, 305–33. Cambridge, U.K.: Cambridge University Press.

Horton, S., and J. Ross. 2003. "The Economics of Iron Deficiency." *Food Policy* 28: 51–75.

Horton, S., M. Shekar, C. McDonald, A. Mahal, and J. Brooks. 2010. *Scaling Up Nutrition: What Will It Cost?* Washington, DC: World Bank.

Horton, S., A. Wesley, and M. V. Mannar. 2011. "Double-Fortified Salt Reduces Anemia, Benefit: Cost Ratio Is Modestly Favorable." *Food Policy* 36 (5): 581–87.

Ip, S., M. Chung, G. Raman, P. Chew, N. Magula, and others. 2007. "Breastfeeding and Maternal and Infant Health Outcomes in Developed Countries." Tufts–New England Medical Center Evidence-Based Practice Center, Boston, MA.

Jain, A., J. Concato, and J. M. Leventhal. 2002. "How Good Is the Evidence Linking Breastfeeding to Intelligence?" *Pediatrics* 109 (6): 1044–53.

Jayachandran, S., and A. Lleras-Muney. 2009. "Life Expectancy and Human Capital Investments: Evidence from Maternal Mortality Declines." *Quarterly Journal of Economics* 124 (1): 349–97.

Jolly, K., L. Ingram, K. S. Khan, J. J. Deeks, N. Freemantle, and others. 2012. "Systematic Review of Peer Support for Breastfeeding Continuation: Meta Regression Analysis of the Effect of Setting, Intensity, and Timing." *BMJ* 344: d8287.

Kinra, S., K. R. Sarma, V. V. R. Mendu, R. Ravikumar, V. Mohan, and others. 2008. "Effect of Integration of Supplemental Nutrition with Public Health Programmes in Pregnancy and Early Childhood on Cardiovascular Risk in Rural Indian Adolescents: Long Term Follow-Up of Hyderabad Nutrition Trial." *BMJ* 337: a605.

Kramer, M. S., F. Aboud, E. Mironova, I. Vanilovich, R. W. Platt, and others. 2008. "Breastfeeding and Child Cognitive Development: New Evidence from a Large Randomized Trial." *Archives of General Psychiatry* 65 (5): 578–84.

Kramer, M. S., and R. Kakuma. 2012. "Optimal Duration of Exclusive Breastfeeding (Review)." *Cochrane Database of Systematic Reviews* 8: CD003517.

Krutikova, S., J. R. Behrman, I. Bennett, J. Escobal, and W. Schott. 2015. "Maternal Mental Health and Child Well-Being." Unpublished, Oxford University, Oxford, U.K.

Levy, S. 2006. *Progress against Poverty: Sustaining Mexico's PROGRESA-Oportunidades Program.* Washington, DC: Brookings Institution.

Levy, S., and E. Rodriguez. 2004. *Economic Crisis, Political Transitions, and Poverty Policy Reform: Mexico's Progresa-Oportunidades Program.* Washington, DC: Inter-American Development Bank.

Lomborg, Bjorn, ed. 2014. *How to Spend $75 Billion to Make the World a Better Place.* 2nd edition. Copenhagen, Denmark: Copenhagen Consensus Center.

Majid, M. F. 2015. "The Persistent Effects of In Utero Nutrition Shocks over the Life Cycle: Evidence from Ramadan Fasting." *Journal of Development Economics* 117: 48–57.

Maluccio, J., J. Hoddinott, J. R. Behrman, R. Martorell, A. R. Quisumbing, and A. D. Stein. 2006. "The Impact of an Experimental Nutritional Intervention in Childhood on Education among Guatemalan Adults." Report 207, International Food Policy Research Institute, Washington, DC.

———. 2009. "The Impact of Improving Nutrition during Early Childhood on Education among Guatemalan Adults." *Economic Journal* 119 (537): 734–63.

Martorell, R., L. K. Khan, and D. G. Schroeder. 1994. "Reversibility of Stunting: Epidemiological Findings in Children from Developing Countries." *European Journal of Clinical Nutrition* 48: S45–57.

Maselko, J., S. Sikander, S. Bhalotra, O. Bangash, N. Ganga, and others. 2015. "Impact of an Early Perinatal Depression Intervention on Long-Term Child Development Outcomes." *Lancet Psychiatry* 2 (7): 9–17.

Nandi, A., A. Ashok, S. Kinra, J. R. Behrman, and R. Laxminarayan. 2016. "Early Childhood Nutrition Is Positively Associated with Adolescent Educational Outcomes: Evidence from the Andhra Pradesh Child and Parents Study (APCAPS)." *Journal of Nutrition* 146 (4): 806–13.

Nilsson, P. 2008. "Does a Pint a Day Affect Your Child's Pay? The Effect of Prenatal Alcohol Exposure on Adult Outcomes." CEMMAP Working Paper CWP22/08, Centre for Microdata Methods and Practice, Institute for Fiscal Studies, London.

Ojukwu, J. U., J. U. Okebe, D. Yahav, and M. Paul. 2009. "Oral Iron Supplementation for Preventing or Treating Anaemia among Children in Malaria-Endemic Areas." *Cochrane Database of Systematic Reviews* 3: CD006589. doi:10.1002/14651858.CD006589.pub2.

Orazem, P., P. Glewwe, and H. Patrinos. 2009. "The Benefits and Costs of Alternative Strategies to Improve Educational Outcomes." In *Global Crises, Global Solutions: Costs and Benefits*, edited by Bjorn Lomborg, 180–214. Cambridge, U.K.: Cambridge University Press.

Pachón, H., R. Spohrer, Z. Mei, and M. K. Serdula. 2015. "Evidence of the Effectiveness of Flour Fortification Programs on Iron Status and Anemia: A Systematic Review." *Nutrition Reviews* 73 (11): 780–95.

Politi, D. 2011. "The Impact of Iodine Deficiency Eradication on Schooling: Evidence from the Introduction of Iodized Salt in Switzerland." Discussion Paper 2010–02, Scottish Institute of Research in Economics, University of Edinburgh.

Prentice, A. M., K. A. Ward, G. R. Goldberg, L. M. Jarjou, S. E. Moore, and others. 2013. "Critical Windows for Nutritional Interventions against Stunting." *American Journal of Clinical Nutrition* 97 (5): 911–18.

Rahman, A., A. Malik, S. Sikander, C. Roberts, and F. Creed. 2008. "Cognitive Behaviour Therapy–Based Intervention by Community Health Workers for Mothers with Depression and Their Infants in Rural Pakistan: A Cluster-Randomised Controlled Trial." *The Lancet* 372 (9642): 902–9.

Rees, D. I., and J. J. Sabia. 2009. "The Effect of Breast Feeding on Educational Attainment: Evidence from Sibling Data." *Journal of Human Capital* 3 (1): 43–72.

Renfrew, M. J., D. Craig, L. Dyson, F. McCormick, S. Rice, and others. 2009. "Breastfeeding Promotion for Infants in Neonatal Units: A Systematic Review and Economic Analysis." *Health Technology Assessment* 13 (40): 1–146.

Rothstein, D. S. 2013. "Breastfeeding and Children's Early Cognitive Outcomes." *Review of Economics and Statistics* 95 (3): 919–31.

Schott, W., B. T. Crookston, E. A. Lundeen, A. D. Stein, J. R. Behrman, and others. 2013. "Child Growth from Ages 1 to 8 Years in Ethiopia, India, Peru and Vietnam: Key Distal Household and Community Factors." *Social Science and Medicine* 97 (2013): 278–87.

Schweinhart, L. J., J. Montie, Z. Xiang, W. S. Barnett, C. R. Belfield, and others. 2005. *Lifetime Effects: The High/Scope Perry Preschool Study through Age 40*. Ypsilanti, MI: High/Scope.

Stein, A. D., J. R. Behrman, A. DiGirolamo, R. Grajeda, R. Martorell, and others. 2005. "Schooling, Educational Achievement, and Cognitive Functioning among Young Guatemalan Adults." *Food and Nutrition Bulletin* 26 (2): S46–S54.

Stratton, K., C. Howe, and F. Battaglia, eds. 1996. *Fetal Alcohol Syndrome: Diagnosis, Epidemiology, Prevention, and Treatment*. Committee to Study Fetal Alcohol Syndrome, Division of Biobehavioral Sciences and Mental Disorders, Institute of Medicine. Washington, DC: National Academies Press.

Venkataramani, A. 2012. "Early Life Exposure to Malaria and Cognition in Adulthood: Evidence from Mexico." *Journal of Health Economics* 31 (5): 767–80.

Victora, C. G. 2000. "Effect of Breastfeeding on Infant and Child Mortality due to Infectious Diseases in Less Developed Countries: A Pooled Analysis." *The Lancet* 355 (9202): 451–55.

Victora, C. G., L. Adair, C. Fall, P. C. Hallal, R. Martorell, and others. 2008. "Maternal and Child Undernutrition: Consequences for Adult Health and Human Capital." *The Lancet* 371 (9609): 340–57.

Victora, C. G., M. de Onis, P. C. Hallal, M. Blössner, and R. Shrimpton. 2010. "Worldwide Timing of Growth Faltering: Revisiting Implications for Interventions." *Pediatrics* 125 (3): e473–80.

Victora, C. G., B. L. Horta, C. L. de Mola, L. Quevedo, R. T. Pinheiro, and others. 2015. "Association between Breastfeeding and Intelligence, Educational Attainment, and Income at 30 Years of Age: A Prospective Birth Cohort Study from Brazil." *The Lancet Global Health* 3 (4): e199–e205.

Weitzman, M., S. Gortmaker, and A. Sobol. 1992. "Maternal Smoking and Behavior Problems of Children." *Pediatrics* 90 (3): 342–49.

WHO (World Health Organization). 2003. *Kangaroo Mother Care: A Practical Guide*. Geneva: WHO.

Wilcox, A. J. 2001. "On the Importance—and the Unimportance—of Birthweight." *International Journal of Epidemiology* 30 (6): 1233–41.

Chapter 28

Postponing Adolescent Parity in Developing Countries through Education: An Extended Cost-Effectiveness Analysis

Stéphane Verguet, Arindam Nandi, Véronique Filippi, and Donald A. P. Bundy

INTRODUCTION

Despite substantial progress in the achievement of Millennium Development Goal 5 to reduce the maternal mortality ratio—the number of maternal deaths per 100,000 live births—by two-thirds between 2000 and 2015, substantial inequalities remain in maternal mortality across countries worldwide (Kassebaum and others 2014; UN 2013; UN MME 2015; Verguet and others 2014). Maternal mortality ratios remain unacceptably high in South Asia and Sub-Saharan Africa, particularly West Africa (Kassebaum and others 2014; UN MME 2015). Together, South Asia and Sub-Saharan Africa account for 86 percent of the world's maternal deaths (WHO and others 2014).

Building on the momentum gathered by the Millennium Development Goals, the post-2015 agenda and its Sustainable Development Goals set the ambitious target of further reducing the maternal mortality ratio, currently about 200 deaths per 100,000 live births globally (UNICEF 2016), to 70 per 100,000 by 2030 (UNW 2016).

Women ages 15–19 years face elevated risks of pregnancy-related mortality and morbidity. In low- and middle-income countries (LMICs), these risks are disproportionately higher (IHME 2013; WHO and others 2014), and the maternal mortality ratios are much larger, on average (Kassebaum and others 2014; UN MME 2015). Furthermore, among girls younger than age 16 years, the relative risk of pregnancy-related mortality is up to five times higher compared with women ages 20–24 years (Huang 2011; Mayor 2004). Although the education of girls has been expanded worldwide (Gakidou and others 2010), early marriages remain common; up to 65 percent and 76 percent of women are married by age 18 years in Bangladesh and Niger, respectively (UNICEF 2016). As a result, the rates of adolescent pregnancies remain very high in many LMICs (Bates, Maselko, and Schuler 2007; Beguy, Ndugwa, and Kabiru 2013; Chloe, Thapa, and Mishra 2004; Dixon-Mueller 2008).

Maternal and adolescent health need to be examined through a wider perspective beyond mortality—notably, morbidity outcomes, such as long-term sequelae for both mothers and their children, and the financial vulnerability of women and adolescents (Ashford 2002; Dale, Stoll, and Lucas 2003; Filippi and others 2006; Langer and others 2015). Pregnant young women present higher chances of school dropout (Lloyd and Mensch 2008; Marteleto, Lam, and Ranchhod 2008; Meekers and Ahmed 1999), and they could face high risks of pregnancy-related impoverishment and

Corresponding author: Stéphane Verguet, Department of Global Health and Population, Harvard T. H. Chan School of Public Health, Boston, MA, United States, verguet@hsph.harvard.edu.

negative economic consequences (Arsenault and others 2013; Ilboudo, Russell, and D'Exelle 2013; Powell-Jackson and Hoque 2012) if they choose to carry their pregnancy to term. Out-of-pocket (OOP) medical payments in LMICs can lead to impoverishment and related coping strategies, such as borrowing money or selling assets, to pay for health care (Kruk, Goldmann, and Galea 2009; Xu and others 2003).

In the absence of other financing mechanisms, such as private health insurance or fee exemptions, household medical expenditures can be catastrophic (Wagstaff 2010), exceeding a specified percentage of total household expenditures. For example, with increased incidence of complicated deliveries owing to pregnancies at young ages, the OOP costs associated with maternal delivery in facilities are likely to be higher and may subsequently put pregnant adolescents at increased risk of medical impoverishment. In particular, this increased likelihood of financial risk would be expected to be greater among poorer socioeconomic groups; these groups have less disposable income and higher rates of adolescent pregnancies (IIPS 2010; INS and ICF International 2013). This hypothesis is one of several that this chapter examines.

Protection from health care financial risks has become a critical component of national strategies in many countries (Boerma and others 2014; WHO 2010, 2013). Reduction of these financial risks is one objective of public sector policies. For example, public investment in education to increase girls' educational levels could reduce adolescent pregnancies and subsequent risks of both mortality and impoverishment, especially among the poorest women.

Health economic evaluations (cost-effectiveness analyses) have traditionally focused on estimating an intervention's cost per health gain (Jamison and others 2006). Extended cost-effectiveness analysis (ECEA) (Verguet, Gauvreau, and others 2015; Verguet, Kim, and Jamison 2016; Verguet, Laxminarayan, and Jamison 2015; Verguet and others 2013; Verguet, Olson, and others 2015) supplements traditional economic evaluation by incorporating evaluation of financial risk protection (FRP)—prevention of medical impoverishment. ECEA quantifies how much FRP, equity, and health can be purchased for a given expenditure. ECEA can provide answers to help policy makers select the optimal policies for increasing FRP and equity and for improving the distribution of health benefits (WHO 2010, 2013).

Many determinants of adolescent pregnancy and fertility have long been reported in the scientific literature, notably by John Bongaarts (Bongaarts 1978; Bongaarts and Potter 1983). In this chapter, we restrict our analysis to one specific underlying factor of fertility—female educational attainment—and examine its impact on adolescent maternal mortality and medical impoverishment associated with complicated delivery in facility. For this purpose, this chapter uses ECEA to measure the potential mortality, FRP, and equity benefits that could be gained through public financing of increased education of adolescent girls in two illustrative country examples: Niger and India.

METHODS

This chapter examines the potential impact on maternal mortality and impoverishment of the increase in the level of female education by one school year for a cohort of adolescent women. Definitions of age groupings and age-specific terminology used in this volume can be found in chapter 1 (Bundy and others 2017).

We consider the population of adolescent women, ages 15–19 years, in Niger and India. Niger has the highest total fertility rate globally (7.6 children per woman of reproductive age) and a high maternal mortality ratio (553 deaths per 100,000 live births), leading to 5,400 maternal deaths annually. India has the largest population in South Asia (1.3 billion), the largest number of maternal deaths worldwide (45,000 deaths), and a high maternal mortality ratio (174 deaths per 100,000 live births) (Alkima and others 2016; UN DESA 2013; UN MME 2015).

General Approach

First, we examine the hypothetical impact of a one-year increase in the education level of adolescent girls. We study the linear relationship between the mean number of years of education among women ages 15–44 years (IHME 2010) and the adolescent pregnancy rate (percentage of women ages 15–19 years who have had children or are currently pregnant) in LMICs with populations greater than 1 million (World Bank 2015). Annex 28A, section 1 provides further details. This approach enables the estimation of the hypothetical impact of increasing education of girls on reducing adolescent pregnancy rates. In these two countries, we assume that the cohort of adolescent women who complete one more year of education would experience a reduction in pregnancy rates in the short term, that is, over the subsequent five years (ages 15, 16, 17, 18, and 19 years).

Second, using this estimated impact of increased education on adolescent pregnancy rates, we use the ECEA framework to estimate the potential reduction in adolescent maternal mortality and impoverishment.

We calculate the number of maternal deaths averted by a decrease in adolescent pregnancies, the amount of out-of-pocket (OOP) costs averted by the prevention of complicated deliveries, and the corresponding number of cases of catastrophic health expenditures averted. The counterfactual scenario corresponds to the case in which female education is maintained at the same level; hence, there would be no change in adolescent pregnancy rates.

ECEA provides a tool for gaining a more complete understanding of the health and financial benefits associated with different health policies and interventions. ECEA combines the traditional health system perspective from cost-effectiveness analysis with the patient perspective, notably by quantifying the benefits associated with avoiding medical impoverishment and assessing the distributional consequences, such as equity, of policies (Verguet, Kim, and Jamison 2016; Verguet, Laxminarayan, and Jamison 2015). This tool helps policy makers make decisions based on the joint benefits and tradeoffs associated with different policies and interventions, specifically in both health gains and FRP and equity benefits. In addition to health benefits, ECEA estimates the impact of policies along three dimensions:

- Household OOP private expenditures averted by the policy
- Financial protection benefits provided
- Distributional consequences, for example, as applied to socioeconomic status or geographical setting

Third, we tentatively assess the costs associated with raising the education level of adolescent girls by one year. To do so, we multiply the entering female adolescent cohort (estimated as the population of women ages 15–19 years divided by five, or about 204,000 per wealth quintile in Niger, for example) by the annual cost of primary education per pupil as estimated by the United Nations Educational, Scientific and Cultural Organization (UNESCO 2015). This approach enables us to quantify the financial resources that may be needed to achieve such an increase in female education. We do not discount the costs and benefits of increased education because the pregnancy events would occur only a few years into the future (annex 28A, section 2).

We rely on secondary data extracted from survey sources, published literature, and estimates from United Nations (UN) agencies. Specifically, we use the following:

- Country maternal mortality ratios and population estimates from the UN

- Percentage of women ages 15–19 years who are pregnant
- Incidence of complicated deliveries
- Skilled birth attendance coverage per income quintile, based on Niger's Demographic and Health Survey and India's District Level Household and Facility Survey, as a proxy for health care utilization

We rely on an estimated increased relative risk of maternal mortality among adolescent women (Huang 2011). In addition, we use data on OOP costs for complicated maternal deliveries and associated transportation costs extracted from the literature for West Africa (Arsenault and others 2013; Storeng and others 2008) and from India's National Sample Survey (NSSO 2004). Finally, we extract adolescent women's incomes from a country income distribution proxied by a gamma distribution supplemented by gross domestic product (GDP) per capita and Gini coefficient (Salem and Mount 1974; World Bank 2015). All of the parameters used in the analysis are shown in table 28.1.

ECEA Outcomes

First, we estimate the number of maternal deaths averted per income quintile owing to a decrease in the adolescent pregnancy rate through increased education. The magnitude of maternal mortality averted depends on the existing burden, the excess relative risk of maternal mortality among adolescent women, the distribution of adolescent pregnancies per income quintile, and the impact of education on reducing adolescent pregnancy rates.

Second, we estimate the amount of OOP expenditures averted related to complicated adolescent maternal deliveries and associated transportation costs. This amount depends on the incidence of complicated maternal deliveries, the relative risk of maternal mortality among adolescent women, the distribution of adolescent pregnancies per income quintile, health care utilization per income quintile, and the impact of education on reducing adolescent pregnancy rates.

Third, we measure FRP by the number of cases of catastrophic health expenditures averted, per income quintile, which depends on individual income, OOP expenditures, and the educational impact. A catastrophic health expenditure for an adolescent woman is defined as OOP expenses higher than 10 percent of income, a commonly used threshold (Pradhan and Rescott 2002; Ranson 2002; Wagstaff and van Doorslaer 2003). Specifically, among adolescent women no longer facing pregnancies, we estimate the number of individuals, per income quintile, for whom the size of OOP expenses

Table 28.1 Parameters Used for the Analysis of Adolescent Maternal Mortality and Impoverishment Averted by Increased Education in India and Niger

Parameter	India	Niger	Sources
Total population (millions)	1,311	20	UN DESA 2015
Population of women ages 15–19 years	58,400,000	1,021,000	UN DESA 2015
Maternal mortality ratio per 100,000 live births	174	553	Alkima and others 2016
Occurrence of complicated maternal delivery among all deliveries (%)	15	15	Authors' assumption based on Prual and others 2000
Relative risk of maternal mortality for women ages 15, 16, 17, 18, and 19 years	4.6, 1.0, 1.0, 1.0, 1.0	4.6, 1.0, 1.0, 1.0, 1.0	Based on Huang 2011
Percentage of women ages 15–19 years who are pregnant, from poorest to richest (income quintiles 1–5)	19; 17; 13; 8; 3	41; 43; 37; 32; 19	INS and ICF International 2013 IIPS 2010
Percentage of women ages 15, 16, 17, 18, and 19 years who are pregnant	1; 3; 5; 9; 12	3; 12; 16; 19; 18	INS and ICF International 2013 IIPS 2010
Health care utilization (percentage of skilled birth attendance coverage), from poorest to richest (income quintiles 1–5)	24; 34; 48; 64; 85	13; 19; 22; 30; 71	INS and ICF International 2013 IIPS 2007
Out-of-pocket direct medical cost (2014 U.S. dollars) of complicated delivery, from poorest to richest (income quintiles 1–5)	58; 62; 70; 81; 108	97; 127; 140; 124; 152	Based on Arsenault and others 2013; NSSO 2004; Storeng and others 2008
Out-of-pocket transportation cost (2014 U.S. dollars), from poorest to richest (income quintiles 1–5)	8; 8; 8; 8; 6	4 for all income quintiles	Based on NSSO 2004; Perkins and others 2009
Gross domestic product per capita (2014 U.S. dollars)	1,596	427	World Bank 2015
Gini index	0.34	0.32	World Bank 2015
Impact of female education on adolescent pregnancy rate	1 additional year of education leads to an 18 percent relative reduction (SE = 2 percent) in adolescent pregnancy rate	1 additional year of education leads to an 18 percent relative reduction (SE = 2 percent) in adolescent pregnancy rate	Annex 28A, section 1 and table S1
Cost of primary education, per pupil per year (2014 U.S. dollars)	258	72	Based on UNESCO 2015

Note: SE = standard error.

(sum of direct medical costs and transportation costs) would have exceeded 10 percent of their income.

The counterfactual scenario corresponds to the situation in which primary education of girls remains at the same level. All costs are expressed in 2014 U.S. dollars. Complete details of the mathematical derivations used for the analysis are given in annex 28A, section 3.

Sensitivity Analysis

Three univariate sensitivity analyses are performed:

- Different thresholds (20 percent and 40 percent of individual income) for the catastrophic health expenditures

- A poverty headcount, estimating the number of individuals falling below the country poverty line because of OOP costs, in lieu of cases of catastrophic health expenditures
- A smaller effect, 11 percent relative reduction (instead of 18 percent) (annex 28A, section 1, table S1), for the impact of a one-year increase in female education on the adolescent pregnancy rate

RESULTS

Costs

The total costs of increasing education of adolescent girls by one school year would be approximately US$15 million in Niger and US$3 billion in India. The number of adolescent women in the two countries, about 1 million in Niger and 58 million in India (table 28.1), is responsible for the large difference in the estimated cost. We observe different orders of magnitude for the size of the maternal deaths averted (160 for Niger and 1,250 for India), OOP payments averted (US$150,000 and US$3 million, respectively), and cases of catastrophic health expenditures averted (1,110 and 5,160, respectively) (tables 28.2 and 28.3).

Adolescent Maternal Deaths Averted

In each country, the extent of adolescent deaths averted, OOP payments averted, and cases of catastrophic health expenditures averted vary significantly across different income quintiles (tables 28.2 and 28.3). In both countries, more adolescent women's lives would be saved in the bottom two quintiles (49 percent in Niger and 61 percent in India), compared with the top two quintiles (30 percent and 20 percent, respectively).

Out-of-Pocket Expenditures Averted

The OOP expenditures averted display a different pattern. In Niger, more OOP expenditures would be averted in the richer income groups; about 54 percent

of total OOP expenditures would be averted in the top two quintiles, in contrast to 27 percent in the bottom two quintiles (table 28.2). This finding occurs largely because richer individuals use more health care than do poorer individuals; it is also partly because richer individuals spend more out of pocket than do poorer individuals (table 28.1).

In India, the OOP expenditures averted are more evenly distributed among the different income groups. About 42 percent of total OOP expenditures averted accrue in the top two quintiles, in contrast to 34 percent in the bottom two quintiles (table 28.3).

Catastrophic Health Expenditures Averted

Catastrophic health expenditures results (FRP) reflect a combination of key drivers, including (1) the distributions of health care utilization and OOP costs among income quintiles and (2) individual income. For example, in Niger a larger number of cases of catastrophic health expenditures are averted among the richer (52 percent in the top two quintiles) than among the poorer (30 percent in the bottom two quintiles). Large inequalities exist in health care utilization (71 percent in the richest quintiles, compared with 13 percent in the poorest). Moreover, Nigerians' income is

Table 28.2 Impact of Increasing Mean Years of Female Education by One Year in Niger

Outcome	Total	Income quintile I	Income quintile II	Income quintile III	Income quintile IV	Income quintile V
Adolescent maternal deaths averted	164	40 (24%)	40 (25%)	34 (22%)	30 (19%)	20 (11%)
Adolescent OOP expenditures averted (2014 U.S. dollars)	152,000	13,000 (9%)	27,000 (18%)	29,000 (19%)	31,000 (20%)	52,000 (34%)
Adolescent cases of catastrophic health expenditures averted[a]	1,100	130 (12%)	200 (18%)	200 (18%)	240 (22%)	330 (30%)

Note: OOP = out-of-pocket.
a. Cases of catastrophic health expenditures are defined as OOP expenses greater than 10 percent of income.

Table 28.3 Impact of Increasing Mean Years of Female Education by One Year in India

Outcome	Total	Income quintile I	Income quintile II	Income quintile III	Income quintile IV	Income quintile V
Adolescent maternal deaths averted	1,260	400 (32%)	360 (29%)	260 (21%)	170 (14%)	70 (6%)
Adolescent OOP expenditures averted (2014 U.S. dollars)	3,050,000	430,000 (14%)	610,000 (20%)	730,000 (24%)	740,000 (24%)	540,000 (18%)
Adolescent cases of catastrophic health expenditures averted[a]	5,160	5,160 (100%)	0	0	0	0

Note: OOP = out-of-pocket.
a. Cases of catastrophic health expenditures are defined as OOP expenses greater than 10 percent of income.

very low, even in the richer socioeconomic groups; GDP per capita is US$427 (table 28.1).

In contrast, in India all the cases of catastrophic health expenditures that are averted are in the poorer quintiles (100 percent in the bottom income quintile); in spite of large inequalities in health care utilization (85 percent in the richest, compared with 24 percent in the poorest), substantial income inequalities remain. GDP per capita is approximately US$1,596, and richer individuals face little risk of catastrophic health expenditures (table 28.1). The difference between India and Niger occurs because the cost of a complicated delivery is higher relative to average income in Niger than in India.

Sensitivity Analyses

When the threshold for estimation of cases of catastrophic health expenditures is raised (to 20 percent or 40 percent), as expected the magnitude of the cases incurred decreases in India and Niger, with a slight alteration of the distribution across quintiles in Niger. Alternatively, when the poverty headcount metric is used, the distribution of induced poverty across quintiles is significantly altered (annex 28A, tables S3 and S4). Finally, when the impact of female education on the adolescent pregnancy rate is reduced (to 11 percent instead of 18 percent), maternal deaths, OOP costs, and induced cases of impoverishment averted were all reduced by 39 percent (annex 28A, tables S5 and S6).

DISCUSSION AND CONCLUSIONS

The use of the ECEA methodology enables the impact of public policies on distributional consequences and their benefits in protecting against impoverishment to be assessed, in addition to the traditional dimension of health benefits. This type of analysis provides critical additional metrics to policy makers inside and outside the health sector when allocating financial resources. We conclude that increased educational attainment for adolescent girls could bring large poverty reduction benefits in addition to significant health benefits by avoiding early pregnancies and maternal deaths. This finding underscores the great economic vulnerability of adolescent women in such settings (Filippi and others 2006; Langer and others 2015).

Our findings align well with a number of expectations. Beyond the large health and financial benefits, the extent of these gains varies significantly across socioeconomic groups. More lives would be saved in the poorer groups because they face higher rates of early pregnancy. However, more OOP expenditures would be averted in the richer groups because they use more health care than

do poorer ones. Finally, individual income and broader country wealth—low income versus middle income— also affect the distribution of the FRP benefits.

Advantages of Analysis

Our approach permits FRP to be incorporated into the economic evaluation of public policies. This enables interventions to be selected on the basis of how much FRP and equity can be bought, in addition to how much health can be bought, per dollar expenditure. This methodology helps policy makers consider all of these dimensions when making financing decisions. It facilitates comparison across sectors, which is essential for ministries of finance and development. We show how the FRP and equity benefits of public policies can be substantial and should be taken into account, critically underscoring the multifaceted nature of maternal and adolescent health.

Limitation of Analysis

Our analysis presents several limitations.

First, we have limited data and rely on secondary data and published literature to estimate impact and costs (table 28.1). Accordingly, this analysis is illustrative. A more comprehensive accounting of incurred expenditures for adolescent women could be included, with detailed accounting of medical costs, transportation and housing costs, and time and wages lost. For simplicity, we use average OOP expenses linked to complicated deliveries, even though OOP expenses might significantly rise with the degree of complication and emergency. In particular, we do not include broader pregnancy-related OOP costs or other potential expenditures incurred by adolescent women. While we attempt to examine the impact of ill health on impoverishment, we do not study the impact of poverty on health, that is, the potential increased maternal mortality and morbidity consequences associated with lower socioeconomic status. Similarly, we do not include the potential lifetime economic consequences of adolescent pregnancy, such as its short-term impact on school attendance and its long-term impact on earnings losses, because of the lack of empirical data. We also do not consider the costs to induce girls to stay in school another year beyond the costs of an additional school year to the public sector.

Second, our analysis focuses on only the mortality consequences of adolescent pregnancy, and we do not account for the potential sequelae to the mothers and their children following complicated delivery; neither do we consider abortion. Delaying childbirth is modeled as a risk displacement to older women; the elevated risk might be a first pregnancy effect or due to an unstable relationship and abortion. Such elevated risk is particularly high at ages younger than 15 years; hence, the deaths averted could be even higher if that age group were considered in the analysis.

Third, we do not pursue a full uncertainty analysis because our purpose is to expose a framework for policy makers, rather than to provide definitive estimates. Similarly, we choose to represent FRP as measured by cases of catastrophic health expenditures averted. Alternatives include a money-metric value of insurance (McClellan and Skinner 2006; Verguet, Laxminarayan, and Jamison 2015), poverty cases averted (Verguet, Olson, and others 2015), and avoided cases of forced borrowing and asset sales. We choose the number of cases of catastrophic expenditures averted metric because of its simplicity. Yet, issues pertain to its use, notably, the choice of a specific threshold—for example, 5 percent, 20 percent, or 40 percent of the capacity to pay (Xu and others 2003)—and the fact that certain individuals may not always be counted in the analysis (Saksena, Hsu, and Evans 2014; Wagstaff 2010).

Fourth, our analysis is narrowly restricted to the impact of education on teenage pregnancy and does not account for the comparative impact of other determinants of fertility (Bongaarts 1978; Bongaarts and Potter 1983) or interventions to reduce unintended pregnancies (DiCenso and others 2002; Hindin and Fatusi 2009). Similarly, we choose a simple modeling approach to examine the impact of one additional school year on teenage pregnancy and do not detail any specific features of education in the two countries studied, including, for example, the quality and impact of educational expenditures or the determinants of educational attainment (Glewwe and Kremer 2006; Heyneman and Loxley 1983).

In summary, our study's primary intent is to demonstrate how increasing levels of female education could potentially decrease rates of adolescent pregnancies and subsequently yield maternal mortality gains, as well as important equity and FRP benefits, to adolescent women.

ANNEX

The annex to this chapter is as follows. It is available at http://www.dcp-3.org/CAHD.

- Annex 28A. Estimation Methods Used in the Extended Cost-Effectiveness Analysis of Postponing Adolescent Parity

NOTES

Portions of this chapter were previously published:

- Verguet, S., A. Nandi, V. Filippi, and D. A. P. Bundy. 2016. "Maternal-Related Deaths and Impoverishment among Adolescent Girls in India and Niger: Findings from a Modelling Study." *BMJ Open* 6: e011586. doi:10.1136 /bmjopen-2016-011586. © COPYRIGHT OWNER Verguet and others. Licensed under Creative Commons Attribution (CC BY 4.0) available at: https://creativecommons.org /licenses/by/4.0/.

World Bank Income Classifications as of July 2014 are as follows, based on estimates of gross national income (GNI) per capita for 2013:

- Low-income countries (LICs) = US$1,045 or less
- Middle-income countries (MICs) are subdivided:
  a) lower-middle-income = US$1,046 to US$4,125
  b) upper-middle-income (UMICs) = US$4,126 to US$12,745
- High-income countries (HICs) = US$12,746 or more.

REFERENCES

Alkima, L., D. Chou, D. Hogan, S. Zhang, A.-B. Moller, and others. 2016. "Global, Regional, and National Levels and Trends in Maternal Mortality between 1990 and 2015, with Scenario-Based Projections to 2030: A Systematic Analysis by the UN Maternal Mortality Estimation Inter-Agency Group." *The Lancet* 387 (10017): 462–74. doi:10.1016 /S0140-6736(15)00838-7.

Arsenault, C., P. Fournier, A. Philibert, K. Sissoko, A. Coulibaly, and others. 2013. "Emergency Obstetric Care in Mali: Catastrophic Spending and Its Impoverishing Effects on Households." *Bulletin of the World Health Organization* 91: 207–16.

Ashford, L. 2002. "Hidden Suffering: Disabilities from Pregnancy and Childbirth in Less Developed Countries." Policy Brief, Population Reference Bureau, Washington, DC.

Bates, L. M., J. Maselko, and S. R. Schuler. 2007. "Women's Education and the Timing of Marriage and Childbearing in the Next Generation: Evidence from Rural Bangladesh." *Studies in Family Planning* 38 (2): 101–12.

Beguy, D., R. Ndugwa, and C. W. Kabiru. 2013. "Entry into Motherhood among Adolescent Girls in Two Informal Settlements in Nairobi, Kenya." *Journal of Biosocial Science* 45 (6): 721–42.

Boerma, T., P. Eozenou, D. Evans, T. Evans, M. P. Kierny, and others. 2014. "Monitoring Progress towards Universal Health Coverage at Country and Global Levels." *PLoS Medicine* 11 (9): e1001731.

Bongaarts, J. 1978. "A Framework for Analyzing the Proximate Determinants of Fertility." *Population and Development Review* 4 (1): 105–32.

Bongaarts, J., and R. G. Potter. 1983. *Fertility, Biology, and Behavior.* New York: Academic Press.

Bundy, D. A. P., N. de Silva, S. Horton, G. C. Patton, L. Schultz, and D. T. Jamison. 2017. "Child and Adolescent Health and Development: Realizing Neglected Potential." In *Disease Control Priorities* (third edition): Volume 8, *Child and Adolescent Health and Development*, edited by D. A. P. Bundy, N. de Silva, S. Horton, D. T. Jamison, and G. C. Patton. Washington, DC: World Bank.

Chloe, M. J., S. Thapa, and V. Mishra. 2004. "Early Marriage and Early Motherhood in Nepal." *Journal of Biosocial Science* 37 (2): 143–62.

Dale, J. R., B. J. Stoll, and A. O. Lucas. 2003. *Improving Birth Outcomes: Meeting the Challenge in the Developing World.* Washington, DC: National Academies Press.

DiCenso, A., G. Guyatt, A. Willan, and L. Griffith. 2002. "Interventions to Reduce Unintended Pregnancies among Adolescents: Systematic Review of Randomized Controlled Trials." *BMJ* 324: 1426.

Dixon-Mueller, R. 2008. "How Young Is 'Too Young'? Comparative Perspectives on Adolescent Sexual, Marital, and Reproductive Transitions." *Studies in Family Planning* 39 (4): 247–62.

Filippi, V., C. Ronsmans, O. M. R. Campbell, W. Graham, A. Mills, and others. 2006. "Maternal Health in Poor Countries: The Broader Context and a Call for Action." *The Lancet* 368 (9546): 1535–41.

Gakidou, E., K. Cowling, R. Lozano, and C. J. L. Murray. 2010. "Increased Educational Attainment and Its Effect on Child Mortality in 175 Countries between 1970 and 2009: A Systematic Analysis." *The Lancet* 376: 959–74.

Glewwe, P., and M. Kremer. 2006. "Schools, Teachers, and Education Outcomes in Developing Countries." In *Handbook of the Economics of Education*, volume 2, edited by E. Hanushek and F. Welch, 945–1018. Amsterdam: North Holland.

Heyneman, S. P., and W. A. Loxley. 1983. "The Effect of Primary-School Quality on Academic Achievement across Twenty-Nine High- and Low-Income Countries." *American Journal of Sociology* 88 (6): 1162–94.

Hindin, M. J., and A. O. Fatusi. 2009. "Adolescent Sexual and Reproductive Health in Developing Countries: An Overview of Trends and Interventions." *International Perspectives on Sexual and Reproductive Health* 35 (2): 58–62.

Huang, W. 2011. "The Impact of Fertility Changes on Maternal Mortality." PhD thesis, London School of Hygiene and Tropical Medicine. http://researchonline.lshtm.ac.uk/682434.

IHME (Institute for Health Metrics and Evaluation). 2010. *Educational Attainment and Child Mortality Estimates by Country 1970–2009.* Seattle, WA: IHME.

———. 2013. *GBD Cause Patterns.* Seattle, WA: IHME. https://vizhub.healthdata.org/gbd-compare.

IIPS (International Institute for Population Sciences). 2007. *National Family Health Survey (NFHS-3), 2005–06: India.* Mumbai: IIPS.

———. 2010. *District Level Household and Facility Survey (DLHS-3), 2007–08.* Mumbai: IIPS.

Ilboudo, P. G. C., S. Russell, and B. D'Exelle. 2013. "The Long Term Economic Impact of Severe Obstetric Complications for Women and Their Children in Burkina Faso." *PLoS One* 8 (11): e80010.

INS (Institut National de la Statistique) and ICF International. 2013. *Enquête Démographique et de Santé et à Indicateurs Multiples du Niger 2012.* Calverton, MD: INS and ICF International.

Jamison, D. T., J. G. Breman, A. R. Measham, G. Alleyne, M. Claeson, D. B. Evans, P. Jha, A. Mills, and P. Musgrove, editors. 2006. *Disease Control Priorities in Developing Countries* (second edition), Washington, DC: World Bank and Oxford University Press.

Kassebaum, N. J., A. Bertozzi-Villa, M. S. Coggeshall, K. A. Shackelford, C. Steiner, and others. 2014. "Global, Regional, and National Levels and Causes of Maternal Mortality during 1990–2013: A Systematic Analysis for the Global Burden of Disease 2013." *The Lancet* 384 (9947): 980–1004.

Kruk, M. E., E. Goldmann, and S. Galea. 2009. "Borrowing and Selling to Pay for Health Care in Low- and Middle-Income Countries." *Health Affairs* 28 (4): 1056–66.

Langer, A., A. Meleis, F. M. Knaul, R. Atun, M. Aran, and others. 2015. "Women and Health: The Key for Sustainable Development." *The Lancet* 386 (9999): 1165–210. doi:10.1016/S0140-6736(15)60497-4.

Lloyd, C. B., and B. S. Mensch. 2008. "Marriage and Childbirth as Factors in Dropping Out from School: An Analysis of DHS Data from Sub-Saharan Africa." *Population Studies* 62 (1): 1–13.

Marteleto, L., D. Lam, and V. Ranchhod. 2008. "Sexual Behavior, Pregnancy, and Schooling among Young People in Urban South Africa." *Studies in Family Planning* 39 (4): 351–68.

Mayor, S. 2004. "Pregnancy and Childbirth Are Leading Causes of Death in Teenage Girls in Developing Countries." *BMJ* 328: 1152.

McClellan, M., and J. Skinner. 2006. "The Incidence of Medicare." *Journal of Public Economics* 90 (1–2): 257–76.

Meekers, D., and G. Ahmed. 1999. "Pregnancy-Related School Dropouts in Botswana." *Population Studies* 53 (2): 195–209.

NSSO (National Sample Survey Organisation). 2004. National Sample Survey Round 60, Ministry of Statistics and Programme Implementation, Government of India, New Delhi.

Perkins, M., E. Brazier, E. Themmen, B. Bassane, D. Diallo, and others. 2009. "Out-of-Pocket Costs for Facility-Based Maternity Care in Three African Countries." *Health Policy and Planning* 24 (4): 289–300.

Powell-Jackson, T., and M. E. Hoque. 2012. "Economic Consequences of Maternal Illness in Rural Bangladesh." *Health Economics* 21 (7): 796–810.

Pradhan, M., and N. Rescott. 2002. "Social Risk Management Options for Medical Care in Indonesia." *Health Economics* 11 (5): 431–46.

Prual, A., M.-H. Bouvier-Colle, L. de Bernis, and G. Bréart. 2000. "Severe Maternal Morbidity from Direct Obstetric Causes in West Africa: Incidence and Case Fatality Rates." *Bulletin of the World Health Organization* 78 (5): 593–602.

Ranson, M. K. 2002. "Reduction of Catastrophic Health Care Expenditures by a Community-Based Health Insurance Scheme in Gujarat, India: Current Experiences and Challenges." *Bulletin of the World Health Organization* 80 (8): 613–21.

Saksena, P., J. Hsu, and D. B. Evans. 2014. "Financial Risk Protection and Universal Health Coverage: Evidence and Measurement Challenges." *PLoS Medicine* 11 (9): e1001701.

Salem, A. B. Z., and T. D. Mount. 1974. "A Convenient Descriptive Model of Income Distribution: The Gamma Density." *Econometrica* 42 (6): 1115–27.

Storeng, K. T., R. F. Baggaley, R. Ganaba, F. Ouattara, M. S. Akoum, and others. 2008. "Paying the Price: The Cost and Consequences of Emergency Obstetric Care in Burkina Faso." *Social Science and Medicine* 66 (3): 545–57.

UN (United Nations). 2013. "Millennium Development Goals and Beyond 2015." United Nations, New York. http://www.un.org/millenniumgoals.

UN DESA (United Nations Department of Economic and Social Affairs). 2015. "2015 Revision of the World Population Prospects." Population Division, Population Estimates and Projections Section (accessed December 4, 2015), http://esa.un.org/wpp/.

UNESCO (United Nations Educational, Scientific and Cultural Organization). 2015. "Pricing the Right to Education: The Cost of Reaching New Targets by 2030." Education for All Global Monitoring Report Policy Paper 18, UNESCO, New York. http://unesdoc.unesco.org/images/0023/002321/232197E.pdf.

UNICEF (United Nations Children's Fund). 2016. "UNICEF Data: Monitoring the Situation of Children and Women." http://data.unicef.org/.

UN MME (United Nations Maternal Mortality Estimation Inter-Agency Group). 2015. "Maternal Mortality." http://data.unicef.org/maternal-health/maternal-mortality.html.

UNW (United Nations Women). 2016. "SDG 3: Ensure Healthy Lives and Promote Well-Being for All at All Ages." http://www.unwomen.org/en/news/in-focus/women-and-the-sdgs/sdg-3-good-health-well-being.

Verguet, S., C. Gauvreau, S. Mishra, M. MacLennan, S. Murphy, and others. 2015. "The Consequences of Tobacco Tax on Household Health and Finances in Rich and Poor Smokers in China: An Extended Cost-Effectiveness Analysis." *The Lancet Global Health* 3 (4): e206–16.

Verguet, S., J. J. Kim, and D. T. Jamison. 2016. "Extended Cost-Effectiveness Analysis for Health Policy Assessment: A Tutorial." *PharmacoEconomics* 34 (9): 913-23.

Verguet, S., R. Laxminarayan, and D. T. Jamison. 2015. "Universal Public Finance of Tuberculosis Treatment in India: An Extended Cost-Effectiveness Analysis." *Health Economics* 24 (3): 318–22.

Verguet, S., S. Murphy, B. Anderson, K. A. Johansson, R. Glass, and others. 2013. "Public Finance of Rotavirus Vaccination in India and Ethiopia: An Extended Cost-Effectiveness Analysis." *Vaccine* 31 (42): 4902–10.

Verguet, S., O. F. Norheim, Z. D. Olson, G. Yamey, and D. T. Jamison. 2014. "Annual Rates of Decline in Child, Maternal, HIV, and Tuberculosis Mortality across 109 Countries of Low and Middle Income from 1990 to 2013: An Assessment of the Feasibility of Post-2015 Goals." *The Lancet Global Health* 2 (12): e698–709.

Verguet, S., Z. D. Olson, J. B. Babigumira, D. Desalegn, K. A. Johansson, and others. 2015. "Health Gains and Financial Risk Protection Afforded by Public Financing of Selected Interventions in Ethiopia: An Extended Cost-Effectiveness Analysis." *The Lancet Global Health* 3 (15): e288–96.

Wagstaff, A. 2010. "Measuring Financial Protection in Health." In *Performance Measurement for Health System Improvement*, edited by P. C. Smith, E. Mossialos, I. Papanicolas, and S. Leatherman, 114–37. Cambridge, U.K.: Cambridge University Press.

Wagstaff, A., and E. van Doorslaer. 2003. "Catastrophe and Impoverishment in Paying for Health Care: With Applications to Vietnam 1993–1998." *Health Economics* 12 (11): 921–34.

WHO (World Health Organization). 2010. *World Health Report 2010: Health Systems Financing: The Path to Universal Coverage.* Geneva: WHO.

———. 2013. *World Health Report 2013: Research for Universal Health Coverage.* Geneva: WHO.

WHO, UNICEF, United Nations Population Fund, World Bank, and United Nations Population Division. 2014. *Trends in Maternal Mortality: 1990 to 2013. Estimates by WHO, UNICEF, UNFPA, The World Bank, and the United Nations Population Division.* Geneva: WHO. http://www.who.int/reproductivehealth/publications/monitoring/maternal-mortality-2013/en/.

World Bank. 2015. *World Development Indicators 2015.* Washington, DC: World Bank.

Xu, K., D. B. Evans, K. Kawabata, R. Zeramdini, J. Klavus, and others. 2003. "Household Catastrophic Health Expenditure: A Multicountry Analysis." *The Lancet* 362 (9378): 111–17.

Chapter 29

Economics of Mass Deworming Programs

Amrita Ahuja, Sarah Baird, Joan Hamory Hicks, Michael
Kremer, and Edward Miguel

INTRODUCTION

Soil-transmitted helminth (STH) and schistosomiasis infections affect more than 1 billion people, mainly in low- and middle-income countries, particularly school-age children. Although light infections can be fairly asymptomatic, severe infections can have significant health effects, such as malnutrition, listlessness, organ damage, and internal bleeding (Bundy, Appleby, and others 2017).[1]

Low-cost drugs are available and are the standard of medical care for diagnosed infections. Because diagnosis is relatively expensive, and treatment is inexpensive and safe, the World Health Organization (WHO) recommends periodic mass treatments in areas where worm infections are greater than certain thresholds (WHO 2015). A number of organizations, including the Copenhagen Consensus, GiveWell, and the Abdul Latif Jameel Poverty Action Lab, which have reviewed the evidence for, and comparative cost-effectiveness of, a wide range of development interventions, have consistently ranked deworming as a priority for investment.[2] However, Taylor-Robinson and others (2015) challenge this policy, accepting that those known to be infected should be treated but arguing that there is substantial evidence that mass drug administration (MDA) has no impact on a range of outcomes.[3]

This chapter discusses the economics of policy choices surrounding public investments in deworming and considers policy choices under two frameworks:

- *Welfare economics or public finance approach.* Individuals are presumed to make decisions that maximize their own welfare, but government intervention may be justified in cases in which individual actions create externalities for others. These externalities could include health externalities from reductions in the transmission of infectious disease, as well as fiscal externalities if treatment increases long-term earnings and tax payments. Evidence on epidemiological and fiscal externalities from deworming will be important for informing decisions under this perspective.

- *Expected cost-effectiveness approach.* Policy makers should pursue a policy if the statistical expectation of the value of benefits exceeds the cost. Future monetary benefits should be discounted back to the present. Policy makers may also value nonfinancial goals, such as weight gain or school participation; they should pursue a policy if the statistical expectation of the benefit achieved per unit of expenditure exceeds that of other policies that policy makers are considering.

Under either framework, the case for government subsidies will be stronger if demand for deworming is sensitive to price. If everyone would buy deworming medicine on their own, without subsidies, then subsidies would yield no benefits; they would generate a deadweight loss of taxation.

The first perspective focuses on individual goals and assumes that consumers will maximize their own welfare. It treats them as rational and informed, and it

Corresponding author: Joan Hamory Hicks, Senior Researcher, Center for Effective Global Action, University of California, Berkeley, jrhamory@berkeley.edu.

abstracts from intrahousehold conflicts. The second perspective does not make these assumptions and seeks simply to inform policy makers about expected benefit-cost ratios or cost-effectiveness metrics, rather than making welfare statements.

This chapter summarizes the public finance case for deworming subsidies, given the evidence on epidemiological externalities[4] and high responsiveness of household deworming to price. It reviews the evidence on the cost-effectiveness of mass school-based deworming and associated fiscal externalities. It argues that the expected benefits of following the WHO's recommendation of mass presumptive deworming of children in endemic regions exceed the costs, even given uncertainty about the magnitude and likelihood of impacts in given contexts.[5] This benefit is realized even when only the educational and economic benefits of deworming are considered. Finally, the chapter maintains that between the two leading policy options for treatment in endemic areas—mass treatment versus screening and treatment of those found to be infected—the former is preferred under both public finance and cost-effectiveness approaches. Definitions of age groupings and age-specific terminology used in this volume can be found in chapter 1 (Bundy, de Silva, and others 2017).

EPIDEMIOLOGICAL EXTERNALITIES

STHs—including hookworm, roundworm, and whipworm—are transmitted via eggs in feces deposited in the local environment, typically through open defecation or lack of proper hygiene after defecating. Schistosomiasis is spread through contact with infected fresh water. School-age children are particularly vulnerable to such infections and prone to transmitting infection (Bundy, Appleby, and others 2017). Treating infected individuals kills the parasites in their bodies and prevents further transmission. Three studies provide evidence on such epidemiological externalities from deworming school-age children and suggest these externalities can be substantial.

Bundy and others (1990) studied a program in the island of Montserrat, West Indies, where all children between ages 2 and 15 years were treated with albendazole, four times over 16 months, to eliminate STH infections. The authors found substantial reductions in infection rates for the targeted individuals (more than 90 percent of whom received treatment), as well as for young adults ages 16–25 years (fewer than 4 percent of whom were treated). These findings suggest large positive epidemiological externalities, although only one geographic unit was examined.

Miguel and Kremer (2004) studied a randomized school-based deworming program in rural western Kenya from 1998 through 1999, where students in treatment schools received albendazole twice a year; in addition, some schools received praziquantel for schistosomiasis infections annually. The authors found large reductions in worm infections among treated individuals, untreated individuals attending treatment schools, and individuals in schools located near treatment schools. The authors estimated an 18 percentage point reduction after one year in the proportion of moderate-to-heavy infections among untreated individuals attending treatment schools, and a 22 percentage point reduction among individuals attending a school within 3 kilometers of a treatment school.[6]

Ozier (2014) studied this same randomized program in Kenya but focused on children who were ages zero to two years and living in catchment areas of participating schools at the time of program launch. These children were not treated, but they could have benefited from positive within-community externalities generated by the mass school-based deworming. Indeed, 10 years after the program, Ozier estimated average test score gains of 0.2 standard deviation units for these individuals. Consistent with the hypothesis that these children benefited primarily through the reduced transmission of worm infections, the effects were twice as large among children with an older sibling in one of the schools that participated in the program.

Bobonis, Miguel, and Puri-Sharma (2006), in contrast, found small and statistically insignificant cross-school externalities of deworming and iron supplementation on nutritional status and school participation of children in India. The authors noted that this finding is unsurprising in this context, given both the lower prevalence and intensity of worm infections and the small fraction of treated individuals.

Together, these studies provide strong evidence for the existence of large, positive epidemiological externality benefits to mass treatment in endemic areas, especially in areas with higher infection loads.[7] Such externality benefits are important to consider in both the public finance and cost-effectiveness decision-making frameworks. Under the first perspective, such benefits cannot be fully internalized by household decision makers and thus provide a potential rationale for government subsidies. Under the second perspective, externalities increase the cost-effectiveness of the intervention by increasing the total benefit achieved for a given amount of expenditure.

IMPACTS OF THE PRICE OF DEWORMING ON TAKE-UP

Assuming that a behavior generates positive externalities—or that under a cost-effectiveness approach, it is valued by policy makers—public finance theory emphasizes that the attractiveness of a subsidy depends on the ratio of marginal consumers (those who will change their behavior in response to a subsidy) to inframarginal consumers (those who would have engaged in the behavior even in the absence of a subsidy). The higher this ratio, the more attractive the subsidy.

Kremer and Miguel (2007) studied the behavioral response to a change in the price of deworming treatment in the Kenyan deworming program. Starting in 2001, a random subset of participating schools was chosen to pay user fees for treatment, with the average cost of deworming per child set at US$0.30, which was about 20 percent of the cost of drug purchase and delivery through this program. This cost-sharing reduced take-up (the fraction of individuals who received treatment) by 80 percent, to 19 percent from 75 percent.

This result is consistent with findings observed for other products for disease prevention and treatment of non-acute conditions, such as bednets for malaria and water treatment. Figure 29.1 displays how the demand for a range of health care products decreases as price increases.[8] Moreover, Kremer and Miguel (2007) found that user fees did not help target treatment to the sickest students; students with moderate-to-heavy worm infections were not more likely to pay for the medications. These results suggest low costs and large benefits from deworming subsidies, important for both the cost-effectiveness and welfare economics perspectives.

IMPACTS OF DEWORMING ON CHILD WEIGHT

In this and subsequent sections we examine the cost-effectiveness of mass deworming in affecting various outcomes potentially valued by policy makers. We focus primarily on economic outcomes rather than health outcomes because the impact of deworming on health is covered in chapter 13 in this volume (Bundy, Appleby, and others 2017). However, we would like to briefly expand upon that discussion to address the cost-effectiveness of deworming in improving child weight. Bundy, Appleby, and others (2017) discuss recent work of Croke and others (2016), who reviewed the literature on the impact of multiple-dose deworming on child weight. Overall, they estimated that MDA increases weight by an average of 0.13 kilograms, with somewhat larger point estimates among populations in which prevalence is greater than the WHO's 20 percent prevalence threshold for MDA, or the 50 percent threshold for multiple-dose MDA.[9] Assuming that an MDA program

Figure 29.1 Response of Consumer Demand to Increase in the Price of Health Products

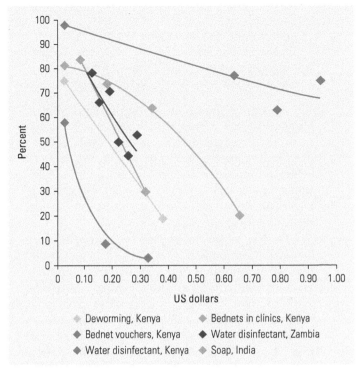

Source: Abdul Latif Jameel Poverty Action Lab 2011.

with two treatments per year costs US$0.60 per person (Givewell 2016), Croke and others (2016) estimated that the cost of deworming MDA per kilogram of weight gain is US$4.48. For comparison with another policy option, a review of school feeding programs by Galloway and others (2009) found that the average of the range associated with a 1 kilogram weight increase for school feeding from evidence from randomized controlled trials is US$182. This finding implies that per dollar of expenditure, mass deworming produces a weight increase 40.62 times that of school feeding. This finding on weight gain suggests that evidence of education and economic impact should not be rejected out of hand based on concern for lack of evidence about mechanisms by which such impacts could be achieved.

IMPACTS OF DEWORMING ON EDUCATION AND LABOR MARKETS

Evidence on the impact of deworming on education and labor market outcomes directly informs the cost-effectiveness perspective, while the fiscal externalities resulting from labor market impacts are important from a welfare economics perspective.

We review publicly available studies of the impact of mass deworming that do the following:

- Use experimental or quasi-experimental methods to demonstrate causal relationships
- Incorporate a cluster design to take into account the potential for infectious disease externalities
- Minimize attrition that could lead to bias.

Most existing studies on deworming randomize at the individual level; they fail to consider the potential for treatment externalities (Bundy and others 2009) and likely underestimate the impact of treatment. We review evidence from three deworming campaigns in different times and contexts—one in the United States in the early twentieth century and two in East Africa at the turn of the twenty-first century.[10]

The first program was launched by the Rockefeller Sanitary Commission (RSC) in 1910 to eradicate hookworm infections in the U.S. South. With baseline hookworm infection rates at 40 percent among school-age children, traveling dispensaries administered treatment to infected individuals in endemic areas and educated local physicians and the public about prevention. The RSC reported a 30 percentage point decrease in infection rates across affected areas 10 or more years after launch of the program (Bleakley 2007).[11]

The second program was a school-based treatment program sponsored by a nongovernmental organization that was phased into 75 schools in a rural district of western Kenya from 1998 through 2001. Baseline helminth infection rates were greater than 90 percent among school children in this area. The nongovernmental organization provided deworming drugs to treat STHs twice per year and schistosomiasis once per year, as well as educational materials on worm prevention. Schools were phased into the program in three groups over four years; each school was assigned to a group through list-randomization, resulting in a cluster randomized stepped-wedge research design.

The third program was delivered by community-based organizations during 2000–03 across 48 parishes in five districts of eastern Uganda.[12] Baseline infection rates were greater than 60 percent in children ages 5–10 years (Kabatereine and others 2001). Treatment was provided during child health days, in which parents were offered multiple health and nutrition interventions for children ages one to seven years. Using a cluster randomization approach, parishes were randomly assigned to receive either the standard intervention of vitamin A supplementation, vaccines, growth monitoring, and feeding demonstrations, or to deworming treatment in addition to the standard package (Alderman and others 2006; Croke 2014).

School Participation

Using a difference-in-difference methodology in his study of the RSC program, Bleakley (2007) compared changes in counties with high baseline worm prevalence to changes in low baseline prevalence counties over the same period. Findings indicate that from 1910 through 1920, counties with higher worm prevalence before the deworming campaign saw substantial increases in school enrollment, both in absolute terms and relative to areas with lower infection rates. A child infected with hookworm was an estimated 20 percentage points less likely to be enrolled in school than a noninfected child and 13 percentage points less likely to be literate. Bleakley's estimates suggest that because of the deworming campaign, a county with a 1910 infection rate of 50 percent would experience an increase in school enrollment of 3 to 5 percentage points and an increase in attendance of 6 to 8 percentage points, relative to a county with no infection problem. This finding remains significant when controlling for a number of potentially confounding factors, such as state-level policy changes and the demographic composition of high- and low-worm load areas. In addition, the author found no significant effects on adult outcomes, which, given the significantly lower infection rates of adults, bolsters the case that deworming was driving these findings.

Miguel and Kremer (2004) provide evidence on the impact of deworming on school participation through their cluster randomized evaluation of the Kenyan school-based deworming program. The authors found substantially greater school participation in schools assigned to receive deworming than in those that had not yet been phased in to the program. Participation increased not only among treated children but also among untreated children in treatment schools and among pupils in schools located near treatment schools. The total increase in school participation, including these externality benefits, was 8.5 percentage points.[13] These results imply that deworming is one of the most cost-effective ways of increasing school participation (Dhaliwal and others 2012). Figure 29.2 shows the cost-effectiveness of deworming in increasing school attendance across a range of development interventions.[14]

Academic Test Scores

In their study of the Kenyan deworming program, Miguel and Kremer (2004) did not find short-term effects on academic test scores.[15] However, the long-term follow-up evaluation of the same intervention (Baird and others 2016) found that among girls, deworming increased the rate of passing the national primary school exit exam by almost 25 percent (9.6 percentage points on

Figure 29.2 Cost-Effectiveness of Development Interventions in Increasing School Attendance

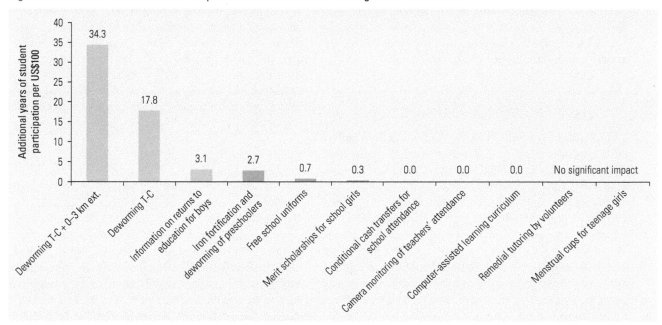

Sources: Hicks, Kremer, and Miguel 2015 based on data from Abdul Latif Jameel Poverty Action Lab.
Note: T–C = the difference between outcomes for those allocated to the deworming treatment group and those allocated to the deworming comparison group; km = kilometers; ext. = externality benefits. Some values are adjusted for inflation but the deworming costs are not. Deworming is costed at US$0.49 per child in Kenya. Some of these programs create benefits beyond school attendance. For example, conditional cash transfers provide income to poor households. The Jameel Poverty Action Lab cost-effectiveness calculations for school participation include conditional cash transfers as program costs.

a base of 41 percent). Ozier (2014) found test-score gains for children younger than age two years at the time of the program.

In the long-term follow-up of the cluster randomized Uganda deworming program, Croke (2014) analyzed English literacy, numeracy, and combined test scores, comparing treatment and control. The study found that children in treatment villages have significantly higher numeracy and combined test scores compared with those in control villages; effect sizes across all three outcomes range from 0.16 to 0.36 standard deviations. The effects were significantly larger for children who were exposed to the program for multiple years.[16]

Labor Market Effects

Bleakley (2007) used data from the 1940 U.S. census to compare adult outcomes among birth cohorts who entered the labor force before and after the deworming campaign in the U.S. South. Adults who had more exposure to deworming as children were significantly more likely to be literate and had higher earnings as adults. The author found a 43 percent increase in adult wages among those exposed to the campaign as children. Given initial infection rates of 30 percent to 40 percent, hookworm eradication would imply a long-term income gain of 17 percent (Bleakley 2010).[17]

Children who were treated for worms in Kenya also had better labor market outcomes later in life. Baird and others (2016) considered women and men separately, given the different set of family and labor market choices they face. They found that Kenyan women who received more deworming treatment are more likely to grow cash crops and reallocate labor time from agriculture to non-agricultural self-employment. Treated men work 17 percent more hours per week, spend more time in entrepreneurial activities, and are more likely to work in higher-wage manufacturing jobs.

Baird and others (2016) estimated the net present value of the long-term educational and economic benefits to be more than 100 times the cost, implying that even policy makers who assume a small subjective probability of realizing these benefits would conclude that the expected benefits of MDA exceed their cost.

Based on these increased earnings, the authors computed an annualized internal rate of return to deworming of 32 percent to 51 percent, depending on whether health spillovers are included. This finding is high relative to other investments, implying that deworming is cost-effective on economic grounds, even without considering health, nutritional, and educational benefits.

Furthermore, because deworming increases the labor supply, it creates a fiscal externality though its impact on tax revenue. Baird and others (2016) estimated that the net present value of increases in tax revenues likely exceeds the cost of the program. The fiscal externalities are sufficiently strong that a government could potentially reduce tax rates by instituting free mass deworming.

EVIDENCE AND POLICY DECISION RULES

This section argues that available evidence is sufficient to support deworming subsidies in endemic regions, even if the magnitude and likelihood of program impacts realized in a given context are uncertain.

When assessing evidence, there will always be some uncertainty about whether an intervention will have benefits in a given context. First, any body of research risks two types of errors: identifying an impact that does not exist (type 1 error), and missing an impact that does exist (type 2). The risk of making a type 1 error is captured by the confidence level (P-value) on estimates of impact. The risk of making a type 2 error is captured by the power of the study. Second, questions about the extent to which a body of research applies to the specific context of interest to policy makers will always arise.

Some (for example, Taylor-Robinson and others 2015) contend that the evidence does not support investments in mass deworming. One area of disagreement is the decision rule used. The decision rule the *Cochrane Review* seems to implicitly apply is that programs should not be implemented unless a meta-analysis (with all its associated assumptions) of randomized controlled trials shows benefits and indicates that the risk of a type 1 error is less than 5 percent. This approach is inconsistent with policy making from both a cost-effectiveness and a public finance perspective.

This decision rule puts no weight on the risk of making a type 2 error, which may be quite important for policy makers who do not want to deny a potentially highly beneficial program to their constituents. Given the statistical tradeoff between type 1 and type 2 errors, the desire to avoid withholding treatment with potentially very high benefits will necessitate being comfortable with less-than-definitive proof about program impact. Note that Taylor-Robinson and others (2015) did not report power, but that Croke and others (2016) found that Taylor-Robinson and others (2015) did not have adequate power to rule out effects that would make deworming cost-effective.

A more reasonable policy rule under uncertainty would be to compare expected costs with expected benefits. Suppose that the costs of the program are known to be C. Suppose policy makers are uncertain about the benefits of the program (relative to not implementing the program) in their circumstances. For simplicity, consider an example in which they believe that the total benefits may be B_1 with probability P_1, B_2 with probability P_2, or B_3 with probability P_3. This framework encompasses the case in which policy makers believe that there is some chance of zero impact because B_3 could equal zero. A risk-neutral policy maker will undertake the program if[18]

$$P_1 \times B_1 + P_2 \times B_2 + P_3 \times B_3 - C > 0.$$

With this framework in mind, from a cost-effectiveness perspective, deworming would still be warranted in many settings on educational and economic grounds alone, even if its benefits were only a fraction of those estimated in the studies discussed. Policy makers would be warranted in moving ahead with deworming, even if they thought benefits were likely to be smaller in their own context or had some uncertainty about whether benefits would be realized at all. In particular, even if the policy maker believes the impact of deworming on school participation is only 10 percent of that estimated in Miguel and Kremer (2004), or equivalently, if the policy maker believes there is a 10 percent chance of an impact of the magnitude estimated by Miguel and Kremer (2004), and a 90 percent chance of zero impact, it would still be among the most highly cost-effective ways of boosting school participation (Ahuja and others 2015). If the impact on weight is even 3 percent of that estimated by Croke and others (2016), then deworming is cost-effective relative to school feeding in increasing weight. If the labor market impact were even 1 percent of that found by Baird and others (2016), then the financial benefits of deworming would exceed the cost. Of course, to the extent that deworming may affect multiple outcomes, deworming will be even more cost-effective.

An analogous expected-value approach would be natural in a welfare economics framework. Labor market effects half as large as those estimated in Baird and others (2016) would be sufficient for deworming to generate enough tax revenue to fully cover its costs.[19] Standard welfare economics criteria for programs being welfare improving are much weaker than for the tax revenue fully covering costs.

From either a cost-benefit or a welfare economics perspective, a sophisticated analysis would be explicitly Bayesian, taking into account policy makers' previous assumptions and their best current assessment of their specific context. Under a Bayesian analysis that places even modest weight on evidence discussed here, mass school-based deworming would be justified in areas with worm prevalence greater than the WHO thresholds.

It is worth noting that a Bayesian policy maker will make current policy decisions based on current information. However, the policy maker would also continue research if the expected benefits outweigh its costs; as new evidence becomes available, it would be systematically combined with the existing best information when making decisions about continuing or modifying the program.

COST OF MASS TREATMENT PROGRAMS VERSUS SCREENED TREATMENT

The WHO recommends mass treatment once or twice a year in regions where worm prevalence is greater than certain thresholds (WHO 2015). Screening, followed by treatment of those testing positive for worms, is far less practical and more costly than mass treatment without diagnostic testing.

School-based mass treatment costs approximately US$0.30 per child per treatment, including delivery costs (GiveWell 2016).[20] Diagnosis of worm infections, in contrast, is far more expensive and complicated. Speich and others (2010) estimate that the cost per child of the Kato-Katz test, the most widely used field test for worm infections, is US$1.88 in 2013 dollars. If the test works perfectly, costs would be more than seven times higher with treatment following screening, compared with mass treatment without screening. Even proponents of the test-and-treat approach acknowledge this huge differential; Taylor-Robinson and others (2015) stated that screening is not recommended by the WHO because screening costs 4–10 times the cost of treatment. Mass treatment is clearly preferred on cost-effectiveness and public finance grounds.

These figures ultimately underestimate the cost of screening, however.[21] First, tests for worms do not identify all infections. Estimates of the specificity for the Kato-Katz method range from approximately 52 percent to 91 percent (Assefa and others 2014; Barda and others 2013). With a specificity of 52 percent, the cost per infection treated would be much higher for screened treatment compared with mass treatment. Second, a large number of infections would remain untreated. With low specificity, many existing infections would be missed; additionally, screened treatment programs need to reach infected children a second time to treat them, and it is unlikely they can reach each child who was tested—making screening even less cost-effective.

In sum, the majority of the 870 million children at risk of worm infections (Uniting to Combat Neglected Tropical Diseases 2014) could be treated each year via mass deworming programs at a cost of less than US$300 million dollars a year, which is feasible given current health budgets. The cost of treating them via screened programs would likely be US$2 billion annually, if not higher, and fewer infections would be treated.

This chapter considers the cost of school-based mass deworming programs, which are particularly inexpensive per person reached. We do not consider the cost-effectiveness of more expensive community-based programs that would include extensive outreach efforts beyond schools. One reasonable hypothesis might be that these more intensive efforts may be most warranted in areas with either high prevalence, and thus likely high intensity, of STHs, or where multiple diseases, such as lymphatic filariasis, onchocerciasis, trachoma, and schistosomiasis, that can be addressed by MDA are endemic (Hotez and others 2007).

CONCLUSIONS

Recent estimates suggest that nearly one-third of children in low- and middle-income countries are treated for worms, many via school- or community-based programs (Uniting to Combat Neglected Tropical Diseases 2014). The most commonly used deworming drugs—albendazole, mebendazole, and praziquantel—have been approved for use by the appropriate regulatory bodies in multiple countries, have been shown to be efficacious against a variety of worm infections, and have minimal side effects (Bundy, Appleby, and others 2017).

The impact of deworming will vary with the local context—including circumstances such as type of worm, worm prevalence and intensity, comorbidity, the extent of school participation in the community, and labor market factors. The decision to expend resources on deworming should be based on a comparison of expected benefits and costs, given the available evidence. Our analysis of evidence from several contexts on the nutritional, educational, and economic impact suggests that the WHO recommendations for mass treatment are justified on both welfare economics and cost-effectiveness grounds. Additional studies will generate further evidence to inform future decisions.

DISCLAIMERS

USAID and the Douglas B. Marshall, Jr. Family Foundation support deworming. Michael Kremer is a former board member of Deworm the World and is currently Scientific Director of Development Innovation Ventures at USAID. Also, Amrita Ahuja is a board member of Evidence Action, a nonprofit organization that supports governments in scaling mass school-based deworming programs; this is a voluntary position with no associated remuneration. None of these organizations had any influence on this chapter.

NOTES

This chapter draws significantly on Ahuja and others (2015).

World Bank Income Classifications as of July 2014 are as follows, based on estimates of gross national income (GNI) per capita for 2014:

- Low-income countries (LICs) = US$1,045 or less
- Middle-income countries (MICs) are subdivided:
  a) lower-middle-income = US$1,046 to US$4,125
  b) upper-middle-income (UMICs) = US$4,126 to US$12,745
- High-income countries (HICs) = US$12,746 or more.

1. For further discussion of biological differences across worms, as well as a broader discussion of deworming, please refer to Bundy, Appleby, and others (2017).
2. See, for example, Hall and Horton (2008), GiveWell (2013), and Abdul Latif Jameel Poverty Action Lab (2012).
3. Bundy, Appleby, and others (2017) provide a discussion of Taylor-Robinson and others (2015).
4. Epidemiological externalities are benefits that accrue to individuals who did not necessarily receive the treatment, for instance, a drug that cures treated individuals, thereby reducing transmission of the disease to others.
5. We do not address the optimality of the WHO prevalence thresholds for MDA.
6. Miguel and Kremer (2014) provide an updated analysis of the data in Miguel and Kremer (2004), correcting some errors in the original paper. Throughout this chapter, we cite Miguel and Kremer (2004) but use the updated numbers, where appropriate.
7. Although they do not explicitly explore externality impacts, several medical studies also show decreases in infection rates among untreated individuals (Miguel and Kremer 2004).
8. See Dupas (2014), Kremer and Glennerster (2011), Kremer and Holla (2009), and Abdul Latif Jameel Poverty Action Lab (2011) for reviews of the literature on the impact of prices on adoption of health interventions.
9. As discussed in more detail in Bundy, Appleby, and others (2017), Croke and others (2016) argued that an influential earlier study (Taylor-Robinson and others 2015) was underpowered to reject the hypothesis that MDA is cost-effective in increasing weight. Croke and others (2016) doubled the sample of 11 estimates of the effect of multiple-dose MDA for worms on weight and updated some of the estimates in Taylor-Robinson and others (2015), for example, by using micro-data provided by the original trial authors.
10. Hall and others (2006) conducted a cluster randomized study of the impact of deworming on health and test score outcomes in Vietnam. Because there is no publicly available version of this paper, we do not discuss this study in detail.

11. This measure includes the direct impact on the treated, as well as indirect impacts accruing to the untreated, population.
12. A parish is an administrative division in Uganda comprising several villages.
13. A two-part reanalysis (Aiken and others 2015; Davey and others 2015) questioned some aspects of this study. However, several independent analysts have cast doubt on the methods and conclusions of the reanalyses, and concluded that the studies leave the case for deworming fundamentally unchanged (see, for instance, Berger 2015; Clemens and Sandefur 2015; Healthcare Triage 2015; and Ozler 2015).
14. Several early studies assessed the impacts of deworming on school attendance, using individually randomized evaluations. For example, Simeon and others (1995) studied treatment among Jamaican children ages 6–12 years; Watkins, Cruz, and Pollitt (1996) studied treatment of children ages 7–12 years in rural Guatemala; and Kruger and others (1996) studied treatment of children ages 6–8 years in South Africa. None of these studies found an impact on school attendance. However, any gains are likely to be underestimated since these are individually randomized studies that do not consider treatment externalities. In addition, attendance in the Watkins, Cruz, and Pollitt (1996) study was measured through the use of school register data, which is unreliable in many low-income countries and which excluded any students who dropped out during the study. Since dropping out is very likely correlated with treatment status, there is a high risk that this gives a biased picture of school participation over time. There is also the potential for school officials to overstate attendance because of their awareness of the program and the data collection.
15. Hall and others (2006) similarly found no impact on test scores of deworming in Vietnam. As noted previously, there is no publicly available version of this paper, so we do not discuss this study further.
16. The original deworming trial was conducted in 48 communities in five districts in Eastern Uganda. Croke (2014) used educational data collected by the Uwezo project. The Uwezo survey randomly sampled communities and households from all five of these districts, creating in effect a random subsample of communities from the original trial. Croke (2014) provided evidence that the sampling of communities by Uwezo was effectively a random sample of the original trial clusters by showing that the communities have no statistically significant differences across a wide range of variables related to adult outcomes. To further support his econometric identification strategy, Croke (2014) explored the pattern of test scores of all children tested in these parishes. The youngest children would have been too young to receive more than two rounds of deworming, while the oldest children, at age 16 years, would have never received the program. One would expect that if effects are truly from the deworming intervention, the impacts would be lower at the two extremes and higher for children in the middle age group, which is what the study found.

17. Two earlier studies looked at the relationship between deworming and labor market outcomes using nonrandomized methods. Using a first-difference research design, Schapiro (1919) found wage gains of 15 percent to 27 percent on Costa Rican plantations after deworming. Weisbrod and others (1973) observed little contemporaneous correlation in the cross-section between worm infections and labor productivity in St. Lucia.

18. This abstracts from curvature of the utility function. Because deworming is inexpensive, and there is no evidence that deworming has serious side effects; because there is evidence for large effects in some cases; and because those with the highest-intensity infections are likely to be poorer than average, risk-averse policy makers or those concerned with equity would be more willing to institute mass deworming than this equation implies.

19. This estimate is conservative, only taking into account direct deworming benefits and ignoring positive externality benefits.

20. GiveWell (2016) calculates the cost of deworming for STHs in India to be US$0.30 per child per treatment, which includes both drug and delivery costs, including the value of staff time.

21. Another screening approach could be to simply ask individuals if they have experienced any of the common side effects of worm infections. Although this screening method is cheaper and potentially useful in environments where stool testing is not practical, it is likely to be very imprecise.

REFERENCES

Abdul Latif Jameel Poverty Action Lab. 2011. "The Price Is Wrong." J-PAL Policy Bulletin, Abdul Latif Jameel Poverty Action Lab, Cambridge, MA.

———. 2012. "Deworming: A Best Buy for Development." J-PAL Policy Bulletin, Abdul Latif Jameel Poverty Action Lab, Cambridge, MA.

Ahuja, A., S. Baird, J. Hamory Hicks, M. Kremer, E. Miguel, and others. 2015. "When Should Governments Subsidize Health? The Case of Mass Deworming." *World Bank Economic Review* 29 (Suppl 1): S9–24.

Aiken, A. M., C. Davey, J. R. Hargreaves, and R. J. Hayes. 2015. "Re-Analysis of Health and Educational Impacts of a School-Based Deworming Programme in Western Kenya: A Pure Replication." *International Journal of Epidemiology* 44 (5): 1572–80. doi:10.1093/ije/dyv127.

Alderman, H., J. Konde-Lule, I. Sebuliba, D. A. P. Bundy, and A. Hall. 2006. "Increased Weight Gain in Preschool Children Due to Mass Albendazole Treatment Given during 'Child Health Days' in Uganda: A Cluster Randomized Controlled Trial." *BMJ* 333: 122–26.

Assefa, L. M., T. Crellen, S. Kepha, J. H. Kihara, S. M. Njenga, and others. 2014. "Diagnostic Accuracy and Cost-Effectiveness of Alternative Methods for Detection of Soil-Transmitted Helminths in a Post-Treatment Setting in Western Kenya." *PLoS Neglected Tropical Diseases* 8 (5): e2843.

Baird, S., J. Hamory Hicks, M. Kremer, and E. Miguel. 2016. "Worms at Work: Long-Run Impacts of a Child Health Investment." *Quarterly Journal of Economics*. doi: 10.1093/qje/qjw022. Working Paper No. 21428, National Bureau of Economic Research, Cambridge, MA. http://qje.oxfordjournals.org/content/early/2016/07/14/qje.qjw022.abstract.

Barda, B., H. Zepherine, L. Rinaldi, G. Cringoli, R. Burioni, and others. 2013. "Mini-FLOTAC and Kato-Katz: Helminth Eggs Watching on the Shore of Lake Victoria." *Parasites and Vectors* 6: 220.

Berger, A. 2015. "New Deworming Reanalyses and Cochrane Review." *The GiveWell Blog*, July 24.

Bleakley, H. 2007. "Disease and Development: Evidence from Hookworm Eradication in the American South." *Quarterly Journal of Economics* 122 (1): 73–117.

———. 2010. "Health, Human Capital, and Development." *Annual Review of Economics* 2 (1): 283–310.

Bobonis, G. J., E. Miguel, and C. Puri-Sharma. 2006. "Anemia and School Participation." *Journal of Human Resources* 41 (4): 692–721.

Bundy, D. A. P., N. de Silva, S. Horton, G. C. Patton, L. Schultz, and D. T. Jamison. 2017. "Child and Adolescent Health and Development: Realizing Neglected Potential." In *Disease Control Priorities* (third edition): Volume 8, *Child and Adolescent Health and Development*, edited by D. A. P. Bundy, N. de Silva, S. Horton, D. T. Jamison, and G. C. Patton. Washington, DC: World Bank.

Bundy, D. A. P., L. Appleby, M. Bradley, K. Croke, T. D. Hollingsworth, and others. 2017. "Mass Deworming Programs in Middle Childhood and Adolescence." In *Disease Control Priorities* (third edition): Volume 8, *Child and Adolescent Health and Development*, edited by D. A. P. Bundy, N. de Silva, S. Horton, D. T. Jamison, and G. C. Patton. Washington, DC: World Bank.

Bundy, D. A. P., M. Kremer, H. Bleakley, M. C. Jukes, and E. Miguel. 2009. "Deworming and Development: Asking the Right Questions, Asking the Questions Right." *PLoS Neglected Tropical Diseases* 3 (1): e362.

Bundy, D. A. P., M. S. Wong, L. L. Lewis, and J. Jorton. 1990. "Control of Geohelminths by Delivery of Targeted Chemotherapy through Schools." *Transactions of the Royal Society of Tropical Medicine and Hygiene* 84 (1): 115–20.

Clemens, M., and J. Sandefur. 2015. "Mapping the Worm Wars: What the Public Should Take Away from the Scientific Debate about Mass Deworming." *The Center for Global Development Blog*, July 30.

Croke, K. 2014. "The Long Run Effects of Early Childhood Deworming on Literacy and Numeracy: Evidence from Uganda." Unpublished.

Croke, K., J. H. Hicks, E. Hsu, M. Kremer, and E. Miguel. 2016. "Does Mass Deworming Affect Child Nutrition? Meta-Analysis, Cost-Effectiveness, and Statistical Power." Working Paper 22382, National Bureau of Economic Research, Cambridge, MA.

Davey, C., A. M. Aiken, R. J. Hayes, and J. R. Hargreaves. 2015. "Re-Analysis of Health and Educational Impacts of a School-Based Deworming Programme in Western Kenya: A Statistical Replication of a Cluster Quasi-Randomized

Stepped-Wedge Trial." *International Journal of Epidemiology* 44 (5): 1581–92. doi:10.1093/ije/dyv128.

Dhaliwal, I., E. Duflo, R. Glennerster, and C. Tulloch. 2012. "Comparative Cost-Effectiveness Analysis to Inform Policy in Developing Countries: A General Framework with Applications for Education." Abdul Latif Jameel Poverty Action Lab, Cambridge, MA.

Dupas, P. 2014. "Getting Essential Health Products to Their End Users: Subsidize, but How Much?" *Science* 345: 1279–81.

Galloway, R., E. Kristjansson, A. Gelli, U. Meir, F. Espejo, and others. 2009. "School Feeding: Outcomes and Costs." *Food and Nutrition Bulletin* 30 (2): 171–82.

GiveWell. 2013. "Top Charities." http://www.givewell.org /charities/top-charities.

———. 2016. "Deworm the World Initiative, led by Evidence Action." http://www.givewell.org/international /top-charities/deworm-world-initiative#sources1155.

Hall, A., and S. Horton. 2008. "Best Practice Paper: Deworming." Copenhagen Consensus Center, Denmark.

Hall, A., L. Nguyen Bao Khanh, D. A. P. Bundy, N. Quan Dung, T. Son Hong, and others. 2006. "A Randomized Trial of Six Monthly Deworming on the Growth and Educational Achievements of Vietnamese School Children." Unpublished.

Healthcare Triage. 2015. "Replication, Re-Analysis, and Worm Wars." https://www.youtube.com/watch?v=9SCFlYlNlLQ.

Hicks, J. H., M. Kremer, and E. Miguel. 2015. "Commentary: Deworming Externalities and Schooling Impacts in Kenya: A Comment on Aiken et al. (2015) and Davey et al. (2015)." *International Journal of Epidemiology* 44 (5): 1593–6. doi:10.1093/ije/dyv129.

Hotez, P. J., D. H. Molyneux, A. Fenwick, J. Kumaresan, S. Ehrlich Sachs, and others. 2007. "Control of Neglected Tropical Diseases." *New England Journal of Medicine* 357: 1018–27.

Kabatereine, N., E. Tukahebwa, S. Brooker, H. Alderman, and A. Hall. 2001. "Epidemiology of Intestinal Helminth Infections among Schoolchildren in Southern Uganda." *East African Medical Journal* 78: 283–86.

Kremer, M., and R. Glennerster. 2011. "Improving Health in Developing Countries: Evidence from Randomized Evaluations." In *Handbook of Health Economics*, Volume 2, edited by M. V. Pauly, T. G. McGuire, and P. P. Barros. Oxford, U.K.: Elsevier Press.

Kremer, M., and A. Holla. 2009. "Pricing and Access: Lessons from Randomized Evaluations in Education and Health." In *What Works in Development: Thinking Big and Thinking Small*, edited by W. Easterly and J. Cohen. Washington, DC: Brookings Institution Press.

Kremer, M., and E. Miguel. 2007. "The Illusion of Sustainability." *Quarterly Journal of Economics* 112 (3): 1007–65.

Kruger, M., C. J. Badenhorst, E.P.G. Mansvelt, J.A. Laubscher, and A.J.S. Benade. 1996. "The Effect of Iron Fortification in a School Feeding Scheme and Anthelminthic Therapy on the Iron Status and Growth of 6–8-Year-Old School Children." *Food and Nutrition Bulletin* 17 (1).

Miguel, E., and M. Kremer. 2004. "Worms: Identifying Impacts on Education and Health in the Presence of Treatment Externalities." *Econometrica* 72 (1): 159–217.

———. 2014. "Guide to Replication of Miguel and Kremer 2004." http://emiguel.econ.berkeley.edu/research/worms -identifying-impacts-on-education-and-health-in-the -presence-of-treatment-externalities.

Ozier, O. 2014. "Exploiting Externalities to Estimate the Long-Term Effects of Early Childhood Deworming." Policy Research Working Paper 7052, World Bank, Washington, DC.

Ozler, B. 2015. "Worm Wars: A Review of the Reanalysis of Miguel and Kremer's Deworming Study." *Development Impact Blog*, July 24.

Schapiro, L. 1919. "The Physical and Economic Benefits of Treatment for Hookworm Disease." *Journal of the American Medical Association* 73: 1507–09.

Simeon, D. T., S. M. Grantham-McGregor, J. E. Callender, and M. S. Wong. 1995. "Treatment of *Trichuris trichiura* Infections Improves Growth, Spelling Scores and School Attendance in Some Children." *Journal of Nutrition* 125 (7): 1875–83.

Speich, B., S. Knopp, K. A. Mohammed, I. S. Khamis, L. Rinaldi, and others. 2010. "Comparative Cost Assessment of the Kato-Katz and FLOTAC Techniques for Soil-Transmitted Helminth Diagnosis in Epidemiological Surveys." *Parasites and Vectors* 3 (71): 1–11.

Taylor-Robinson, D. C., N. Maayan, K. Soares-Weiser, S. Donegan, and P. Garner. 2015. "Deworming Drugs for Soil-Transmitted Intestinal Worms in Children: Effects on Nutritional Indicators, Haemoglobin, and School Performance." *Cochrane Database of Systematic Reviews* 7: CD000371. doi:10.1002/14651858.CD000371 .pub6.

Uniting to Combat Neglected Tropical Diseases. 2014. "Delivering on Promises and Driving Progress." http:// unitingtocombatntds.org/sites/default/files/document /NTD_report_04102014_v4_singles.pdf.

Watkins, W. E., J. R. Cruz, and E. Pollitt. 1996. "The Effects of Deworming on Indicators of School Performance in Guatemala." *Transactions of the Royal Society of Tropical Medicine and Hygiene* 90 (2): 156–61.

Weisbrod, B. A., R. L. Andreano, R. E. Baldwin, and A. C. Kelley. 1973. *Disease and Economic Development: The Impact of Parasitic Diseases in St. Lucia*. Madison: University of Wisconsin Press.

WHO (World Health Organization). 2015. "Deworming to Combat the Health and Nutritional Impact of Helminth Infections." e-Library of Evidence for Nutrition Actions (eLENA), WHO, Geneva. http://www.who.int/elena/titles /deworming/en.

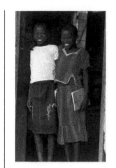

Chapter 30

The Effects of Education Quantity and Quality on Child and Adult Mortality: Their Magnitude and Their Value

Elina Pradhan, Elina M. Suzuki, Sebastián Martínez,
Marco Schäferhoff, and Dean T. Jamison

INTRODUCTION

This chapter analyzes the economic returns to education investments from a health perspective.[1] It estimates the effects of education on under-five mortality, adult mortality, and fertility. It calculates the economic returns to education resulting from declines in under-five mortality and adult mortality, while considering the effects of education investments on income. It also develops policy-relevant recommendations to help guide education investments.

Our study adds to the evidence that education is a crucial mechanism for enhancing the health and well-being of individuals. The relationship between education and health is bidirectional, because poor health could affect educational attainment (Behrman 1996; Case, Fertig, and Paxson 2005; Currie and Hyson 1999; Ding and others 2009). Historical findings in the education and health literature have highlighted the strong association between education and health. Recent literature has exploited natural experiments to provide causal evidence of the impact of education on health. Studies show that education plays a critical role in reducing the transmission of human immunodeficiency virus/acquired immune deficiency syndrome (HIV/AIDS) in women by improving prevention and treatment. Keeping adolescent girls in secondary school significantly attenuates the risk of HIV/AIDS infection

(Baird and others 2012; Behrman 2015; De Neve and others 2015). Early child development has a lifelong impact on the mental and physical health of individuals.[2] Other studies have demonstrated that progress in education can increase positive health-seeking behaviors (such as accessing preventive care) and reduce overall dependency on the health system (Cutler and Lleras-Muney 2010; Feinstein and others 2006; Kenkel 1991; Sabates and Feinstein 2006).

Previous literature on education, health, and economic productivity suggests that the impact of education is more significant in times of rapid technological progress (Preston and Haines 1991; Schultz 1993). The morbidity and mortality differentials across levels of schooling are significant in the presence of increasing scientific knowledge about diseases and behaviors, as well as access to medicines and vaccines. Additionally, analysis by Jamison, Murphy, and Sandbu (2016) shows that most variation in under-five mortality can be explained by heterogeneities in the speed at which countries adopt low-cost health technologies to increase child survival.

Different studies that have assessed the effects of education on mortality and fertility show an association between educational attainment and reductions in both outcomes.[3] This chapter goes beyond previous work by using improved and updated data, and by controlling

Corresponding author: Elina Pradhan, Harvard T. H. Chan School of Public Health, Boston, Massachusetts, United States; epradhan@mail.harvard.edu.

tightly for country-specific effects in both levels and rates of change of mortality. Although several studies have examined the effects of female schooling on child mortality, we are aware of only one other cross-national study (Wang and Jamison 1998) that estimated the macro effects of schooling on adult mortality. Other studies have focused on the relationship between schooling and adult health, but they primarily do so for a single country or small set of countries.[4] Some key findings from our study are highlighted in box 30.1.

Our study comes at a critical juncture for education and health, as the global community moves forward in the context of the Sustainable Development Goals, which stress the importance of taking into account the cross-sectoral nature of global development challenges.

This chapter is organized into three broad sections:

- The first section presents the results of our regression analysis, which examines the effects of increases in mean years of schooling, as well as schooling quality, on under-five mortality, adult female mortality, adult male mortality, and fertility. We also decompose the changes in mortality between 1970 and 2010, and estimate the mortality impact of education gains in the Millennium Development Goal (MDG) period. The findings from our regression inform the subsequent sections, which use the estimated effect size to determine the rates of return to and benefit-cost ratios (BCRs) of education.
- The second section explores the effects of augmenting the traditional rates of return analysis for education

with its mortality-related health effects. We also estimate the BCR of education from earnings-only and health-inclusive perspectives, and address the question: What would be the returns to investing US$1 in education in low-, lower-middle-, and upper-middle-income countries?

- Finally, we discuss our findings, present recommendations, and consider the next steps the global education community might take to ensure that all countries make substantial progress toward global education targets.

MODELING THE EFFECTS OF EDUCATIONAL ATTAINMENT ON HEALTH

Data and Methods

We estimated the effects of educational attainment over time, measured in mean years of schooling for ages 25 years and older. This age group was selected to ensure that the data were unlikely to contain censored observations.[5] Data on mean years of schooling were obtained through the Barro and Lee (2013) dataset, which includes 92 low- and middle-income countries (LMICs), each of which included observations at five-year intervals between 1970 and 2010. Mortality rates were defined as the probability of dying between age 0 and age 5 years for under-five mortality, and the probability of dying between age 15 and age 60 years for adult mortality. The United Nations (UN) World Population Prospects (2015 revision) was used for all fertility and mortality estimates (table 30.1). Annex 30A contains a full list of countries included in

---

Box 30.1

Key Findings

Of the impressive reductions in mortality seen in low- and middle-income countries (LMICs) between 1970 and 2010, we estimate that 14 percent of the reductions in under-five mortality, 30 percent of the reductions in adult female mortality, and 31 percent of the reductions in adult male mortality can be attributed to gains in female schooling. Quality (as measured by standardized test scores) also has a substantial effect on health outcomes.

Gains in educational attainment during the Millennium Development Goals period saved an

estimated 7.3 million lives in LMICs between 2010 and 2015.

The health benefits of additional schooling are higher for earlier years of schooling. The marginal impact of schooling at the primary level is higher compared with the impact at the secondary level.

Every dollar invested in schooling would return US$10 in low-income and US$3.8 in lower-middle-income countries. These values reflect increased earnings plus the value of reductions in under-five and adult mortality.

Table 30.1 Sources of Data in the Study

Variable	Description	Data sources
Educational attainment (mean years of schooling)	Mean years of total schooling among the population ages 25 years and older. Both overall and gender-specific estimates were used.	Barro and Lee (2013) dataset, version 2.0
Standardized achievement test scores	Aggregate standardized test scores, developed by Angrist, Patrinos, and Schlotter (2013) on the basis of global and regional achievement tests.	World Bank EdStats Global Achievement database
Under-five mortality	Probability of dying between birth and exact age five years, expressed as deaths per 1,000 live births.	UN World Population Prospects 2015
Adult mortality	Expressed as deaths under age 60 years per 1,000 alive at age 15 years, calculated at current age-specific mortality rates. Both overall and sex-specific estimates were used.	UN World Population Prospects 2015
Male and female deaths, by broad age group	Number of male/female deaths by five-year age groups.	UN World Population Prospects 2015
Fertility	Total fertility rate (children per woman).	UN World Population Prospects 2015
GDP per capita	Per capita expenditure-side real GDP (PPP-adjusted).	Penn World Tables, version 8.1 (April 2015) (Feenstra, Inklaar, and Timmer 2015)

Note: GDP = gross domestic product; PPP = purchasing power parity; UN = United Nations.

the analysis. Definitions of age groupings and age-specific terminology used in this volume can be found in chapter 1 (Bundy and others 2017).

Regression Models

We modeled the effects of educational attainment (female schooling, male schooling, and overall schooling) on under-five mortality, adult female mortality, and adult male mortality controlling for time and income (gross domestic product [GDP] per capita) using hierarchical linear models (HLMs) as in equation (30.1). Jamison, Murphy, and Sandbu (2016) provide a range of comparative models on under-five mortality and assess their statistical properties. They concluded that the HLM structure has the best fit to macro-level data to determine the macro-level impact of education on mortality, and we therefore develop their modeling approach here.

$$y_{it} = \beta_0 + \beta_1 educ_{it} + \sum_{a=1}^{t} \beta_{2a} time_t$$
$$+ \beta_3 Log(GDP_{PC}) + \beta_{2i} time_t + u_i + \in_{it}$$
(30.1)

The under-five mortality model estimates the impact of adult education (education of those ages 25 years and older) on the mortality of those under age 5 at each time period *t*, while the adult mortality models estimate the impact of adult education on aggregate adult mortality or self and peer mortality, adjusting for income, any technological advancements, and secular time trends. Time is specified as a categorical variable that indicates

five-year increments from 1970 to 2010, and is a proxy variable for measuring technological progress over the study period. Annex 30B contains descriptive statistics for countries included in the regression, including means and standard deviations for mortality and fertility rates, years of schooling, and test scores.

Preston (1975, 2007) shows that national income plays a critical role in improving health outcomes. He further argues that factors exogenous to income have played a crucial role in improving mortality. An influential paper by Pritchett and Summers (1996) pointed to education as well as income as being among the important factors influencing mortality decline. As highlighted by Jamison, Murphy, and Sandbu (2016), technological progress, which includes research, development and implementation advances in vaccines, sanitation, clinical care, and disease control, has played a driving role in improving health outcomes in recent years. In line with these authors, we also loosened the assumption of homogeneity of technical advancements across countries. By allowing the impact of time or technological progress to vary every five years, and by allowing for a country-specific impact of technological progress on mortality in addition to controlling for GDP, we provide conservative estimates of the impact of education on mortality and fertility. Annex 30C provides additional details on the model, and annex 30D tabulates all regression results in detail.

Decomposition Analysis

Results from the regressions were then used to decompose the changes in under-five, adult male, and female mortality between 1970 and 2010. In this analysis, we first calculate the difference in mean covariates in the sample in 2010 compared with 1970. Then, we calculate the overall reduction in mortality when education increases by the difference in mean from 2010 to 1970, which is the impact estimate from the HLM model multiplied by the difference in the mean of that covariate. The fraction attributable to any particular covariate is then the overall reduction in mortality attributable to the changes in that particular covariate, divided by the overall change in mortality over the period. For example, equation (30.2) illustrates the estimation process for the fraction attributable to education, $\Delta Mort_{ed}$, where $\Delta Educ = \overline{Educ_{2010}} - \overline{Educ_{1970}}$ and β_{ed} = the estimate of impact of education on mortality from the HLM model.

$$\Delta Mort_{ed} = \frac{\beta_{ed} \times \Delta Educ}{\beta_{ed} \times \Delta Educ + \beta_{gdp} \times \Delta GDP + \beta_{2010} \times \Delta T}$$

(30.2)

Estimating the Mortality Impact of Education Gains in the MDG Period

To understand the impact of education gains during the MDG period on under-five and adult mortality, we also estimate the number of excess deaths that could have

occurred had educational attainment stayed at the 1990 levels. In this analysis, we model the counterfactual scenario of the number of additional deaths during 2010–15 had education stagnated at 1990 levels, where we apply the increases in education in low-income countries (LICs) and lower-middle-income countries to the coefficient from our HLM results to calculate the excess deaths. Annex table 30C.2 provides estimation details.

Results

Effects of Schooling on Adult and Under-Five Mortality and Fertility

We modeled the effects of education based on three different schooling variables: mean years of schooling for girls, boys, and both genders. The results of our analysis, which examined female and male adult mortality separately, make an important contribution to the existing evidence base. Very few studies have focused on any potential impacts that educational attainment may have on adult mortality at the macro level. To the best of our knowledge, the most recent cross-country study that specifically assessed the macro effects of schooling on adult mortality is from 1998 (Wang and Jamison 1998).

Table 30.2 shows the results of our hierarchical models; each column represents the results for the five dependent variables—overall adult mortality, adult male mortality, adult female mortality, under-five mortality,

Table 30.2 Impact of Schooling on Health Outcomes: Results from Hierarchical Linear Models

	Dependent Variables				
	Ln[Adult mortality rate], both sexes	Ln[Adult mortality rate], male	Ln[Adult mortality rate], female	Ln[Under-five mortality rate]	Ln[Total fertility rate]
Independent variables					
Panel A:					
Mean years of schooling, both sexes	−0.030***	−0.025**	−0.031***	−0.033**	−0.024***
Ln[GDP per capita]	−0.057***	−0.040**	−0.083***	−0.13***	−0.047***
Panel B:					
Mean years of schooling (female)	−0.030***	−0.022**	−0.037***	−0.042***	−0.024***
Schooling ratio (male:female)	0.016	0.019*	0.010	−0.009	−0.011
Ln[GDP per capita]	−0.052**	−0.034*	−0.079***	−0.13***	−0.047***
Panel C:					
Mean years of schooling (male)	−0.015	−0.014	−0.010	−0.015	−0.015*
Schooling ratio (male:female)	0.018*	0.020**	0.013	−0.008	−0.011
Ln[GDP per capita]	−0.058***	−0.039**	−0.084***	−0.13***	−0.047***

Note: GDP = gross domestic product. Ln[x] denotes natural log of variable x. Period: 1970–2010. Countries: 80. Observations: 688. Standard errors and goodness of fit measures reported in annex 30D.
*p < .10; **p < .05; ***p < .01.

and fertility. Panel A shows results for models in which we consider the impact of average male and female schooling on the five health outcomes. Panels B and C show the impact of female and male schooling, respectively, while controlling for the ratio of male to female years of schooling. The schooling ratio is included to control for any differential impact of male and female schooling in panels B and C, respectively.

Table 30.2 demonstrates that improvements in female educational attainment drove declines in mortality and fertility in LMICs between 1970 and 2010: A one-year increase in a country's mean years of schooling (both sexes) is associated with a 2.5 percent reduction in male adult mortality and 3.1 percent reduction in female adult mortality, a 3.3 percent reduction in under-five mortality, and a 2.4 percent reduction in the total fertility rate (TFR), in LMICs (panel A of table). The effect of male schooling on adult and under-five mortality and TFR is small and often not significant. In contrast, improvements in female schooling are associated with large declines in both female and male adult mortality, accounting for much of the observed effects of education on health. A one-year increase in mean years of schooling for girls (panel B of table) is associated with reductions in female and male adult mortality of 3.7 percent and 2.2 percent, respectively; under-five mortality declines by 4.2 percent, and the TFR by 2.4 percent. The comparison of the effect of male (panel C of table) and female schooling (large effect) on adult mortality, under-five mortality, and fertility clearly shows that the education-related declines in mortality between 1970 and 2010 in LMICs are strongly linked to increases in female schooling.[6]

Decomposition Analysis: Reductions in Adult and Under-Five Mortality Rates from Gains in Female Schooling, 1970 2010

Based on the results of our HLM, we developed estimates of the proportion of mortality reductions between 1970 and 2010 that can be attributed to improvements in female schooling. Adult female, adult male, and under-five mortality all saw impressive reductions over this period, with particularly dramatic improvements seen in under-five mortality. Between 1970 and 2010, the global under-five mortality rate declined by 64 percent, from 139 deaths under age five years per 1,000 live births to 50 in 2010. In LICs, gains have been particularly strong since 1990: under-five mortality declined by more than 50 percent, from 186 deaths per 1,000 live births to 91, during this 20-year span. The adult mortality rate, that is, the probability that a person dies (expressed per thousand persons) between age 15 and age 60 at prevailing mortality rates, also recorded a notable decline between 1970 and 2010, falling 38 percent globally, from 247 to 153. Reductions in

adult female mortality were particularly substantial, declining by 43 percent over the 40-year period.

Our decomposition analysis suggests that of the reductions in mortality seen in LICs and middle-income countries (MICs) between 1970 and 2010, 14 percent of reductions in under-five mortality, 30 percent of reductions in adult female mortality, and 31 percent of reductions in adult male mortality can be attributed to gains in female schooling (figure 30.1, panel A). This panel shows that technological progress, and to a much lesser extent income, affected mortality over this period, a finding in line with other studies (Jamison, Murphy, and Sandbu 2016).

Mortality Impact of Increases in Educational Attainment during the MDG Period

A complementary way of assessing the magnitude of education's impact on mortality is to look at the reduction in the number of deaths resulting from a given increase in education levels. We take as an example the increase in female education in LMICs during the MDG period from 1990 to 2015. This increase was 1.5 years in LICs and 2.4 years in MICs. We ask the question: Based on the results of our model (table 30.2), how many more deaths would have occurred in children under age 5 years and in adults ages 15–59 years if education levels had remained at their 1990 levels? Panel B of figure 30.1 shows the results. We estimate that a total of 7.3 million under-five and adult deaths were averted between 2010 and 2015 because of increases in educational attainment since 1990. Total deaths averted in MICs were substantially higher than in LICs because the population exposed to mortality risk is about six times larger in MICs compared with LICs, and MICs saw a greater increase in average years of female schooling during the MDG period than did LICs.

Effects of Different Levels of Schooling on Mortality and Fertility

In addition to analyzing the overall impact of increasing average schooling by one year in a country, we considered whether differential effects accrue at different levels of schooling (table 30.3). We conducted a quadratic analysis that relaxes the assumption that each additional year of schooling has the same impact on health, hence allowing the relative change in mortality with changing years of attainment to be evaluated.[7] Our analysis indicates that additional years of schooling have sustained effects on all the health outcomes we examined. The coefficient on the squared years of female schooling term is positive and significant for all health outcomes, indicating that the

Figure 30.1 Education's Contribution to Mortality Decline

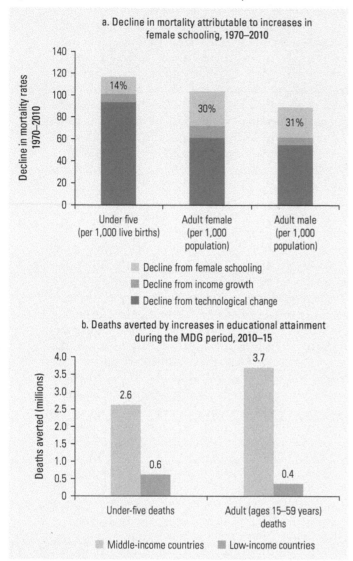

a. Decline in mortality attributable to increases in female schooling, 1970–2010

Decline from female schooling

Decline from income growth

Decline from technological change

b. Deaths averted by increases in educational attainment during the MDG period, 2010–15

Middle-income countries

Low-income countries

Note: MDG = Millennium Development Goal.

relative effect of education on health outcomes declines with increasing years of educational attainment. This result means that the marginal impact of schooling at the primary level is higher compared with the impact at the secondary level.

Effects of Educational Quality

In addition to the effect of years of schooling on health, we evaluated the effects of educational quality on health outcomes. This analysis proved challenging for a variety of reasons. Most fundamentally, cross-country data on educational quality are extremely limited, particularly for LICs and lower-middle-income countries. Researchers have used results from global or regional achievement tests (such as PISA, TIMSS, SACMEQ, PASEC, and LLECE[8]) to standardize estimates of educational quality, based on country performance on such exams. However, significant gaps remain in both longitudinal and country coverage, and concerns have been raised about the validity of using results from a limited set of tests as a proxy for educational quality.

Because of the limited number of LMICs with longitudinal data on quality, we expanded our analysis to include high-income countries (HICs) with data on quality in the Barro and Lee (2013) dataset. Annex 30A provides a full list of countries used in the HLM regressions on quality.

To evaluate the impact of education quality on health, we ran an augmented version of the HLM in table 30.2, panel B, to which we added a variable measuring schooling quality (standardized achievement test scores).

Our findings largely underscore the robustness of the impact of years of schooling on health outcomes, and further suggest that quality can have an additive and substantial impact on health outcomes (table 30.4).

Table 30.3 Impact of Schooling Levels on Health Outcomes

	Dependent Variables				
	Ln[Adult mortality rate], both sexes	Ln[Adult mortality rate], male	Ln[Adult mortality rate], female	Ln[Under-five mortality rate]	Ln[Total fertility rate]
Independent variables					
Mean years of female schooling (linear)	−0.081***	−0.071***	−0.089***	−0.14***	−0.10***
Mean years of female schooling (quadratic)	0.005***	0.005***	0.005***	0.010***	0.008***
Ln[GDP per capita]	−0.043**	−0.026	−0.070***	−0.11***	−0.032**

Note: GDP = gross domestic product. Ln[x] denotes natural log of variable x. Period: 1970–2010. Countries: 80. Observations: 688. Standard errors and goodness of fit measures reported in annex 30D.
*$p < .10$; **$p < .05$; ***$p < .01$.

Table 30.4 Impact of School Quality on Health Outcomes: Results from Hierarchical Linear Models

| | Dependent variables | | | | | |
| | Ln[Adult mortality rate], both sexes | | Ln[Under-five mortality rate] | | Ln[Total fertility rate] | |
Independent variables	(A)	(B)	(A)	(B)	(A)	(B)
Mean years of schooling (female)	–0.017*	–0.016*	–0.057***	–0.058***	–0.031***	–0.031***
Schooling ratio (male:female)	–0.013	–0.019	0.19***	0.18***	0.20***	0.20***
Ln[GDP per capita]	–0.020***	–0.20***	–0.45***	–0.46***	–0.16***	–0.16***
Test scores		–0.0025**		–0.0035**		–0.00024

Note: GDP = gross domestic product. Ln[x] denotes natural log of variable x. Period: 1970–2010. Countries: 103. Observations: 362. Standard errors and goodness of fit measures reported in annex 30D.
*p < .10; **p < .05; ***p < .01.

Table 30.5 Impact on Health Outcomes of a One Standard Deviation Change in Education Quantity and Quality

| | Dependent Variables | | | | |
Independent variables	Ln[Adult mortality rate], both sexes	Ln[Adult mortality rate], male	Ln[Adult mortality rate], female	Ln[Under-five mortality rate]	Ln[Total fertility rate]
Test scores	–0.024**	–0.02*	–0.023**	–0.034**	–0.002
Mean years of schooling (female)	–0.048*	–0.033	–0.072**	–0.18***	–0.093***
Ratio (years:test scores)	2.0	1.7	3.1	5.2	40

Note: Appendix 30B, table 30B.5 tabulates the mean and standard deviation of the test scores and years of schooling used in this analysis. Ln[x] denotes natural log of variable x. Period: 1970–2010. Countries: 103. Observations: 362.
*p < .10; **p < .05; ***p < .01.

Column (B) under each dependent variable shows the results of the HLM model with education quality proxied by the composite test scores. Comparison of the returns to mean years of schooling in column (B) as compared to column (A), where the HLM model does not control for quality, shows that the impact of returns to schooling is about the same with or without controlling for test scores. In fact, improvements in test scores are predicted to reduce mortality and fertility further, above and beyond the improvements in years of schooling.

Given the substantial difference in a one-unit change between educational attainment (one year of schooling) and test scores (a one-point increase in scores), we also present the results of both quantity and quality by using a one standard deviation change above their mean values to enable better comparability between the two (table 30.5). The results of this analysis suggest that the impact of quality is substantial. A one standard deviation change in educational quality, measured by standardized achievement scores, is associated with a 2.4 percent decline in the overall adult mortality rate, a 2.3 percent decrease in adult female mortality, and a 3.4 percent decrease in under-five mortality. In all cases, however, the impact of female educational attainment remains larger than the impact of educational quality. For the three health outcomes for which both years of schooling and test scores are significant—overall adult mortality, female mortality, and under-five mortality—the impact of female years of schooling ranges from 2 to 5.2 times the impact of quality.

Our estimates of the magnitude of the effect of education quality on under-five mortality substantially exceed those of Jamison, Jamison, and Hanushek (2007), perhaps because (1) we estimate the impact on under-five mortality rather than on infant mortality, and (2) we have more observations from LMICs than these authors. However, our sample would still benefit from additional observations for LICs, lower-middle-income countries, and upper-middle-income countries (UMICs).

Our findings show that the impact of school quality on health outcomes is considerable and merits further scrutiny. It also highlights the limitations of the data, a challenge that should be considered when interpreting these results. Of the 103 countries included in the analysis, 59 countries have fewer than four years of observations. Of those with four or more observations, 35—or 80 percent of the sample—are HICs. Further work is needed to develop robust measures of education quality that are comparable across countries and tracked over time.

CALCULATING HEALTH-INCLUSIVE RATES OF RETURN TO EDUCATION AND BENEFIT-COST RATIOS

Previous analyses have estimated the returns to education. Using household and labor market survey data, Montenegro and Patrinos (2013, 2014) have estimated the private returns accruing from increased schooling. They note that three major findings have held across analyses:

- Private returns to schooling tend to remain in the range of 10 percent per year of schooling.
- Returns are, on average, higher in LMICs.
- Returns to primary schooling are higher than returns to secondary schooling.

When estimating private returns to education, researchers assume that costs of schooling are absorbed by the government and that the only costs to students are the opportunity costs of forgone earnings; any gains reflect the income differential between the earnings earned by students with different levels of educational attainment. The term *social rates of return* refers to the rate of return to education when the full cost of schooling is incorporated. In an analysis of 15 LMICs, Psacharopoulos, Montenegro, and Patrinos (2017) further considered the full cost of schooling. They found that the social rates of return to primary education were higher than those to secondary and tertiary education for both LICs and lower-middle-income countries.[9]

Our analysis makes an important contribution to existing research on the rates of return to education by expanding the traditional focus on earnings returns to consider some health-related (nonmarket) externalities associated with increased educational attainment (Lochner 2011; Oreopoulos and Salvanes 2011). By capturing reductions in mortality, our analysis provides a more comprehensive evaluation of returns to schooling and strengthens the investment case for education by quantifying health returns in addition to earnings returns.

Methods

The empirical work conducted as a first step in this analysis generated coefficients for the effect of one additional year of female education on under-five mortality, adult female mortality, and adult male mortality. In this section, we use these coefficients to generate the valuation of these changes in monetary terms. Earlier research by our team, funded by the Norwegian government, reviewed available evidence on the effects of education and then estimated the economic returns resulting from the reduction in under-five mortality attributable to increases in female education (Schäferhoff and others 2015). Our analysis follows the general approach used in this previous study, but improves the methodology and expands it to incorporate the monetary value of both under-five and adult mortality reductions.[10]

The literature in economics of education typically reports its benefit-cost analyses as internal rates of return, namely, the value of the discount rate that makes equal the present values of the cost and benefit streams. We calculate both the rate of return and more standard benefit to cost ratios.

Estimating both internal rates of return and BCRs involved the following four broad steps:

First, we used the effects of education on under-five mortality, adult male mortality, and adult female mortality from our cross-country regressions as the basis for our health-inclusive rate-of-return (RoR) and BCR analysis. From the regressions, we obtained the level of mortality reductions resulting from one more year of female schooling for each income group. For example, the average years of schooling in lower-middle-income countries is six years; our RoR and BCR calculations for these countries then estimated the rate of return to increasing female schooling from six years, on average, to seven years.

Second, applying methods similar to Global Health 2035 (Jamison and others 2013a, 2013b) and our Norwegian Agency for Development Cooperation (Norad) study, we placed dollar values on these mortality reductions. We calculated the expected health value at age a, expressed in dollars, associated with the assumed one-year increase in education level using the information on dollar value of mortality reductions combined with status quo mortality rates and fertility rates. The value-of-a-life-year (VLY) methodology used here underestimates the VLY in LICs compared with UMICs. While there is some evidence in the literature to support this assumption because the economic component of the VLY is dependent on the economic productivity of a country, there is limited reason to assume that the social VLY would differ by a country's economic productivity (Stenberg and others 2016). We applied a conservative value of a statistical life (VSL) estimate in our study, and provide upper and lower bounds of RoR estimates and BCRs in annex 30D to illustrate the uncertainty around life year valuations.

Third, we calculated the earnings value for an increment in education. We received smoothed age-earnings profiles for LICs, lower-middle-income countries, and UMICs from Psacharopoulos, Montenegro, and Patrinos (2017) for different levels of schooling. We then estimated the marginal increase in earnings at each age across each schooling level (as in our example, where we estimated the expected level of mortality reductions resulting from one additional year of schooling for individuals with a starting level of six years). The earnings value of this increment in education for a person of age a is simply the difference between the age-earnings profiles of a secondary school graduate and a primary school graduate divided by the number of years of secondary schooling.

Fourth, we drew on cost data from the International Commission on Financing Global Education Opportunity, which provides estimates of the direct cost (c_1) for schooling at the respective grade levels in each income group (table 30.6). The direct cost is the cost of teacher time, implicit rent on facilities, and consumables such as textbooks. We assumed that if children are in school, they forgo earnings, so the earning value of a person of age a will be negative at the age of entry for the additional year of schooling (A). The direct cost of schooling at ages greater than A is assumed to be zero. Similarly, the opportunity cost (c_2) of attending one more year of school was calculated as the earnings forgone by attending one more year of school. Similar to direct costs, the opportunity costs of schooling at ages greater than A is also zero. Annex 30E discusses our approach in estimating the direct and opportunity costs of schooling in detail, and it tabulates the costs used in our analysis.

Table 30.6 Direct per-pupil annual costs of schooling (unweighted), in 2012 US$

	Low income	Lower middle income	Upper middle income
Primary	$68	$230	$1,300
Lower secondary	$140	$300	$1,400
Upper secondary	$300	$430	$1,300

Note: The table includes the estimated average (unweighted) per pupil costs by income group (YR2012, in 2012 US$). These cost estimates were provided by the International Commission on Financing Global Education Opportunity and were also used by Psacharopoulos, Patrinos, and Montenegro (2017).

Estimating Internal Rate of Return

Equation (30.3) expresses the net present value of costs and benefits ($ePVNR[r_s]$), in a standard RoR (r_s) analysis:

$$ePVNR(r_s) = \sum_{a=A}^{65} \frac{ev(a) - c_1(a) - c_2(a)}{(1+r_s)^{a-A}}. \quad (30.3)$$

The standard RoR (r_s) is simply the value of r_s such that the net present value of earnings ($ePVNR[r_s]$) is zero. Standard RoRs calculated are then compared with the health-inclusive RoRs, which we label hRoRs. Equation (30.4) gives the present value of net benefits when the benefit stream is augmented by the value of education's health effect:

$$hPVNB(r_h) = \sum_{a=A}^{65} \frac{ev(a) + hv(a) - c_1(a) - c_2(a)}{(1+r_h)^{a-A}}. \quad (30.4)$$

The health-inclusive RoR (r_h), hRoR, is simply that value of r_h such that the health-inclusive net present value ($hPVNR(r_h)$) is zero.

Estimating Benefit-Cost Ratios

To calculate the health-inclusive BCRs, we simply apply the annual discount rate of 3 percent to all costs and benefits. The health-inclusive BCR at discount rate (r), $hBCR(r)$, is listed below in equation (30.5), and the earnings-only BCR, $eBCR(r)$ in equation (30.6).

$$hBCR(r) = \frac{\sum_{a=A}^{65} \left[ev(a)(1+r)^{A-a} + hv(a)(1+r)^{A-a} \right]}{\sum_{a=A}^{65} \left[c_1(a)(1+r)^{A-a} + c_2(a)(1+r)^{A-a} \right]}$$

$$(30.5)$$

$$eBCR(r) = \frac{\sum_{a=A}^{65} \left[ev(a)(1+r)^{A-a} \right]}{\sum_{a=A}^{65} \left[c_1(a)(1+r)^{A-a} + c_2(a)(1+r)^{A-a} \right]}$$

$$(30.6)$$

Annex 30D provides the detailed methods used for RoR and BCR calculations, and an example of how benefits to reductions in under-five and adult male and female mortalities are valued.

Results

Health-Inclusive Rate of Return from Investments in Education

The standard social rate of return or earnings return is the rate of return to schooling considering direct costs, opportunity costs, and earnings benefits from schooling. Our initial calculations suggest that the earnings return of investing in an additional year of schooling in LICs is 11 percent (table 30.7). These standard social rates of return, however, do not consider other social benefits of schooling. Here, we consider the added benefit of schooling on potential reductions in under-five mortality, adult male mortality, and adult female mortality.

Including the health benefits due to an additional year of schooling, the rate of return to investing in an additional year of schooling in LICs increases to 16 percent (14 percent to 18 percent).[11] This means that the rate of return to education increases significantly when the returns to education resulting from reductions in adult mortality and under-five mortality are added to the standard rate of return.

Figure 30.2 demonstrates that the health benefits accruing from education are comparable to and at certain ages even exceed earnings benefits in LICs. This is particularly true during early adulthood (ages 20–40 years), when the benefits of reduced adult and under-five mortality are 20 percent larger than the earnings benefits. The protective benefit of education for reducing under-five mortality is particularly impressive in these settings, where under-five mortality rates remain high.

The health-inclusive social rate of return calculations that consider health benefits show that the returns resulting from lower mortality are high in lower-middle-income countries, where the updated social returns with health, at 9.3 percent (8.4 percent to 10 percent) are 34 percent (21 percent to 46 percent) of the standard social rate of return (see table 30.7 and figure 30.3).

In addition to calculating rates of return for LICs and lower-middle-income countries, we estimate that the standard social rate of return of increasing schooling by a year in UMICs is 3.0 percent (table 30.7 and figure 30.4). The health-inclusive RoR is 4.7 percent (4.1 percent to 5.3 percent), which is approximately 55 percent (36 percent to 74 percent) of the returns from earnings.

The results tabulated in the chapter consider the VSL to be 130 times GDP per capita, which is a conservative estimate compared with the Global Health 2035 series and our previous Norad report. The estimated health-inclusive rates of return are sensitive to the VSL assigned to mortality reductions. In annex figure 30F.1, we also present the estimated internal rates of return at VSLs of 80 to 180 times GDP per capita. At 14 percent and 8.5 percent rates of return, the health-inclusive returns to education are high in LICs and lower-middle-income countries, respectively, even with the lowest VSL multiplier used.

The health-inclusive rates of return are relatively larger in lower-middle-income countries, compared with UMICs, because of higher mortality in lower-middle-income countries. In particular, the returns to reductions in under-five mortality are higher in lower-middle-income countries than in UMICs, where under-five mortality rates are less than half those in lower-middle-income countries. As shown in figure 30.4, the earnings benefits of schooling are consistently higher than the health benefits across all ages in UMICs. In addition, compared with lower-middle-income countries, the absolute value of health benefits and earnings benefits are higher in UMICs because of differences in GDP and VSL valuations across these two income groups.

Table 30.7 Rate of Return of One Additional Year of Schooling in LICs, Lower-Middle-Income Countries, and UMICs

percent

	Standard private rate of return	Without health benefits (standard social rate of return)	Health-inclusive social rate of return
IRR			
LICs	16	11	16
Lower-middle-income countries	9.0	7.0	9.3
UMICs	5.0	3.0	4.7
Benefits and costs included			
Health benefits	No	No	Yes
Earnings benefits	Yes	Yes	Yes
Direct cost of an additional year of schooling	No	Yes	Yes
Opportunity cost of attending an additional year of schooling	Yes	Yes	Yes

Note: IRR = internal rate of return; LICs = low-income countries; UMICs = upper-middle-income countries.

Benefit-Cost Analysis

In addition to the internal rate of return, the returns to education can alternatively be conceptualized in the form of a benefit-cost analysis. Our results suggest that there is an enormous payoff to investing in education when investments are assessed from a health perspective. Every dollar invested in female schooling in LICs and lower-middle-income countries would return US$10 and US$3.8, respectively, in earnings and reductions in under-five and adult mortality.

For our analysis, we assumed a discount rate of 3.0 percent, which is consistent with the discount rate used in other benefit-cost calculations in public health, including the 2013 *Lancet* Commission on Investing in Health. Although benefits exceed costs for all income groups even when taking into account only the earnings effects of education, the additional benefits from health are significant, particularly in LICs and lower-middle-income countries.

As with RoR estimates, the BCRs are also estimated with some uncertainty. We present sensitivity analyses of the ratios in annex figure 30F.1 where we estimate BCRs for a VSL ranging from 80 to 180 times GDP per capita. In annex figure 30F.2 we present the range of BCR estimates for discount rates from 1.0 percent to 5.0 percent. Similar to internal rate of return results, we find that the health-inclusive benefit of an additional year of schooling is substantial for LICs and lower-middle-income countries even at the lowest VSL multiplier used, with returns of US$8.3 and US$3.3, respectively, for every dollar spent.

In LICs, the health benefits of education represent an impressive 92 percent increase over the earnings-only BCR; in lower-middle-income countries, health augments the traditional BCR by 44 percent. Put in other terms, 48 percent (US$4.7) of returns would come from the effect of schooling on mortality in LICs, while 31 percent (US$1.1) of the returns to education in lower-middle-income countries result from the effect on adult and under-five mortality. Even in UMICs, where lower mortality rates and higher educational attainment might suggest smaller gains, the BCR increases by 47 percent when health is taken into account, with health gains representing 32 percent (US$0.47) of the health-inclusive BCR (table 30.8).

DISCUSSION

Our results on under-five mortality are broadly consistent with previous robust analyses of the effect of schooling on under-five mortality, including that of Jamison, Murphy, and Sandbu (2016), who found that a one-year increase in female education was associated with a 3.6 percent decline in under-five mortality among 95 LMICs between 1970 and 2004. Our study, and other tightly

Figure 30.2 Benefit Stream for LICs from One Additional Year of Schooling

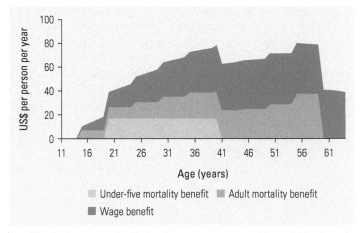

Note: LICs = low-income countries. The benefit streams are per person with one additional year of schooling. Our models assume that the health benefits accrue only to female schooling but that the wage benefits accrue to both males and females. Hence, the estimates of the dollar value of health benefits is a weighted average with the weight depending on the fraction of the educated cohort that is female. The calculations assume the cohort is 50 percent female.

Figure 30.3 Benefit Stream for Lower-Middle-Income Countries from One Additional Year of Schooling

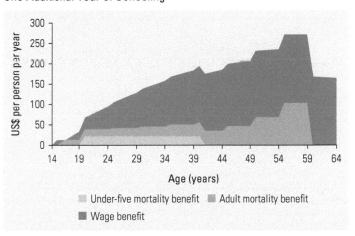

Note: The benefit streams are per person with one additional year of schooling. Our models assume that the health benefits accrue only to female schooling but that the wage benefits accrue to both males and females. Hence, the estimates of the dollar value of health benefits is a weighted average with the weight depending on the fraction of the educated cohort that is female. The calculations assume the cohort is 50 percent female.

controlled studies like Jamison, Murphy, and Sandbu (2016), yield estimates of education's effects on under-five mortality that fall well below what is often reported in the literature.

Our previous analyses have also established a clear link between schooling and improved under-five health. A meta-analysis, conducted as part of our previous study for the Oslo Summit on Education, found that one additional year of female schooling was associated with a decrease in under-five mortality of between 3.6 percent and 9.9 percent (Schäferhoff and others 2015). This finding shows that our estimate on under-five mortality, while still substantial, is at the bottom end of the range of previous studies. Even this lower estimate of effect size yields a quantitatively important effect on mortality and, as we have shown, is a significant addition to the estimated economic rate of return to education. Additionally, our results show that educational quality affects health above and beyond years of schooling, but better data and further research are needed to better understand the relationship, particularly in LMICs.

The strong impact that education has on female mortality is striking and contributes further evidence on the beneficial impacts of education to women's well-being. Schools are frequently used as channels for health information, notably, education on sexual and reproductive health. More-educated people have better access to and understanding of healthy behavior and practices. Moreover, the impact of education on women's empowerment and decision-making power is well documented (International Center for Research on Women 2005; World Bank 2014). Hence, educated women not only have increased access to health services and information, but they are better able to make healthier choices because of their increased bargaining and decision-making power within their households.

Gains in female educational attainment have been impressive over the past 40 years. The mean years of schooling attained by girls in low- and middle-income countries have increased from about 2 in 1970 to more than 6 in 2010; the ratio of male-to-female educational attainment has increased from 67 percent to 86 percent. As our analysis shows, these gains in female schooling were pivotal in reducing under-five mortality and adult mortality. However, women's educational attainment continues to lag behind men's. In the LICs included in our analysis, mean educational attainment for women remained only 2.8 years in 2010, suggesting that many girls either do not attend or at least fail to complete primary school. Further reductions in mortality can be achieved with health-focused policies, as well as education policies that address out-of-school children, especially out-of-school girls.

Our analysis is limited by the paucity of data. The VLY estimates used in the health-inclusive rate of return and BCR analysis are based on evidence mostly from developed economies. Given the range of literature from LMICs, UMICs, and HICs and the uncertainty around VLY, the results presented in this chapter are based on a conservative estimate. Further sensitivity analysis using a

Figure 30.4 Benefit Stream for UMICs from One Additional Year of Schooling

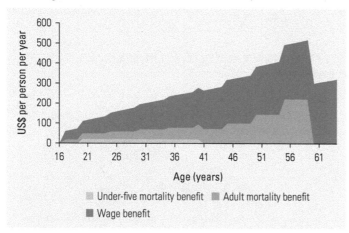

Note: UMICs = upper-middle-income countries. The benefit streams are per person with one additional year of schooling. Our models assume that the health benefits accrue only to female schooling but that the wage benefits accrue to both males and females. Hence, the estimates of the dollar value of health benefits is a weighted average with the weight depending on the fraction of the educated cohort that is female. The calculations assume the cohort is 50 percent female.

Table 30.8 Benefit-Cost Ratios of One Additional Year of Schooling in LICs, Lower-Middle-Income Countries, and UMICs

Income group		Earnings-only BCR	Health-inclusive BCR	% difference (health-inclusive versus earnings-only)
LICs		5.3	10	92
Lower-middle-income countries		2.6	3.8	44
UMICs		1.0	1.5	47
Benefits and costs included	Health benefits	No	Yes	
	Earnings benefits	Yes	Yes	
	Direct cost	Yes	Yes	
	Opportunity cost	Yes	Yes	

Note: BCR = benefit-cost ratio; LICs = low-income countries; UMICs = upper-middle-income countries.

range of VLY estimates is presented in annex 30F. Additionally, the rate of return analyses use modeled costs of schooling given the lack of comprehensive country data on private and public expenditures on schooling. While estimating the impact of schooling on health outcomes, we recognize that the bidirectionality of the relationship between education and health could bias our estimates. Our models on adult mortality estimate the relationship between education and self and peer mortality—poor health especially during school years could limit schooling, which in turn could affect health in adult years. It would be important to continue empirical research to precisely quantify this relationship. Investments in data are also needed to understand education quality—our analyses on education quality were severely restricted by the lack of data on education quality for LICs and lower-middle-income countries.

This study shows that the existing estimates of the rate of return to education are quantitatively important underestimates. This finding results from the systematic inclusion of the dollar value of education's favorable effect on health. Although investments in education are not undertaken specifically to improve health, they produce substantial health returns. In fact, returns to education investments on health are likely to be larger than reported in this study. To the best of our knowledge, our study is the most comprehensive assessment of the monetized health benefits resulting from education, but it underestimates the full effects of education on health. This is the case because it is focused on the impact of education on adult mortality and under-five mortality. Other health outcomes—most important, the effects of education on morbidity—are not considered in our study.

Nevertheless, a BCR that takes into account the health impact of increases in education provides a forceful rationale for a much stronger cross-sectoral collaboration between the education and health sectors.

CONCLUSIONS

This study shows that although investments in education are not undertaken specifically to improve health, they produce substantial health returns. Returns are particularly high in LICs and lower-middle-income countries. Our evidence also exemplifies the important determinants of health that lie outside the health sector. Addressing these determinants requires cross-sectoral collaboration and links between education and health. Other research has shown that improved health is also linked to better education.

The need for cross-sectoral work is captured in the Sustainable Development Goals, and certain funders

have already begun to strengthen the links between the two sectors. The Global Fund to Fight AIDS, Tuberculosis and Malaria has begun to finance education by supporting conditional cash transfers to keep girls in school in four Sub-Saharan African countries with high HIV/AIDS prevalence and incidence, with the objective of reducing HIV transmission. The government of Norway has strengthened cross-sectoral links through its global health and education Vision 2030 initiative. Other donors could rethink their strategies, which in many cases still reflect separate approaches to education and health.

Based on our results, we conclude the following:

- Returns to education are substantially higher than generally understood, and it is important for donors and countries to reflect this in their investment decisions.
- The results strongly indicate that female education matters more than male education in achieving health outcomes. Investments targeted to girls' education yield a substantial return on health. Increased efforts are needed to close remaining gender gaps.
- It is important to get children into school because of the substantial health effects resulting from school attendance, even while awaiting further improvements in quality, which our analysis also show to be important.
- The highly positive BCR that takes into account the health impact of education provides a compelling rationale for much stronger cross-sectoral collaboration between the education and health sectors.
- Despite the recent shift in the global dialogue on quality of education in LMICs, substantial gaps remain in the availability of data on the quality of education and learning, among other data and knowledge gaps. These gaps are largely the result of limited donor investments in global public goods for education. Increased donor support would facilitate better research and progress measurement.

ANNEXES

The online annexes to this chapter are as follows. They are available at http://www.dcp-3.org/CAHD.

- Annex 30A. Countries Included in the Regression Analysis
- Annex 30B. Descriptive Statistics
- Annex 30C. Technical Annex: Hierarchical Linear Model
- Annex 30D. Incorporating Education's Effect on Mortality into Internal Rates of Return

DISCLAIMER

This paper was initially prepared for the International Commission on Financing Global Education Opportunity as a background paper for the report, "The Learning Generation: Investing in Education for a Changing World." The views and opinions in this background paper are those of the author(s) and are not endorsed by the Education Commission or its members. For more information about the Commission's report, please visit http://report.educationcommission.org.

ACKNOWLEDGMENTS

We would like to thank George Psacharopoulos and Susan Horton for their helpful feedback, and Austen Peter Davis, Desmond Bermingham, and Tore Godal for directions on an earlier analysis. We are grateful to Harry Patrinos, Claudio Montenegro, and George Psacharopoulos for sharing data on age-earnings profiles aggregated by income groups.

We thank the International Commission on Financing Global Education Opportunity, which funded this study. We also thank Norad for supporting an initial study of the economic returns of education resulting from reductions in under-five mortality, which was prepared for the Oslo Summit on Education for Development (July 2015).

NOTES

World Bank Income Classifications as of July 2015 are as follows, based on estimates of gross national income (GNI) per capita for 2014:

- Low-income countries (LICs) = US$1,045 or less
- Middle-income countries (MICs) are subdivided:
  a) lower-middle-income = US$1,046 to US$4,125
  b) upper-middle-income (UMICs) = US$4,126 to US$12,735
- High-income countries (HICs) = US$12,736 or more.

Since the chapter was written, the income classifications of some countries have changed. As of July 2016, Cambodia is a lower-middle-income country; Senegal is a low-income country; Tonga is a lower-middle-income country, and República Bolivariana de Venezuela is an upper-middle-income country.

1. See Schäferhoff and others (2015) for an initial study of the economic results of education from reductions in under-five mortality commissioned by Norad.
2. The foundations of lifelong health are built in early childhood. Center on the Developing Child at Harvard University (http://www.developingchild.harvard.edu).
3. For a systematic meta-analysis, see Schäferhoff and others (2015). See also, for example, Caldwell (1980); Wagstaff (1993); Filmer and Pritchett (1999); Grossman (2006); Gakidou and others (2010); Gupta and Mahy (2003); Kuruvilla and others (2014); Jamison and others (2013); Jamison, Murphy, and Sandbu (2016); Wang and others (2014).
4. Matsumura and Gubhaju (2001) on Nepal; Shkolnikov and others (1998) on the Russian Federation; Hurt, Ronsmans, and Saha (2004) on Bangladesh; Yamano and Jayne (2005) on Kenya; de Walque and others (2005) on Uganda; Lleras-Muney (2005) on the United States; Rowe and others (2005) on Nepal.
5. For example, years of schooling for students age 15 years would underestimate their full educational attainment because they are still in school.
6. Our results on the effects of schooling on fertility are in line with other cross-country studies that show declines in TFR as women's educational level rises (Bongaarts 2010; Martin and Juarez 1995; Mboup and Saha 1998; Muhuri, Blanc, and Rutstein 1994).
7. Conducting a categorical levels analysis would have required data on the length of each level of schooling for each country in each time period (year). For example, one country may define primary school as having a five-year duration, while another may define it as seven years; furthermore, country definitions of levels of schooling change over time. Because we lacked accurate data on levels over time, it was not possible to run such an analysis.
8. Program for International Student Assessment (PISA) (OECD 2012); Trends in International Mathematics and Science Study (TIMSS) (Mullis and Martin 2013); Southern and Eastern Africa Consortium for Monitoring Educational Quality (SACMEQ) (Hungi 2011); Program for the Analysis of CONFEMEN Education Systems (PASEC) (PASEC 2015); Latin American Laboratory for Assessment of the Quality of Education: Regional Comparative and Explanatory Study (LLECE) (UNESCO 2015).
9. The authors noted that this characterization of rates of return overlooks many of the important returns that might also be associated with improved educational attainment. Furthermore, the social rates of return were highest for tertiary education in UMICs. The authors note that given almost universal primary completion rates in UMICs, there is an unsatisfactory control group of noncompleters to compare with, likely understating returns at the primary level (Psacharopoulos, Montenegro, and Patrinos 2017).
10. Our methods build on those used by *The Lancet Commission on Investing in Health*, which used existing literature to propose a standardized approach to placing dollar values on mortality change. See Cropper, Hammitt, and Robinson (2011); Jamison and others (2013a, 2013b); Viscusi (2015).
11. All figures were calculated using a VSL of 130 times GDP per capita. We conducted additional analyses using a VSL of 80 times GDP per capita (lower bound) and 180 times GDP per capita (upper bound). The figures in parentheses refer to these lower- and upper-bound estimates.

REFERENCES

Angrist, N., H. A. Patrinos, and M. Schlotter. 2013. "An Expansion of a Global Data Set on Educational Quality: A Focus on Achievement in Developing Countries." Policy Research Working Paper 6356, World Bank, Washington, DC.

Baird, S. J., R. S. Garfein, C. T. McIntosh, and B. Özler. 2012. "Effect of a Cash Transfer Programme for Schooling on Prevalence of HIV and Herpes Simplex Type 2 in Malawi: A Cluster Randomised Trial." *The Lancet* 379 (9823): 1320–29.

Barro, R., and J. W. Lee. 2013. "A New Data Set of Educational Attainment in the World, 1950–2010." *Journal of Development Economics* 104 (September): 184–98.

Behrman, J. A. 2015. "The Effect of Increased Primary Schooling on Adult Women's HIV Status in Malawi and Uganda: Universal Primary Education as a Natural Experiment." *Social Science and Medicine Journal* 127: 108–15.

Behrman, J. R. 1996. "The Impact of Health and Nutrition on Education." *World Bank Research Observer* 11 (1): 23–37.

Bongaarts, J. 2010. "The Causes of Educational Differences in Fertility in Sub-Saharan Africa." *Vienna Yearbook of Population Research* 8: 31–50.

Bundy, D. A. P., N. de Silva, S. Horton, G. C. Patton, L. Schultz, and D. T. Jamison. 2017. "Child and Adolescent Health and Development: Realizing Neglected Potential." In *Disease Control Priorities* (third edition): Volume 8, Child and Adolescent Health and Development, edited by D. A. P. Bundy, N. de Silva, S. Horton, D. T. Jamison, and G. C. Patton. Washington, DC: World Bank.

Caldwell, J. C. 1980. "Mass Education as a Determinant of the Timing of Fertility Decline." *Population and Development Review* 6 (2): 225–55.

Case, A., A. Fertig, and C. Paxson. 2005. "The Lasting Impact of Childhood Health and Circumstance." *Journal of Health Economics* 24 (2): 365–89.

Cropper, M., J. K. Hammitt, and L. A. Robinson. 2011. "Valuing Mortality Risk Reductions: Progress and Challenges." *Annual Review of Resource Economics, Annual Reviews* 3 (1): 313–36.

Currie, J., and R. Hyson. 1999. "Is the Impact of Health Shocks Cushioned by Socioeconomic Status? The Case of Low Birthweight." *American Economic Review* 89 (2): 245–50.

Cutler, D. M., and A. Lleras-Muney. 2010. "Understanding Differences in Health Behaviors by Education." *Journal of Health Economics* 29 (1): 1–28.

De Neve, J. W., G. Fink, S. V. Subramanian, S. Mayo, and J. Bar. 2015. "Length of Secondary Schooling and Risk of HIV Infection in Botswana: Evidence from a Natural Experiment." *The Lancet Global Health* 3 (8): e470–77.

de Walque, D., J. S. Nakiyingi-Miiro, J. Busingye, and J. A. Whitworth. 2005. "Changing Association between Schooling Levels and HIV-1 Infection over 11 Years in a Rural Population Cohort in South-West Uganda." *Tropical Medicine and International Health* 10 (10): 993–1001.

Ding, W., S. F. Lehrer, J. N. Rosenquist, and J. Audrain-McGovern. 2009. "The Impact of Poor Health on Academic Performance: New Evidence Using Genetic Markers." *Journal of Health Economics* 28 (3): 578–97.

Feenstra, R. C., R. Inklaar, and M. P. Timmer. 2015. "The Next Generation of the Penn World Table." *American Economic Review* 105 (10): 3150–82.

Feinstein, L., R. Sabates, T. M. Anderson, A. Sorhaindo, and C. Hammond. 2006. "What Are the Effects of Education on Health?" In *Measuring the Effects of Education on Health and Civic Engagement: Proceedings of the Copenhagen Symposium*, 171–354. Paris: Organisation for Economic Co-operation and Development. http://www.oecd.org/edu /innovation-education/37425753.pdf.

Filmer, D., and L. Pritchett. 1999. "Child Mortality and Public Spending on Health: How Does Money Matter?" *Social Science and Medicine* 49 (10): 1309–23.

Gakidou, E., K. Cowling, R. Lozano, and C. J. Murray. 2010. "Increased Educational Attainment and Its Effect on Child Mortality in 175 Countries between 1970 and 2009: A Systematic Analysis." *The Lancet* 376 (9745): 959–74.

Grossman, M. 2006. "Education and Nonmarket Outcomes." *Handbook of the Economics of Education*, 577–633. Amsterdam: Elsevier.

Gupta, N., and M. Mahy. 2003. "Adolescent Childbearing in Sub-Saharan Africa: Can Increased Schooling Alone Raise Ages at First Birth?" *Demographic Research* 8 (4): 93–106.

Hungi, N. 2011. "Accounting for Variations in the Quality of Primary School Education." Working Paper, Southern and Eastern Africa Consortium for Monitoring Educational Quality. http://www.sacmeq.org/sites/default/files/sacmeq /publications/07_multivariate_final.pdf.

Hurt, L. S., C. Ronsmans, and S. Saha. 2004. "Effects of Education and Other Socioeconomic Factors on Middle Age Mortality in Rural Bangladesh." *Journal of Epidemiology and Community Health* 58 (4): 315–20.

International Center for Research on Women. 2005. "A Second Look at the Role Education Plays in Women's Empowerment." International Center for Research on Women, Washington, DC. http://www.icrw.org/files /publications/A-Second-Look-at-the-Role-Education-Plays -in-Womens-Empowerment.pdf.

Jamison, D. T., P. Jha, V. Malhotra, and S. Verguet. 2013. "Human Health: The Twentieth-Century Transformation of Human Health: Its Magnitude and Value." In *How Much Have Global Health Problems Cost the World?* edited by B. Lomborg, 207–46. Cambridge, U.K.: Cambridge University Press.

Jamison, D. T., S. Murphy, and M. Sandbu. 2016. "Why Has Under-5 Mortality Decreased at Such Different Rates in Different Countries?" *Journal of Health Economics* 48 (July): 16–25.

Jamison, D. T., L. H. Summers, G. Alleyne, K. J. Arrow, S. Berkley, and others. 2013a. "Global Health 2035: A World Converging within a Generation." *The Lancet* 382 (9908): 1898–955.

———. 2013b. "Global Health 2035: A World Converging within a Generation." Summary appendix 3. *The Lancet*

382 (9908): 1898–955. http://www.thelancet.com/cms/attachment/2010532020/2032648078/mmc3.pdf.

Jamison, E. A., D. T. Jamison, and E. A. Hanushek. 2007. "The Effects of Education Quality on Income Growth and Mortality Decline." *Economics of Education Review* 26 (6): 772–89.

Kenkel, D. S. 1991. "Health Behavior, Health Knowledge, and Schooling." *Journal of Political Economy* 99 (2): 287–305.

Kuruvilla, S., J. Schweitzer, D. Bishai, S. Chowdhury, D. Caramani, and others. 2014. "Success Factors for Reducing Maternal and Child Mortality." *Bulletin of the World Health Organization* 92 (7): 533–54.

Lleras-Muney, A. 2005. "The Relationship between Education and Adult Mortality in the United States." *Review of Economic Studies* 72: 189–221.

Lochner, L. 2011. "Nonproduction Benefits of Education: Crime, Health, and Good Citizenship." *Handbook of the Economics of Education* Vol. 4, 183–274. Amsterdam: Elsevier.

Martin, T. C., and F. Juarez. 1995. "The Impact of Women's Education on Fertility in Latin America: Searching for Explanations." *International Family Planning Perspectives* 21 (2): 52–57.

Matsumura, M., and B. Gubhaju. 2001. "Women's Status, Household Structure and the Utilization of Maternal Health Services in Nepal." *Asia-Pacific Population Journal* 16 (1): 24–44.

Mboup, G., and T. Saha. 1998. "Fertility Levels, Trends, and Differentials." DHS Comparative Studies 28, Macro International, Calverton, MD

Montenegro, C. E., and H. A. Patrinos. 2013. "Returns to Schooling around the World." Background paper for World Development Report 2013, World Bank, Washington, DC.

———. 2014. "Comparable Estimates of Returns to Schooling around the World." Policy Research Working Paper 7020, World Bank, Washington, DC.

Muhuri, P. K., A. K. Blanc, and S. O. Rutstein. 1994. "Socioeconomic Differentials in Fertility." DHS Comparative Studies 13, Macro International, Calverton, MD.

Mullis, I. V. S., and M. O. Martin. 2013. *TIMSS 2015 Assessment Frameworks*. Chestnut Hills, MA: TIMSS and PIRLS International Study Center, Boston, College. http://timssandpirls.bc.edu/timss2015/downloads/T15_Frameworks_Full_Book.pdf.

OECD (Organisation for Economic Co-operation and Development). 2012. *PISA 2012 Results in Focus: What 15-Year-Olds Know and What They Can Do with What They Know*. Paris: OECD. https://www.oecd.org/pisa/keyfindings/pisa-2012-results-overview.pdf.

Oreopoulos, P., and K. Salvanes. 2011. "Priceless: The Nonpecuniary Benefits of Schooling." *Journal of Economic Perspectives* 25 (2): 159–84.

PASEC. 2015. *PASEC 2014 Performances des systèmes éducatifs en Afrique subsaharienne francophone*. Dakar: PASEC. http://www.dgessmena.org/IMG/pdf/-9.pdf.

Preston, S. H. 1975. "The Changing Relation between Mortality and Level of Economic Development." *Population Studies* 29 (2): 231–48.

———. 2007. "The Changing Relation between Mortality and Level of Economic Development." *International Journal of Epidemiology* 36 (3): 484–90.

Preston, S. H., and M. R. Haines. 1991. *Fatal Years: Child Mortality in Late Nineteenth-Century America*. Princeton, NJ: Princeton University Press.

Pritchett, L., and L. Summers. 1996. "Wealthier Is Healthier." *Journal of Human Resources* 31 (4): 841–68.

Psacharopoulos, G., C. E. Montenegro, and H. A. Patrinos. 2017. "Education Financing Priorities in Developing Countries." *Journal of Educational Planning and Administration* 31 (1): 5–16.

Rowe, M., B. K. Thapa, R. Levine, S. Levine, and S. K. Tuladhar. 2005. "How Does Schooling Influence Maternal Health Practices? Evidence from Nepal." *Comparative Education Review* 49 (4): 512–33.

Sabates, R., and L. Feinstein. 2006. "The Role of Education in the Uptake of Preventative Health Care: The Case of Cervical Screening in Britain." *Social Science and Medicine* 62 (12): 2998–3010.

Schultz, T. W. 1993. *Origins of Increasing Returns*. Oxford, U.K.: Blackwell Publishers.

Schäferhoff, M., D. Evans, N. Burnett, P. Komaromi, J. Kraus, and others. 2015. "Estimating the Costs and Benefits of Education from a Health Perspective." Prepared for the Oslo Summit on Education for Development, July 6–7.

Shkolnikov, V. M., D. A. Leon, S. Adamets, E. Andreev, and A. Deev. 1998. "Educational Level and Adult Mortality in Russia: An Analysis of Routine Data 1979 to 1994." *Social Science and Medicine* 47 (3): 357–69.

Stenberg, K., K. Sweeny, H. Axelson, M. Temmerman, and P. Sheehan. 2016. "Returns on Investment in the Continuum of Care for Reproductive, Maternal, Newborn, and Child Health." In *Disease Control Priorities* (third edition): Volume 2, *Reproductive, Maternal, Newborn, and Child Health*, edited by R. Black, R. Laxminarayan, M. Temmerman, and N. Walker. Washington, DC: World Bank.

UNESCO (United Nations Educational, Scientific and Cultural Organization). 2015. "Initial Background Information: Latin American Laboratory for Assessment of the Quality of Education." UNESCO, Paris. http://unesdoc.unesco.org/images/0024/002439/243980e.pdf.

United Nations, Department of Economic and Social Affairs, Population Division. 2015. "World Population Prospects: The 2015 Revision." DVD edition.

Viscusi, W. K. 2015. "The Role of Publication Selection Bias in Estimates of the Value of a Statistical Life." *American Journal of Health Economics* 1 (1): 27–52.

Wagstaff, Adam. 1993. "The Demand for Health: An Empirical Reformulation of the Grossman Model." *Health Economics* 2 (2): 189–98.

Wang, H., C. A. Liddell, M. M. Coates, M. D. Mooney, C. E. Levitz, and others. 2014. "Global, Regional, and National Levels of Neonatal, Infant, and Under-5 Mortality during 1990–2013: A Systematic Analysis for the Global

Burden of Disease Study 2013." *The Lancet* 384 (9947): 957–79.

Wang, J., and D. T. Jamison. 1998. "Regression Residuals as Performance Measures: An Assessment of Robustness in the Context of Country-Level Data. Draft." Presented at the Annual Meeting of the American Educational Research Association, San Diego, CA, April 13–17.

World Bank. 2014. *Voice and Agency: Empowering Women and Girls for Shared Prosperity*. Washington, DC: World Bank. http://www.worldbank.org/content/dam/Worldbank /document/Gender/Voice_and_agency_LOWRES.pdf.

Yamano, T., and T. S. Jayne. 2005. "Working-Age Adult Mortality and Primary School Attendance in Rural Kenya." *Economic Development and Cultural Change* 53 (3): 619–53.

DCP3 Series Acknowledgments

Disease Control Priorities, third edition *(DCP3)* compiles the global health knowledge of institutions and experts from around the world, a task that required the efforts of over 500 individuals, including volume editors, chapter authors, peer reviewers, advisory committee members, and research and staff assistants. For each of these contributions we convey our acknowledgment and appreciation. First and foremost, we would like to thank our 32 volume editors who provided the intellectual vision for their volumes based on years of professional work in their respective fields, and then dedicated long hours to reviewing each chapter, providing leadership and guidance to authors, and framing and writing the summary chapters. We also thank our chapter authors who collectively volunteered their time and expertise to writing over 170 comprehensive, evidence-based chapters.

We owe immense gratitude to the institutional sponsor of this effort: The Bill & Melinda Gates Foundation. The Foundation provided sole financial support of the Disease Control Priorities Network (DCPN). Many thanks to Program Officers Kathy Cahill, Philip Setel, Carol Medlin, and (currently) Damian Walker for their thoughtful interactions, guidance, and encouragement over the life of the project. We also wish to thank Jaime Sepúlveda for his longstanding support, including chairing the Advisory Committee for the second edition and, more recently, demonstrating his vision for *DCP3* while he was a special advisor to the Gates Foundation. We are also grateful to the University of Washington's Department of Global Health and successive chairs King Holmes and Judy Wasserheit for providing a home base for the *DCP3* Secretariat, which included intellectual collaboration, logistical coordination, and administrative support.

We thank the many contractors and consultants who provided support to specific volumes in the form of economic analytical work, volume coordination, chapter drafting, and meeting organization: the Center for Disease Dynamics, Economics & Policy; Center for Chronic Disease Control; Centre for Global Health Research; Emory University; Evidence to Policy Initiative; Public Health Foundation of India; QURE Healthcare; University of California, San Francisco; University of Waterloo; University of Queensland; and the World Health Organization.

We are tremendously grateful for the wisdom and guidance provided by our advisory committee to the editors. Steered by Chair Anne Mills, the advisory committee ensures quality and intellectual rigor of the highest order for *DCP3*.

The National Academies of Sciences, Engineering, and Medicine, in collaboration with the Interacademy Medical Panel, coordinated the peer-review process for all *DCP3* chapters. Patrick Kelley, Gillian Buckley, Megan Ginivan, Rachel Pittluck, and Tara Mainero managed this effort and provided critical and substantive input.

World Bank Publishing provided exceptional guidance and support throughout the demanding production and design process. We would particularly like to thank Carlos Rossel, Mary Fisk, Nancy Lammers, Rumit Pancholi, Deborah Naylor, and Sherrie Brown for their diligence and expertise. Additionally, we thank Jose de Buerba, Mario Trubiano, Yulia Ivanova, and Chiamaka Osuagwu of the World Bank for providing professional counsel on communications and marketing strategies.

Several U.S. and international institutions contributed to the organization and execution of meetings that supported the preparation and dissemination of *DCP3*. We would like to express our appreciation to the following institutions:

- University of Bergen, consultation on equity (June 2011)
- University of California, San Francisco, surgery volume consultations (April 2012, October 2013, February 2014)
- Institute of Medicine, first meeting of the Advisory Committee to the Editors (March 2013)
- Harvard Global Health Institute, consultation on policy measures to reduce incidence of noncommunicable diseases (July 2013)
- National Academy of Medicine, systems strengthening meeting (September 2013)
- Center for Disease Dynamics, Economics & Policy (Quality and Uptake meeting, September 2013; reproductive and maternal health volume consultation, November 2013)
- National Cancer Institute, cancer consultation (November 2013)
- Union for International Cancer Control, cancer consultation (November 2013, December 2014)
- Harvard T. H. Chan School of Public Health, economic evaluation consultation (September 2015)
- University of California, Berkeley School of Public Health, and Stanford Medical School, occupational and environmental health consultations (December 2015).

Carol Levin provided outstanding governance for cost and cost-effectiveness analysis. Stéphane Verguet added valuable guidance in applying and improving the extended cost-effectiveness analysis method. Elizabeth Brouwer, Kristen Danforth, Nazila Dabestani, Shane Murphy, Zachary Olson, Jinyuan Qi, and David Watkins provided exceptional research assistance and analytic assistance. Brianne Adderley ably managed the budget and project processes, while Jennifer Nguyen, Shamelle Richards, and Jennifer Grasso contributed exceptional project coordination support. The efforts of these individuals were absolutely critical to producing this series, and we are thankful for their commitment.

Volume and Series Editors

VOLUME EDITORS

Donald A. P. Bundy

Donald A. P. Bundy contributed to the seminal *World Development Report 1993: Investing in Health* and to the three subsequent editions of *Disease Control Priorities* (1993, 2006, and 2017) that followed from it. After two decades pursuing academic studies of how to control the impact of infectious disease on child development in poor populations, he left the University of Oxford to join the Human Development team at the World Bank. He achieved leadership roles in both the health and the education sectors and their interaction, supporting governments in 77 low- and middle-income countries to apply scientific rigor to the design, implementation, and evaluation of their national programs. His focus on alleviating poverty and inequity led to coordinating the World Bank's response to neglected tropical diseases (NTDs), including managing support for the African Programme for Onchocerciasis Control (APOC), which treated more than 100 million people annually in 31 countries. He now leads the Bill & Melinda Gates Foundation's global strategy to eliminate NTDs. He has published more than 350 books and scientific articles and produced several documentary films, including a series broadcast on PBS.

Nilanthi de Silva

Nilanthi de Silva holds the Chair in Parasitology in the Faculty of Medicine at the University of Kelaniya, Sri Lanka, where she has lectured since 1993 and presently serves as the Dean. She is the Chair of the World Health Organization (WHO) Strategic and Technical Advisory Group on Neglected Tropical Diseases, as well as the Chair of the WHO Working Group on Access to Assured Quality,

Essential Medicines for Neglected Tropical Diseases. Over the past decade, she has also served as a member of a WHO reference group on food-borne diseases epidemiology, and on advisory boards for Children Without Worms and the Partnership for Child Development.

Susan Horton

Susan Horton is Professor at the University of Waterloo and holds the Centre for International Governance Innovation (CIGI) Chair in Global Health Economics in the Balsillie School of International Affairs there. She has consulted for the World Bank, the Asian Development Bank, several United Nations agencies, and the International Development Research Centre, among others, in work carried out in over 20 low- and middle-income countries. She led the work on nutrition for the Copenhagen Consensus in 2008, when micronutrients were ranked as the top development priority. She has served as associate provost of graduate studies at the University of Waterloo, vice-president academic at Wilfrid Laurier University in Waterloo, and interim dean at the University of Toronto at Scarborough.

Dean T. Jamison

Dean T. Jamison is Emeritus Professor in Global Health Sciences at the University of California, San Francisco, and the University of Washington. He previously held academic appointments at Harvard University and the University of California, Los Angeles. Prior to his academic career, he was an economist on the staff of the World Bank, where he was lead author of the World Bank's *World Development Report 1993: Investing in Health*. He serves as lead editor for *DCP3* and was lead editor for the previous two editions. He holds a PhD in economics from Harvard University and is an elected member of the Institute of Medicine of the U.S. National Academies. He recently served as Co-Chair and Study Director of *The Lancet's* Commission on Investing in Health.

George C. Patton

George C. Patton is a Professorial Fellow in Adolescent Health Research at the University of Melbourne and a Senior Principal Research Fellow with Australia's National Health and Medical Research Council. He has led long-term longitudinal studies dealing with health and social development from childhood into adulthood and into the next generation. He has also led large-scale prevention trials promoting the health, well-being, and social development of adolescents in community and school settings. Globally, he has led two special series in adolescent health for *The Lancet* and was the Chair of a *Lancet* Commission on Adolescent Health and Wellbeing.

SERIES EDITORS

Dean T. Jamison

See the list of volume editors.

Rachel Nugent

Rachel Nugent is Vice President for Global Noncommunicable Diseases at RTI International. She was formerly a Research Associate Professor and Principal Investigator of the DCPN in the Department of Global Health at the University of Washington. Previously, she served as Deputy Director of Global Health at the Center for Global Development, Director of Health and Economics at the Population Reference Bureau, Program Director of Health and Economics Programs at the Fogarty International Center of the National Institutes of Health, and senior economist at the Food and Agriculture Organization of the United Nations. From 1991 to 1997, she was associate professor and department chair in economics at Pacific Lutheran University.

Hellen Gelband

Hellen Gelband is an independent global health policy expert. Her work spans infectious disease, particularly malaria and antibiotic resistance, and noncommunicable disease policy, mainly in low- and middle-income countries. She has conducted policy studies at Resources

for the Future, the Center for Disease Dynamics, Economics & Policy, the (former) Congressional Office of Technology Assessment, the Institute of Medicine of the U.S. National Academies, and a number of international organizations.

Susan Horton

See the list of volume editors.

Prabhat Jha

Prabhat Jha is the founding director of the Centre for Global Health Research at St. Michael's Hospital and holds Endowed and Canada Research Chairs in Global Health in the Dalla Lana School of Public Health at the University of Toronto. He is lead investigator of the Million Death Study in India, which quantifies the causes of death and key risk factors in over two million homes over a 14-year period. He is also Scientific Director of the Statistical Alliance for Vital Events, which aims to expand reliable measurement of causes of death worldwide. His research includes the epidemiology and economics of tobacco control worldwide.

Ramanan Laxminarayan

Ramanan Laxminarayan is Director of the Center for Disease Dynamics, Economics & Policy in Washington, DC. His research deals with the integration of epidemiological models of infectious diseases and drug resistance into the economic analysis of public health problems. He was one of the key architects of the Affordable Medicines Facility–malaria, a novel financing mechanism to improve access and delay resistance to antimalarial drugs. In 2012, he created the Immunization Technical Support Unit in India, which has been credited with improving immunization coverage in the country. He teaches at Princeton University.

Charles N. Mock

Charles N. Mock, MD, PhD, FACS, has training as both a trauma surgeon and an epidemiologist. He worked as a surgeon in Ghana for four years, including at a rural hospital (Berekum) and at the Kwame Nkrumah University of Science and Technology (Kumasi). In 2005–07, he served as Director of the University of Washington's Harborview Injury Prevention and Research Center. In 2007–10, he worked at the WHO headquarters in Geneva, where he was responsible for developing the WHO's trauma care activities. In 2010, he returned to his position as Professor of Surgery (with joint appointments as Professor of Epidemiology and Professor of Global Health) at the University of Washington. His main interests include the spectrum of injury control, especially as it pertains to low- and middle-income countries: surveillance, injury prevention, prehospital care, and hospital-based trauma care. He was President (2013–15) of the International Association for Trauma Surgery and Intensive Care.

Contributors

Amina Abubakar
Centre for Geographic Medicine Research–Coast, KEMRI/ Wellcome Trust Research Programme, Kilifi, Kenya

Amrita Ahuja
Douglas B. Marshall, Jr., Family Foundation, Houston, Texas, United States

Harold Alderman
International Food Policy Research Institute, Washington, DC, United States

Nicholas Allen
Department of Psychology, University of Oregon, Eugene, Oregon, United States

Laura Appleby
Partnership for Child Development, London, United Kingdom

Elisabetta Aurino
Partnership for Child Development, London, United Kingdom

Peter Azzopardi
Senior Health Specialist, Center for Adolescent Health, University of Melbourne, Melbourne, Victoria, Australia

Sarah Baird
Department of Global Health, George Washington University, Washington, DC, United States

Louise Banham
Global Partnership for Education, Washington, DC, United States

Jere Behrman
Department of Economics, University of Pennsylvania, Philadelphia, Pennsylvania, United States

Habib Benzian
College of Dentistry, New York University, New York, New York, United States

Sonia Bhalotra
Department of Economics, University of Essex, Colchester, United Kingdom

Zulfiqar Bhutta
Division of Women and Child Health, Aga Khan University Hospital, Karachi, Pakistan

Maureen M. Black
RTI International, Washington, DC, United States

Paul Bloem
World Health Organization, Geneva, Switzerland

Chris Bonell
Department of Social & Environmental Health Research, London School of Hygiene & Tropical Medicine, London, United Kingdom

Mark Bradley
GlaxoSmithKline, London, United Kingdom

Sally Brinkman
Telethon Kids Institute, West Perth, Western Australia, Australia

Jere Behrman
University of Pennsylvania, Pennsylvania, United States

Simon Brooker
Bill & Melinda Gates Foundation, Seattle, Washington, United States

Carmen Burbano
World Food Programme, Rome, Italy

Nicholas Burnett
Results for Development, Washington, DC, United States

Tania Cernuschi
World Health Organization, Geneva, Switzerland

Sian Clarke
Department of Disease Control, London School of Hygiene & Tropical Medicine, London, United Kingdom

Carolyn Coffey
Murdoch Childrens Research Institute, Melbourne, Victoria, Australia

Peter Colenso
Independent consultant, Brighton, United Kingdom

Kevin Croke
World Bank, Washington, DC, United States

Amy Daniels
Simons Foundation, New York, New York, United States

Elia de la Cruz Toledo
School of Social Work, Columbia University, New York, New York, United States

Anil Deolalikar
Department of Economics, University of California, Riverside, Riverside, California, United States

Damien de Walque
World Bank, Washington, DC, United States

Lesley Drake
Partnership for Child Development, London, United Kingdom

Lia Fernald
School of Public Health, University of California, Berkeley, Berkeley, California, United States

Meena Fernandes
Partnership for Child Development, Brussels, Belgium

Deepika Fernando
Department of Parasitology, Faculty of Medicine, University of Colombo, Colombo, Sri Lanka

Veronique Filippi
Department of Infectious Disease Epidemiology, London School of Hygiene & Tropical Medicine, London, United Kingdom

Günther Fink
Department of Global Health and Population, Harvard University, Boston, Massachusetts, United States

Rae Galloway
Independent consultant, Washington, DC, United States

Renu Garg
World Health Organization, New Delhi, India

Aulo Gelli
International Food Policy Research Institute, Washington, DC, United States

Andreas Georgiadis
Oxford Department for International Development, University of Oxford, Oxford, United Kingdom

Paul Gertler
Haas School of Business, University of California, Berkeley, Berkeley, California, United States

Caroline Gitonga
Measure Evaluation, Nairobi, Kenya

Boitshepo Giyose
Food and Agriculture Organization of the United Nations, Rome, Italy

Paul Glewwe
Department of Applied Economics, University of Minnesota, St. Paul, Minnesota, United States

Joseph Gona Nzovu
KEMRI-Wellcome Trust Research Programme, Kilifi, Kenya

Amber Gove
RTI International, Washington, DC, United States

Natasha Graham
United Nations Children's Fund, New York, New York, United States

Brian Greenwood
Faculty of Infectious and Tropical Diseases, London School of Hygiene and Tropical Medicine, London, United Kingdom

Elena Grigorenko
Department of Psychology, University of Houston, Houston, Texas, United States

Cai Heath
Partnership for Child Development, London, United Kingdom

Joan Hamory Hicks
Center for Effective Global Action, University of California, Berkeley, Berkeley, California, United States

Melissa Hidrobo
International Food Policy Research Institute, Washington, DC, United States

Kenneth Hill
Stanton-Hill Research, Moultonborough, New Hampshire, United States

Tara Hill
Results for Development, Washington, DC, United States

T. Deirdre Hollingsworth
Mathematics Institute, University of Warwick, Coventry, United Kingdom

Elissa Kennedy
Burnett Institute, Melbourne, Victoria, Australia

Imran Khan
Sightsavers, Washington, DC, United States

Josephine Kiamba
Partnership for Child Development, Johannesburg, South Africa

Jane Kim
T. H. Chan School of Public Health, Harvard University, Boston, Massachusetts, United States

Michael Kremer
Department of Economics, Harvard University, Cambridge, Massachusetts, United States

D. Scott LaMontagne
PATH, Seattle, Washington, United States

Zohra Lassi
School of Medicine, University of Adelaide, Adelaide, South Australia, Australia

Ramanan Laxminarayan
Center for Disease Dynamics, Economics & Policy, Washington, DC, United States

Jacqueline Mahon
United Nations Population Fund, New York, New York, United States

Lu Mai
Development Research Foundation, Beijing, China

Sebastián Martínez
SEEK Development, Berlin, Germany

Sergio Meresman
Inter American Institute on Disability and Inclusive Development, Montevideo, Uruguay

Katherine A. Merseth
RTI International, Washington, DC, United States

Edward Miguel
Department of Economics, University of California, Berkeley, Berkeley, California

Arlene Mitchell
Global Child Nutrition Foundation, Seattle, Washington, DC

Sophie Mitra
Department of Economics, Fordham University, New York, New York,

Anoosh Moin
Department of Paediatrics, Aga Khan University, Karachi, Pakistan

Ali Mokdad
Institute for Health Metrics and Evaluation, University of Washington, Washington, United States

Bella Monse
GIZ German Development Cooperation, Manila, the Philippines

Daniel Mont
Center for Inclusive Policy, Washington, DC, United States

Arindam Nandi
Tata Centre for Development, University of Chicago, Chicago, Illinois, United States

Joaniter Nankabirwa
Department of Medicine, Makerere University College of Health Sciences, Kampala, Uganda

Daniel Plaut
Results for Development, Washington, DC, United States

Elina Pradhan
T. H. Chan School of Public Health, Harvard University, Boston, Massachusetts

Rachel Pullan
Department of Disease Control, London School of Hygiene & Tropical Medicine, London, United Kingdom

Nicola Reavley
Department of Population and Global Health, University of Melbourne, Melbourne, Victoria Australia

John Santelli
Mailman School of Public Health, University of Columbia, New York, New York

Bachir Sarr
Partnership for Child Development, Ottawa, Canada

Susan M. Sawyer
Department of Paediatrics, University of Melbourne, Melbourne, Victoria, Australia

Marco Schaferhöff
SEEK Development, Berlin, Germany

David Schellenberg
Department of Disease Control, London School of Hygiene & Tropical Medicine, London, United Kingdom

Linda Schultz
World Bank, Washington, DC, United States

Andy Shih
Autism Speaks, New York, New York, United States

Elina Suzuki
Organisation for Economic Co-operation and Development, Paris, France

Nicole Stauf
The Health Bureau Ltd., Buckingham, United Kingdom

Milan Thomas
Results for Development, Washington, DC, United States

Hugo C. Turner
School of Public Health, Imperial College London, London, United Kingdom

Benoit Varenne
World Health Organization, Brazzaville, Republic of Congo

Stéphane Verguet
T. H. Chan School of Public Health, Harvard University, Boston, Massachusetts, United States

Russell Viner
Institute of Child Health, University College London, London, United Kingdom

Jane Waldfogel
School of Social Work, Columbia University, New York, New York, United States

Susan Walker
Tropical Medical Research Institute, University of the West Indies, Mona, Kingston, Jamaica

Kristie Watkins
Department of Infectious Disease Epidemiology, Imperial College London, London, United Kingdom

Deborah Watson-Jones
Faculty of Infectious and Tropical Diseases, London School of Hygiene & Tropical Medicine, London, United Kingdom

Kristine West
Department of Economics, St. Catherine's University, St. Paul, Minnesota, United States

Jordan Worthington
Results for Development, Washington, DC, United States

Kin Bing Wu
World Bank (retired), Menlo Park, California, United States

Ahmadu Yakubu
World Health Organization, Geneva, Switzerland

Linnea Zimmerman
Department of Population, Family and Reproductive Health, Johns Hopkins University, Baltimore, Maryland, United States

Advisory Committee to the Editors

Reviewers

Yoko Akachi
United Nations University World Institute for
Development Economics Research, Helsinki, Finland

Harold Alderman
International Food Policy Research Institute,
Washington, DC, United States

Sarah Baird
Department of Global Health, George Washington
University, Washington, DC, United States

W. Stephen Barnett
National Institute for Early Education Research, Rutgers
University, New Brunswick, New Jersey, United States

Samuel Berlinski
Inter-American Development Bank, Washington, DC,
United States

Michael J. Boivin
College of Osteopathic Medicine, Michigan State
University, Ann Arbor, Michigan, United States

Judith Rafaelita B. Borja
Office of Population Studies Foundation, University of
San Carlos, Cebu City, the Philippines

Cecilia Breinbauer
Department of Global Health, University of
Washington, Seattle, Washington, United States

Claire Brindis
Philip R. Lee Institute for Health Policy Studies,
University of California, San Francisco, San Francisco,
California, United States

V. Chandra-Mouli
Department of Reproductive Health and Research,
World Health Organization, Geneva, Switzerland

Lois K. Cohen
National Institute of Dental and Craniofacial Research,
National Institutes of Health, Bethesda, Maryland,
United States

Phaedra S. Corso
College of Public Health, University of Georgia, Athens,
Georgia, United States

Joy Miller Del Rosso
Save the Children, Fairfield, Connecticut, United States

Angela Diaz
Departments of Pediatrics and Preventive Medicine
Icahn School of Medicine, Mount Sinai, New York,
New York, United States

Dolores Dickson
Camfed Ghana, Accra, Ghana

Le Thuc Duc
Vietnam Academy of Social Sciences, Hanoi, Vietnam

Maureen Durkin
School of Medicine and Public Health, University of
Wisconsin, Madison, Wisconsin, United States

Aulo Gelli
International Food Policy Research Institute,
Washington, DC, United States

Amanda Glassman
Center for Global Development, Washington, DC,
United States

Rachel Glennerster
Abdul Latif Jameel Poverty Action Lab, Massachusetts
Institute of Technology, Boston, Massachusetts,
United States

Policy Forum Participants

The following individuals provided valuable insights to improve this volume's key findings through participation in the Disease Control Priorities-World Health Organization, Eastern Mediterranean Regional Office policy forum on Child and Adolescent Health and Development, in Geneva, Switzerland, on May 20, 2016. The forum was organized by Dr. Ala Alwan, Regional Director, World Health Organization, and member of the DCP3 Advisory Committee to the Editors.

Simon Abiramia
Member of the Lebanese Parliament; President of the Parliamentary Committee of Youth and Sports; President of the Board of Directors, OKO; General Manager, LIFRA and NVMD Beirut, Lebanon

Hala Abou-Ali
Secretary General, National Council for Childhood and Motherhood; Member of House of Representatives, Cairo, Arab Republic of Egypt

Nawal Al Hamad
Deputy Director, Public Authority for Food and Nutrition, Ministry of Health, Safat, Kuwait

Ahmed bin Mohamed bin Obaid Al-Saidi
Minister of Health, Muscat, Oman

Suleiman Nasser Al Shehri
Consultant, Public Health and Pediatrics; Director General, School Health Ministry of Health, Riyadh, Saudi Arabia

Sheikh Mohammed Hamad J. Al-Thani
Director, Public Health Department, Supreme Council of Health, Doha, Qatar

Ala Alwan
Regional Director Emeritus, World Health Organization, Regional Office for the Eastern Mediterranean, Cairo, Arab Republic of Egypt

Assad Hafeez
Director General, Ministry of National Health Services, Regulation, and Coordination Islamabad, Pakistan

Moushira Mahmoud Khattab
Ambassador; Former Minister of Family and Population, Cairo, Arab Republic of Egypt

Elizabeth Mason
Honorary Fellow; Institute of Global Health, University College London, London, United Kingdom

Samira Merai
Minister for Women, Family, and Childhood, Ministry of Women, Family, and Children Tunis, Tunisia

Africa Regional Roundtable Participants

The following individuals provided valuable feedback on the volume's essential packages through participation in the Africa Regional Roundtable on Child and Adolescent Health and Development, held at the African Union in Addis Ababa, Ethiopia, March 7–8, 2016. The forum was organized by Dr. Lesley Drake, Executive Director of Partnership for Child Development and contributor to DCP3 Child and Adolescent Health and Development Volume 8.

Oluyemisi Omobolanle Ayoola
Assistant Director, Federal Ministry of Health, Nigeria

Berhanu Moreda Birbissa
Adviser, State Minister of General Education, Ministry of Education, Ethiopia

Nana-Kwadwo Amanikwaa Duku Biritwum
Project Manager, NTDs, Ghana Health Service, Ghana

Joseph Jide Dada
Assistant Director and Desk Officer, School Health, Federal Ministry of Education, Federal Secretariat, Nigeria

Tina Eyaru
Deputy Director, Technical Education and Nutrition, Federal Ministry of Education, Federal Secretariat, Nigeria

Markos Tigist Fekadu
Lecturer, Hawassa University, Ethiopia

Amaya Gillespie
Coordinator, UNICEF, United States

Abdi Sheikh Abdullahi Habat
Director, Ministry of Education, Kenya

Ahma Kebede
Director General, Ethiopia Public Health Institute, Ethiopia

Judith Ongaji Kimiywe
Professor, Kenyatta University, Kenya

Laila Lokosang
Senior CAADP Adviser, Food and Nutrition, Directorate of Rural Economy and Agriculture, African Union Commission, Ethiopia

Catherine Gakii Murungi
Senior Lecturer, Kenyatta University, Kenya

Kate Beverly Quarshie
Deputy Chief Nutrition Officer, Nutrition Department, Ghana Health Service, Ghana

Kokou Sename
Project Officer, Department of Human Resources, Science and Technology, African Union, Ethiopia

Matilda Steiner-Asiedu
Dean, School of Biological Sciences, University of Ghana, Department of Nutrition and Food Science, Ghana

Anta Tal–Dia
Head of the Health and Development Institute,
Universite Cheikh Anta Diop, Senegal

Alemayehu Tekelemariam
Associate Professor, Addis Ababa University,
Ethiopia

Askale Teklu
Team Leader, World Food Program, Ethiopia

Esiet Uwemedimo Uko
Director, Action Health Incorporated, Nigeria

Bain Worku
Girl Effect, Ethiopia

Thomas Yanga
Director, World Food Program, Ethiopia

Index

Boxes, figures, maps, notes, and tables are indicated by b, f, m, n, and t following the page number.

in early childhood, 38–39, 38f, 38t
malaria and, 186–187
in men (15–49 years), 41, 42f
prevalence, 330–332
soil-transmitted helminth infections and, 173
in women (15–49 years), 41, 42f
Angold, A., 111
anorexia, 140–141
anxiety, 111
Appleby, Laura J., 165
Aurino, Elisabetta, 147, 228, 355
Australia
adolescent health interventions in, 372–373
burden of disease in, 57, 62
disability prevalence in, 224, 225t
Austria, binge drinking in, 63
autism spectrum disorders, 231–232
Azerbaijan, overweight/obesity prevalence in, 40
Azzopardi, Peter, 57, 239

B
Bains, K., 136
Baird, Sarah, 413
Baltussen, Naus and Limburg, 228
Bangladesh
adolescent pregnancy in, 139
cash transfers programs in, 331, 332, 333
early marriage in, 65
mobile health in, 300
nutrition in, 389
preprimary school education in, 262
school feeding programs in, 139, 158
stunting in, 83
Banham, Louise, 269
Banister, J., 27
Barooah, B., 153, 155
BCRs. *See* benefit-cost ratios
Beaver, P. C., 173
Behrman, Jere R., 79, 88, 91, 93, 385
Belgium
burden of disease in, 63
education in, 49
benefit-cost ratios (BCRs)
adolescence interventions, 277–279, 278f, 278t,
371–379, 372–373t, 375–377t
cash transfers, 334–335
defined, 13
disability interventions, 227–228
early childhood interventions, 83–84, 84t, 88–89,
91–92, 343–346, 345–346t, 348
education interventions, 318b, 424, 430–433,
431–432t, 433–434f, 434t
HPV vaccinations, 204–206, 204t

malaria interventions, 192–193
middle childhood interventions, 83–84, 84t, 88–89,
91–92, 277–279, 278f, 278t, 361
nutrition interventions, 87–89, 88–89t, 385, 389,
392–397, 394t
oral health interventions, 359–360, 362
school feeding programs, 157–158, 157t, 158f
tetanus vaccinations, 203–204
Benin
adolescence interventions in, 279, 281
middle childhood interventions in, 279, 281, 357
nutrition in, 135, 137
Benzian, Habib, 211
Berlinski, S., 92, 94
Bernal, R., 91–92
Best, C., 154
Bhalotra, Sonia, 385
Bhutan, 203–204, 223, 273
Bhutta, Zulfiqar, 87, 89, 133, 140
binge drinking, 63, 66–67m. *See also* alcohol use
Bin Ghouth, S., 184–185
Bin Mohanna, M. A., 184–185
Black, Maureen M., 253, 343
Bleakley, H., 93
Bloem, Paul, 199
BMI. *See* body mass index
Bobonis, G. J., 93
body mass index (BMI). *See also* overweight/obesity;
underweight
in adolescence, 63, 69, 108, 133, 135–137, 244
cash transfers programs and, 327, 329, 331
deworming programs and, 173
in early childhood, 387
in middle childhood, 133, 135–137
nutrition outcomes and, 37, 39–41
Bolivia, early childhood development in, 91, 344–346,
348–349
Bonell, Chris, 287
Botswana, burden of disease in, 63
Bradley, Mark, 165
brain development, 6–7, 119–131
in adolescence, 75, 109, 240
anatomical maturation, 119–121, 120f
early environment and attachment, 125
environmental experiences and, 123–124
functional development, 121–122
genome-environome dynamics, 122–125,
123–124f
language development, 125–126
literacy skills, 126, 127f
neuroplasticity, 124–125
numeracy skills, 126–127
nutritional requirements, 122–123

Egypt
  middle childhood interventions in, 357
  nutrition in, 135–136, 389
  overweight/obesity prevalence in, 40
  underweight prevalence in, 39
  vaccinations in, 203
El Salvador, cash transfers programs in, 328, 332
EMA (European Medicines Agency), 192, 201
Engle, P. L., 85, 90, 92
ESPs. *See* education sector plans
Ethiopia
  adolescence interventions in, 101, 273,
    279, 281, 297
  deworming programs in, 171
  early childhood interventions in, 90
  middle childhood interventions in, 90, 101,
    273, 279, 281, 362
  nutrition in, 39–40, 42–43, 139, 392
  oral health in, 213
  underweight prevalence in, 40
Europe and Central Asia. *See also specific countries*
  adolescence interventions in, 108
  burden of disease in, 63
  deworming programs in, 169
  disability in, 224, 228
  early childhood interventions in, 87
  education in, 49
  malaria in, 185
  middle childhood interventions in, 87
  mortality rates in, 26–28, 31, 33–34
  nutrition in, 40–41
European Medicines Agency (EMA), 192, 201
European School Survey Project on Alcohol and
    Other Drugs, 61
executive control, 110–111

F
Fall, C. H. D., 139
Fernald, Lia, 79, 325
Fernandes, Meena, 147, 307, 355
Fernández, C., 91–92
Fernando, Deepika, 183, 187, 189
Fiji, underweight prevalence in, 63
Filippi, Véronique, 403
Filmer, D., 226
financial risk protection (FRP), 404–405
Fink, Günther, 99, 101
Fit for School Action Framework, 215, 215b
Fjell, A. M., 110
fluoride interventions, 216, 216b
Focusing Resources on Effective School Health
    (FRESH), 169, 171, 214, 230, 270, 276,
    279–281, 280–281f

Framework Convention on Tobacco Control, 245
France, illicit substance use in, 63
FRESH. *See* Focusing Resources on Effective School
    Health
FRP (financial risk protection), 404–405

G
Galiani, S., 92, 94
Galloway, Rae, 37
The Gambia
  adolescence interventions in, 279
  burden of disease in, 63
  education in, 310
  malaria in, 12, 183
  middle childhood interventions in, 279
Garg, Renu, 211
GBD. *See* Global Burden of Disease study
Gelli, Aulo, 147, 160n4
gender equity
  in adolescence, 240, 274–276, 275–276f
  in early childhood, 256
  in middle childhood, 274–276, 275–276f
genome-environome dynamics of brain development,
    122–125, 123–124f
Georgiadis, Andreas, 99, 101, 102
Germany
  adolescence interventions in, 372
  burden of disease in, 63
  education in, 49
Gertler, Paul, 91, 325
Ghana
  adolescence interventions in, 275,
    277–279, 281
  cash transfers programs in, 328–330, 333
  middle childhood interventions in, 275, 277–279,
    281, 357, 361–362
  nutrition in, 135–137, 150–153, 156, 158–159
  school feeding programs in, 150–153, 156, 158–159
Gilligan, D., 153, 154
Gitonga, Caroline W., 183
Giyose, Boitshepo, 147
Glewwe, Paul, 79, 93, 102, 228
Global Burden of Disease (GBD) study, 32, 60, 107.
    See also burden of disease
Global School-Based Student Health
    Survey, 58, 217
Global Youth Tobacco Survey, 58, 217
Golden, M. H. N., 100, 102
Gona, Joseph, 231
Gove, Amber, 253
governance, 258–259
Graber, J. A., 111
Graham, Natasha, 221

Van Praag, M., 94n2
Varenne, Benoit, 211
Vargas-Barón, E., 256
vector control for malaria, 190–191
Verguet, Stéphane, 403
Vermeersch, C., 153
Vietnam
   burden of disease in, 69
   disability in, 225–226, 229, 230t
   early childhood interventions in, 90
   education in, 49, 317
   middle childhood interventions in, 101
   nutrition in, 43, 154, 158
   vaccinations in, 202, 204–205
Vijverberg, W., 94n2
Viner, Russell M., 107
violence
   adolescence and, 111, 242–243
   early child development and, 4b
vision correction, 13, 228–229
Vitor-Silva, S., 185

W
Waldfogel, Jane, 369
Walker, Susan, 79, 93
Wang, H., 25
Washington Group on Disability Statistics,
   222, 229b
wasting, 87
Watkins, Kristie L., 99
Watson-Jones, Deborah, 199
West, Kristine, 228
whipworm, 165–166. *See also* deworming programs
WHO. *See* World Health Organization
WHO and World Bank, 221–222, 225–226
Woessmann, L., 47
women. *See also* gender equity
   anemia in, 41, 42f
   overweight/obesity in, 40–41, 41f
   underweight in, 40–41, 41f
*World Development Report 2007: Development and
   the Next Generation* (World Bank), 5
World Education Forum, 169, 214, 230, 270, 279
World Health Assembly, 61, 171
World Health Organization (WHO)
   on adolescence interventions, 61–62, 242–243,
      291–293, 379–380

on anemia prevalence, 38, 38t
on deworming programs, 171–172, 413–415, 419
on early childhood interventions, 256, 259
Global Health Estimates (GHE), 32, 33–34t
on malaria, 185–186, 189–190
on middle childhood interventions, 10, 357
on mortality causes, 25
on nutrition, 135, 153–154
on oral health, 213
on soil-transmitted helminth (STH)
   infections, 179b
World Population Prospects (WPP), 32
Worthington, Jordan, 307
Worthman, C. M., 111
Wu, Kin Bing, 47

Y
Yakubu, Ahmadu, 199
Yamasaki, I., 223, 226
Yemen
   early childhood interventions in, 90
   malaria in, 184
   nutrition in, 392
   underweight prevalence in, 63
Yin, Y. N., 140
Youth for Road Safety (YOURS), 300

Z
Zambia
   adolescence interventions in, 279
   cash transfers programs in, 327–328,
      331–332, 334
   disability in, 226
   middle childhood interventions in, 279
   sexual and reproductive health in, 65
Zanzibar
   adolescence interventions in, 281
   disability in, 228, 230
   early childhood interventions in, 261
   middle childhood interventions in, 281
Zimbabwe
   adolescence interventions in, 279
   disability in, 226
   health and education outcomes in, 16
   middle childhood interventions in, 279
   nutrition in, 39–40, 42
Zimmerman, Linnea, 25, 26, 32

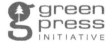